Cardiovascular Ultrasound: A Practical Guide

Cardiovascular Ultrasound: A Practical Guide

Editor: Jared Peters

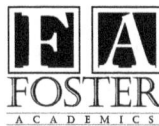

FOSTER ACADEMICS

www.fosteracademics.com

www.fosteracademics.com

FA FOSTER
ACADEMICS

Cataloging-in-Publication Data

Cardiovascular ultrasound : a practical guide / edited by Jared Peters.
    p. cm.
Includes bibliographical references and index.
ISBN 978-1-63242-627-7
1. Echocardiography. 2. Intravascular ultrasonography. 3. Cardiovascular system--Diseases.
I. Peters, Jared.
RC683.5.U5 C37 2019
616.120 754 3--dc23

Foster Academics,
118-35 Queens Blvd., Suite 400,
Forest Hills, NY 11375, USA

ISBN 978-1-63242-627-7 (Hardback)

Contents

Preface

An echocardiogram or a cardiovascular ultrasound is a sonogram of the heart that is developed using 2D, 3D and Doppler ultrasound. Echocardiography is one of the most popular diagnostic tests used in cardiology for the management, diagnosis and follow-up care of patients ailing from any known or suspected heart condition. It provides useful information pertaining to the shape and size of the heart, its pumping capacity, and the positioning and extent of tissue damage, if any. An echocardiogram also offers estimates of the cardiac output, diastolic function and ejection fraction. The most significant advantage of echocardiography is its non-invasiveness and lack of side effects. Some of the common types of echocardiogram are transthoracic echocardiogram, stress echocardiogram and transesophageal echocardiogram, besides others. 3D echocardiography is also possible by using a matrix array of ultrasound probes and processing system. This book is a valuable compilation of topics, ranging from the basic to the most complex advancements in cardiovascular ultrasonography. From theories to research to practical applications, case studies related to all contemporary topics of relevance in this field have been included herein. It will prove to be immensely beneficial to students and researchers working in this field.

This book is the end result of constructive efforts and intensive research done by experts in this field. The aim of this book is to enlighten the readers with recent information in this area of research. The information provided in this profound book would serve as a valuable reference to students and researchers in this field.

At the end, I would like to thank all the authors for devoting their precious time and providing their valuable contribution to this book. I would also like to express my gratitude to my fellow colleagues who encouraged me throughout the process.

Editor

Total average diastolic longitudinal displacement by colour tissue doppler imaging as an assessment of diastolic function

Martina Chantal de Knegt[1*], Tor Biering-Sørensen[1], Peter Søgaard[2], Jacob Sivertsen[1], Jan Skov Jensen[1] and Rasmus Møgelvang[3]

Abstract

Background: The current method for a non-invasive assessment of diastolic dysfunction is complex with the use of algorithms of many different echocardiographic parameters. Total average diastolic longitudinal displacement (LD), determined by colour tissue Doppler imaging (TDI) via the measurement of LD during early diastole and atrial contraction, can potentially be used as a simple and reliable alternative.

Methods: In 206 patients, using GE Healthcare Vivid E7 and 9 and Echopac BT11 software, we determined both diastolic LD, measured in the septal and lateral walls in the apical 4-chamber view by TDI, and the degree of diastolic dysfunction, based on current guidelines. Of these 206 patients, 157 had cardiac anomalies that could potentially affect diastolic LD such as severe systolic heart failure ($n = 45$), LV hypertrophy ($n = 49$), left ventricular (LV) dilation ($n = 30$), and mitral regurgitation ($n = 33$). Intra and interobserver variability of diastolic LD measures was tested in 125 patients.

Results: A linear relationship between total average diastolic LD and the degree of diastolic dysfunction was found. A total average diastolic LD of 10 mm was found to be a consistent threshold for the general discrimination of patients with or without diastolic dysfunction. Using linear regression, total average diastolic LD was estimated to fall by 2.4 mm for every increase in graded severity of diastolic dysfunction ($\beta = -0.61$, *p-value* <0.001). Patients with LV hypertrophy had preserved total average diastolic LD despite being classified as having diastolic dysfunction. Reproducibility of LD measures was acceptable.

Conclusions: There is strong evidence suggesting that patients with a total average diastolic LD under 10 mm have diastolic dysfunction.

Keywords: Echocardiography, Colour tissue Doppler imaging, Diastolic function, Diastolic longitudinal displacement

Background

There is no simple means of reliably diagnosing left ventricular (LV) diastolic dysfunction: The current method for a non-invasive assessment of diastolic function requires the use of algorithms primarily based on a pulsed Doppler measurement of early mitral inflow velocity (E) and a colour tissue Doppler imaging (TDI) assessment of early mitral annular velocity (e'), thereby giving an indirect assessment of LV filling pressures (E/e'), as determined by the Bernouili principle and Laplace law [1]. Other parameters include an assessment of early and atrial mitral inflow patterns (E/A), deceleration time (DT), and left atrial (LA) volume [2]. Using these parameters, LV diastolic dysfunction is traditionally classified as grade 1: abnormal relaxation; grade 2: pseudonormal relaxation, or grade 3: restrictive filling pattern.

* Correspondence: martinadeknegt@gmail.com
[1]Herlev and Gentofte Hospital, Department of Cardiology, Faculty of Health Sciences, University of Copenhagen, Copenhagen, Denmark
Full list of author information is available at the end of the article

Even though it is agreed that no single current echocardiographic measure is sufficient for a diagnosis of LV diastolic dysfunction, the use of algorithms of many different echocardiographic parameters is also problematic as a situation of "one size fits all" arises. Additionally, the fundamental use of velocity based parameters in these algorithms is deficient as the use of velocities as a determinant of diastolic function only takes one snapshot of imaging into consideration, thereby making an accurate depiction of severity difficult to obtain, especially in patients with atrial fibrillation. Lastly, the echocardiographic parameters used in these algorithms are only estimates of LV filling pressures and are subject to limitations of the imaging technique, such as angle dependency, sample volume, and tethering artifacts as well as to shortcomings inherent to derivation of pressures from inflow or re-extension signals [1].

Furthermore, the reliability, feasibility, and practical utility of the individual markers of diastolic dysfunction have been questioned and concordance has been shown to be poor [3, 4]. With regards to e', septal and lateral measurements differ and it has, therefore, been recommended that averages be used [5]. e' can also be reduced inaccurately by mitral annular calcification, surgical rings, or prosthetic valves [1]. With regards to E/e', pulsed Doppler velocities have been shown to overestimate colour TDI velocities, thereby, potentially leading to error in the assessment of LV diastolic function [6]. The use of E/e' has also been questioned in patients with hypertrophic and dilated cardiomyopathy and in decompensated patients with resynchronization therapy [7, 8]. Moreover, E/e' >15 is associated with an elevated LV filling pressure and E/e' <8 is evidence of normal filling pressure - there is, therefore, a big gap (between E/e' 8-15) for which additional investigations are required to obtain a LV filling pressure estimate [1]. The use of E/A and DT is also problematic as both measures are bimodal and a situation with pseudo-normalisation occurs, making it difficult to discern between a patient with normal diastolic function and a patient with a relatively severe grade of diastolic dysfunction.

Our group has previously shown that a combined assessment of both early and late diastolic velocities by colour TDI is a strong prognostic marker of acute myocardial infarction, heart failure, and cardiovascular death in the general population [9]. This indicates that an assessment of both early and late diastole is important for a meaningful assessment of true LV diastolic function. Total diastolic longitudinal displacement (LD) calculated via the integration of the early (E) and atrial (A) velocity waves, obtained by colour TDI, is a potentially new measurement of diastolic function that avoids the major drawbacks associated with the current velocity based assessment, namely an independent measurement that

has a linear relationship with the degree of diastolic dysfunction, i.e. non-biphasic, and a measurement that takes the whole diastolic process into consideration, i.e. not just a snapshot of imaging.

The aims of this study are to investigate: 1) The potential of colour TDI determined total diastolic LD in the determination of diastolic function in the healthy and dysfunctional heart, 2) The ability of total diastolic LD to predict adverse outcomes, 3) To assess reproducibility of total diastolic LD.

Methods
Data source
The Department of Cardiology, Herlev and Gentofte Hospital, University of Copenhagen performs routine echocardiograms according to a standardised protocol and these echocardiograms are stored on a local server.

Study population
A total of 486 consecutive patients were retrieved from the echocardiogram database. To obtain a representation of structural heart disease (no cardiac abnormalities; severe systolic heart failure; LV hypertrophy; LV dilation; and mitral regurgitation), the echocardiograms were analysed in accordance with the following criteria:

Inclusion criteria:

- No cardiac abnormalities: Eyeball LVEF >50 % and normal cardiac dimensions.
- Severe systolic heart failure: Eyeball LVEF <30 %.
- LV hypertrophy: LV mass/body surface area ≥113 g/m^2 for women and ≥131 g/m^2 for men.
- LV dilation: LV internal dimension at end-diastole/body surface area ≥3.8 cm/m^2 for women and ≥3.7 cm/m^2 for men.
- Mitral regurgitation: ≥grade 2.

Exclusion criteria:

- Overlapping diseases of the above mentioned, for example, mitral regurgitation in a patient with LV hypertrophy. Exceptions: patients with a dilated LV, hypertrophic LV, or mitral regurgitation may have had a LVEF under 30 %.
- Incomplete examinations.
- Bundle branch block.
- Atrial fibrillation.
- Unsuitability for colour TDI, i.e. indistinguishable E- and A-wave.

A total of 89 patients fulfilled inclusion criteria for "no cardiac abnormalities"; 138 patients fulfilled inclusion criteria for "severe systolic heart failure"; 117 patients fulfilled criteria for "LV hypertrophy"; 75 patients fulfilled inclusion criteria for "LV dilation"; and 67 patients fulfilled criteria for "mitral regurgitation". After application of exclusion criteria, the final study population consisted of 206 patients, 49 of whom were classified as having normal cardiac dimensions and function. The 157 remaining patients all had heart anomalies that could potentially affect diastolic LD such as severe systolic heart failure ($n = 45$), LV hypertrophy ($n = 49$), LV dilation ($n = 30$), and mitral regurgitation ($n = 33$). Diastolic function was assessed and participants were graded as having a normal relaxation ($n = 76$), abnormal relaxation ($n = 75$), pseudonormal relaxation ($n = 44$), or restrictive filling pattern ($n = 11$).

Echocardiographic analyses

All echocardiograms were obtained using Vivid E7 and Vivid 9 ultrasound systems (GE Healthcare, Horten Norway) and all images were stored digitally on a central server. All participants were examined with conventional two-dimensional echocardiography, m-mode, pulsed-wave TDI, colour TDI and two-dimensional strain imaging. All the echocardiographic analyses in the present study were performed de novo and offline (blinded to other clinical data) using Echopac BT11 software (GE Healthcare, Horten Norway).

Conventional echocardiography

LV end-diastolic dimensions (interventricular septum wall thickness (IVS), LV internal dimension (LVID), and LV posterior wall thickness (PWT)) and LA diameter were obtained from the parasternal long-axis view at the mitral valve leaflet tips. Pulsed wave Doppler was used to record mitral inflow between the tips of the mitral leaflets. LVEF was obtained using modified Simpson's biplane method in the 4-chamber and 2-chamber view [10]. LA volume was estimated by the area-length method [10]. LV mass index was calculated as the anatomic mass (LV mass = 0.8x(1.04[(IVSd + LVIDd + PWTd)3 – LVIDd3]) + 0.6 g) [11], divided with body surface area. All measurements were acquired from the parasternal approach and measured at the level of the mitral valve at end-diastole. Relative wall thickness was calculated as $(2 \times LV\ PWT)/(LVID)$ and the subgroup of patients with LV hypertrophy was sub-categorized with regards to concentric or eccentric hypertrophy in accordance with current American Society of Echocardiography Committee recommendations [10]. Severity of mitral regurgitation was determined according to current guidelines [12]. All chamber quantifications are in accordance with the American Society of Echocardiography Committee recommendations [10].

Tissue Doppler Imaging (TDI)

Colour TDI loops were obtained in the apical 4-chamber view. Peak longitudinal systolic velocities (s') as well as early diastolic (e') and late diastolic (a') velocities were measured in the septal and lateral wall using a 5 mm circular sample volume placed in the left ventricular myocardial just proximal to the mitral annular level. Total average systolic and diastolic LD was determined by calculating the area under the curve, using tissue tracking software, of the systolic, early and late diastolic waves, respectively, and averaging septal and lateral findings (Fig. 1). Potential L-waves between the early and late diastolic waves were not included in the assessment of total average diastolic displacement. Systolic displacement was measured as the maximal displacement between aortic valve opening and aortic valve closure and post-systolic contraction was not included in systolic displacement measurements.

Pulsed wave TDI tracings, used to measure peak myocardial velocities, were obtained with the range gate placed at the septal and lateral mitral annular segments in the 4-chamber view. The average of septal and lateral e' by pulsed wave TDI was used to calculate E/e'.

M-mode

Mitral annular plane systolic excursion (MAPSE) was determined in the septal and lateral walls in the apical four-chamber view in all participants. This was done by placing the M-mode cursor in the septal and lateral borders in the mitral annular plane. In doing so, an image of either septal or lateral mitral annular displacement was obtained. MAPSE was measured from the lowest to the highest point of contraction, excluding post-systolic contractions, i.e. measurements were obtained between aortic valve opening and aortic valve closure.

Two-dimensional Strain Imaging (2DSI)

Using 2-dimensional speckle tracking derived strain imaging, the left ventricular myocardial wall was traced in the 4-chamber view with the basal septal and lateral segments starting at the mitral annular level. By the tracking of speckles from frame-to-frame, myocardial deformation was assessed. The average of regional measurements in a 6-segment model from the apical 4-chamber view was used as an estimate of longitudinal displacement (LD), longitudinal strain (LS) and longitudinal strain rate (LSR). Regional basal longitudinal displacement, strain, and strain rate was calculated as the average of the basal septal and lateral segments in the apical 4-chamber view.

TDI and strain measurements are reported as absolute values.

Determination of degree of diastolic dysfunction

Patients were graded as having either normal diastolic function or abnormal diastolic function grade 1–3 according to current EAE/ASE recommendations [2].

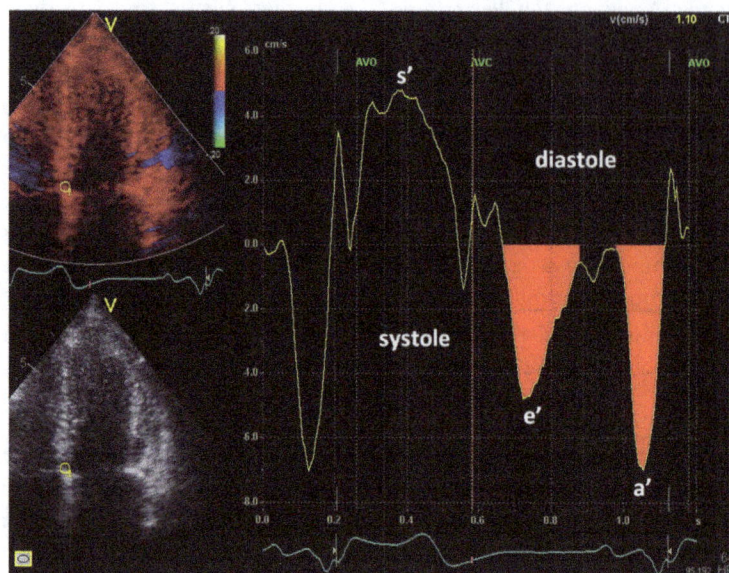

Fig. 1 Image of colour tissue Doppler imaging with septal longitudinal displacement measurements depicted as area under the curve in early and late diastole. *s', peak mitral annular systolic velocity; e', peak early mitral annular diastolic velocity; a', peak atrial mitral annular diastolic velocity; AVO, aortic valve opening; AVC, aortic valve closing*

Prognostics study

Data on mortality (primary endpoint) was obtained using the unique personal identification number in the Central Office of Civil Registration and the Danish National Board of Health's National Patient Registry.

Statistical analysis

All statistical analyses were done using SPSS version 20 (SPSS, Inc, Chicago, IL). In Table 1, continuous Gaussian distributed variables and proportions were compared using Student's t-test and $\chi 2$-test, respectively. Pearsons correlation was used to determine any associations between the degree of diastolic dysfunction and total average diastolic LD as well as between total average diastolic LD and individual parameters used in the assessment of diastolic and systolic function. Using logistic regressions, odds ratios for unadjusted and adjusted models were calculated to establish the association between peak velocities and diastolic LD and the primary endpoint (death). Interactions with the subgroup type were tested for. Bland-Altman analysis was used to evaluate intraobserver and interobserver variability and was expressed as mean difference ± 1.96 standard deviation (SD) and as coefficient of variation (CV) [13]. P-values <0.05 in two-sided tests were considered statistically significant.

Results

Patient characteristics

Main characteristics of the study population are presented in Table 1. Parameters of advanced echocardiography are

presented in Table 2. Compared to controls, patients with structural heart disease had both reduced early and active diastolic function as assessed by various echocardiographic techniques such as TDI and speckle tracking. Of the 49 patients with LV hypertrophy, 32 (65 %) had concentric hypertrophy; 17 (35 %) had eccentric hypertrophy.

Total average diastolic longitudinal displacement and degree of diastolic dysfunction

A linear relationship, also after adjustment for age and gender, between total average diastolic LD and the degree of diastolic dysfunction was found (Fig. 2). This linear relationship is due to a fall in TT-e' in the mild stages of diastolic dysfunction and TT-a' which only starts to diminish at more severe degrees of diastolic dysfunction (Additional file 1: Figure S1 and S2). This linear relationship indicates the value of total average diastolic LD as an indicator of LV diastolic function and a total average diastolic LD of 10 mm was found to be a consistent threshold for the general discrimination of patients with or without diastolic dysfunction. This threshold was chosen on the basis of findings in Fig. 3 where the vast majority of controls with normal diastolic function had a total average diastolic LD above 10 mm. Pearson correlation was calculated to be −0.61 with a *p-value* <0.001. Using linear regression, total average diastolic LD was estimated to fall by 2.4 mm for every increase in graded severity of diastolic dysfunction ($\beta = -0.61$, *p-value* <0.001). A similar relationship was found when investigating total average diastolic velocity (e' + a') and degree of diastolic function (Pearson

Table 1 Characteristics of the patients studied

	Controls (n = 49)	Severe Systolic HF (n = 45)	LV Hypertrophy (n = 49)	LV Dilation (n = 30)	Mitral Regurgitation (n = 33)
Age, y	58 ± 15	65 ± 15*	69 ± 15***	76 ± 9***	71 ± 11***
Male sex, % (n)	43 (21)	93 (42)	47 (23)	57 (17)	55 (18)
Height, cm	173 ± 9	177 ± 9*	171 ± 10	167 ± 7**	171 ± 9
Weight, kg	76 ± 16	82 ± 15	73 ± 14	65 ± 14**	72 ± 15
LVIDd, cm	4.7 ± 0.6	5.6 ± 0.7***	5.2 ± 0.7**	6.8 ± 0.8***	5.0 ± 0.9
BSA, m²	1.9 ± 0.2	2.0 ± 0.2*	1.8 ± 0.2	1.7 ± 0.2***	1.8 ± 0.2
LVIDd/BSA, cm/m²	2.5 ± 0.3	2.9 ± 0.4***	2.8 ± 0.4***	4.0 ± 0.2***	2.7 ± 0.5*
LVEF, %	64 ± 7	30 ± 9***	60 ± 7*	25 ± 12***	53 ± 16***
IVS, cm	0.9 ± 0.2	0.9 ± 0.2	1.2 ± 0.2***	1.0 ± 0.2	1.0 ± 0.3
LVPWd, cm	0.9 ± 0.2	0.9 ± 0.2	1.2 ± 0.2***	1.0 ± 0.1	1.0 ± 0.3
LVM/BSA, g/m²	70 ± 16	102 ± 19***	130 ± 23***	171 ± 42***	103 ± 37**
DDF 0, % (n)	74 (36)	24 (11)	35 (17)	0 (0)	36 (12)
DDF 1, % (n)	22 (11)	51 (23)	39 (19)	47 (14)	24 (8)
DDF 2, % (n)	4 (2)	11 (5)	27 (13)	47 (14)	30 (10)
DDF 3, % (n)	0 (0)	13 (6)	0 (0)	7 (2)	9 (3)
E/A	1.2 ± 0.5	1.2 ± 0.8	1.1 ± 0.5	1.4 ± 1.0	1.5 ± 0.6**
DT, ms	221 ± 57	191 ± 98	236 ± 59	218 ± 66	223 ± 93
LAV, ml/m²	24.5 ± 9.0	33.8 ± 10.5***	39.6 ± 13.7***	45.5 ± 18.2***	46.5 ± 16.5***
E/e'	8.6 ± 3.6	12.3 ± 6.4**	12.4 ± 5.4***	17.0 ± 7.9***	19.3 ± 14.9***
Known IHD, % (n)	18 (9)	69 (31)	4 (2)	17 (5)	21 (7)

HF heart failure, *LV* Left ventricular, *LVIDd* LV internal dimension in diastole, *BSA* body surface area, *LVEF* LV ejection fraction, *IVS* interventricular septum, *LVPWd* LV posterior wall in diastole, *LVM* LV mass, *DDF* degree of diastolic dysfunction, *E/A* early inflow velocity/atrial inflow velocity, *DT* deceleration time, *LAV* left atrial volume, *E/e'* early inflow velocity/early diastolic tissue velocity, *IHD* ischemic heart disease
*P <0.05 compared with the control group
**P <0.01 compared with the control group
***P <0.001 compared with the control group

correlation 0.63, *p-value* <0.001), although a cutoff of 12 cm/s is appropriate here (Additional file 1: Figure S3).

Total average diastolic longitudinal displacement in various heart conditions

Figure 3 illustrates findings of total average diastolic LD in various heart conditions in comparison to the degree of diastolic dysfunction. Median values of all participants classified as having normal diastolic function had a total average diastolic LD above 10 mm, except for patients with severe systolic heart failure. A closer examination of the patients with severe systolic heart failure with normal diastolic function as determined by current guidelines [2] revealed that patients with a diastolic LD ≥10 mm had reduced markers of systolic function (mean LS = −11.5 ± 7.1 %; mean LSR = −0.85 ± 0.2 s^{-1}; and mean systolic LD by TDI (TT-s') = 10.7 ± 1.5 mm). Systolic function of individuals with severe systolic heart failure, normal diastolic function, and a diastolic LD <10 mm was also reduced, but to a greater degree (LS = −9.9 ± 5.7 %, LSR = −0.68 ± 0.32 s^{-1}, TT-s' = 7.0 ± 1.7 mm).

Generally, median values of mean diastolic LD fell with increasing severity of diastolic dysfunction for all subgroups except for the control group and patients with LV hypertrophy, who both had a preserved total average diastolic LD ≥10 mm despite being categorised as having an abnormal relaxation pattern. Median values of all participants classified as having either a pseudo-normal or restrictive filling pattern had a total average diastolic LD <10 mm. Table 3 shows the configuration of the E- and A-waves in controls and in patients with LV hypertrophy and an abnormal relaxation pattern. In both groups, peak velocities for the A-wave were greater than for the E-wave but displacement in the E- and A-waves for each was roughly equal, indicating that these two groups had low, broad E-waves and tall, narrow A-waves.

A further analysis of controls with grade 1 diastolic dysfunction and a diastolic LD ≥10 mm revealed that the sole reason for these individuals being classified as having grade 1 diastolic dysfunction was a lateral e' <10 cm/s or septal e' <8 cm/s and not enlarged atriums (LA volume <34 ml/m²).

Table 4 shows the correlation of average diastolic and systolic LD measures with peak average diastolic and systolic velocities for subjects with LV hypertrophy and

Table 2 Advanced echocardiographic parameters within subgroups

	Controls (n = 49)	Severe Systolic HF (n = 45)	LV Hypertrophy (n = 49)	LV Dilation (n = 30)	Mitral Regurgitation (n = 33)
TDI					
s′, cm/s	6.2 ± 1.4	3.8 ± 1.2***	5.4 ± 1.1**	2.9 ± 1.1***	5.3 ± 2.3
e′, cm/s	−7.6 ± 2.3	−4.4 ± 1.6***	−5.9 ± 2.2***	−3.6 ± 1.7***	−5.3 ± 2.5***
a′, cm/s	−7.6 ± 1.8	−5.7 ± 2.3***	−6.8 ± 1.7*	−4.3 ± 2.0***	−5.6 ± 2.6***
e′ + a′, cm/s	−15.2 ± 2.7	−10.1 ± 2.5***	−12.7 ± 2.2***	−7.9 ± 2.7***	−11.0 ± 4.6***
TT-s′, mm	11.4 ± 2.0	6.5 ± 2.3***	10.8 ± 2.0	4.7 ± 2.5***	9.3 ± 4.3*
TT-e′, mm	7.3 ± 2.2	3.6 ± 1.8***	5.6 ± 2.1***	2.6 ± 1.2***	4.8 ± 2.6***
TT-a′, mm	5.2 ± 1.5	4.0 ± 1.7***	5.2 ± 1.5	3.1 ± 1.6***	4.2 ± 1.9**
TT-e′ + TT-a′, mm	12.6 ± 2.3	7.5 ± 2.2***	10.8 ± 2.2***	5.7 ± 1.9***	9.0 ± 4.0***
M-mode					
MAPSE, mm	12.3 ± 2.4	7.4 ± 2.1***	11.3 ± 2.0*	5.4 ± 2.2***	10.4 ± 4.1*
2D strain					
LS, %	−14.8 ± 3.8	−9.1 ± 4.5***	−12.0 ± 3.8**	−6.6 ± 4.3***	−12.1 ± 4.8**
LD, mm	15.4 ± 2.6	7.7 ± 3.0***	15.8 ± 3.0	6.1 ± 3.8***	12.7 ± 5.7*
s, cm/s	6.5 ± 1.5	4.0 ± 1.0***	5.7 ± 1.0**	2.5 ± 2.0***	5.0 ± 1.9***
e, cm/s	−6.5 ± 2.8	−3.8 ± 1.6***	−5.4 ± 2.1*	−2.3 ± 1.9***	−5.3 ± 2.7
a, cm/s	−7.4 ± 1.7	−5.3 ± 1.9***	−6.5 ± 2.0*	−4.1 ± 1.8***	−5.4 ± 2.2***
e + a, cm/s	−13.9 ± 3.2	−9.1 ± 2.3***	−11.9 ± 2.6**	−6.5 ± 3.0***	−10.7 ± 4.3**
s, s^{-1}	−1.0 ± 0.3	−0.8 ± 0.2***	−0.9 ± 0.4	−0.8 ± 0.3**	−1.0 ± 0.4
e, s^{-1}	1.3 ± 0.4	0.9 ± 0.5***	1.0 ± 0.3**	0.7 ± 0.4***	1.1 ± 0.4*
a, s^{-1}	1.2 ± 0.4	0.9 ± 0.4***	1.1 ± 0.5	0.9 ± 0.5**	1.1 ± 0.4
e + a, s^{-1}	2.5 ± 0.5	1.8 ± 0.6***	2.2 ± 0.7*	1.6 ± 0.8***	2.1 ± 0.7**

TDI tissue Doppler Imaging, *s′* systolic tissue velocity by TDI measured at the mitral annulus, *e′* early diastolic tissue velocity by TDI measured at the mitral annulus, *a′* late diastolic tissue velocity by TDI measured at the mitral annulus, *TT-s′* systolic displacement measured at the mitral annulus, *TT-e′* early diastolic displacement measured at the mitral annulus, *TT-a′* late diastolic displacement measured at the mitral annulus, *MAPSE* M-mode derived mitral annular plane systolic excursion, *LS* longitudinal strain by 2D strain imaging, *LD* longitudinal displacement by 2D strain imaging, *s* systolic tissue velocity/strain rate by 2D strain imaging measured at the basal septal and lateral segments, *e* early diastolic tissue velocity/strain rate by 2D strain imaging measured at the basal septal and lateral segments, *a* late diastolic tissue velocity/strain rate by 2D strain imaging measured at the basal septal and lateral segments
*P <0.05 compared with the control group
**P <0.01 compared with the control group
***P <0.001 compared with the control group

varying degrees of diastolic dysfunction. A moderate correlation was found between total average systolic LD and total average diastolic LD as well as between peak longitudinal systolic velocity by TDI (s') and total average diastolic LD, especially in patients with normal diastolic function and in patients with abnormal relaxation. An examination of parameters of systolic function in patients with LV hypertrophy indicates preserved systolic function (LVEF = 60 ± 7 %, LSR = −0.92 ± 0.35 s^{-1}, LS = 12.0 ± 3.8, TT-s' = 10.8 ± 2.0 mm, s' = 5.38 ± 1.14 cm/s).

Left ventricular ejection fraction and total average diastolic longitudinal displacement
Figure 4 illustrates the relationship of total average diastolic LD with LVEF. Participants are clustered into two main groups: a group with a total average diastolic LD <10 mm and a LVEF <50 % and a group with a total average diastolic LD >10 mm and a LVEF >50 %, and

two smaller groups: a group with total average diastolic LD <10 mm and an LVEF >50 % and a group with a total average diastolic LD >10 mm and an LVEF <50 %.

By examining the colour combinations of subjects in Fig. 4, it can be seen that the vast majority of subjects with no diastolic dysfunction have a LVEF >50 % and a diastolic LD >10 mm while the vast majority of subjects with grade 3 diastolic dysfunction have a LVEF <50 % and a diastolic LD <10 mm.

Regarding subjects with a LVEF >50 % and a diastolic LD <10 mm, it can be seen that almost all subjects have some degree of diastolic dysfunction. A comparison of longitudinal systolic function of these subjects, i.e. patients with LVEF >50 % and diastolic LD <10 mm (n = 32), compared to subjects with LVEF >50 % and diastolic LD >10 mm (n = 88) revealed that systolic function was reduced in this group: LS = −12.3 ± 4.1 %, LSR = −0.86 ± 0.33 s^{-1}, TT-s' = 9.2 ± 1.8 mm and s' = 4.8 ± 1.0 cm/s

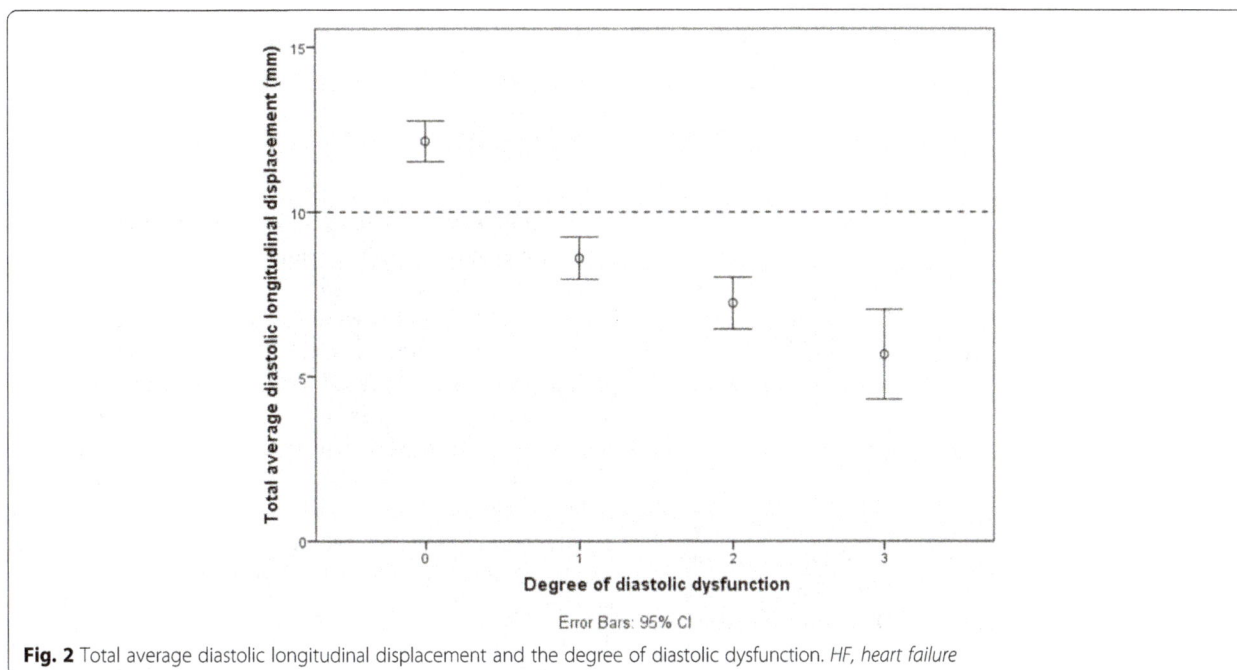

Fig. 2 Total average diastolic longitudinal displacement and the degree of diastolic dysfunction. *HF, heart failure*

compared to LS = -13.9 ± 3.9 %, LSR = -1.05 ± 0.32 s^{-1}, TT-s' = 11.9 ± 2.2 mm and s' = 6.3 ± 1.4 cm/s.

An examination of systolic function of the 4 individuals with a LVEF <50 % and a diastolic LD >10 mm revealed a LS of -11.5 ± 7.1 %, LSR = -0.78 ± 0.17 s^{-1}, TT-s' = 10.8 ± 1.5 mm and s' = 5.3 ± 1.2 cm/s. An analysis of the comorbidities of these patients revealed that they all suffered from ischemic heart disease.

Correlations

Pearsons correlation was used to determine the association of average diastolic LD with a variety of other echocardiographic parameters (Table 5). With regards to the entire population, strong associations were found when comparing LD in early diastole (TT-e') with early mitral annular velocity (e'), LD in late diastole (TT-a') with late mitral annular velocity (a'), total average

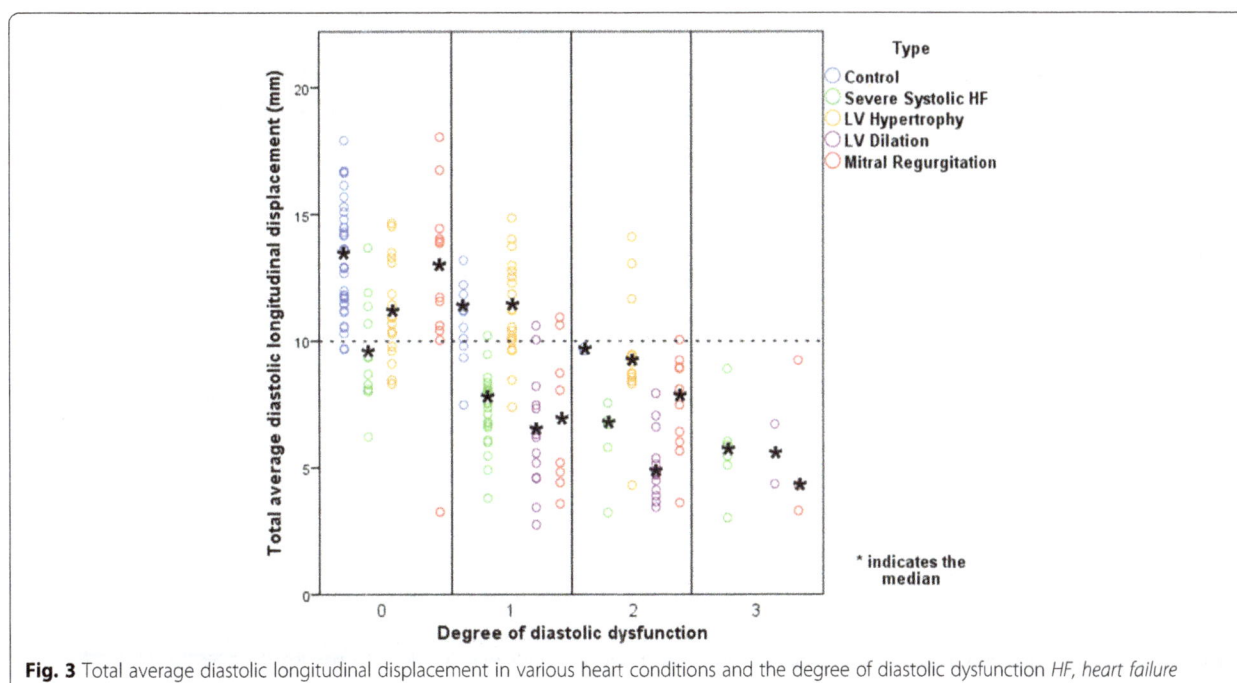

Fig. 3 Total average diastolic longitudinal displacement in various heart conditions and the degree of diastolic dysfunction *HF, heart failure*

Table 3 The configuration of the early and atrial waves in controls and in subjects with left ventricular hypertrophy and an abnormal relaxation pattern

Configuration	Controls Mean ± SD	LV hypertrophy Mean ± SD
e' (cm/s)	5.44 ± 1.46	5.11 ± 1.56
a' (cm/s)	7.27 ± 2.41	7.86 ± 1.22
TT-e' (mm)	5.44 ± 1.20	5.02 ± 1.51
TT-a' (mm)	5.31 ± 1.71	6.24 ± 0.91

e' early diastolic tissue velocity by TDI measured at the mitral annulus, *a'* late diastolic tissue velocity by TDI measured at the mitral annulus, *TT-e'* early diastolic displacement measured at the mitral annulus, *TT-a'* late diastolic displacement measured at the mitral annulus

diastolic LD (TT-e' + TT-a') with e' + a', and the ratio of diastolic LD between the early and atrial wave (TT-e'/TT-a') with peak velocities for the early and atrial wave (e'/a'). When considering systolic displacement measured by TDI, M-mode, and 2D strain imaging and TDI derived total average diastolic LD, strong correlations were found. Weaker correlations were found when comparing total average diastolic LD to other systolic measures, such as LVEF, LS and LSR. A comparison of associations between groups (Table 5) reveals that the strongest associations were seen when comparing diastolic LD measurements with diastolic velocity measurements. A weaker association was seen when comparing average diastolic LD with systolic LD and velocity, and was weakest for patients with LV hypertrophy. The biggest fluctuations and weakest correlations between groups were seen when determining the association of average diastolic LD with markers of systolic function such as LVEF, LS and LSR.

Agreement with echocardiographic parameters
Figure 5 depicts the mean differences (bias) of total average systolic and diastolic measurements plotted against the mean of the two average LD measurements,

(Bland-Altman plot). The mean difference was calculated to −0.58 mm indicating that average systolic LD underestimates total average diastolic LD. The limits of agreement were calculated to ±3.46 mm and a coefficient of variation (CV) of 19 % was found.

Total average diastolic longitudinal displacement as a predictor of adverse cardiac outcomes
There were 33 events (death) during 2.6 ± 1.2 years follow-up. Odds ratios were calculated to determine the predictive capabilities of total diastolic LD in comparison to diastolic colour TDI velocities with regards to all-cause mortality: per unit decrease, risk of death increased in a similar pattern for e' + a' and TT-e' + TT-a' (Table 6). Following adjustment for covariates (first multivariate analysis adjusted for age and gender and second multivariate analysis adjusted for age, gender, LVEF, LV internal dimension in diastole/body surface area, LV mass index, and LS), e' + a' and TT-e' + TT-a' remained significant predictors of death. LA volume was also shown to be a significant predictor of death, also after adjustment in multivariate analyses. The calculation of area under the curve in ROC curves (Fig. 6) showed similar results.

Reproducibility
Intraobserver variability for septal and lateral LD measurements of the E-wave and A-wave was relatively low, as is shown by the mean difference being close to zero (Additional file 1: Figure S4). Limits of agreement are, however, fairly wide and the largest variability, as indicated by CV, was seen in lateral A-wave LD measurements.

Interobserver variability findings were found to be similar to intraobserver variability. All mean differences were close to zero. The greatest variability was seen in E-wave LD measurements in comparison to A-wave LD

Table 4 Correlations of total average diastolic longitudinal displacement with peak average diastolic velocities and average systolic longitudinal displacement for subjects with LV hypertrophy and no diastolic dysfunction and a first and second degree of diastolic dysfunction

Comparison	DDF 0		DDF 1		DDF 2	
	Pearson Correlation	*P-value*	Pearson Correlation	*P-value*	Pearson Correlation	*P-value*
e' and TT-e'	0.92	<0.001	0.77	<0.001	0.67	<0.05
a' and TT-a'	0.89	<0.001	0.81	<0.001	0.88	<0.001
e' + a' and TT-e' + TT-a'	0.81	<0.001	0.81	<0.001	0.88	<0.001
TT-e'/TT-a' and e'/a'	0.95	<0.001	0.75	<0.001	0.76	<0.001
TT-s' and TT-e' + TT-a'	0.53	<0.05	0.62	<0.05	0.79	<0.001
TT-e' + TT-a' and s'	0.46	0.06	0.40	0.09	0.80	<0.001

e' early diastolic tissue velocity by TDI measured at the mitral annulus, *a'* late diastolic tissue velocity by TDI measured at the mitral annulus, *s'* systolic tissue velocity by TDI measured at the mitral annulus, *TT-e'* early diastolic displacement measured at the mitral annulus, *TT-a'* late diastolic displacement measured at the mitral annulus, *TT-s'* systolic displacement measured at the mitral annulus

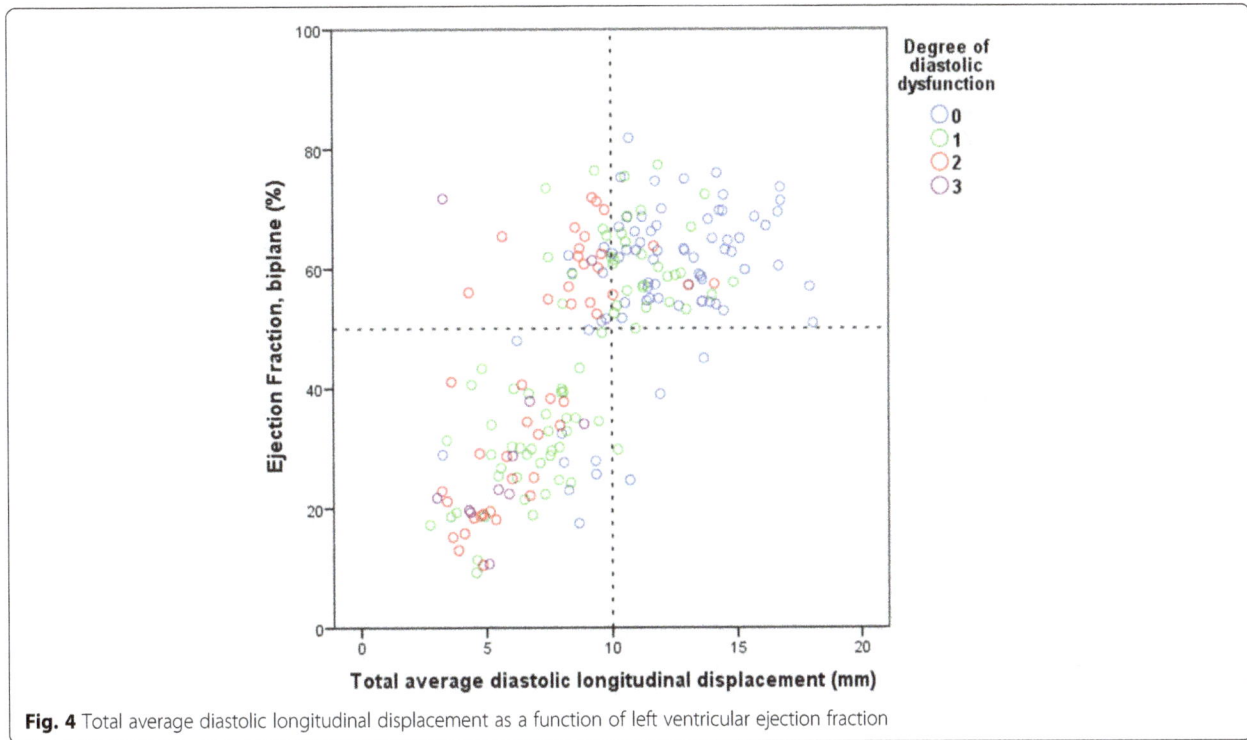

Fig. 4 Total average diastolic longitudinal displacement as a function of left ventricular ejection fraction

measurements, as is indicated by the larger limits of agreement and larger CV.

Discussion

This is the first study, to our knowledge, to investigate total average diastolic LD determined by colour TDI as a potential new parameter for the determination of LV

diastolic dysfunction. Our findings on the predictive capabilities and reproducibility of this parameter are important with regards to its utilisation in clinical practice.

Tissue Doppler Imaging

TDI is a useful echocardiographic technique to evaluate global and regional systolic and diastolic function in a

Table 5 Correlations of average diastolic longitudinal displacement with peak average diastolic velocities, average systolic longitudinal displacement and other measures of systolic function for all subjects and between subgroups

Comparison	All subjects		Control		Severe systolic HF		LV hypertrophy		LV dilation		Mitral regurgitation	
	r	p-value	r	p-value	r	p-value	r	p-value	r	p-value	r	p-value
e′ and TT-e′	0.93	<0.001	0.90	<0.001	0.89	<0.001	0.88	<0.001	0.91	<0.001	0.95	<0.001
a′ and TT-a′	0.92	<0.001	0.87	<0.001	0.94	<0.001	0.89	<0.001	0.90	<0.001	0.92	<0.001
e′ + a′ and TT-e′ + TT-a′	0.94	<0.001	0.84	<0.001	0.89	<0.001	0.85	<0.001	0.88	<0.001	0.96	<0.001
TT-e′/TT-a′ and e′/a′	0.90	<0.001	0.92	<0.001	0.87	<0.001	0.94	<0.001	0.94	<0.001	0.86	<0.001
TT-e′/TT-a′ and E/A	0.67	<0.001	0.83	<0.001	0.79	<0.001	0.87	<0.001	0.52	<0.001	0.62	<0.001
TT-s′ and TT-e′ + TT-a′	0.88	<0.001	0.82	<0.001	0.73	<0.001	0.66	<0.001	0.76	<0.001	0.88	<0.001
s′ and TT-e′ + TT-a′	0.85	<0.001	0.73	<0.001	0.70	<0.001	0.56	<0.001	0.78	<0.001	0.89	<0.001
e′ + a′ and s′	0.82	<0.001	0.74	<0.001	0.74	<0.001	0.43	<0.001	0.75	<0.001	0.87	<0.001
LVEF and TT-e′ + TT-a′	0.71	<0.001	−0.03	0.83	0.52	<0.001	0.01	0.94	0.81	<0.001	0.58	<0.001
LS and TT-e′ + TT-a′	−0.60	<0.001	−0.06	0.67	−0.50	<0.001	−0.18	0.21	−0.57	<0.001	−0.64	<0.001
LSR and TT-e′ + TT-a′	−0.41	<0.001	0.05	0.73	−0.29	0.05	−0.31	<0.05	−0.40	<0.05	−0.52	<0.001
LD and TT-e′ + TT-a′	0.76	<0.001	0.52	<0.001	0.31	<0.05	0.33	<0.05	0.75	<0.001	0.78	<0.001
MAPSE and TT-e′ + TT-a′	0.82	<0.001	0.63	<0.001	0.54	<0.001	0.37	<0.01	0.83	<0.001	0.84	<0.001

HF heart failure, *LV* left ventricular, *e′* early mitral annular diastolic velocity, *TT-e′* displacement in early diastole, *a′* late mitral annular diastolic velocity, *TT-a′* displacement in late diastole, *TT-e′ + TT-a′* total average diastolic displacement; *s′*, mitral annular systolic velocity, *TT-s′* total average systolic displacement, *LVEF* left ventricular ejection fraction, *LS* longitudinal strain derived from the 4-chamber view, *LSR* longitudinal strain rate derived from the 4-chamber view, *LD* longitudinal displacement derived from strain imaging in the 4-chamber view, *MAPSE* M-mode derived mitral annular plane systolic excursion

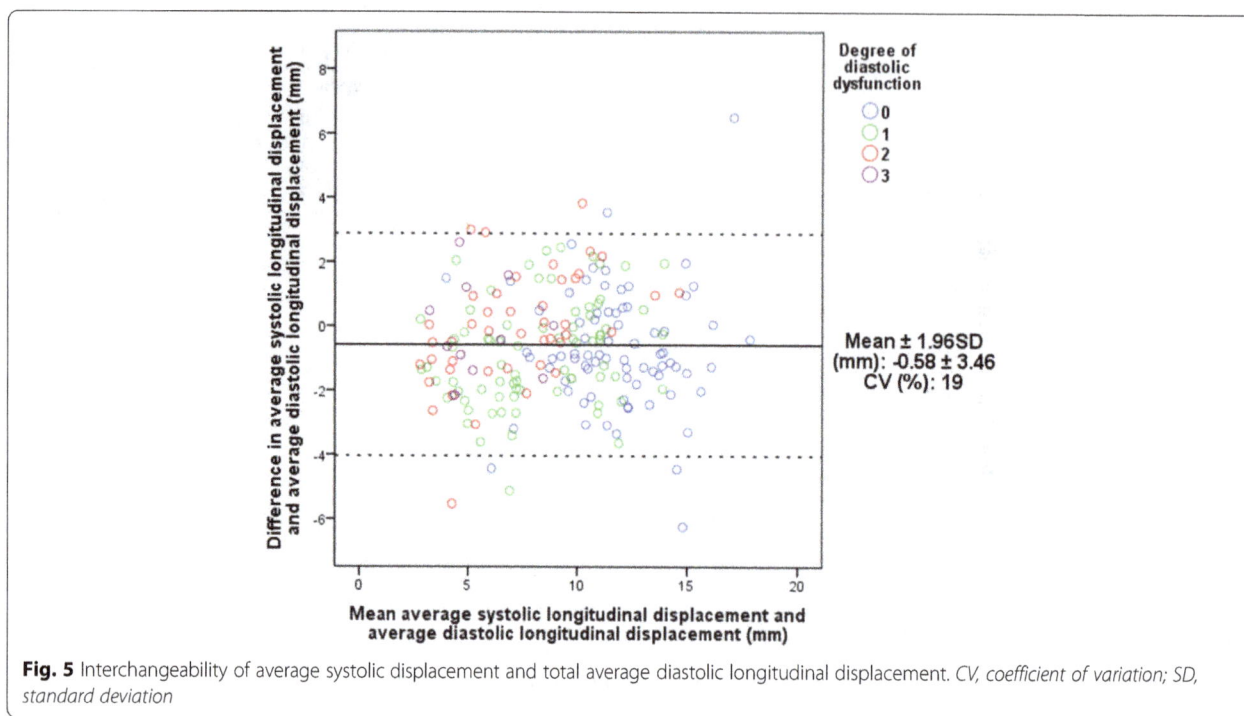

Fig. 5 Interchangeability of average systolic displacement and total average diastolic longitudinal displacement. *CV, coefficient of variation; SD, standard deviation*

variety of different cardiac conditions [14]. Even though it is reproducible, widespread, and allows for extensive off-line analysis [15], it is underutilised in clinical practice. Limitations of TDI include angle dependency with possible underestimations of tissue velocities if the angle of interrogation exceeds 20° [14] and overestimations when using excessive gain [16]. Furthermore, difficulties in estimating diastolic tissue velocities and displacement arise in patients with non-discernible E and A waves, i.e. patients with atrial fibrillation.

Total average diastolic longitudinal displacement and degree of diastolic dysfunction

One of the major drawbacks of current diastolic parameters is that there often is a biphasic element involved, as is seen with E/A and DT. This results in difficulty in discerning between a patient with normal diastolic function and a patient with a relatively severe grade of diastolic dysfunction. As depicted in Fig. 2, total average diastolic LD has a linear relationship with the degree of diastolic dysfunction, thereby eliminating this risk of misinterpretation. This linear relationship is due to a fall in TT-e' in the mild stages of diastolic dysfunction and TT-a' which only starts to diminish at more severe degrees of diastolic dysfunction (Additional file 1: Figure S1 and S2). A total average diastolic LD of 10 mm was found to be a consistent threshold for the general discrimination of patients with or without diastolic dysfunction and this can potentially be used in a clinical situation as an independent marker for the general

evaluation of a patient's overall diastolic function. Furthermore, total average diastolic LD considers the shape of the E- and A-wave and not just peak velocity values. Theoretically, this must provide a more reliable measurement in comparison to single snapshot based parameters, see below.

Total average diastolic longitudinal displacement in various heart conditions

Total average diastolic LD is a potentially superior parameter for the true evaluation of diastolic dysfunction in comparison to current velocity based echocardiographic parameters: total average diastolic LD looks at the entire diastolic process as it takes the shape of the E and A diastolic waves, and not just peak values, into consideration. This is illustrated in Fig. 3 where controls and patients with LV hypertrophy have a preserved total average diastolic dysfunction despite being classified as having abnormal relaxation. A compensatory mechanism that is not measured by current diastolic evaluation methods could, potentially, be at work. An analysis of the configuration of the E- and A-waves in controls and in patients with LV hypertrophy and an abnormal relaxation pattern (Table 3) reveals that preserved diastolic LD is not due to a compensatory increase in overall A-wave size, as one might anticipate, but is due to E-waves being low and broad in shape and A-waves being high and narrow in shape, a situation that is not taken into consideration when just looking at peak velocities.

Table 6 Unadjusted and adjusted univariable and multivariable odds ratios

	Unadjusted model:		Multivariable model adjusted for age and gender:		Multivariable model adjusted for age, gender, LVEF, LVIDd/BSA, LVMI, LS:	
	Odds ratio (95 % CI)	P-value	Odds ratio (95 % CI)	P-value	Odds ratio (95 % CI)	P-value
TT-e' + TT-a' per 1 mm decrease	1.47 (1.26–1.71)	<0.001	1.33 (1.13–1.57)	<0.01	1.35 (1.04–1.74)	<0.05
TT-e' per 1 mm decrease	1.63 (1.30–2.04)	<0.001	1.39 (1.07–1.80)	<0.05	1.18 (0.82–1.69)	0.374
TT-a' per 1 mm decrease[a]	1.59 (1.26–2.03)	<0.001	1.51 (1.16–1.95)	<0.01	1.38 (1.01–1.88)	<0.05
TT-s' per 1 mm decrease	1.31 (1.16–1.48)	<0.001	1.18 (1.03–1.36)	<0.05	1.05 (0.83–1.33)	0.703
-e' per 1 cm/s decrease	1.70 (1.34–2.15)	<0.001	1.41 (1.07–1.85)	<0.05	1.24 (0.90–1.72)	0.192
-a' per 1 cm/s decrease[a]	1.45 (1.20–1.73)	<0.001	1.35 (1.10–1.65)	<0.01	1.25 (0.99–1.58)	0.066
-e' + a' per 1 cm/s decrease	1.42 (1.24–1.62)	<0.001	1.30 (1.12–1.51)	<0.01	1.27 (1.04–1.55)	<0.05
Per degree of DDF:						
• No DDF	-	-	-	-	-	-
• DDF 1	2.26 (0.80–6.38)	0.124	0.76 (0.22–2.58)	0.658	0.39 (0.10–1.50)	0.171
• DDF 2	5.44 (1.91–15.52)	<0.01	1.59 (0.48–5.26)	0.451	0.80 (0.21–3.02)	0.744
• DDF 3	1.17 (0.13–10.72)	0.892	0.59 (0.06–5.94)	0.652	0.21 (0.02–2.51)	0.216
E/e' per 1 unit decrease	1.09 (1.04–1.14)	<0.001	1.05 (1.01–1.09)	<0.05	1.04 (1.00–1.09)	0.058
E/A per 1 unit decrease	1.04 (0.61–1.79)	0.881	1.43 (0.78–2.60)	0.248	1.28 (0.69–2.37)	0.432
DT per 1 ms decrease	1.00 (1.00–1.01)	0.921	1.00 (0.99–1.00)	0.535	1.00 (1.00–1.01)	0.997
LAD per 1 cm decrease	1.56 (0.53–4.63)	0.420	1.85 (0.42–8.19)	0.420	-	-
LA volume per 1 ml/m² decrease	1.05 (1.02–1.08)	<0.001	1.04 (1.01–1.07)	<0.05	1.05 (1.01–1.09)	<0.05
Per change in patient subgroup:						
• Control	-	-	-	-	-	-
• Cardiac dysfunction	9.08 (1.07–77.08)	<0.05	3.75 (0.39–36.30)	0.253	1.01 (0.07–15.01)	0.993
• LV hypertrophy	5.46 (0.61–48.53)	0.128	1.89 (0.19–18.79)	0.586	1.06 (0.09–12.34)	0.966
• LV dilation	27.79 (3.35–230.35)	<0.01	7.49 (0.83–67.96)	0.073	0.75 (0.03–18.18)	0.859
• Mitral regurgitation	18 (2.15–150.46)	<0.01	7.19 (0.79–65.87)	0.081	3.88 (0.39–38.60)	0.248

DDF Degree of diastolic dysfunction, *e'* early mitral annular diastolic velocity, *TT-e'* displacement in early diastole, *a'* late mitral annular diastolic velocity, *TT-a'* displacement in late diastole, *TT-e' + TT-a'* total average diastolic displacement, *s'* mitral annular systolic velocity, *TT-s'* total average systolic displacement, *DT* deceleration time, *LAD* left atrial diameter, *LA* left atrial
[a]Interaction with subgroup type

An analysis of the various heart conditions of the patients included in this study reveals that total average diastolic LD is a potential indicator of diastolic dysfunction irrespective of the primary heart condition, as discussed below:

With regards to the control group, as expected, the majority of patients are categorised as having either normal diastolic function or grade 1 diastolic dysfunction. An unexpected finding, however, is that the majority of control patients with grade 1 diastolic dysfunction have a diastolic LD >10 mm. On further analysis, these individuals did not have enlarged left atriums and the sole reason for these individuals being classified as having grade 1 diastolic dysfunction was a LA volume <34 ml/m². The majority of these patients also had an E/A ratio <0.8.

With regard to patients with severe systolic heart failure, it is questionable how a patient with severely reduced systolic function (eyeball LVEF <30 %) can have

a preserved diastolic function as, with regards to conventional understanding, a reduced systolic function should result in a reduced diastolic function and vice versa. A closer inspection of these patients revealed that the individuals with a diastolic LD >10 mm had reduced markers of systolic function, though greater than individuals with a diastolic LD <10 mm.

With regards to patients with LV hypertrophy, a preserved total average diastolic LD is seen despite patients being categorised as having an abnormal relaxation pattern, indicating that total average diastolic LD may not be optimal for the discernment of diastolic dysfunction in this patient group. As described above, an analysis of the E- and A-waves of these patients (Table 3) reveals broad E-waves and tall, narrow A-waves. For subjects with LV hypertrophy and grade 1 and 2 diastolic dysfunction (Table 4), a moderate correlation was found between total average systolic LD and total average diastolic LD as well as between s' and total average

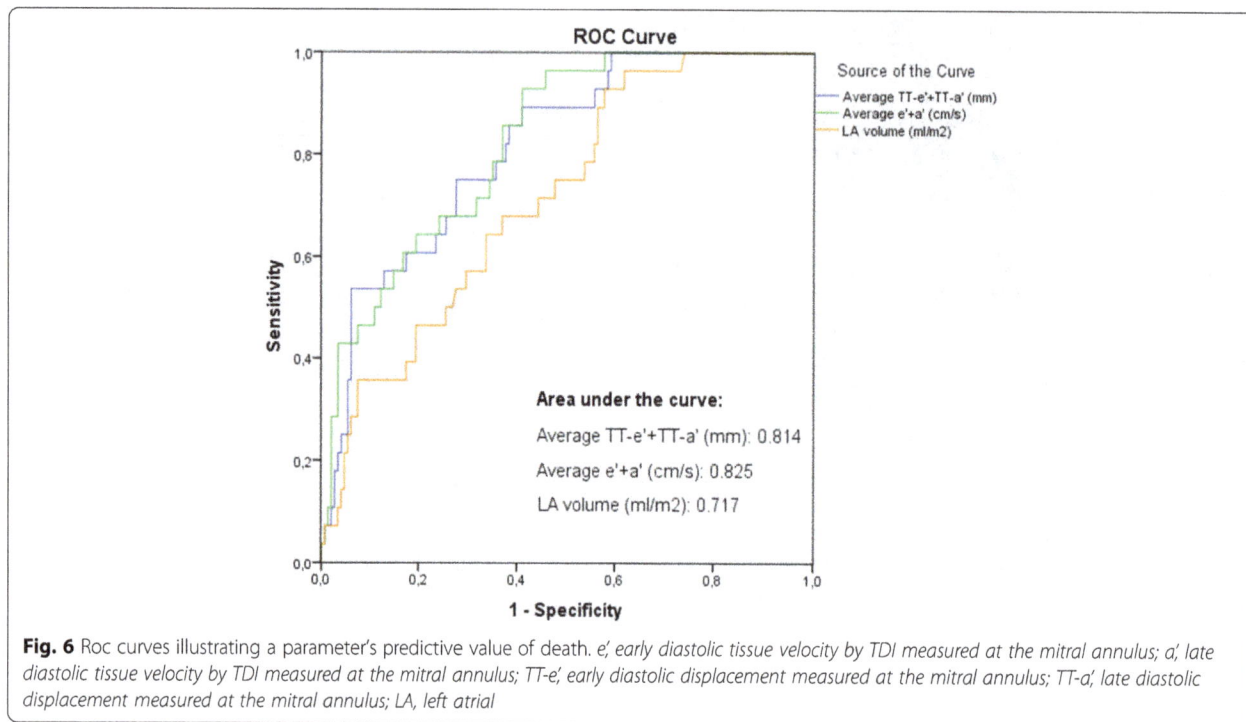

Fig. 6 Roc curves illustrating a parameter's predictive value of death. *e', early diastolic tissue velocity by TDI measured at the mitral annulus; a', late diastolic tissue velocity by TDI measured at the mitral annulus; TT-e', early diastolic displacement measured at the mitral annulus; TT-a', late diastolic displacement measured at the mitral annulus; LA, left atrial*

diastolic LD indicating a potentially preserved systolic function and reduced diastolic function, as would be expected in patients with LV hypertrophy. An examination of parameters of systolic function indicates slightly reduced systolic function.

With regards to patients with LV dilation and mitral regurgitation, the expected pattern of falling diastolic LD with increasing grades of diastolic dysfunction is seen. No patients with LV dilation have normal diastolic function, as is to be expected.

Systolic and diastolic function

LV systolic dysfunction is commonly differentiated from LV diastolic dysfunction by the presence of a reduced LVEF [17, 18]. This differentiation is potentially erroneous as abnormalities of contractile function and diastolic dysfunction have been shown to coexist, and diastolic dysfunction often has its genesis in systole [19]. The idea of isolated diastolic function can, therefore, be questioned and it can be suggested that heart failure should be viewed as an individual disease where systolic and diastolic dysfunction are the extremes on a spectrum of different phenotypes of the same disease [19, 20]. In this study, systolic and diastolic function are shown to go hand-in-hand, i.e. a patient with poor systolic function is also shown to have poor diastolic function. This relationship is clearly depicted when using total average diastolic LD as a marker of diastolic dysfunction (Fig. 4), indicating that LD is a potentially valid substitute for present velocity-based determinations of diastolic dysfunction.

Likewise, it is relevant to test the correlation between average systolic LD and total average diastolic LD as, intuitively, heart LD in systole must equal heart LD in diastole if the heart is to remain the same overall size. Good associations were found with regards to total average diastolic LD and measurements of systolic heart function such as peak systolic velocity (s'), systolic LD (TT-s'), M-mode derived MAPSE and 2D strain derived LD (Table 5). This finding, as well as the relationship seen between LVEF and total average diastolic dysfunction in Fig. 4, also challenges the concept of isolated diastolic dysfunction. It would be correct to classify patients with reduced diastolic function and preserved LVEF as patients with heart failure with preserved ejection fraction (HFPEF) but incorrect to assume that these patients have isolated diastolic dysfunction as we found that systolic function, determined by longitudinal deformation measurements such as s' and LS, was reduced in these patients despite a preserved LVEF. This indicates that diastolic LD may additionally be a marker of systolic function that is more sensitive than LVEF.

Despite acceptable correlations between total average diastolic LD and measurements of systolic heart function (Table 5), it can be seen that echocardiographic systolic measurements are not identical to diastolic measurements. This may be partially due to the presence of L-waves which were not included in the assessment of diastolic LD as only E- and A-waves were evaluated. L-waves are often observed in mid-diastole and indicate continued pulmonary vein flow through the left atrium into the left ventricle after the E-wave [21]. Furthermore, the discrepancy between total average diastolic LD and systolic heart function may indicate that the relationship between early and late diastole may reveal aspects of heart pump function that cannot be revealed by an assessment of systolic function alone.

Interchangeability and reproducibility of displacement measurements

Average systolic LD was found to slightly underestimate total average diastolic LD by approximately 0.6 mm (Fig. 5). Even though limits of agreement are wide (±3.46 mm), a CV of 19 % suggests that these two parameters are potentially interchangeable.

Furthermore, as is shown in Table 5, the correlation between average diastolic peak velocity measurements and total average diastolic LD was very good and a similar relationship of e' + a' with the degree of diastolic dysfunction compared to TT-e' + TT-a' and the degree of diastolic function was found, albeit a cut-off of 12 cm/s is more appropriate here instead of 10 mm (Additional file 1: Figure S3). Furthermore, area under the curve illustrating the predictive value of TT-e' + TT-a' and e' + a' was very similar. As total average diastolic LD is a little tricky and time consuming to measure, average diastolic peak velocity measurements seems to be a valid substitute.

Reproducibility of displacement measurements of E- and A-waves was reasonable, taking into consideration that this is the first time that diastolic LD by colour TDI has been validated, and was fairly equal in the determination of both intra and interobserver variability. Limits of agreement were fairly wide and the largest variability was seen in the determination of displacement of the lateral A-wave.

Prediction of adverse cardiac outcomes

An analysis of death as an endpoint, using odds ratios and ROC curve analyses, showed that risk of death per unit decrease in both average diastolic LD (TT-e' + TT-a') and average peak diastolic velocities (e' + a') was similar, even after adjustment for covariates.

Clinical implications

Total average diastolic LD has the potential to revolutionise the way in which we look at diastolic function. It looks at the entire diastolic process, therefore, making it a promising and sensitive marker of diastolic function. Furthermore, it has the potential to be used in a clinical setting as a quick and effective determinant of patients with and without diastolic dysfunction.

Study limitations

A variety of limitations in this study have to be addressed:

Firstly, the validity of total average diastolic LD was measured against determinants from current guidelines for the non-invasive determination of diastolic dysfunction as the golden standard. Future research with the use of invasive diastolic measurements is, therefore, required.

Secondly, only the septal and lateral wall in the 4-chamber view was assessed. A truer (but also much more time-consuming) depiction of global longitudinal diastolic performance would be obtained if the anterior, inferior, posterior and anteroseptal mitral annular sites were included.

Thirdly, all-cause mortality was the only primary endpoint evaluated in this study. An assessment of more endpoints, including cardiovascular death, may show the prognostic value of total average diastolic LD to be even higher.

Conclusions

Total average diastolic LD is a promising alternative to current algorithm-based evaluations. It has a linear relationship with the degree of diastolic dysfunction assessed by current guidelines and a 10 mm threshold in total average diastolic LD can potentially be used independently to evaluate patients with and without diastolic dysfunction in a variety of different heart conditions with reasonable intra and interobserver reproducibility.

Abbreviations
2DSI: Two-dimensional strain imaging; A: Atrial mitral inflow velocity; a': Atrial mitral annular diastolic velocity; A-wave: Atrial mitral annular diastolic velocity wave; CV: Coefficient of variation; DT: Deceleration time; E: Early mitral inflow velocity; e': Early mitral annular diastolic velocity; E-wave: Early mitral annular diastolic velocity wave; LA: Left atrial; LD: Longitudinal displacement; LS: Longitudinal strain; LSR: Longitudinal strain rate; LV: Left ventricle; LVEF: Left ventricular ejection fraction; TDI: Tissue Doppler imaging; TT-a': Mean atrial diastolic longitudinal displacement; TT-e': Mean early diastolic longitudinal displacement; TT-e' + TT-a': Total average diastolic longitudinal displacement; TT-s': Mean systolic longitudinal displacement

Funding
The Division of Clinical Cardiovascular Research, Department of Cardiology, Herlev and Gentofte Hospital.

Authors' contributions
MK made substantial contributions to the conception or design of the work, the acquisition, analysis, interpretation of data, drafting the work and revising it critically for important intellectual content, performed final approval of the version to be published, and agree to be accountable for all aspects of the work in ensuring that questions related to the accuracy or integrity of any part of the work are appropriately investigated and resolved. RM and JSJ made substantial contributions to the conception, acquisition, and interpretation of data, revising it critically for important intellectual content, performed final approval of the version to be published, and agree to be accountable for all aspects of the work in ensuring that questions related to the accuracy or integrity of any part of the work are appropriately investigated and resolved. TBS, JS and PS made substantial contributions to acquisition, and interpretation of data, revising it critically for important intellectual content, performed final approval of the version to be published, and agree to be accountable for all aspects of the work in ensuring that questions related to the accuracy or integrity of any part of the work are appropriately investigated and resolved. All authors read and approved the final manuscript.

Competing interests

All authors report no support from any organisation for the submitted work; no financial relationships with any organisations that might have an interest in the submitted work; no other relationships or activities that could appear to have influenced the submitted work.

Author details

[1]Herlev and Gentofte Hospital, Department of Cardiology, Faculty of Health Sciences, University of Copenhagen, Copenhagen, Denmark. [2]Department of Cardiology, Centre for Cardiovascular Research, Aalborg University Hospital, Aalborg, Denmark. [3]Rigshospitalet, Department of Cardiology, Faculty of Health Sciences, University of Copenhagen, Copenhagen, Denmark.

References

1. Tschöpe C, Paulus WJ. Is echocardiographic evaluation of diastolic function useful in determining clinical care? Doppler echocardiography yields dubious estimates of left ventricular diastolic pressures. Circulation. 2009;120(9):810–20. discussion 820.
2. Nagueh SF, Smiseth OA, Appleton CP, Byrd BF, Dokainish H, Edvardsen T, et al. Recommendations for the evaluation of left ventricular diastolic function by echocardiography: an update from the American society of echocardiography and the European association of cardiovascular imaging. J Am Soc Echocardiogr. 2016;29(4):277–314.
3. Little WC, Oh JK. Echocardiographic evaluation of diastolic function can be used to guide clinical care. Circulation. 2009;120(9):802–9.
4. Petrie MC, Hogg K, Caruana L, McMurray JJV. Poor concordance of commonly used echocardiographic measures of left ventricular diastolic function in patients with suspected heart failure but preserved systolic function: is there a reliable echocardiographic measure of diastolic dysfunction? Heart. 2004;90(5):511–7.
5. Paulus WJ, Tschöpe C, Sanderson JE, Rusconi C, Flachskampf FA, Rademakers FE, et al. How to diagnose diastolic heart failure: a consensus statement on the diagnosis of heart failure with normal left ventricular ejection fraction by the Heart Failure and Echocardiography Associations of the European Society of Cardiology. Eur Heart J. 2007;28(20):2539–50.
6. McCulloch M, Zoghbi WA, Davis R, Thomas C, Dokainish H. Color tissue Doppler myocardial velocities consistently underestimate spectral tissue Doppler velocities: impact on calculation peak transmitral pulsed Doppler velocity/early diastolic tissue Doppler velocity (E/Ea). J Am Soc Echocardiogr. 2006;19(6):744–8.
7. Geske JB, Sorajja P, Nishimura RA, Ommen SR. Evaluation of left ventricular filling pressures by Doppler echocardiography in patients with hypertrophic cardiomyopathy: correlation with direct left atrial pressure measurement at cardiac catheterization. Circulation. 2007;116(23):2702–8.
8. Mullens W, Borowski AG, Curtin RJ, Thomas JD, Tang WH. Tissue Doppler imaging in the estimation of intracardiac filling pressure in decompensated patients with advanced systolic heart failure. Circulation. 2009;119(1):62–70.
9. Mogelvang R, Biering-Sørensen T, Jensen JS. Tissue Doppler echocardiography predicts acute myocardial infarction, heart failure, and cardiovascular death in the general population. Eur Heart J Cardiovasc Imaging. 2015;16(12):1331–7.
10. Lang RM, Badano LP, Mor-Avi V, Afilalo J, Armstrong A, Ernande L, et al. Recommendations for cardiac chamber quantification by echocardiography in adults: an update from the American Society of Echocardiography and the European Association of Cardiovascular Imaging. Eur Heart J Cardiovasc Imaging. 2015;16(3):233–70.
11. Devereux RB, Alonso DR, Lutas EM, Gottlieb GJ, Campo E, Sachs I, et al. Echocardiographic assessment of left ventricular hypertrophy: comparison to necropsy findings. Am J Cardiol. 1986;57(6):450–8.
12. Zoghbi WA, Enriquez-Sarano M, Foster E, Grayburn PA, Kraft CD, Levine RA, et al. Recommendations for evaluation of the severity of native valvular regurgitation with two-dimensional and Doppler echocardiography. J Am Soc Echocardiogr. 2003;16(7):777–802.
13. Hanneman SK. Design, analysis and interpretation of method-comparison studies. AACN Adv Crit Care. 2008;19(2):223–34.
14. Kadappu KK, Thomas L. Tissue Doppler imaging in echocardiography: value and limitations. Heart Lung Circ. 2015;24(3):224–33.
15. de Knegt MC, Biering-Sorensen T, Sogaard P, Sivertsen J, Jensen JS, Mogelvang R. Concordance and reproducibility between M-mode, tissue Doppler imaging, and two-dimensional strain imaging in the assessment of mitral annular displacement and velocity in patients with various heart conditions. Eur Heart J Cardiovasc Imaging. 2014;15(1):62–9.
16. Marwick TH. Clinical applications of tissue Doppler imaging: a promise fulfilled. Heart. 2003;89(12):1377–8.
17. De Keulenaer GW, Brutsaert DL. Diastolic heart failure: a separate disease or selection bias? Prog Cardiovasc Dis. 2007;49(4):275–83.
18. Yu C-M, Lin H, Yang H, Kong S-L, Zhang Q, Lee SW-L. Progression of systolic abnormalities in patients with "isolated" diastolic heart failure and diastolic dysfunction. Circulation. 2002;105(10):1195–201.
19. Brutsaert DL, De Keulenaer GW. Diastolic heart failure: a myth. Curr Opin Cardiol. 2006;21(3):240–8.
20. Shah AM, Solomon SD. Phenotypic and pathophysiological heterogeneity in heart failure with preserved ejection fraction. Eur Heart J. 2012;33(14):1716–7.
21. Kerut EK. The Mitral L-Wave: a relatively common but ignored useful finding. Echocardiography. 2008;25(5):548–50.

2

Myocardial performance index in female athletes

Zahraa Alsafi[1*], Andreas Malmgren[1], Petri Gudmundsson[2], Martin Stagmo[3] and Magnus Dencker[1]

Abstract

Background: Long-term intensive training leads to morphological and mechanical changes in the heart generally known as "athlete's heart". Previous studies have suggested that the diastolic and systolic function of the ventricles is unaltered in athletes compared to sedentary.

The purpose of this study was to investigate myocardial performance index (MPI) by pulsed wave Doppler (PWD) and by tissue Doppler imaging (TDI) in female elite athletes compared to sedentary controls.

Methods: The study consisted of 32 athletes (mean age 20 ± 2 years) and 34 sedentary controls (mean age 23 ± 2 years). MPI by PWD and TDI were measured in the left (LV) and right ventricle (RV) in both groups. Moreover, comparisons of MPI by the two methods and between the LV and RV within the two groups were made.

Results: There were no significant differences in MPI between athletes and controls ($p > 0.05$), whereas the LV had significantly higher MPI compared to RV ($p < 0.001$, in athletes and controls). The agreement and the correlation between the two methods measuring MPI showed low agreement and no correlation (athletes RV $r = -0.027$, LV $r = 0.12$; controls RV $r = 0.20$, LV $r = 0.30$).

Conclusion: The global function of the LV and RV measured by MPI with PWD and TDI is similar in female athletes compared to sedentary controls. Conversely, both MPI by PWD and by TDI shows a significant difference between the LV and RV. However, the agreement and correlation between conventional methods of measuring MPI by PWD compared to MPI by TDI is very poor in both these populations.

Keywords: Athlete's heart, Diastolic function, Echocardiography, Left ventricle, Myocardial performance index, Right ventricle, Systolic function

Background

Persistent vigorous training increases the need for oxygenated blood to metabolic tissues in the body leading to morphological and mechanical changes in the heart generally known as "athlete's heart" [1–9]. The function of the athlete's heart has not been extensively studied, with regard to different sports and female gender. Moreover, the function of the left ventricle (LV) has been examined more than the right ventricle (RV) [9–12].

Sports can be divided into different categories but can be classified in three main groups; dynamic, static or combined (dynamic and static) sports [4, 9]. Morphologic changes of the athlete's heart are related to the type of sport practised by the athlete but it is also related to gender [6].

Myocardial performance index (MPI) is an easily measured index for the assessment of global heart function, combining both systolic and diastolic components. It can be derived from both pulsed wave Doppler (PWD) and tissue Doppler imaging (TDI) and is defined as the sum of the isovolumic contraction time (ICT) and the isovolumic relaxation time (IRT) divided by the ejection time (ET) [10, 13–24]. MPI has been shown to be independent of HR, blood pressure, loading conditions and the geometry of the ventricles [11, 17, 20, 21] and can be used to evaluate the function of both the RV and the LV [22].

No studies up till now have, to our knowledge, investigated MPI in both RV and LV in female athletes. For this reason, the aim of this study was to gain further understanding of the function of female athlete's heart by

* Correspondence: Zahraa.alsafi@hotmail.com
[1]Department of Medical Imaging and Physiology, Skåne University Hospital, Lund University, Malmö, Sweden
Full list of author information is available at the end of the article

evaluating differences in conventional MPI and MPI by TDI in elite female team-handball players compared to a sedentary group of females.

Methods
Study population
The study consisted of 35 female elite team-handball players (mean age 20 ± 2 years) and 34 sedentary controls (mean age 23 ± 2 years). Of the 35 handball players, two were excluded because of cardiovascular disease, one because of a bicuspid aortic valve and one because of a recent hospitalization of suspected myocarditis. Another handball player was excluded due to insufficient quality of echocardiographic image recording. Hence, the final study population included a total of 32 female elite team-handball players. The females included in the control group did not perform any or only slight physical activity, less than two hours a week and were a similar age to the handball players. Weight and height were measured with participants dressed in light clothing. Body mass index (BMI) was calculated as the weight in kilograms divided by the height in meters squared (kg/m^2). The formula by Du Bois and Du Bois [25] was used for the calculation of BSA. Systolic (SBP) and diastolic (DBP) blood pressure was measured in a supine position in the right arm after 10 min rest (Omron M8 Comfort, Omron Healthcare, Kyoto, Japan). All participants were given a written questionnaire to define their amount of training during a week. The female elite handball players trained in average 10.8 ± 2.3 h per week, whereas 1.7 h were strength training and another 1.8 h per week were fitness training. The remaining of the training time was used for team-game handball training. Two of the participants in the control group were smokers, while none of the athletes were smokers. All participants gave their written informed consent to take part in the study. The study was approved by the Regional Ethical Review Board of Lund University in Sweden.

Echocardiography
Participants were examined using an iE33 (Philips Medical systems, Andover, MA, USA) ultrasound equipment, with an S3 transducer, according to current guidelines by American Society of Echocardiography [26] as previously described [27]. The study was performed with the participants resting in a left lateral decubitus position. All measurements were performed three times on separate cardiac cycles and averaged. One experienced echocardiographer performed all examinations and measurements were performed off-line by another single observer using Xcelera (Philips Medical systems, Andover, MA, USA).

Conventional pulsed wave Doppler
To derive MPI of RV (MPIRV) by conventional PWD, an apical four-chamber view was obtained and the sample volume was placed between the tips of the leaflets of the tricuspid valve. An interval "a" was measured from the end to the onset of tricuspid inflow and it represents the sum of ICT, IRT and ET. The right ventricular ejection time (RVET) was obtained from the short-axis view and the sample volume was placed below the pulmonary valve. The interval "b" that represents the RVET was measured from the onset to the end of the RV outflow.

MPI of LV (MPILV) was measured from the apical four-chamber view by placing the sample volume at the tips of the mitral valve leaflets. From the end to the onset of mitral inflow "a" interval was measured. From the apical five-chamber view with the sample volume placed below the aortic valve, "b" interval was measured between onset and end of LV outflow. MPI was later calculated as (a-b)/b, representing (ICT + IRT)/ET [26]. The mean differences of MPI by PWD and TDI were tested between the two groups. Moreover, MPILV and MPIRV were tested within each group.

Tissue Doppler imaging
MPI by TDI (TDMPI) was obtained from the apical four-chamber view by placing the sample volume at the lateral mitral annulus, lateral tricuspid annulus and septal annulus. Measurements of TDI isovolumic contraction time (tICT) were obtained by measuring from the end of a′-wave (atrial-contraction wave) to the onset of s-wave (myocardial systolic wave); TDI isovolumic relaxation time (tIRT) was obtained by measuring between the end of the S-wave and the onset of the e′-wave (early-diastolic wave); TDI ejection time (tET) was measured from onset to the end of s-wave (Fig. 1). TDMPI was then calculated as (tICT + tIRT)/tET [26]. A mean value was additionally calculated between TDMPI at lateral mitral annulus (TDMPIlm) and TDMPI at septal annulus (TDMPIs) that was named (mTDMPIm/s), and also between TDMPI at lateral tricuspid annulus (TDMPIlt) and TDMPIs, (mTDMPIt/s).

A comparison was made between all TDMPI parameters, where TDMPIlm was compared to TDMPIs and to TDMPIlt. Furthermore, TDMPIs was compared to TDMPIlt and finally mTDMPIm/s compared to mTDMPIt/s. The comparisons were made within each group but also the same comparisons were made in both groups combined.

Because the echocardiographic measurements were performed by one observer, intra variability measurements were made in 5 subjects in the athletes group and 5 subjects in the sedentary control group. The intra variability measurements in the athlete group in MPIRV was 7,6%, MPILV 9,2%, TDMPIlm 6,4%, TDMPIs 7,3%, TDMPIlt 4,4%, TDMPIm/s 5% and TDMPIt/s 5,6%. In the sedentary group MPIRV was

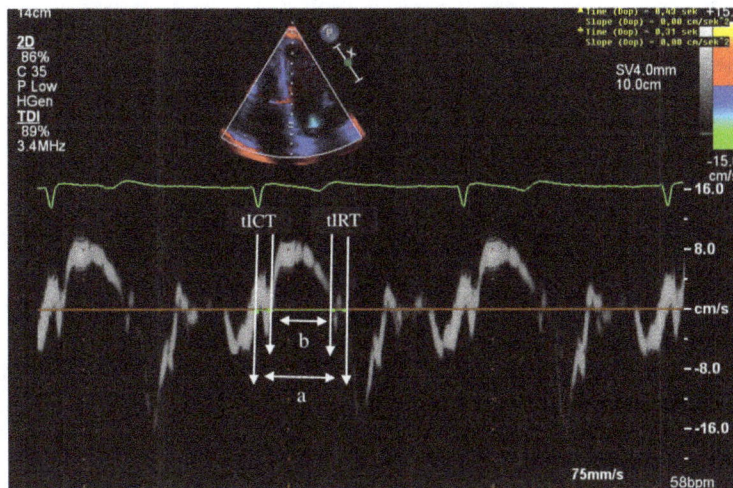

Fig. 1 Myocardial performance index measured by tissue Doppler imaging. Time intervals by tissue Doppler imaging derived from septal annulus. tICT, tissue isovolumic contraction time; tIRT, tissue isovolumic relaxation time; a = isovolumic contraction time + isovolumic relaxation time + ejection time; b = ejection time. MPI = (a-b)/b

8%, MPILV 3,4%, TDMPIlm 3,7%, TDMPIs 2,8%, TDMPIlt 3,2%, TDMPIm/s 1,6% and TDMPIt/s was 2,0%.

Statistical analysis

All statistical analyses were performed using standard statistical software (SPSS version 22.0, Inc., Chicago, IL, USA). Data are expressed as mean ± standard deviation (SD). The data was tested for normal distribution, by a visual analysis of histograms and by a Q-Q plot, which showed a normal distributed material. The independent Student's t-test was used to test for mean differences between the two groups. The paired Student's t-test was used to test for mean differences between different parameters within a group. Bland-Altman plots were used to test the agreement between the conventional MPI by PWD and TDMPI. The correlation between the two methods was tested with Pearson's correlation coefficient. Values were considered statistically significant at a *p*-value below 0.05.

Results

The acquired images were of good quality in all subjects, which made all planned measurements possible. All demographics and subject characteristics are presented in Table 1. The study population consisted of totally 66 participants, 32 athletes and 34 sedentary controls. Age, length, weight, BMI, BSA, DBP and HR were significantly different between the two groups. There were no significant differences in SBP and MPI data between athletes and controls.

MPIRV compared to MPILV showed a significant difference in the athletes group as well as in the sedentary group. The results are displayed in Table 2.

Table 1 Demographics and echocardiographic data of the athletes and the sedentary controls

	Athletes (*n* = 32)	Sedentary (*n* = 34)	*p*-value
Age (years)	20.4 ± 2.0	23.2 ± 1.7	< 0.001
Length (cm)	175 ± 7	171 ± 5	0.02
Weight (kg)	73.1 ± 8.0	64.3 ± 8.5	< 0.001
BMI (kg/m^2)	23.9 ± 2.1	22.0 ± 2.8	0,002
BSA (m^2)	1.88 ± 0.13	1.75 ± 0.12	< 0.001
Heart rate (beats/min)	56 ± 8	70 ± 13	< 0.001
SBP (mm Hg)	121 ± 8	121 ± 11	ns
DBP (mm Hg)	67 ± 6	71 ± 7	0.004
MPIRV	0.23 ± 0.13	0.20 ± 0.12	ns
MPILV	0.35 ± 0.07	0.32 ± 0.08	ns
TDMPIlm	0.47 ± 0.06	0.49 ± 0.08	ns
TDMPIs	0.52 ± 0.07	0.54 ± 0.09	ns
TDMPIlt	0.44 ± 0.07	0.45 ± 0.08	ns
mTDMPIm/s	0.50 ± 0.05	0.51 ± 0.07	ns
mTDMPIt/s	0.48 ± 0.06	0.50 ± 0.07	ns

Data values are presented as mean ± SD
Body mass index (BMI), Body surface area (BSA), Diastolic blood pressure (DBP), Systolic blood pressure (SBP), Mean value of tissue Doppler myocardial performance index derived from lateral mitral annulus and septum (mTDMPIm/s), Mean value of tissue Doppler myocardial performance index derived from lateral tricuspid annulus and septum (mTDMPIt/s), Conventional myocardial performance index of left ventricle (MPILV), Conventional myocardial performance index of right ventricle (MPIRV), Myocardial performance index by tissue Doppler of lateral mitral annulus (TDMPIlm), Myocardial performance index by tissue Doppler of lateral tricuspid annulus (TDMPIlt), Myocardial performance index by tissue Doppler of septum (TDMPIs)

Table 2 Myocardial performance index derived from conventional pulsed Doppler in athletes and sedentary

Participant	MPIRV	MPILV	p-value
Athlete (n = 32)	0.23 ± 0.13	0.35 ± 0.07	<0.001
Sedentary (n = 34)	0.20 ± 0.12	0.32 ± 0.08	<0.001

Data values are presented as mean ± SD
Conventional myocardial performance index of left ventricle (MPILV).
Conventional myocardial performance index or right ventricle (MPIRV)

All TDMPI parameters were compared to each other in both groups and all parameters showed a significant difference except for two in the athletes group, TDMPIlm compared to TDMPIlt. Likewise, TDMPIm/s compared to TDMPIt/s in the athletes group did not show any difference. When both athletes group and sedentary group were put together, all parameters showed a significant difference. All results are displayed in Tables 3 and 4.

The Bland and Altman analysis illustrated in Fig. 2 shows a clinically important disagreement between the conventional MPI by PWD and MPI by TDI. Figure 2 demonstrates a comparison between MPIRV and TDMPIRV in athletes (the mean difference was 0.21 and 95% limits of agreement from −0.08 to 0.29) and in the sedentary controls MPIRV compared to TDMPIRV showed a mean difference of 0.25 (95% limits of agreement from −0.018 to 0.50). A comparison between MPILV and TDMPILV in athletes (the mean difference was 0.12 and 95% limits of agreement from −0.06 to 0.29) and in the sedentary controls MPILV compared to TDMPILV showed a mean difference of 0.17 (95% limits of agreement from −0.015 to 0.35).

We found no statistically significant correlation between the two methods measured in both RV ($r = -0.027$) and LV ($r = 0.12$) in the athletes group and RV ($r = 0.20$) and LV ($r = 0.30$) in the sedentary controls.

Table 3 Comparison of myocardial performance index by tissue Doppler in athletes and sedentary

Tissue Doppler MPI	Athletes: (n = 32)	Sedentary (n = 34)
	Mean ± SD	Mean ± SD
A) TDMPIlm	0.47 ± 0.06	0.49 ± 0.08
B) TDMPIs	0.52 ± 0.07	0.54 ± 0.09
C) TDMPIlt	0.44 ± 0.07	0.45 ± 0.08
D) mTDMPIm/s	0.50 ± 0.05	0.51 ± 0.07
E) mTDMPIt/s	0.48 ± 0.06	0.50 ± 0.07

Data values are presented as mean ± SD
Mean value of tissue Doppler myocardial performance index derived from lateral mitral annulus and septum (mTDMPIm/s), Mean value of tissue Doppler myocardial performance index derived from lateral tricuspid annulus and septum (mTDMPIt/s), Myocardial performance index by tissue Doppler of lateral mitral annulus (TDMPIlm), Myocardial performance index by tissue Doppler of lateral tricuspid annulus (TDMPIlt), Myocardial performance index by tissue Doppler of septum (TDMPIs)
Athletes: A vs B $p = 0.001$, A vs C $p = 0.16$, B vs C $p = < 0.001$, D vs E $p = 0.15$.
Sedentary: A vs B $p = 0.001$, A vs C $p = 0.045$, B vs C $p = < 0.001$, D vs E $p = 0.03$

Table 4 Comparison of myocardial performance index by tissue Doppler in the combined group of athletes and sedentary controls (n = 66)

Tissue Doppler MPI	Mean ± SD
A) TDMPIlm	0.48 ± 0.07
B) TDMPIs	0.53 ± 0.08
C) TDMPIlt	0.45 ± 0.08
D) mTDMPIm/s	0.50 ± 0.06
E) mTDMPIt/s	0.49 ± 0.07

Data values are presented as mean ± SD
Mean value of tissue Doppler myocardial performance index derived from lateral mitral annulus and septum (mTDMPIm/s), Mean value of tissue Doppler myocardial performance index derived from lateral tricuspid annulus and septum (mTDMPIt/s), Myocardial performance index by tissue Doppler of lateral mitral annulus (TDMPIlm), Myocardial performance index by tissue Doppler of lateral tricuspid annulus (TDMPIlt), Myocardial performance index by tissue Doppler of septum (TDMPIs)
A vs B $p = < 0.001$, A vs C $p = 0.01$, B vs C $p = < 0.001$, D vs E $p = 0.01$

Discussion

This is the first report, to our knowledge, on MPI in female athletes and also the first to measure MPI in both LV and RV. This study has demonstrated that there is no significant difference in conventional MPI by PWD and TDMPI between female elite team-handball players and sedentary controls. We have also shown that conventional MPI by PWD is significantly higher in LV compared to RV in both groups.

Team-handball is classified as a highly dynamic and moderate static sport, thus combining static and dynamic training, which has more morphological/structural effects on the heart compared to other sports [4]. The cardiac dimensions of our study population have previously been examined by Malmgren and co-workers [27], who showed a significant enlargement of cardiac dimensions in female elite team-handball players compared to sedentary controls. Thus, showing that cardiac remodelling appears in elite female handball players as it does in athletes practicing endurance or team game sports [27]. Hence, our findings are supported in the study of Dzudie et al. [3] that included 21 male team-handball players and 21 male controls showing morphological changes between the group of athletes compared to the control group but no difference in the LV diastolic function or ejection fraction (EF) between the two groups. In the meta-analysis by Pluim et al. [1] no relation between cardiac geometry and cardiac systolic and diastolic function could be found in athletes. Furthermore, no differences in cardiac systolic and diastolic function between athletes and sedentary controls were demonstrated [1]. Additionally, Butz and co-workers [28] studied the morphologic cardiac changes by echocardiography in 100 male professional handball players and reported a degree of hypertrophy and increased LV mass and end diastolic diameter in their study population [28]. However, they could not show

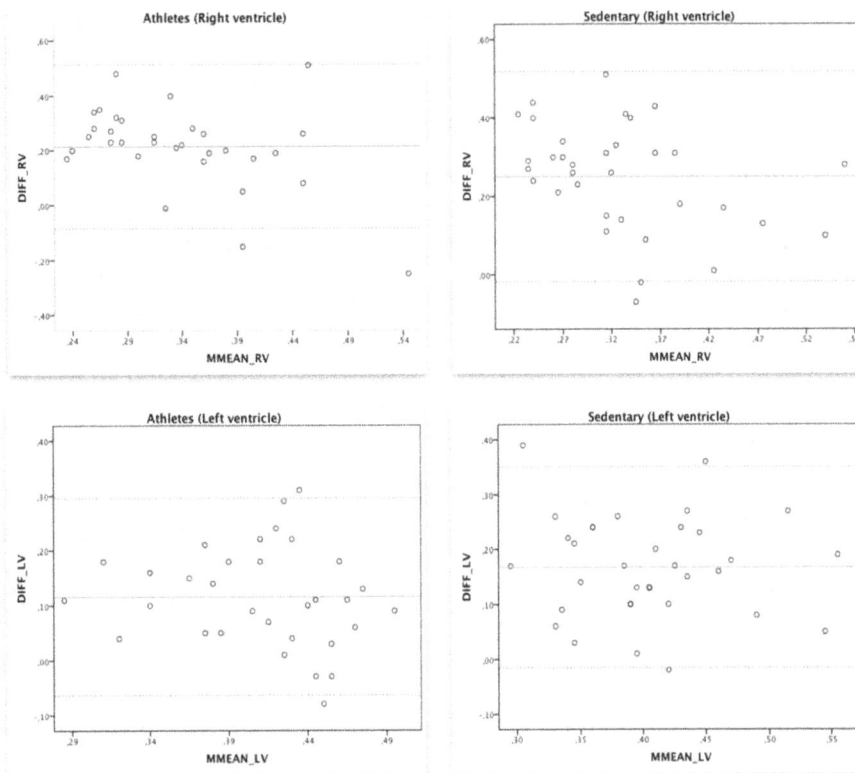

Fig. 2 Bland-Altman plot for conventional myocardial performance index (MPI) and myocardial performance index by tissue Doppler. Bland-Altman plot for conventional myocardial performance index (MPI) by pulsed wave Doppler and myocardial performance index by tissue Doppler TDMPI of right ventricle (upper left) and left ventricle (lower left) in the athletes group and the right ventricle (upper right) and left ventricle (lower left) in the sedentary group. The mean value of the two methods is displayed on the x-axis and the difference between the methods is displayed on the y-axis. The two dotted lines represent a 95% confidence interval and the solid line represents the mean difference between the measurements

any differences in diastolic function, nor in systolic or early diastolic velocities. Hence the results of the mentioned studies are similar to ours showing no significant difference in MPI between athletes and controls.

This current study did not show any difference in MPILV nor MPIRV between the two groups, which is in disagreement with the study by Kasikcioglu et al. [29] that involved 52 male athletes whereas 30 athletes were runners and 32 wrestlers, and a group of 43 sedentary controls. The study stated a significant difference in MPIRV between the athletes and the controls, showing a lower MPI at the RV of athletes compared to controls. Moreover, the study of Tüzün and co-workers [30] that included 66 elite male athletes (36 sprinters and 30 endurance athletes) and 33 sedentary controls were able to demonstrate a significant difference in MPILV between athletes and controls. MPI was reported as 0.37 ± 0.07 in sprinters and 0.36 ± 0.05 in endurance athletes and these results corresponds to our value of MPILV in athletes, which was reported as 0.35 ± 0.07. However, the value of MPI in the sedentary controls in both studies mentioned [29, 30] is much higher and does

not correspond to ours. Also, their results does not correspond to earlier studies where the normal range for MPI was reported as 0.34 ± 0.04 in healthy volunteers by Moller et al. [31]. Previous studies have reported more effect on male athlete's heart compared to females [6, 7]. Furthermore, this present study consisted of a lower number of participants compared to the study by Kasikcioglu et al. [29], which may be a limitation in the possibility of reporting a significant difference between the two groups. Besides, the male athletes in the mentioned study [29] trained as a minimum 10 h per week for at least 8 years. The athletes in our study had been training at elite level from 0 to 8 years. The significant difference in RV in the male athletes could have been caused by training for a longer period of time compared to the female athletes of this current study.

In both athletes and sedentary controls there is a significant difference in MPI by PWD between LV and RV. This difference may exist due to the different shape and geometry between the LV and the RV. The size of the RV is about two-thirds the size of the LV [32] and the RV wall is thinner (2–5 mm) compared to the wall of the LV (7–11 mm) [33]. Also, the LV has a twisting and rotating motion when contracting, while the twisting and rotating motion does not contribute to the contraction of the RV [34]. Besides, the pressure in the RV reaches an early peak compared to the LV and also a rapid decline in pressure. This is due to the low pulmonary artery diastolic pressure that the RV needs to exceed while contracting and therefore the ICT is shorter in RV compared to LV. The filling in RV starts before the LV and finishes after and also the IRT is shorter in RV compared to LV [34]. All of these different characters of LV and RV may be a reason of the significant difference between the ventricles seen in MPI by PWD. However, even though there are differences between the ventricles, they still generally pump the same effective stroke volume [34].

When TDMPI parameters were compared to one another in each group separately, all comparisons showed a significant difference in the sedentary control group. Although in the athletes group the TDMPIlm compared to TDMPIlt did not show any significant difference, neither did mTDMPIm/s compared to mTDMPIt/s. As seen in Table 3 the p-values in both groups follow the same pattern, whereas the p-value of TDMPIlm compared to TDMPIlt and mTDMPIm/s compared to mTDMPIt/s shows a weak significance in the sedentary controls. Consequently, since all other result were similar between both groups as well as the fact that all participants are young healthy subjects, they were all merged as a group to make the same comparisons. The results of this analysis are presented in Table 4 showing a significant difference between all TDMPI parameters. This indicates that TDMPI measured at the mitral, tricuspid and septal annulus is significantly different in all young and healthy subjects. These findings are similar to our findings presented from the conventional MPI by PWD that showed a difference in MPI between the two ventricles. Both LV and RV affect the septal annulus and therefore a significant difference is seen when comparing mTDMPIm/s and mTDMPIt/s. The different characters mentioned previously between the ventricles, also support these results showing a difference between LV and RV. The study by Rojo et al. [18] that included 77 patients with a previous myocardial infarction and a control group of 20 healthy young subjects, TDMPI was measured at septal annulus and lateral mitral annulus and additionally a mean value between those two measurements was calculated. In the healthy control group TDMPIlm compared to TDMPIs did not show any significant difference while in the present study there is a significant difference. The current study has a larger number of subjects included, which may be an explanation of that.

The results of this study have not been adjusted for age even though there was a significant difference in age between the athletes and the sedentary controls. Normally, the vascular stiffening is increased from the age of 30 and onward in both male and females [35]. The stiffening mostly affects the diastolic function of the LV, whereas the early diastolic filling rate decreases after the age of 20, so that by the age of 80, the early diastolic filling rate is declined to nearly 50% [35]. Since both groups are healthy young people, mostly in their early twenties, the adjustment for age was not considered to be of any significance.

The HR of athletes was significantly lower compared to the sedentary controls, but no adjustment for HR was made in this study. The reason is that MPI has been established to be independent of HR in a study by Tei et al. [11] consisting of 37 normal subjects and 26 patients with primary pulmonary hypertension. In that study, HR was correlated with each Doppler parameter in normal subjects and patients with primary pulmonary hypertension. The results showed a significant correlation between HR and ICT, IRT and ET. Though, there was no significant association between HR and MPI [11].

Keser et al. [15] showed a good correlation between the two methods measuring MPI and suggested the use of TDI when measuring MPI. This is due to the superiority of the methods' sensitivity in not being affected by HR fluctuations. Also Harada et al. [17] showed very good correlation between the two methods. However, more recent studies have presented moderate to low correlation between the conventional way of measuring MPI and the modified method by TDI. Rojo et al. [18] suggested that the modified MPI by TDI is not possible to be used as an alternative to the conventional MPI by PWD due to the weak correlation between the two methods. The present study consisting of a higher number of participants compared to previously mentioned studies did not show any correlation between the two methods of measuring MPI and the agreement between the methods was shown to be low. Our findings are similar to those of Rojo et al. [18] that showed poor agreement between the methods due to longer systolic intervals and shorter diastolic intervals when measuring with TDI.

Furthermore, the Bland-Altman plots in Fig. 2 shows that the TDI measurements always show higher MPI values compared to measuring with PWD. These findings can be supported by the fact that the upper reference limit of MPI by PWD is 0.40, while the upper reference limit of TDMPI is 0.55 [26]. The difference between the two methods is that TDMPI is measured in one cardiac cycle, while the inflow and outflow velocities in left ventricle outflow tract and right ventricle outflow tract measured by the PWD are not possible to measure from the same cardiac cycle [26]. This might explain that no correlation was seen between the two methods.

Moreover, newer echocardiographic methods exist to evaluate LV and RV function in athletes. Vitarelli and co-workers [36] used TDI, speckle-tracking imaging

(STI) and three-dimensional echocardiography to assess systemic ventricular-vascular function and RV function in athletes. They showed that ventricular and vascular response in athletes underlie different adaptations of ventricular volumes and arterial stiffness. STI was also used by Oxborough et al. [37] to estimate RV structure and function in ultra-endurance athletes and determine whether changes in the RV are correlated with alterations in LV function. The study could demonstrate that there is a RV dilatation and dysfunction in the recovery after an ultra-marathon. Likewise LV systolic and diastolic function also is reduced after an ultramarathon which is believed to be a result of a combination of essential reduction in function and RV interaction. Additionally, Knackstedt et al. [38] used STI in former world class swimmers to evaluate the cardiac function, employing longitudinal strain and circumferential strain. The results of their study are in concordance with ours, showing that there is no definite LV or RV dysfunction in athletes using modern imaging modalities.

Limitations
The limitation of measuring MPI in the conventional way by PWD is that the inflow and outflow velocities are measured separately. The reproducibility of the method is therefore reduced and is also affected by fluctuations in the HR during the examination. This makes the calculation of the index more complex, because several cardiac cycles have to be obtained to average the measurements.

Conclusion
The global function of the LV and RV measured by MPI with PWD and TDI is similar in female elite team-handball players compared to sedentary controls. Conversely, both MPI by PWD and TDMPI shows a significant difference between LV and RV, whereas LV has higher MPI compared to RV. However, the agreement and correlation between conventional methods of measuring MPI by PWD compared to TDMPI is not good and therefore TDMPI should not be used interchangeably with MPI by PWD.

Abbreviations
BMI: Body Mass Index; BSA: Body surface area; EF: Ejection fraction; ET: Ejection time; HR: Heart rate; ICT: Isovolumic contraction time; IRT: Isovolumic relaxation time; LV: Left ventricle; MPI: Myocardial performance index; MPI_LV: Myocardial performance index of left ventricle; MPI_RV: Myocardial performance index of right ventricle; MRI: Magnetic resonance imaging; mTDMPI_m/s: mean value of myocardial performance index by tissue Doppler measured at lateral mitral annulus and septal annulus; mTDMPI_t/s: mean value of myocardial performance index by tissue Doppler measured at lateral tricuspid annulus and septal annulus; PWD: Pulsed wave Doppler; RV: Right ventricle; RVET: Right ventricular ejection time; SD: Standard deviation; STI: Speckle tracking imaging; SV: Stroke volume; TDI: Tissue Doppler imaging; TDMPI: Myocardial performance index by tissue Doppler; TDMPI_lm: Myocardial performance index by tissue Doppler at lateral mitral annulus; TDMPI_lt: Myocardial performance index by tissue Doppler at lateral tricuspid annulus; TDMPI_s: Myocardial performance index by tissue Doppler at septal annulus; tET: Ejection time by tissue Doppler; tICT: Isovolumic contraction time by tissue Doppler; tIRT: Isovolumic relaxation time by tissue Doppler

Acknowledgements
Not applicable.

Funding
Not applicable.

Authors' contributions
The authors' contributions were as follows: All authors designed the study. AM was responsible for recruiting the subjects and performed all examinations on both groups. ZA made all measurements on the echocardiographic images and interpreted the patient data to evaluate the global heart function using PWD and TDI and made all statistical calculations. ZA wrote the first draft of the manuscript. AM, PG, MD and MS were major contributors in writing the manuscript. All authors made critical revisions of the manuscript. All authors read and approved the final manuscript.

Consent for publication
Not applicable.

Competing interests
The authors declare that they have no competing interests.

Author details
[1]Department of Medical Imaging and Physiology, Skåne University Hospital, Lund University, Malmö, Sweden. [2]Department of Biomedical Science, Malmö University, Malmö, Sweden. [3]Department of Cardiology, Skåne University Hospital, Lund University, Lund, Sweden.

References
1. Pluim BM, Zwinderman AH, van der Laarse A, van der Wall EE. The athlete's heart. A meta-analysis of cardiac structure and function. Circulation. 2000; 101(3):336–44.
2. Wernstedt P, Sjostedt C, Ekman I, Du H, Thuomas KA, Areskog NH, et al. Adaptation of cardiac morphology and function to endurance and strength training. A comparative study using MR imaging and echocardiography in males and females. Scand J Med Sci Sports. 2002;12(1):17–25.
3. Dzudie A, Menanga A, Hamadou B, Kengne AP, Atchou G, Kingue S. Ultrasonographic study of left ventricular function at rest in a group of highly trained black African handball players. Eur J Echocardiogr. 2007;8(2):122–7.
4. Mitchell JH, Haskell W, Snell P, Van Camp SP. Task Force 8: classification of sports. J Am Coll Cardiol. 2005;45(8):1364–7.
5. Pelliccia A, Maron BJ, Di Paolo FM, Biffi A, Quattrini FM, Pisicchio C, et al. Prevalence and clinical significance of left atrial remodeling in competitive athletes. J Am Coll Cardiol. 2005;46(4):690–6.
6. Sharma S. Athlete's heart–effect of age, sex, ethnicity and sporting discipline. Exp Physiol. 2003;88(5):665–9.
7. Pelliccia A, Culasso F, Di Paolo FM, Maron BJ. Physiologic left ventricular cavity dilatation in elite athletes. Ann Intern Med. 1999;130(1):23–31.
8. Pelliccia A, Maron BJ, Spataro A, Proschan MA, Spirito P. The upper limit of physiologic cardiac hypertrophy in highly trained elite athletes. N Engl J Med. 1991;324(5):295–301.
9. Barbier J, Ville N, Kervio G, Walther G, Carre F. Sports-specific features of athlete's heart and their relation to echocardiographic parameters. Herz. 2006;31(6):531
10. Miller D, Farah MG, Liner A, Fox K, Schluchter M, Hoit BD. The relation between quantitative right ventricular ejection fraction and indices of tricuspid annular motion and myocardial performance. J Am Soc Echocardiogr. 2004;17(5):443–7.
11. Tei C, Dujardin KS, Hodge DO, Bailey KR, McGoon MD, Tajik AJ, et al. Doppler echocardiographic index for assessment of global right ventricular function. J Am Soc Echocardiogr. 1996;9(6):838–47.
12. Pagourelias ED, Kouidi E, Efthimiadis GK, Deligiannis A, Geleris P, Vassilikos V. Right atrial and ventricular adaptations to training in male Caucasian athletes: an echocardiographic study. J Am Soc Echocardiogr. 2013;26(11):1344–52.
13. Su HM, Lin TH, Voon WC, Lee KT, Chu CS, Lai WT, et al. Differentiation of left ventricular diastolic dysfunction, identification of pseudonormal/restrictive mitral inflow pattern and determination of left ventricular filling pressure by Tei index obtained from tissue Doppler echocardiography. Echocardiography. 2006;23(4):287–94.

14. Tei C, Nishimura RA, Seward JB, Tajik AJ. Noninvasive Doppler-derived myocardial performance index: correlation with simultaneous measurements of cardiac catheterization measurements. J Am Soc Echocardiogr. 1997;10(2):169–78.

15. Keser N, Yildiz S, Kurtog N, Dindar I. Modified TEI index: a promising parameter in essential hypertension? Echocardiography. 2005;22(4):296–304.

16. Tei C, Ling LH, Hodge DO, Bailey KR, Oh JK, Rodeheffer RJ, et al. New index of combined systolic and diastolic myocardial performance: a simple and reproducible measure of cardiac function–a study in normals and dilated cardiomyopathy. J Cardiol. 1995;26(6):357–66.

17. Harada K, Tamura M, Toyono M, Yasuoka K. Comparison of the right ventricular Tei index by tissue Doppler imaging to that obtained by pulsed Doppler in children without heart disease. Am J Cardiol. 2002;90(5):566–9.

18. Rojo EC, Rodrigo JL, Perez de Isla L, Almeria C, Gonzalo N, Aubele A, et al. Disagreement between tissue Doppler imaging and conventional pulsed wave Doppler in the measurement of myocardial performance index. Eur J Echocardiogr. 2006;7(5):356–64.

19. Gaibazzi N, Petrucci N, Ziacchi V. Left ventricle myocardial performance index derived either by conventional method or mitral annulus tissue-Doppler: a comparison study in healthy subjects and subjects with heart failure. J Am Soc Echocardiogr. 2005;18(12):1270–6.

20. Carluccio E, Biagioli P, Alunni G, Murrone A, Zuchi C, Biscottini E, et al. Improvement of myocardial performance (Tei) index closely reflects intrinsic improvement of cardiac function: assessment in revascularized hibernating myocardium. Echocardiography. 2012;29(3):298–306.

21. Tei C, Dujardin KS, Hodge DO, Kyle RA, Tajik AJ, Seward JB. Doppler index combining systolic and diastolic myocardial performance: clinical value in cardiac amyloidosis. J Am Coll Cardiol. 1996;28(3):658–64.

22. Vonk MC, Sander MH, van den Hoogen FH, van Riel PL, Verheugt FW, van Dijk AP. Right ventricle Tei-index: a tool to increase the accuracy of non-invasive detection of pulmonary arterial hypertension in connective tissue diseases. Eur J Echocardiogr. 2007;8(5):317–21.

23. Arnlov J, Lind L, Andren B, Riserus U, Berglund L, Lithell H. A Doppler-derived index of combined left ventricular systolic and diastolic function is an independent predictor of cardiovascular mortality in elderly men. Am Heart J. 2005;149(5):902–7.

24. Lind L, Andren B, Arnlov J. The Doppler-derived myocardial performance index is determined by both left ventricular systolic and diastolic function as well as by afterload and left ventricular mass. Echocardiography. 2005;22(3):211–6.

25. Du Bois D, Du Bois EF. A formula to estimate the approximate surface area if height and weight be known. 1916. Nutrition. 1989;5(5):303–11.

26. Rudski LG, Lai WW, Afilalo J, Hua L, Handschumacher MD, Chandrasekaran K, et al. Guidelines for the echocardiographic assessment of the right heart in adults: a report from the American Society of Echocardiography endorsed by the European Association of Echocardiography, a registered branch of the European Society of Cardiology, and the Canadian Society of Echocardiography. J Am Soc Echocardiogr. 2010;23(7):685–713.

27. Malmgren A, Dencker M, Stagmo M, Gudmundsson P. Cardiac dimensions and function in female handball players. J Sports Med Phys Fitness. 2015;55(4):320–8.

28. Butz T, van Buuren F, Mellwig KP, Langer C, Oldenburg O, Treusch KA, et al. Systolic and early diastolic left ventricular velocities assessed by tissue Doppler imaging in 100 top-level handball players. Eur J Cardiovasc Prev Rehabil. 2010;17(3):342–8.

29. Kasikcioglu E, Oflaz H, Akhan H, Kayserilioglu A. Right ventricular myocardial performance index and exercise capacity in athletes. Heart Vessel. 2005;20(4):147–52.

30. Tuzun N, Ergun M, Alioglu E, Edem E, Tengiz I, Aytemiz F, et al. TEI Index in elite sprinters and endurance athletes. J Sports Med Phys Fitness. 2015;55(9):988–94.

31. Moller JE, Poulsen SH, Egstrup K. Effect of preload alternations on a new Doppler echocardiographic index of combined systolic and diastolic performance. J Am Soc Echocardiogr. 1999;12(12):1065–72.

32. Bleeker GB, Steendijk P, Holman ER, Yu CM, Breithardt OA, Kaandorp TA, et al. Assessing right ventricular function: the role of echocardiography and complementary technologies. Heart. 2006;92(Suppl 1):i19–26.

33. Auger DA, Zhong X, Epstein FH, Spottiswoode BS. Mapping right ventricular myocardial mechanics using 3D cine DENSE cardiovascular magnetic resonance. J Cardiovasc Magn Reson. 2012;14:4.

34. Haddad F, Hunt SA, Rosenthal DN, Murphy DJ. Right ventricular function in cardiovascular disease, part I: anatomy, physiology, aging, and functional assessment of the right ventricle. Circulation. 2008;117(11):1436–48.

35. Hollingsworth KG, Blamire AM, Keavney BD, Macgowan GA. Left ventricular torsion, energetics, and diastolic function in normal human aging. Am J Physiol Heart Circ Physiol. 2012;302(4):H885–92.

36. Vitarelli A, Capotosto L, Placanica G, Caranci F, Pergolini M, Zardo F, et al. Comprehensive assessment of biventricular function and aortic stiffness in athletes with different forms of training by three-dimensional echocardiography and strain imaging. Eur Heart J Cardiovasc Imaging. 2013; 14(10):1010–20.

37. Oxborough D, Shave R, Warburton D, Williams K, Oxborough A, Charlesworth S, et al. Dilatation and dysfunction of the right ventricle immediately after ultraendurance exercise: exploratory insights from conventional two-dimensional and speckle tracking echocardiography. Circ Cardiovasc Imaging. 2011;4(3):253–63.

38. Knackstedt C, Hildebrandt U, Schmidt K, Syrocki L, Lang A, Bjarnason-Wehrens B, et al. Analysis of right and left ventricular deformation in former world class swimmers: evaluation using speckle tracking. J Sports Med Phys Fitness. 2015;55(9):978–87.

3

Quantification of the relative contribution of the different right ventricular wall motion components to right ventricular ejection fraction: the ReVISION method

Bálint Lakatos[1†], Zoltán Tősér[2†], Márton Tokodi[1], Alexandra Doronina[1], Annamária Kosztin[1], Denisa Muraru[3], Luigi P. Badano[3], Attila Kovács[1*] and Béla Merkely[1†]

Abstract

Three major mechanisms contribute to right ventricular (RV) pump function: (i) shortening of the longitudinal axis with traction of the tricuspid annulus towards the apex; (ii) inward movement of the RV free wall; (iii) bulging of the interventricular septum into the RV and stretching the free wall over the septum. The relative contribution of the aforementioned mechanisms to RV pump function may change in different pathological conditions.

Our aim was to develop a custom method to separately assess the extent of longitudinal, radial and anteroposterior displacement of the RV walls and to quantify their relative contribution to global RV ejection fraction using 3D data sets obtained by echocardiography.

Accordingly, we decomposed the movement of the exported RV beutel wall in a vertex based manner. The volumes of the beutels accounting for the RV wall motion in only one direction (either longitudinal, radial, or anteroposterior) were calculated at each time frame using the signed tetrahedron method. Then, the relative contribution of the RV wall motion along the three different directions to global RV ejection fraction was calculated either as the ratio of the given direction's ejection fraction to global ejection fraction and as the frame-by-frame RV volume change ($\Delta V/\Delta t$) along the three motion directions.

The ReVISION (Right VentrIcular Separate wall motIon quantificatiON) method may contribute to a better understanding of the pathophysiology of RV mechanical adaptations to different loading conditions and diseases.

Keywords: 3D echocardiography, Right ventricle, Decomposed wall motion

Introduction

During the last decades the right side of the heart has gained more and more attention. Compared to the relatively simple conical shape of the left ventricle, the right ventricle (RV) shows a more complex anatomical structure. When viewed from anterior-lateral view it shows a triangular shape, whereas when it is viewed from a short axis cross-section it has a crescent shape, partially wrapping the left ventricle. Anatomically, the RV is traditionally divided into three parts: the inlet portion, which consists of the tricuspid valve, chordae tendinae and the papillary muscles, the apical part with trabeculated muscle, and the outlet portion, also called the infundibulum with the pulmonary valve, which seperates the ventricle from the pulmonary trunk [1]. In contrast with the predominantly oblique arrangement of the left ventricular myocytes, the RV free wall has two layers: in the subepicardium the myocardial fibres are oriented circumferentially, whereas in the subendocardium they are directed longitudinally [1]. Finally, the RV shows a distinctive, peristaltic-like contraction pattern: the activation starts from the inlet portion and ends at the outlet [2].

Three main mechanisms contribute to RV pump function: (i) shortening of the longitudinal axis with traction of the tricuspid annulus towards the apex; (ii) inward

---

* Correspondence: attila.kovacs@cirg.hu

†Equal contributors

[1]MTA-SE Cardiovascular Imaging Research Group, Heart and Vascular Center, Semmelweis University, Városmajor St. 68, H-1122 Budapest, Hungary

Full list of author information is available at the end of the article

movement of the RV free wall; (iii) bulging of the inter-ventricular septum into the RV during the left ventricu-lar contraction and stretching the free wall of the RV over the septum [3]. Since the relative contribution of the three mechanism may vary in different cardiac con-ditions [4], the availability of a technique able to assess the relative contribution of these three components to the global RV pump function will help to clarify the pathophysiology and the mechanical adaptations of the RV in different loading conditions.

Shortcomings of current imaging techniques in the evaluation of the RV

The complexity of RV geometry and mechanics may in part explain current difficulties in the assessment of its function using conventional tomographic techniques. The most widely used two-dimensional transthoracic echocardiography provides several parameters, however, the majority of the conventional measures refer only to the longitudinal contraction of the chamber [5]. Three-dimensional (3D) echocardiography offers a unique op-portunity to map the whole endocardial surface of the RV independent on any assumption about its shape and to display its motion using surface rendering modalities [6]. Since the RV pump function is the result of several different mechanisms, just measuring the RV ejection fraction may not be sensitive enough to characterize the different pathological conditions. The relative contribu-tion of the three aforementioned mechanisms to global RV function may be different in certain diseases affecting the RV and therefore, being able to obtain a separate quantification of the relative contribution of each of them could hold diagnostic and prognostic information.

Accordingly, our aim was to develop a custom method to separately quantify the extent of longitudinal, radial and anteroposterior displacement of the RV walls and their relative contribution to the global RV ejection fraction using 3D data sets of the RV obtained by echocardiography.

Material and methods

Image acquisition and 3D model reconstruction

Current matrix-array transducers permit the acquisition of 3D volumetric data of the RV during routine trans-thoracic echocardiographic examinations [7]. Dedicated software (4D RV-Function 2, TomTec Imaging GmbH, Unterschleissheim, Germany) is commercially available to generate a 3D surface rendering model (beutel) of the RV by a semi-automated algorithm [8, 9]. Time series of this 3D model (i.e. series of polygon meshes) can be exported volume-by-volume throughout the cardiac cycle (Additional file 1).

Novel method for decomposing the motion of the RV

We developed the ReVISION (Right VentrIcular Separate wall motIon quantificatiON) method using the Unity3D engine to decompose the motion of the exported RV beutel along three orthogonal axes and calculate the respective volume at each time frame. Note that the Euclidean axes in the dedicated software's output corres-pond to the anatomically relevant ones (longitudinal, ra-dial and anteroposterior). We decomposed the movement of the RV wall in a vertex-based manner (e.g. for the longi-tudinal motion we took into account only the movement of the vertices along the Y axis) (Figs. 1 and 2; Additional files 2, 3 and 4). That is for each $m_1,...,m_n$ series of meshes where $m_i = \left\{ \left(x_1^i, y_1^i, z_1^i \right), ..., \left(x_k^i, y_k^i, z_k^i \right) \right\}$

$$m_i^y := \left\{ \left(x_1^i, y_j^i, z_1^i \right) \mid \left(x_j^i, y_j^i, z_j^i \right) \in m_i \right\}$$

The volumes of the beutels accounting for the RV wall motion in only one direction (either longitudinal, radial, or anteroposterior) were calculated at each time frame using the signed tetrahedron method [10] (Fig. 3). No triangulation step was necessary, as all the polygons of the RV beutel were already triangles.

Let P be the set triangles of an m_i^y mesh. For each $p \in P$ let $p = \{(x_1 y_1, z_1), ..., (x_3 y_3, z_3)\}$ The volume of tetrahe-dron bounded by the vertices of p and the origin:

$$V_p := \frac{1}{6}(-x_3 y_2 z_1 + x_2 y_3 z_1 + x_3 y_1 z_2 - x_1 y_3 z_2 - x_2 y_1 z_3 + x_1 y_2 z_3)$$

Note that V_p is signed, meaning that the values may be negative in case the normal vector of the polygon points towards the origin (when the dot product of a position vector of one of its vertices and the normal vec-tor of the polygon is negative). The volume of the mesh is the sum of the signed V_p volumes:

$$V = \sum_{p \in P} V_p$$

Novel parameters of RV function

Ejection fraction is the most common measure of RV pump function and it is defined as the difference between end-diastolic and end-systolic volumes indexed to end-diastolic volume. Using the ReVISION method, volume changes due to the RV wall motion along the three directions can be separately quantified and the corresponding ejection frac-tion value can be calculated (i.e. radial ejection fraction). The relative contribution of the RV wall motion along the three different directions to global RV ejection fraction can be expressed by the ratio of the given direction's ejec-tion fraction to global ejection fraction. It may be also clinically relevant to evaluate the frame-by-frame RV volume change along the three motion directions. By

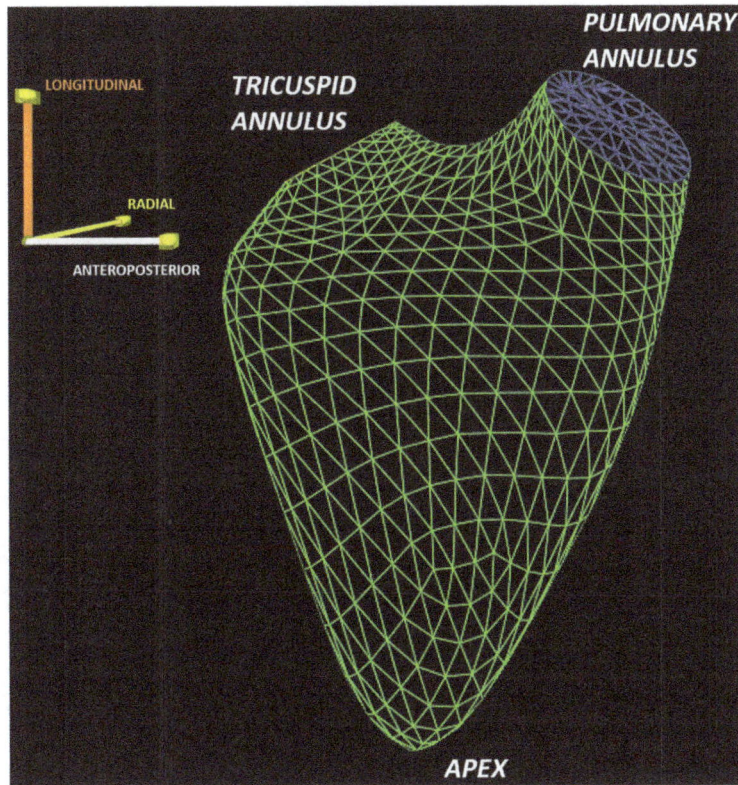

Fig. 1 Example of the exported mesh (*right ventricular beutel*) using the wireframe surface rendering display method. The model is positioned to correspond to the three anatomically relevant axes (longitudinal, radial and anteroposterior)

calculating the difference quotients between the given frames (ΔV/Δt), we were able to estimate the relative contribution of longitudinal, radial and anteroposterior motion to systolic, and also to diastolic RV function (Fig. 4). It is important to note, that these parameters are measured in a completely automated way, therefore, the ReVISION method implies no intra- or interobserver variability.

Discussion

We have shown that, using surface rendered data sets of the RV obtained with transthoracic 3D echocardiography, it is possible to decompose the displacement of the RV wall in a vertex-based manner. The volumes of the beutels accounting for the RV wall motion in only one direction (either longitudinal, radial, or anteroposterior) can be calculated at each time frame using the

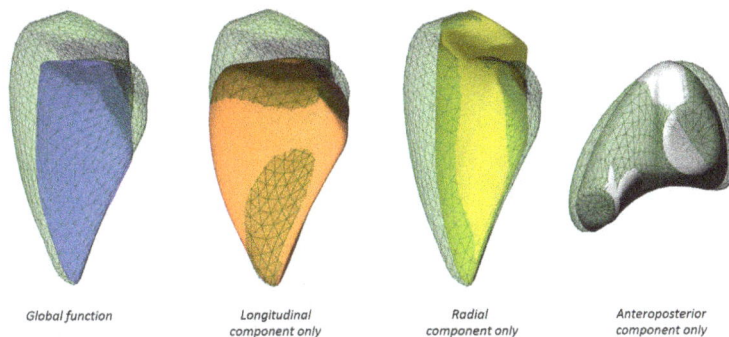

Fig. 2 The motion of the right ventricular wall during the cardiac cycle can be decomposed along three anatomically relevant axes (longitudinal, radial and anteroposterior) and the change of the volume during the cardiac cycle can be measured for each axis

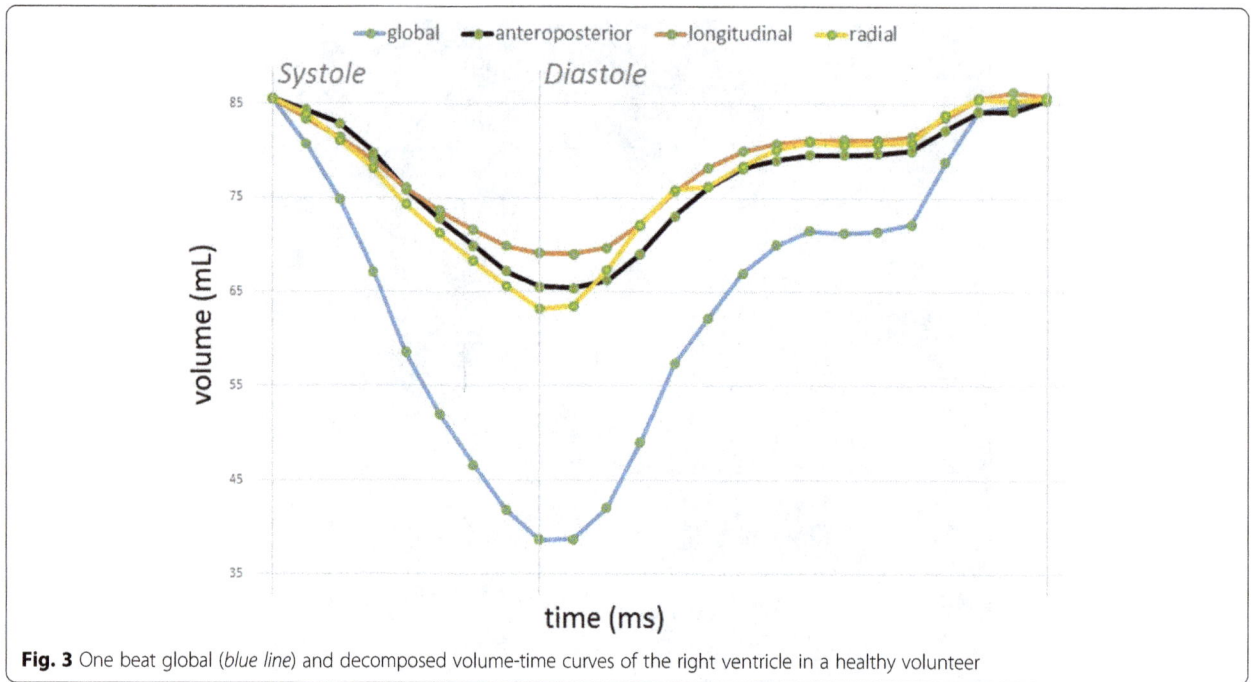

Fig. 3 One beat global (*blue line*) and decomposed volume-time curves of the right ventricle in a healthy volunteer

signed tetrahedron method. Using the ReVISION, we can compute novel parameters of RV function (the relative contribution of the different RV wall motions to global RV ejection fraction and the frame-by-frame RV volume change ($\Delta V/\Delta t$) along the three aforementioned directions). These parameters may help to improve our understanding of the pathophysiology of RV mechanical adaptations to different loading conditions and diseases (Table 1).

The RV is a significant contributor to global heart function and therefore, a better understanding of its functional pattern may be of high clinical interest. Despite the fact that the relative contribution of the longitudinal shortening, radial displacement and septal

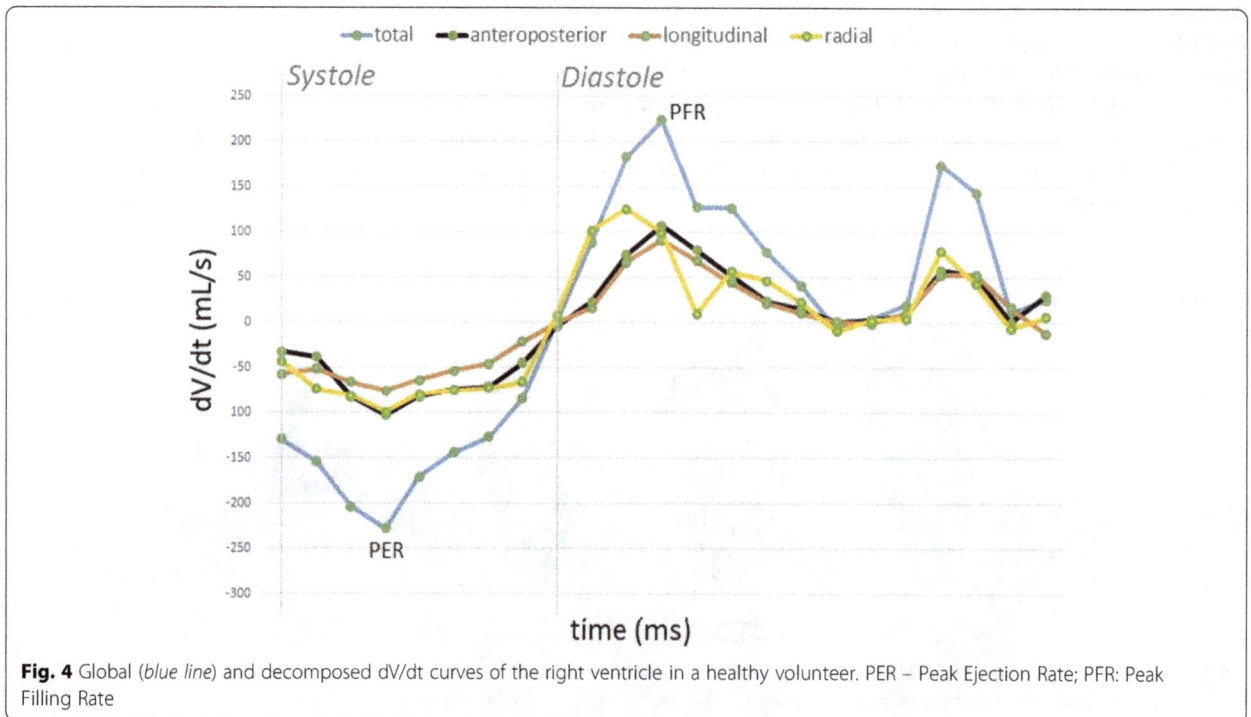

Fig. 4 Global (*blue line*) and decomposed dV/dt curves of the right ventricle in a healthy volunteer. PER – Peak Ejection Rate; PFR: Peak Filling Rate

Table 1 Potential clinical applications of the ReVISION method

Scenarios of clinical interest and suggested functional alterations	
Healthy subjects	Normal contribution of the three components
Post-cardiac surgery patients	Potential predominance of radial displacement
Heart transplanted patients	Long-term predominance of radial displacement
Pressure overload conditions (pulmonary hypertension, acute pulmonary embolism)	Potential reduction of radial displacement
Volume overload conditions (pulmonary regurgitation, atrial septal defect)	Potential reduction of longitudinal displacement
Athlete's heart	Effects of regular and acute exhaustive exercise
Right ventricular ischemia	Regional and/or global abnormalities
Arrhythmogenic right ventricular dysplasia	Regional and/or global abnormalities
Congenital heart diseases	Depending on the pathology

thickening to global RV function may change in different diseases affecting the RV [5], there is no established method to evaluate their importance to global RV ejection fraction.

Conventional echocardiographic parameters of the RV

Echocardiography is a widely used, non-invasive imaging modality to describe cardiac morphology and function. However, ultrasonic assessment of the RV is challenging due to the complex anatomy of the chamber. Conventional two-dimensional acquisition protocols require to obtain several imaging views using the parasternal, apical and subcostal approaches. The most commonly used echocardiographic measures to characterize RV morphology are simple linear diameters, while functional aspects are mainly investigated by measuring the tricuspid annular plane systolic excursion (TAPSE) and the RV fractional area change (FAC) [11]. The latter parameters have shown their correlation with RV ejection fraction measured by cardiac magnetic resonance imaging (MRI) [12] and proven their prognostic value as well [13–16]. Nevertheless, several limitations have to be taken into consideration, especially in certain pathological conditions. TAPSE is an easy-to-obtain M-mode parameter of RV function, referring solely to longitudinal motion of RV free wall (Fig. 5). However, since the reference is outside of the heart, TAPSE measures not only the shortening of the RV free wall but also the traction of the RV resulting from left ventricular contraction and the effects of the heart translation within the chest [4]. FAC incorporates both the radial displacement of the RV free wall and the longitudinal motion of the tricuspid annulus toward the apex, assessed on a single tomographic apical

four-chamber view and therefore, suffers from the inherent limitations of the limited RV myocardial mass included in this measurement (Fig. 6). These shortcomings of TAPSE and FAC can be overcome by the acquisition of a 3D data set including the whole RV using echocardiography.

Relative contribution of the different mechanisms in certain cardiac conditions

Using 3D echocardiographic datasets, RV volumes and global ejection fraction can be measured with a good correlation with MRI results [8, 9]. However, we still lack data about the relative contribution of longitudinal, radial and anteroposterior component of RV wall motion to global ejection. During physiological conditions, the longitudinal shortening was suggested to account for the majority of RV pump function, however, larger normative studies are needed to characterize potential age and gender related alterations [3]. Moreover, there are several diseases and clinical scenarios, where the normal ratio between the different mechanisms can change. Clinical interest includes post-cardiac surgery patients, heart transplanted patients (with evidently reduced TAPSE values without signs and symptoms of right heart failure; Fig. 7), pulmonary hypertension patients (with often severe symptoms and dilated RV along with preserved TAPSE; Fig. 8), congenital heart diseases, elite athletes, etc. Evidence suggests that RV longitudinal component measured by TAPSE is markedly reduced in post-cardiac surgery patients despite the absence of global RV ejection fraction decrease [17]. Recent studies with MRI suggest that RV function is reflected better by radial rather than longitudinal wall displacement in pulmonary hypertension patients [18, 19]. Pettersen and coworkers demonstrated that, after the Senning procedure (which transforms the RV to the systemic pump of the circulation), the patients have more pronounced radial component of RV function [20]. As a special case of RV overload, physiological or even detrimental effects of regular and/or acute exhaustive physical exercise may be of clinical interest [21, 22]. After an endurance race, conventional parameters suggest a less pronounced decrease of longitudinal shortening compared to ejection fraction, which also refers to a post-race functional shift [23]. Moreover, there is a growing interest in separated evaluation of longitudinal and radial RV function in pediatric cardiology patients [24]. These studies have shown the importance of the varying contribution of longitudinal and radial component in certain conditions, but did not provide distinct quantitative assessment for these phenomena. The ReVISION method may be the first to answer these questions by quantifying all major mechanisms using a single 3D dataset obtained by the easily accessible and non-invasive transthoracic echocardiography.

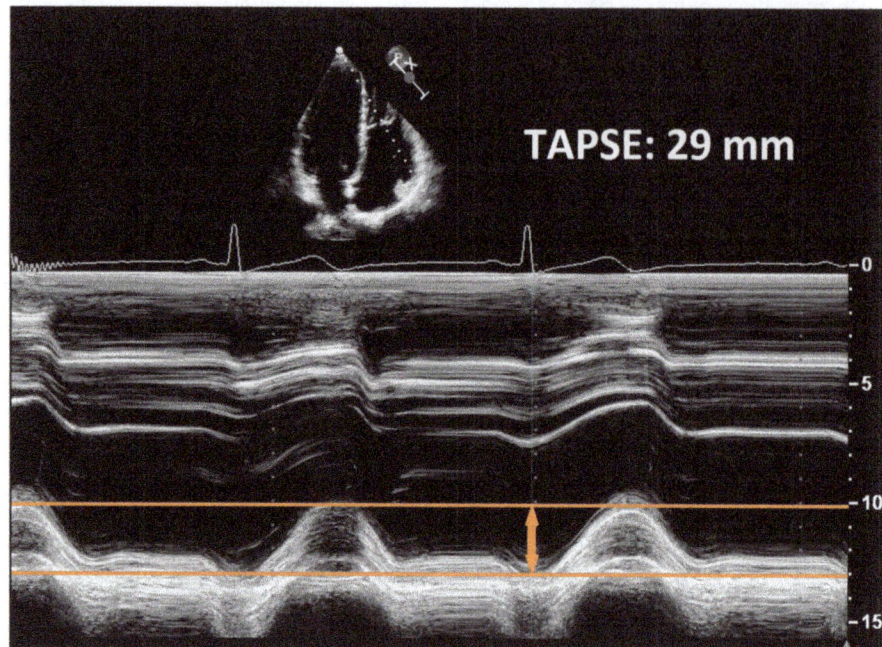

Fig. 5 M-mode tracing of the Tricupid Annular Plane Systolic Excursion (TAPSE). Note that this parameter reflects only the longitudinal motion of the right ventricle

Rationale of the functional shift

The underlying causes of the varying relative contribution of these mechanisms to global RV function in different cardiac conditions remain to be clarified. Beyond the mechanical effects of volume and/or pressure overload, there are several other and often overlapping factors that may be responsible for these findings. Several research groups hypothesized that the myocardial fiber architecture of the RV can change in certain conditions. Classical anatomical dissections revealed that in patients with congenital heart malformations such as Tetralogy of Fallot, pulmonary or tricuspid atresia, significant changes can be observed in the myocardial fiber arrangement within the RV wall. These changes include the more oblique orientation of the longitudinal layer, and also the presence of a middle circumferential layer which is absent from physiological conditions [25, 26]. Pressure overload has been proven to induce changes in RV fiber orientation as well, with a relative dominance of the circumferential fiber direction within the RV wall [27]. These effects may manifest in changes of RV shape, which can be severely deformed in pulmonary hypertension patients [28] and may also induce functional remodeling. Radial shortening, which is usually generated by the circumferential fibers in the subepicardial layer of the free wall, may reflect RV pump function better in this scenario than longitudinal shortening [18]. Considering that RV function has shown to be a powerful predictor of the prognosis of pulmonary hypertension [29], the possibility of a distinct quantification of the radial and longitudinal contribution to global RV ejection fraction may provide valuable information about the early

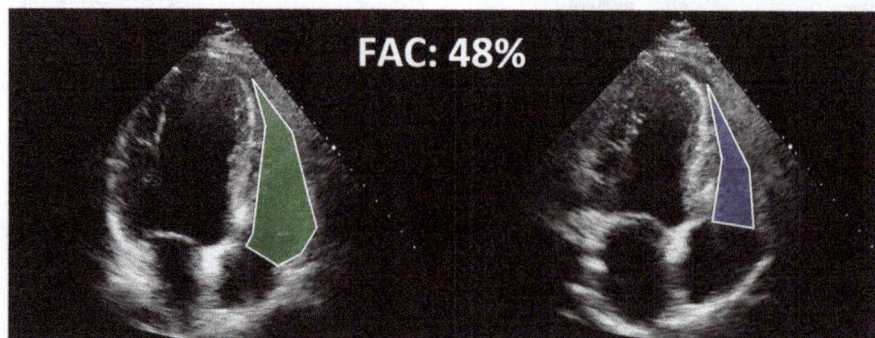

Fig. 6 Fractional Area Change (FAC) measurement of the right ventricle

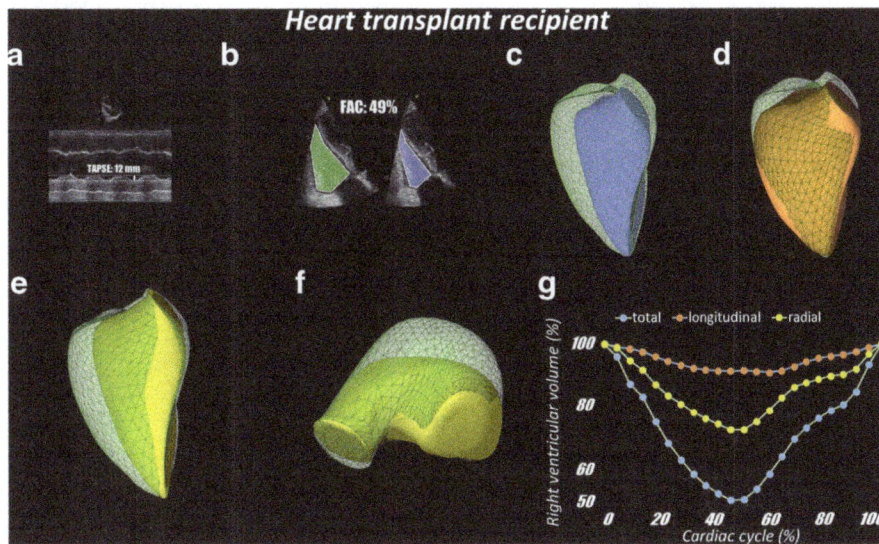

Fig. 7 Representative heart transplant recipient. Panel **a**: TAPSE (12 mm) is reduced indicating moderate RV systolic dysfunction. Panel **b**: FAC (49%) is preserved indicating normal RV systolic function. Panel **c**: RV end-diastolic (90 ml) and end-systolic (44 ml) volumes as well as RV ejection fraction (51%) obtained from 3D echocardiography data sets show normal RV systolic function. Panel D: RV longitudinal displacement is markedly reduced. Panel **e** and **f**: By removing the longitudinal and anteroposterior components of RV volume change allows the appreciation of the increased extent of radial displacement of RV wall. Panel **g**: Quantitative analysis of the relative contribution of longitudinal and radial RV wall displacement to global RV volume change confirms the significant reduction of longitudinal displacement and an increase of radial displacement as the main mechanism to preserve RV stroke volume and ejection fraction (patient 144 days after the transplantation)

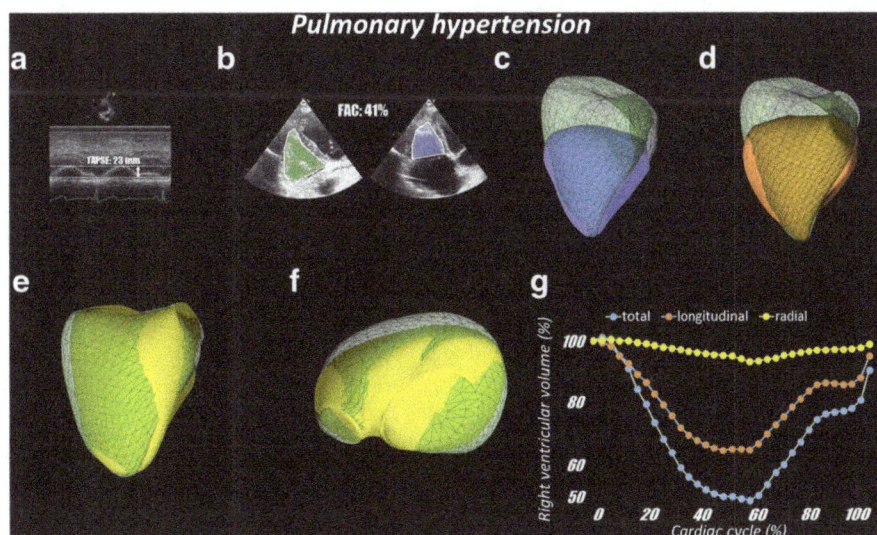

Fig. 8 Representative pulmonary hypertension patient. Panel **a**: TAPSE (23 mm) was normal. Panel **b**: FAC (41%) was also normal indicating preserved RV systolic function. Panel **c**: RV end-diastolic (92 ml) and end-systolic (48 ml) volumes as well as RV ejection fraction (48%) obtained from 3D echocardiography data sets showed normal RV systolic function. Panel **d**: the longitudinal displacement appears supernormal. Panel **e** and **f**: By removing the longitudinal and anteroposterior components of RV volume change, the radial displacement of RV wall appears dramatically reduced. Panel **g**: Quantitative analysis of the relative contribution of longitudinal and radial RV wall displacement to global RV volume change confirms the significant reduction of radial displacement and an increase of longitudinal displacement as the main mechanism to preserve RV stroke volume and ejection fraction in chronic, compensated RV pressure overload pathophysiology (pulmonary artery systolic pressure: 69 mmHg)

detection of impaired RV myocardial function (e.g. when global ejection fraction is still normal) and RV functional remodeling during the follow-up of these patients. Moreover, there are very limited data on the subclinical stages of the disease, and distinct quantification of the radial and longitudinal contribution to global RV ejection fraction may serve as a screening method to detect initial RV involvement in patients with systemic sclerosis, idiopathic pulmonary fibrosis, etc. The function of the interventricular septum accounts for a significant part of global RV ejection fraction, mainly by its longitudinal shortening [3]. Some authors emphasize the detrimental effect of interventricular septal abnormal motion, which occurs in cardiothoracic operations that involve cardiopulmonary bypass [30, 31]. Pericardial constraint and ventricular interdependence can be hampered by the opening of the pericardial sac, which may result in RV functional alterations [32, 33]. However, left ventricular contraction contributes to RV function also by stretching the RV free wall over the interventricular septum. Importantly, this component may be at least partly characterized by the third (e.g. the anteroposterior) component of RV wall motion. No data exist on the functional significance of RV wall anteroposterior motion, which can be quantified by our novel method as well. Loss of innervation may be another important factor which may affect global RV function in patients undergoing heart transplantation. Evidence suggests that the transplanted heart can be reinnervated by both sympathetic and parasympathetic fibers [34, 35], and the re-gain of autonomic nervous control can result in the recovery of RV longitudinal shortening over time.

ΔV/Δt analysis

Current literature is scarce about the clinical value of RV peak ejection rate and peak filling rate due to their previously complicated measurements with radionuclide ventriculography [36, 37]. 3D echocardiography offers an easier way to measure them, allowing also the decomposition of the different contributions of the different RV wall motion directions that may provide additional physiological and pathological insights into the systolic and also diastolic dynamics of the RV. Considering that the fiber orientation of the RV varies in different regions and also transmurally [1], this method may be a marker of heterogeneous contraction and relaxation pattern in certain cardiovascular conditions.

Conclusions

Since the possibility to quantify the relative contribution of the different components of right ventricular wall motion to global right ventricular ejection fraction would be of high clinical interest in both physiological and pathological cardiac conditions, we developed the ReVISION

method to obtain these components separately from 3D data sets of the right ventricle by echocardiography. Since there is no reference method to test the accuracy of our measurements, only prospective outcome studies can assess the clinical value of our approach.

The ReVISION software can be freely downloaded for scientific purposes from www.revisionmethod.com

Acknowledgement
None.

Funding
This study was supported by the National Research, Development and Innovation Office (NKFIH) of Hungary (K120277 and NVKP_16-1-2016-0017 to B. M.) and by the Arrhythmia Foundation.

Authors' contributions
BL analyzed and interpreted the preliminary data and was a major contributor in writing the manuscript. ZT designed the practical implementation of the method described in the manuscript, and had a major contribution in writing. MT helped in the software development and in the data analysis. AD helped in literature analysis, reviewed the manuscript. AK helped in data analysis and literature search, reviewed the manuscript. DM and LPB provided the rationale of the technique and had a major role in manuscript preparation. AK was a major developer of the method described, drafted the manuscript. BM provided the institutional background of the research, reviewed the manuscript. All authors read and approved the final manuscript.

Competing interests
The authors declare that they have no competing interest.

Consent for publication
Not applicable.

Author details
[1]MTA-SE Cardiovascular Imaging Research Group, Heart and Vascular Center, Semmelweis University, Városmajor St. 68, H-1122 Budapest, Hungary. [2]Department of Software Technology and Methodology, Eötvös Loránd University, Budapest, Hungary. [3]Department of Cardiac, Thoracic and Vascular Sciences, University of Padova, Padova, Italy.

References
1. Ho SY, Nihoyannopoulos P. Anatomy, echocardiography, and normal right ventricular dimensions. Heart. 2006;92 Suppl 1:i2–13.
2. Dell'Italia LJ. The right ventricle: anatomy, physiology, and clinical importance. Curr Probl Cardiol. 1991;16(10):653–720.
3. Buckberg G, Hoffman JI. Right ventricular architecture responsible for mechanical performance: unifying role of ventricular septum. J Thorac Cardiovasc Surg. 2014;148(6):3166–71. e3161-3164.
4. Badano LP, Ginghina C, Easaw J, Muraru D, Grillo MT, Lancellotti P, Pinamonti B, Coghlan G, Marra MP, Popescu BA, et al. Right ventricle in pulmonary arterial hypertension: haemodynamics, structural changes, imaging, and proposal of a study protocol aimed to assess remodelling and treatment effects. Eur J Echocardiogr. 2010;11(1):27–37.
5. Rudski LG, Lai WW, Afilalo J, Hua L, Handschumacher MD, Chandrasekaran K, Solomon SD, Louie EK, Schiller NB. Guidelines for the echocardiographic assessment of the right heart in adults: a report from the American Society of Echocardiography endorsed by the European Association of Echocardiography, a registered branch of the European Society of Cardiology, and the Canadian Society of Echocardiography. J Am Soc Echocardiogr. 2010;23(7):685–713. quiz 786-688.

6.   Jenkins C, Bricknell K, Hanekom L, Marwick TH. Reproducibility and accuracy of echocardiographic measurements of left ventricular parameters using real-time three-dimensional echocardiography. J Am Coll Cardiol. 2004;44(4):878–86.

7.   Lang RM, Badano LP, Tsang W, Adams DH, Agricola E, Buck T, Faletra FF, Franke A, Hung J, De Isla LP, et al. EAE/ASE recommendations for image acquisition and display using three-dimensional echocardiography. J Am Soc Echocardiogr. 2012;25(1):3–46.

8.   Medvedofsky D, Addetia K, Patel AR, Sedlmeier A, Baumann R, Mor-Avi V, Lang RM. Novel Approach to Three-Dimensional Echocardiographic Quantification of Right Ventricular Volumes and Function from Focused Views. J Am Soc Echocardiogr. 2015;28(10):1222–31.

9.   Muraru D, Spadotto V, Cecchetto A, Romeo G, Aruta P, Ermacora D, Jenei C, Cucchini U, Iliceto S, Badano LP. New speckle-tracking algorithm for right ventricular volume analysis from three-dimensional echocardiographic data sets: validation with cardiac magnetic resonance and comparison with the previous analysis tool. Eur Heart J Cardiovasc Imaging. 2015;17:1279–89.

10. Cha Z, Tsuhan C. Efficient feature extraction for 2D/3D objects in mesh representation. Image Processing, 2001 Proceedings 2001 International Conference. 2001;933:935–8.

11. Lang RM, Badano LP, Mor-Avi V, Afilalo J, Armstrong A, Ernande L, Flachskampf FA, Foster E, Goldstein SA, Kuznetsova T, et al. Recommendations for cardiac chamber quantification by echocardiography in adults: an update from the American Society of Echocardiography and the European Association of Cardiovascular Imaging. J Am Soc Echocardiogr. 2015;28(1):1–39. e14.

12. Corona-Villalobos CP, Kamel IR, Rastegar N, Damico R, Kolb TM, Boyce DM, Sager AE, Skrok J, Shehata ML, Vogel-Claussen J, et al. Bidimensional measurements of right ventricular function for prediction of survival in patients with pulmonary hypertension: comparison of reproducibility and time of analysis with volumetric cardiac magnetic resonance imaging analysis. Pulm Circ. 2015;5(3):527–37.

13. Kjaergaard J, Akkan D, Iversen KK, Kober L, Torp-Pedersen C, Hassager C. Right ventricular dysfunction as an independent predictor of short- and long-term mortality in patients with heart failure. Eur J Heart Fail. 2007;9(6-7):610–6.

14. Guazzi M, Bandera F, Pelissero G, Castelvecchio S, Menicanti L, Ghio S, Temporelli PL, Arena R. Tricuspid annular plane systolic excursion and pulmonary arterial systolic pressure relationship in heart failure: an index of right ventricular contractile function and prognosis. Am J Physiol Heart Circ Physiol. 2013;305(9):H1373–1381.

15. Brown SB, Raina A, Katz D, Szerlip M, Wiegers SE, Forfia PR. Longitudinal shortening accounts for the majority of right ventricular contraction and improves after pulmonary vasodilator therapy in normal subjects and patients with pulmonary arterial hypertension. Chest. 2011;140(1):27–33.

16. Nagy VK, Szeplaki G, Apor A, Kutyifa V, Kovacs A, Kosztin A, Becker D, Boros AM, Geller L, Merkely B. Role of Right Ventricular Global Longitudinal Strain in Predicting Early and Long-Term Mortality in Cardiac Resynchronization Therapy Patients. PLoS ONE. 2015;10(12), e0143907.

17. Tamborini G, Muratori M, Brusoni D, Celeste F, Maffessanti F, Caiani EG, Alamanni F, Pepi M. Is right ventricular systolic function reduced after cardiac surgery? A two- and three-dimensional echocardiographic study. Eur J Echocardiogr. 2009;10(5):630–4.

18. Kind T, Mauritz GJ, Marcus JT, van de Veerdonk M, Westerhof N, Vonk-Noordegraaf A. Right ventricular ejection fraction is better reflected by transverse rather than longitudinal wall motion in pulmonary hypertension. J Cardiovasc Magn Reson. 2010;12:35.

19. Swift AJ, Rajaram S, Capener D, Elliot C, Condliffe R, Wild JM, Kiely DG. Longitudinal and transverse right ventricular function in pulmonary hypertension: cardiovascular magnetic resonance imaging study from the ASPIRE registry. Pulm Circ. 2015;5(3):557–64.

20. Pettersen E, Helle-Valle T, Edvardsen T, Lindberg H, Smith HJ, Smevik B, Smiseth OA, Andersen K. Contraction pattern of the systemic right ventricle shift from longitudinal to circumferential shortening and absent global ventricular torsion. J Am Coll Cardiol. 2007;49(25):2450–6.

21. Stefani L, Pedrizzetti G, De Luca A, Mercuri R, Innocenti G, Galanti G. Real-time evaluation of longitudinal peak systolic strain (speckle tracking measurement) in left and right ventricles of athletes. Cardiovasc Ultrasound. 2009;7:17.

22. Olah A, Nemeth BT, Matyas C, Horvath EM, Hidi L, Birtalan E, Kellermayer D, Ruppert M, Merkely G, Szabo G, et al. Cardiac effects of acute exhaustive exercise in a rat model. Int J Cardiol. 2015;182:258–66.

23. La Gerche A, Burns AT, Mooney DJ, Inder WJ, Taylor AJ, Bogaert J, Macisaac AI, Heidbuchel H, Prior DL. Exercise-induced right ventricular dysfunction and structural remodelling in endurance athletes. Eur Heart J. 2012;33(8): 998–1006.

24. Hashimoto I, Watanabe K. Alternation of right ventricular contraction pattern in healthy children-shift from radial to longitudinal direction at approximately 15 mm of tricuspid annular plane systolic excursion. Circ J. 2014;78(8):1967–73.

25. Sanchez-Quintana D, Anderson RH, Ho SY. Ventricular myoarchitecture in tetralogy of Fallot. Heart. 1996;76(3):280–6.

26. Sanchez-Quintana D, Climent V, Ho SY, Anderson RH. Myoarchitecture and connective tissue in hearts with tricuspid atresia. Heart. 1999;81(2):182–91.

27. Tezuka F, Hort W, Lange PE, Nurnberg JH. Muscle fiber orientation in the development and regression of right ventricular hypertrophy in pigs. Acta Pathol Jpn. 1990;40(6):402–7.

28. Addetia K, Maffessanti F, Yamat M, Weinert L, Narang A, Freed BH, Mor-Avi V, Lang RM. Three-dimensional echocardiography-based analysis of right ventricular shape in pulmonary arterial hypertension. Eur Heart J Cardiovasc Imaging. 2016;17(5):564–75.

29. Humbert M, Sitbon O, Chaouat A, Bertocchi M, Habib G, Gressin V, Yaici A, Weitzenblum E, Cordier JF, Chabot F, et al. Survival in patients with idiopathic, familial, and anorexigen-associated pulmonary arterial hypertension in the modern management era. Circulation. 2010;122(2):156–63.

30. Reynolds HR, Tunick PA, Grossi EA, Dilmanian H, Colvin SB, Kronzon I. Paradoxical septal motion after cardiac surgery: a review of 3,292 cases. Clin Cardiol. 2007;30(12):621–3.

31. Buckberg G, Athanasuleas C, Saleh S. Septal myocardial protection during cardiac surgery for prevention of right ventricular dysfunction. Anadolu Kardiyol Derg. 2008;8 Suppl 2:108–16.

32. Santamore WP, Dell'Italia LJ. Ventricular interdependence: significant left ventricular contributions to right ventricular systolic function. Prog Cardiovasc Dis. 1998;40(4):289–308.

33. Unsworth B, Casula RP, Kyriacou AA, Yadav H, Chukwuemeka A, Cherian A, Stanbridge Rde L, Athanasiou T, Mayet J, Francis DP. The right ventricular annular velocity reduction caused by coronary artery bypass graft surgery occurs at the moment of pericardial incision. Am Heart J. 2010;159(2):314–22.

34. Buendia-Fuentes F, Almenar L, Ruiz C, Vercher JL, Sanchez-Lazaro I, Martinez-Dolz L, Navarro J, Bello P, Salvador A. Sympathetic reinnervation 1 year after heart transplantation, assessed using iodine-123 metaiodobenzylguanidine imaging. Transplant Proc. 2011;43(6):2247–8.

35. Bernardi L, Bianchini B, Spadacini G, Leuzzi S, Valle F, Marchesi E, Passino C, Calciati A, Vigano M, Rinaldi M, et al. Demonstrable cardiac reinnervation after human heart transplantation by carotid baroreflex modulation of RR interval. Circulation. 1995;92(10):2895–903.

36. Bai HT, Fujitani K, Fukuzaki H. Impaired right ventricular filling in old myocardial infarction. Jpn Heart J. 1987;28(4):479–94.

37. Zavadovsky KV, Krivonogov NG, Lishmanov YB. The usefulness of gated blood pool scintigraphy for right ventricular function evaluation in pulmonary embolism patients. Ann Nucl Med. 2014;28(7):632–7.

4

Prenatal screening of fetal ventriculoarterial connections: benefits of 4D technique in fetal heart imaging

Yu Wang[1], Miao Fan[2], Faiza Amber Siddiqui[3], Meilian Wang[3,4], Wei Sun[1], Xue Sun[1], Wenjia Lei[1] and Ying Zhang[1*]

Abstract

Background: Identification of prenatal ventriculoarterial connections in fetuses with conotruncal anomalies (CTA) remains one of the greatest challenges for sonographers performing screening examinations. Herein, we propose a novel protocol of 4D volume analysis that identifies ventriculoarterial connections and evaluate its clinical utility in routine screenings.

Methods: Twenty-nine cases of transposition of the great arteries (TGA), 22 cases of double-outlet right ventricle (DORV), 36 cases of tetralogy of Fallot (TOF), 14 cases of truncus arteriosus (TCA), and randomly selected 70 normal fetuses were reviewed in this study. All cases were evaluated using 2D data alone (2D method), post-processing volumes with no exact algorithm (4D-1 method), or with the proposed algorithm (4D-2 method), or using the 2D and 4D data together (combined method). Comparisons were made to evaluate the detection rate of ventriculoarterial connections for these different methods.

Results: During 18–28 gestational weeks, the detection rate of 4D-2 modality was satisfactory. The detection rate of the combined method was significantly higher than 2D method in the identification of TGA, TOF, and TCA. The detection rate of 4D-1 method was significantly lower than 4D −2 modality for CTA fetuses. During late pregnancy, the detection rate for both 4D modalities was very low due to the poor quality of the 4D volumes.

Conclusions: We proposed a detailed protocol, which allowed the examiner to identify fetal ventriculoarterial connections by 4D volumes. Inclusion of blood information into the volumes improved diagnosis. Our findings suggest that the incorporation of 4D STIC into routine screenings could improve the detection for TGA, TOF, and TCA.

Keywords: Fetal echocardiography, Conotruncal anomalies, 4D, Spatiotemporal image correlation, STIC

Background

Congenital heart disease (CHD), accounting for about 2.4 to 13.7 per 1000 live births [1], is the most common congenital malformation leading to perinatal morbidity and mortality and is considered the leading cause of death in newborn with congenital anomalies [2, 3]. Of all CHDs, up to 10–30% are conotruncal anomalies (CTA), which are characterized by a defect in the conotruncal septum arising from an abnormal cardiac neural crest cell migration [4–7]. As a result of errors during embryogenesis, a spectrum of various malformations could result, among which the most common include tetralogy of Fallot (TOF), transposition of the great arteries (TGA), double-outlet right ventricle (DORV) and truncus arteriosus (TCA).

Fetal two-dimensional echocardiography (2DE) and color Doppler echocardiography (CDE) are currently the primary techniques for the diagnosis of fetal CHD. During the past 20 years, the prenatal diagnostic ability of CHD has been promoted dramatically due to the high resolution 2D ultrasound and the advances in Doppler technology [8]. But as far as some complex CTA are concerned, the examiner needs to perform a thorough fetal echo to visualize the outflow tracts and the great arteries in detail, which often goes beyond the

* Correspondence: baogoubei@hotmail.com
[1]Department of Sonography, Shengjing Hospital of China Medical University, Heping District, Shenyang, China
Full list of author information is available at the end of the article

capability of sonographers performing routine prenatal ultrasound [9–11].

The introduction of 4D ultrasound provides an additional method to evaluate fetal cardiac structures [12]. New modalities for motion-gated cardiac scanning and application of spatiotemporal image correlation (STIC) technique allow the post-processing of the 4D volume datasets and subsequently evaluate cardiac anatomy with the use of multi-planar slicing or surface rendering of 4D volumes [13–16]. This single 4D volume technique allows the identification of different cardiac planes and often times, cardiac structures that are not demonstrated by 2DE techniques [17]. Various reports [18, 19] have demonstrated the value of 4D STIC in the diagnosis of fetal CHDs; however, its application has been limited mainly because of the difficulty in the post analysis of 4D volumes.

The primary objective of this report was to propose a novel protocol of 4D volume analysis in identification of fetal ventriculoarterial connections. We also investigated whether the 4D modality could help in improving the detection for fetal CTA in routine screenings.

Methods
Population study
This was a retrospective study. Fetal echocardiograms at Shengjing Hospital of China Medical University from Jan 2010 to Dec 2016 were reviewed to search the cases of DORV, TGA, TOF, and TCA. All TGA fetuses included in the study complicated with ventricular septal defect (VSD). Fetuses with complex CHDs were excluded from the current study. Cases without confirmation were also excluded. In total, 29 cases of TGA, 22 cases of DORV, 36 cases of TOF, and 14 cases of TCA were included in the study. For DORV fetuses, parallel great arteries (aorta on the left/left-anterior/right-anterior to the pulmonary artery) were found in 18 cases, while orthogonal great arteries were demonstrated in the other 4 cases. Gestational age ranged from 18 to 36 (median, 27.8) weeks. All cases were confirmed by the result of follow-up, including postnatal echocardiography, computed tomographic angiography, and the postmortem findings. Randomly selected 70 fetuses with normal cardiac structures were also included in the study. Intracardiac anatomy of all fetuses were confirmed by postnatal echocardiogram. Gestational age ranged from 18 to 36 (median, 26.4) weeks. All the normal and CHD fetuses were singletons. As the gestational age might affect the detection of fetal cardiac structures for 4D modality, the fetuses were divided into two groups according to gestational age (gestational weeks, GW: 18–28 and 29–36). Fetal traditional echocardiography (including 2DE and CDE) and 4D volume acquisition

were performed in all the fetuses and the data were saved as video clips and 4D volumes.

Ultrasonography technique
The patients were examined using either a 4D ultrasound system (Voluson 730 Expert, GE Healthcare, Kretztechnik, Zipf, Austria) or a 4D ultrasound system (Voluson E8, GE Healthcare, Kretztechnik, Zipf, Austria). They were equipped with a 4-8 MHz transabdominal transducer and STIC respectively. Traditional 2DE and CDE was performed on all fetuses and four chamber view (4CV), left and right outflow tract view, and the three-vessel and trachea view were acquired and stored as digital video clips. STIC volume acquisition was performed when a clear 4CV was identified with apical or lateral insonation of the fetal heart. STIC volumes were acquired using both gray-scale and color. If the condition was not satisfied, the patient was asked to walk for 30 min and then return to the examination. Usually, the echo window for the scanning is suitable for STIC acquisition. The woman was asked to hold her breath during each of three STIC volume acquisitions, which were performed with an automatic sweep using the motorized curved-array transducer. The acquisition time ranged from 10 to 15 s, and the sweep angle ranged from 25 to 40°. This increased with gestational age. The volume datasets included the upper fetal mediastinum and the gastric vacuole. The STIC volumes were reconstructed immediately and displayed in a cine loop and then stored for later offline analysis with the PC software (4D Viewer, version 14.0; GE Medical Systems, Zipf, Austria).

Volume quality classification
Each volume was evaluated and classified on a scale of 1 to 5 adapted from Goncalves et al. [20], according to image quality (1, unacceptable; 2, marginal; 3, acceptable; 4, good; 5, excellent). The main determinants of image quality were the fetal motion artifact, shadowing artifact, and the sharpness of the image.

4D volume datasets analysis to identify ventriculoarterial connections
STIC volume datasets analysis was made to access the originating, coursing and spatial relationship of the two great arteries. All volume datasets were displayed using the multi-planar modality. Three orthogonal planes (Panel A represented the transverse view, Panel B represented the sagittal view, and Panel C represented the coronal view) were displayed simultaneously. We then used two protocols in evaluating ventriculoarterial connections by post-processing the 4D volumes.

Protocol A (4D-1 modality): Post-processing 4D volumes of gray-scale only

In this protocol, the sonographer was not required to use specific steps to post-process the 4D volumes. Instead, they could adjust the slice position (moving forward or backward) in Panel A, B, and C, to show cardiac structures they determined to be interesting, or they could rotate the images in the x-, y-, and z-axes in the three Panels to obtain the views which could help the diagnosis.

Protocol B (4D-2 modality): Post-processing 4D volumes of both gray-scale and blood flow.

For the STIC volumes with gray-scale, the cardiac apex in the 4CV was oriented upwards and then the reference point was placed in the crux of the heart in Panel A. The reference point to the ventricles was moved (at the lower part of the ventricle, near the position of the outflow tracts). Navigating the reference point slowly from left to right in Panel A and one or two arteries could be visualized in Panel B. Moving the reference point to the valve and then navigating along the artery in Panel B, we could identify whether aorta or the pulmonary artery originated from one or two ventricles in Panel A. The originating and spatial relationships of the two great arteries were then identified. The processes of navigation of the reference point were described in detail in figures and video clips in a case of normal fetus (Fig. 1, Additional file 1: Movie S1 and Additional file 2: Movie S2), TGA (Fig. 2, Additional file 3: Movie S3), DORV (Fig. 3, Additional file 4: Movie S4 and Additional file 5: Movie S5), TOF (Fig. 4, Additional file 6: Movie S6), and TCA (Fig. 5, Additional file 7: Movie S7), respectively. The time for 4D volume post analysis was recorded. The number of corrected evaluation of ventriculoarterial connections was recorded.

For the STIC volumes with blood flow information, adjusting the images in Panel A was done to show the outlet of the ventricles, and the rendered 4D images showing the great arteries were then displayed in Panel D. Reducing the size of ROI in Panel B facilitated the images in Panel D. A combination of smooth surface and gradient light algorithms and post-processing adjustments were used to improve the image quality.

2D video clips interpretation and 4D volume data analysis (4D-1 modality and 4D-2 modality) was carried out by sonographers A, B, and C, respectively. The sonographers were blinded to the patients' information, prior sonographic imaging reports, and the findings of the follow-up visit. All the 2D and 4D image data were randomly ordered to analyze. The 2D video clips and the 4D data were then prepared in pairs for each patient. Sonographer C assessed ventriculoarterial connections and made the diagnosis using both the 2D and the 4D data (the combined method). Inter-observer agreement of the 4D methods (4D-1 and 4D-2) for diagnostic accuracy of ventriculoarterial connections was determined by two other sonographers (sonographer A, and D) who reanalyzed 4D volumes, respectively, in all the fetuses. Intra-observer variability of 4D-1 and 4D-2 was determined by reanalysis of 4D volumes by sonographer B and sonographer C, respectively, in all fetuses 30 days later. All the sonographers were screening sonographers with 1-year clinical experience. Furthermore, sonographer C and D were trained for 2 weeks in the proposed protocol (4D-2 modality) for 4D volume post-processing analysis.

Statistical analysis

The detection rate of ventriculoarterial connections in fetal TGA, DORV, TCA, and TOF was determined as the number of cases in whom 2D or 4D method correctly identified ventriculoarterial connections, expressed as a percentage of the total number of cases of TGA, DORV, TCA, and TOF, respectively. The detection rate of ventriculoarterial connections for different methods were compared via McNemar analysis. The volume quality scores of different gestational periods were compared via independent t-test. P-values < 0.05 were considered statistically significant. All statistical analyses were performed using commercially available software (SPSS, release 17.0).

Results

In the current study, we used different methods to identify fetal ventriculoarterial connections for both CTA fetuses and the normal fetuses. For normal fetuses, ventriculoarterial connections could be identified by traditional 2D method in all fetuses during the full gestation period (18–36 GW). For 4D-2 modality, the detection rate was 100% during the second trimester and decreased dramatically (11 of 20; 55%) during late pregnancy. The detection rate for 4D-1 modality was apparently lower as it varied from 82% (41 of 50) to 35% (7 of 20) for the second and third trimester, respectively. During the third trimester, acoustic shadows often appeared when navigating the reference point in the volumes, which led to invisible of origination of the great arteries. These cases were defined as "unclear" or "uncertain" of ventriculoarterial connections.

The mean time for volume post analysis was 8.4 ± 3.3 min and 9.2 ± 4.1 min for 4D-2 and 4D-1 modality, respectively. The inter-observer and intra-observer variability was 3.3 and 5% for 4D-2, respectively. For 4D-1 modality, the inter-observer and intra-observer variability was 15.7 and 13.3%, respectively.

In total, 101 fetuses with TGA, DORV, TOF, and TCA fetuses were included in the current study. The outcomes of CTA fetuses were summarized in Table 1. We then made comparisons of the different methods in evaluation of ventriculoarterial connections (Table 2).

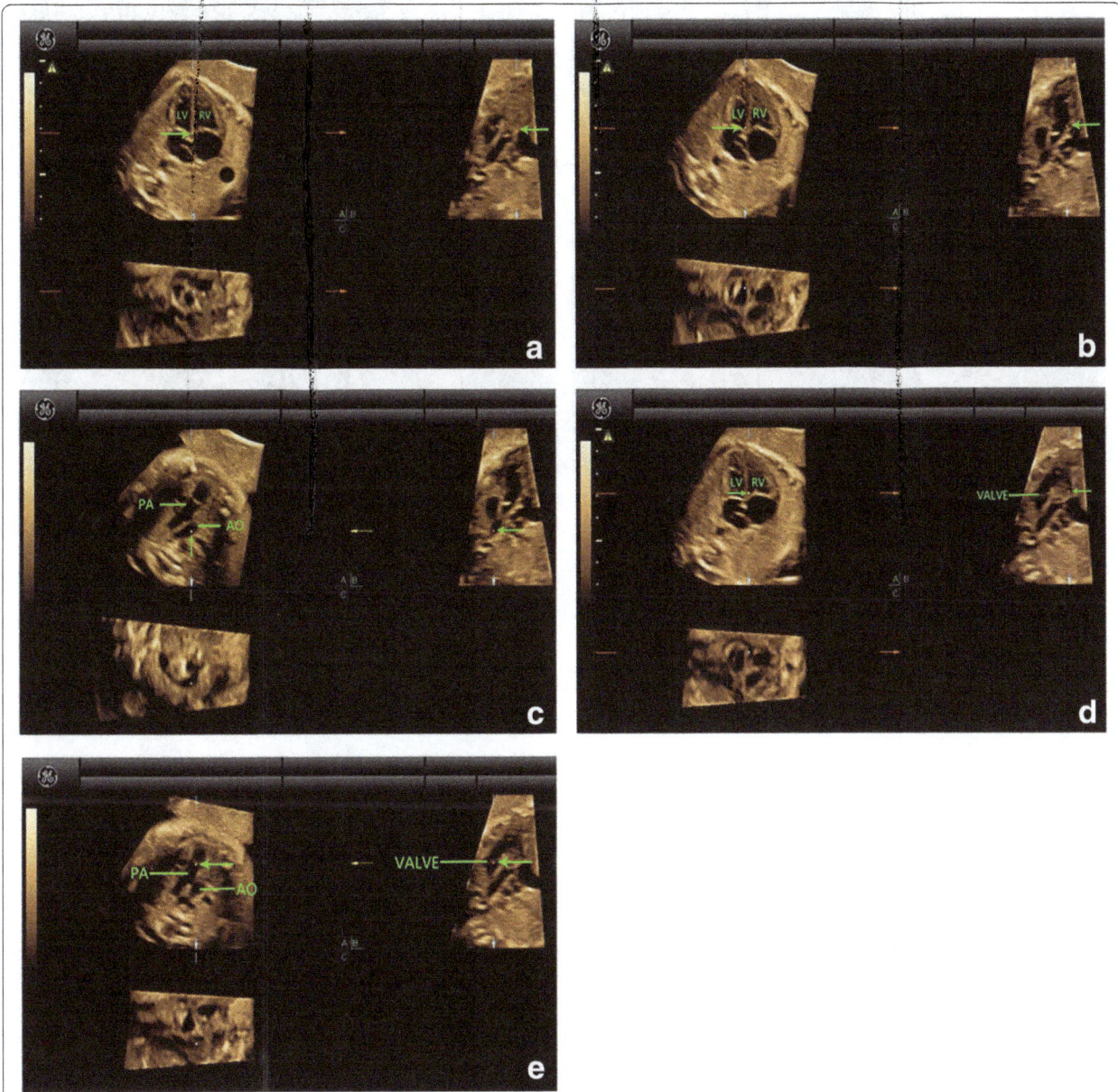

Fig. 1 Multiplanar slicing of a fetus with normal cardiac structure of 19 gestational weeks. Panels **a**, **b**, and **c** represent three orthogonal planes (A, transverse; B, sagittal; and C, coronal). The cardiac apex in the 4CV was oriented upwards and the reference point (indicated by the *green* arrow) was placed in the crux of the heart in Panel **a** (A). Move the reference point to the left ventricle in Panel **a**. By adjusting the position of the reference point in Panel **a**, near the position of the outflow tract (at the basal part of the left ventricle, near the crux of the heart), a great artery with clear course could be visualized in Panel **b** (B). Moving the reference point to this artery and then navigating along the course of the artery in Panel B, we could demonstrate a round (transverse) cross section of one great artery and a longitudinal section of the other great artery (characterized by the short trunk with bifurcation) (C). They were aorta and the pulmonary artery. As the reference point was located at the aorta, it could be confirmed that aorta was originated from the left ventricle. Back to the initial state in Panel **a** (A). Move the reference point to the right ventricle in Panel **a**. By adjusting the position of the reference point in Panel A, near the position of the outflow tract (at the basal part of the right ventricle, near the crux of the heart), a great artery with its valve could be clearly visualized in Panel **b** (D). Moving the reference point to the valve in Panel **b**, two great arteries with cross section and longitudinal section respectively could be visualized in Panel **a** (E). As the reference point was located at the pulmonary artery, it could be confirmed that the pulmonary artery was originated from the right ventricle. AO, aorta; LV, left ventricle; PA, pulmonary artery; RV, right ventricle

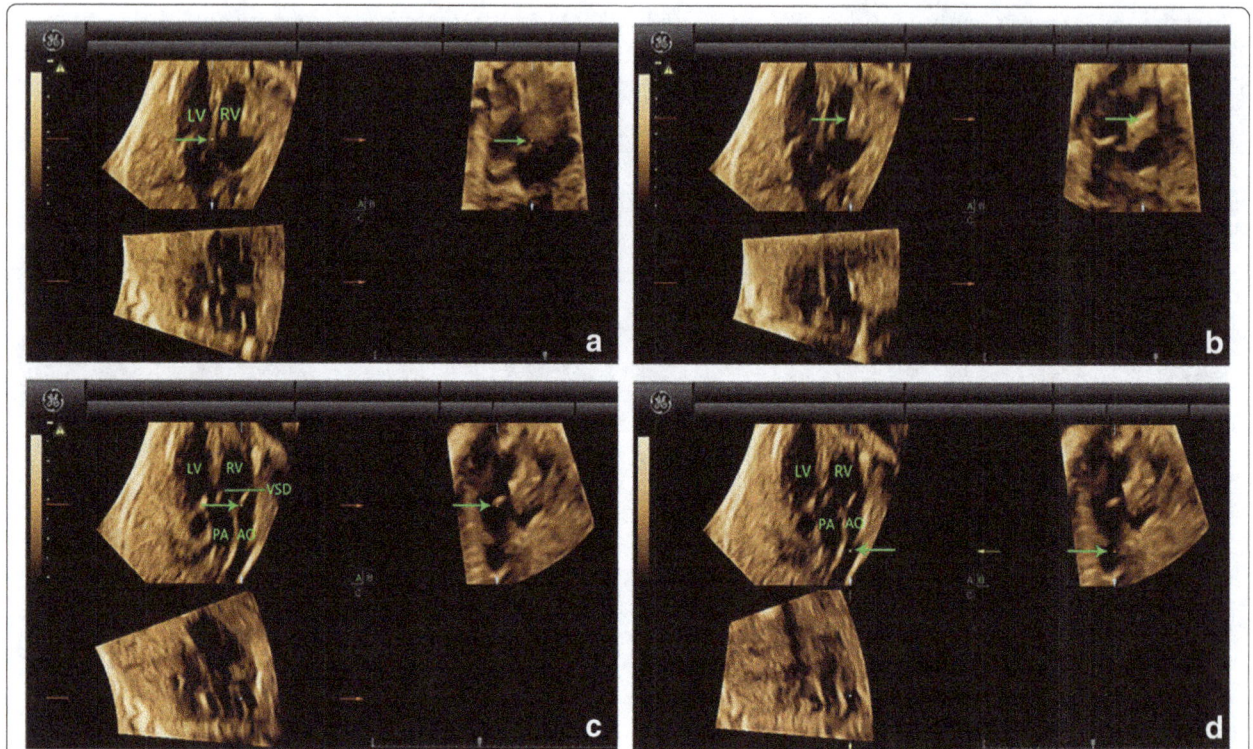

Fig. 2 Multiplanar slicing of TGA in a fetus of 25 gestational weeks. Panels **a**, **b**, and **c** represent three orthogonal planes (A, transverse; B, sagittal; and C, coronal). The cardiac apex in the 4CV was oriented upwards and the reference point (indicated by the *green* arrow) was placed in the crux of the heart in Panel **a** (*A*). Move the reference point to the right ventricle in Panel **a**. By adjusting the position of the reference point in Panel **a**, a great artery connecting to the right ventricle could be visualized in Panel **b** (*B*). Moving the reference point to the valve (*C*) and then navigating along the artery (*D*) in Panel **b**, we could then confirm that aorta was originated from the right ventricle and the pulmonary artery (characterized by the short trunk with bifurcation) from the left in Panel **a**. The parallel relationship of the two great arteries was also demonstrated. In addition, a VSD in large size could also be identified. AO, aorta; LV, left ventricle; PA, pulmonary artery; RV, right ventricle; TGA, transposition of the great arteries; VSD, ventricular septal defect

During the second trimester, the results showed that both the 2D and 4D-2 modalities provided a satisfactory detection rate for all CTA fetuses. For TGA fetuses, 6 cases were diagnosed as VSD without identification of the discordant of ventriculoarterial connections by 2D method. By navigating the reference point when processing the volumes, the sonographer could clearly visualize the full length of the outflow tracts in all cases. In addition, the 4D–rendered images of the great arteries disclosed parallel-like great arteries (Fig. 6a) which were obviously different from the normal arrangement (Fig. 6b). Statistical analysis showed a significantly higher detection rate for the 4D-2 modality when compared with traditional 2D method.

For DORV fetuses, 12 cases were successfully identified by the traditional 2D method, in which aorta was on the left or left-anterior to the pulmonary artery and the two great arteries lay in parallel. The other 3 cases were misdiagnosed as TOF because the two great arteries were wrapped in relationship. The detection rate of the 4D-2 method was similar to the 2D modality, as the arterial conical connections

were not discerned by screening sonographers by either 2D or the 4D modality.

VSD was identified in 6 of 26 cases of TOF, while the overriding of aorta was not identified by the 2D modality. In 1 of the missed 6 cases, 4D-2 modality made the correct diagnosis as the overriding of aorta could be identified when navigating the reference point in the volumes. At the same time, the origination of aorta from both ventricles and the right ventricle gave off the pulmonary artery, which was clearly visualized by the 4D–rendered image (Fig. 7). It was notable that most cases were identified using the combined method, when the sonographers processing the volumes after reviewing the 2D images (the combined method). Statistical analysis showed a significantly higher detection rate for the combined method than traditional 2D modality.

In 4 of 10 TCA fetuses, the final diagnosis was not reached by the 2D modality, as the origination of the pulmonary artery could not be identified. 4D-2 modality performed better as the 4D rendered images clearly delineated the origination of the pulmonary arteries (Fig. 8). It was interesting that the detection rate was significantly

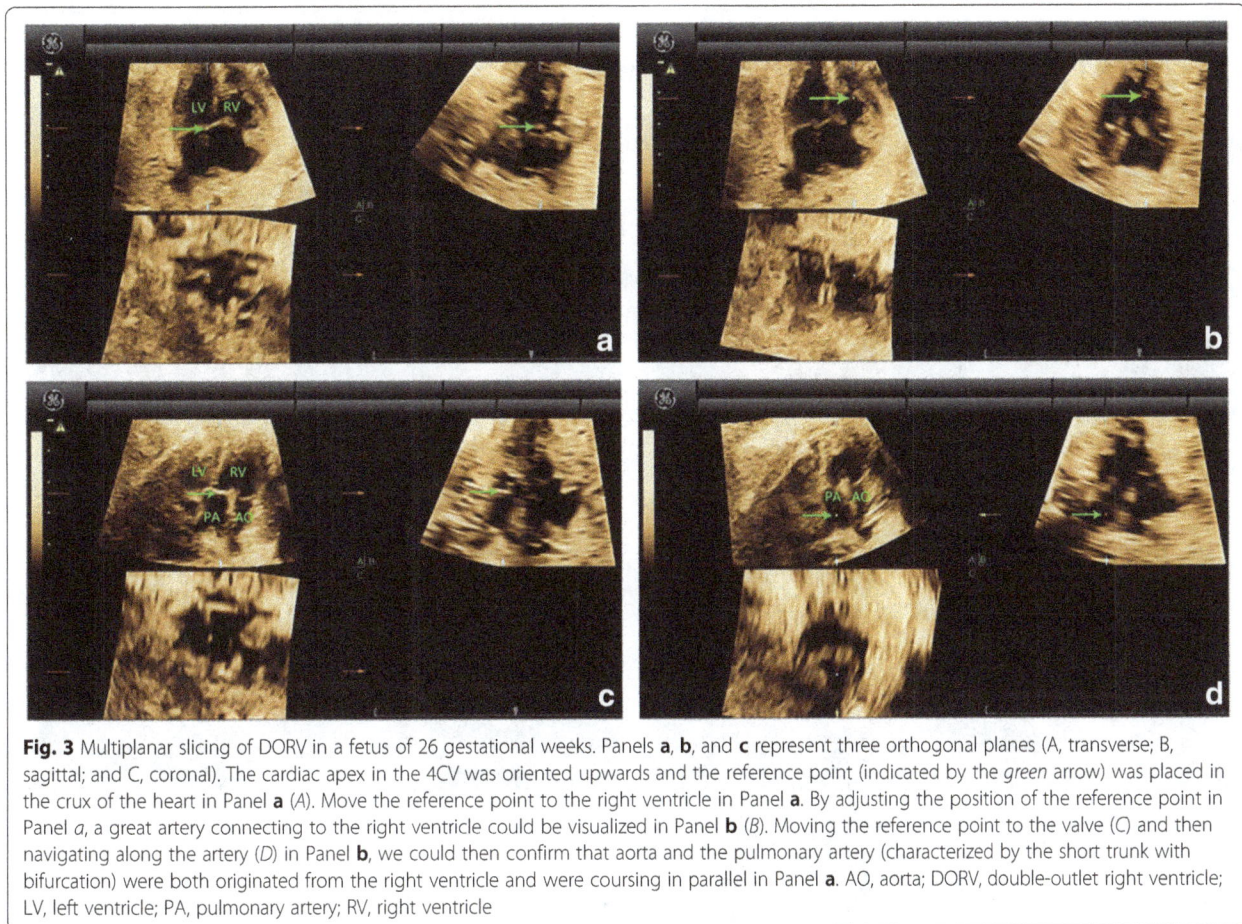

Fig. 3 Multiplanar slicing of DORV in a fetus of 26 gestational weeks. Panels **a**, **b**, and **c** represent three orthogonal planes (A, transverse; B, sagittal; and C, coronal). The cardiac apex in the 4CV was oriented upwards and the reference point (indicated by the *green* arrow) was placed in the crux of the heart in Panel **a** (A). Move the reference point to the right ventricle in Panel **a**. By adjusting the position of the reference point in Panel *a*, a great artery connecting to the right ventricle could be visualized in Panel **b** (B). Moving the reference point to the valve (C) and then navigating along the artery (D) in Panel **b**, we could then confirm that aorta and the pulmonary artery (characterized by the short trunk with bifurcation) were both originated from the right ventricle and were coursing in parallel in Panel **a**. AO, aorta; DORV, double-outlet right ventricle; LV, left ventricle; PA, pulmonary artery; RV, right ventricle

improved compared with traditional 2D method, when the sonographers processed the volumes after reading the 2D images (the combined method).For 4D-1 modality, the detection rate of ventriculoarterial connections was unsatisfactory, as it varied from 30 to 57.7%. The detection rate of ventriculoarterial connections was significantly lower for 4D-1 modality than 4D-2 method.

During the late gestation period, the detection rates of ventriculoarterial connections for both 4D modalities decreased significantly and were lower than 2D modality. The combination of 4D data with 2D data did not improve diagnosis.

The mean time for volume post-analysis was 12.5 ± 4.7 min and 20.5 ± 9.1 min for 4D-2 and 4D-1, respectively. For 4D-2 modality, the sonographer was required to post-process volumes for both gray-scale and color. However, the time needed for post-processing 4D-2 modality was apparently shorter than 4D-1 modality in the detection of CTA fetuses, which confirmed that the proposed protocol could be easily adapted by screening sonographers. The inter-observer and intra-observer variability was 8.2 and 6.8% for 4D-2 modality, respectively. For 4D-1 modality, the inter-observer and intra-observer variability was 18.2 and 15.4%,

respectively. The results suggested that 4D-2 modality showed better reproducibility than 4D-1.

For the 4D-2 modality, we evaluated the relationship of quality of the acquired volumes and the detection rate of ventriculoarterial connections for CTA fetuses. The visualization rate for ventriculoarterial connections correlated with the volume quality. When the quality of volumes was classified as 1, only 18.5% CTA cases were successfully identified, whereas when the volume quality was between 2 and 5, the detection rate was between 92.9 and 100%. The distribution of the volumes quality was shown in Fig. 9. The mean score for volume quality during the second trimester was significantly higher than during late pregnancy (2.86 ± 1.09 vs. 1.40 ± 0.56; $P < 0.01$). The results suggested that the low detection rate for CTA fetuses by the 4D modality during the late pregnancy was caused by the low quality of 4D volumes acquired.

Discussion

Perinatal care particularly in the case of ductus-dependent congestive heart diseases (CHDs) remains a challenge; therefore, early diagnosis of CTA is important to reduce morbidity and mortality [5, 21, 22]. According

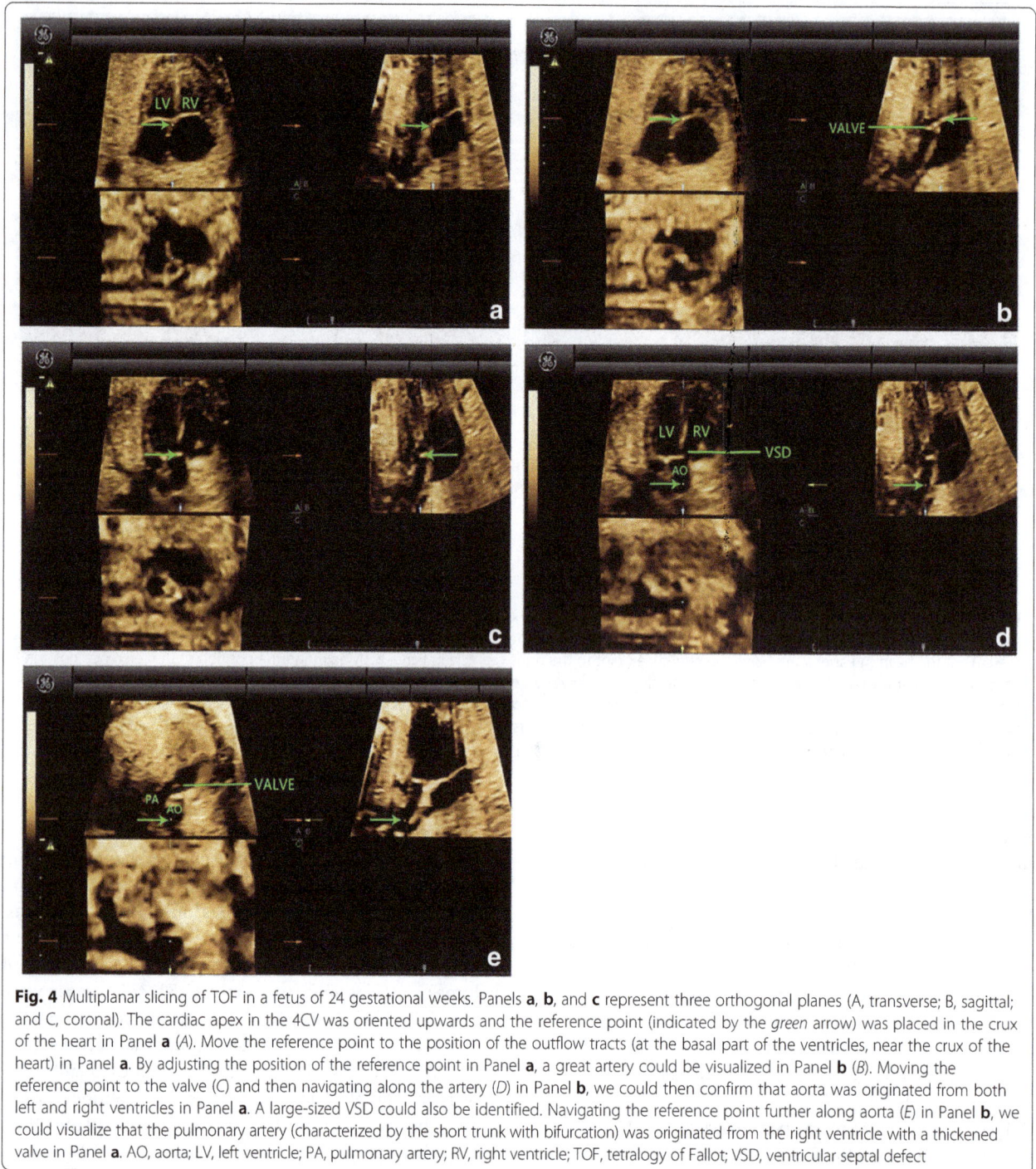

Fig. 4 Multiplanar slicing of TOF in a fetus of 24 gestational weeks. Panels **a**, **b**, and **c** represent three orthogonal planes (A, transverse; B, sagittal; and C, coronal). The cardiac apex in the 4CV was oriented upwards and the reference point (indicated by the *green* arrow) was placed in the crux of the heart in Panel **a** (A). Move the reference point to the position of the outflow tracts (at the basal part of the ventricles, near the crux of the heart) in Panel **a**. By adjusting the position of the reference point in Panel **a**, a great artery could be visualized in Panel **b** (B). Moving the reference point to the valve (C) and then navigating along the artery (D) in Panel **b**, we could then confirm that aorta was originated from both left and right ventricles in Panel **a**. A large-sized VSD could also be identified. Navigating the reference point further along aorta (E) in Panel **b**, we could visualize that the pulmonary artery (characterized by the short trunk with bifurcation) was originated from the right ventricle with a thickened valve in Panel **a**. AO, aorta; LV, left ventricle; PA, pulmonary artery; RV, right ventricle; TOF, tetralogy of Fallot; VSD, ventricular septal defect

to the American Institute of Ultrasound in Medicine (AIUM), 4CV combined with two outflow tract views should be evaluated in routine prenatal screening examinations [23]. However, outflow tracts are not carefully examined in many screening programs. Many CTA fetuses that undergo routine prenatal ultrasound will have four symmetric chambers and the investigation always stops there; at most, two great arteries arising from two

ventricles are visualized without ascertainment at to which of the arteries is the aorta versus the pulmonary artery. Furthermore, the examiner does not always visualize the full length of the outflow tract vessels. Therefore, it is challenging for a screening sonographer or an obstetric sonographer to obtain qualified cardiac images, especially for an inexperienced technician. In addition, interpretation must be done in real-time, either during the

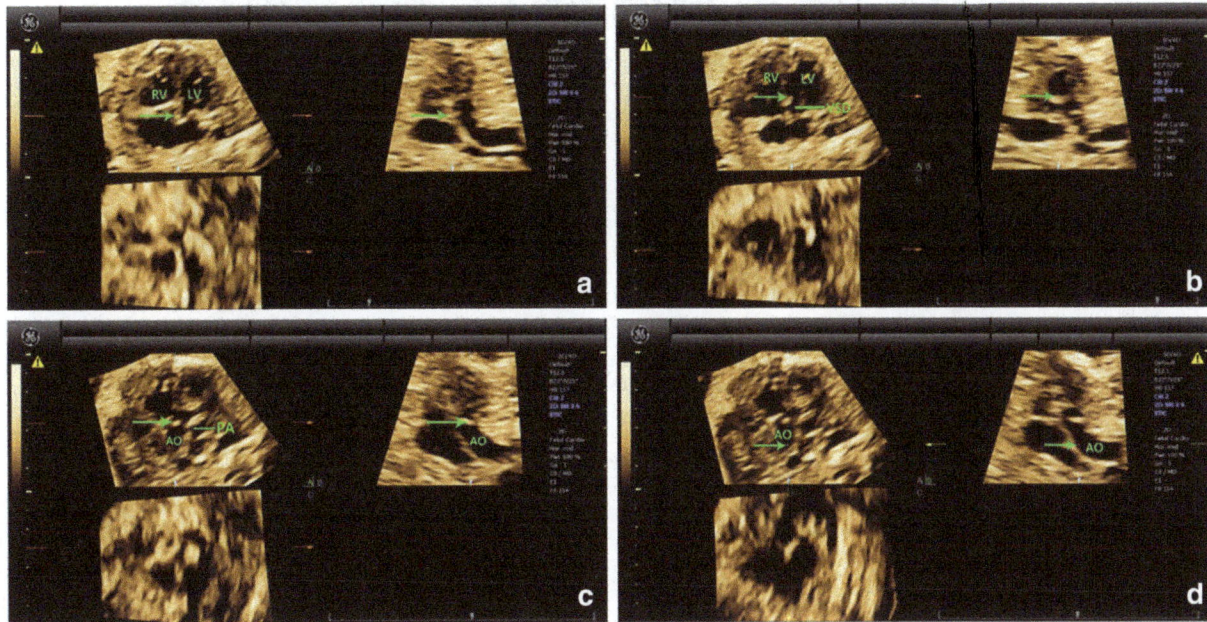

Fig. 5 Multiplanar slicing of TCA in a fetus of 28 gestational weeks. Panels **a**, **b**, and **c** represent three orthogonal planes (A, transverse; B, sagittal; and C, coronal). The cardiac apex in the 4CV was oriented upwards and the reference point (indicated by the *green* arrow) was placed in the crux of the heart in Panel **a** (A). Move the reference point to the position of the outflow tracts (at the basal part of the ventricles, near the crux of the heart) in Panel **a**. By adjusting the position of the reference point in Panel **a**, a great artery could be visualized in Panel **b**. A VSD could also be identified (B). Moving the reference point to the valve (C) and then navigating along the artery (D) in Panel **b**, we could then confirm that only one great artery arising from both ventricles (mainly from the right ventricle) in Panel **a**. This great artery is aorta. The pulmonary artery was visualized arising from the root of aorta in Panel **a**. AO, aorta; LV, left ventricle; PA, pulmonary artery; RV, right ventricle; TCA, truncus arteriosus; VSD, ventricular septal defect

examination or after reviewing video clips, which also challenges most screening sonographers. The aforementioned challenges are underlying reasons for the low detection of CTA during routine screenings. Our study emphasized the necessity for identifying ventriculoarterial connections during prenatal screening and may provide some ideas to improve current screening methods.

STIC is not a new technique, but it has been shown to provide additional information for clinical evaluation of fetal cardiac anatomy [24]. Volume datasets are acquired from the fetal heart to enable appropriate post-processing. Images are acquired by a single automatic volume sweep, followed by the process of systematic analysis of image data according to their spatial and

Table 1 Outcomes of the 101 fetuses with conotruncal cardiac anomalies in our study

CHD	n	TOP		IUFD		NND		NNA	
		n	%	n	%	n	%	n	%
TGA	29	6	20.7%	1	3.4%	2	6.9%	20	70%
DORV	22	8	36.4%	2	9.1%	3	13.6%	9	40.9%
TOF	36	3	8.3%	0	-	2	5.6%	31	86.1%
TCA	14	6	42.9%	1	7.1%	1	7.1%	6	42.9%
Total	101	23	22.8%	4	4%	8	7.9%	66	65.3%

All fetuses of TOP and IUFD were confirmed by autopsy findings. All NND and NNA were confirmed by postnatal echocardiography. Computed tomographic angiography was performed in parts of neonates

CHD congenital heart disease, *DORV* double-outlet right ventricle, *IUFD* intrauterine fetal death, *NNA* neonatal alive, *NND* neonatal death, *TCA* truncus arteriosus, *TGA* transposition of the great arteries, *TOF* tetralogy of Fallot, *TOP* termination of pregnancy

Table 2 The detection rate of ventriculoarterial connections by different methods

CHD (n)	2D (n)	4D-1 (n)	4D-2 (n)	Combined (n)
18–28 GW				
TGA (20)	70% (14)	50% (10)	100%[#] (20)	100%[#] (20)
DORV (15)	80% (12)	53.3% (8)	80% (12)	80% (12)
TOF (26)	76.9% (20)	57.7% (15)	80.8% (21)	96.2%[*] (25)
TCA (10)	60% (6)	30% (3)	80% (8)	100%[*] (10)
29–36 GW				
TGA (9)	66.7% (6)	22.2% (2)	55.6% (5)	66.7% (6)
DORV (7)	85.7% (6)	28.6% (2)	42.9% (3)	85.7% (6)
TOF (10)	80% (8)	20% (2)	50% (5)	80% (8)
TCA (4)	75% (3)	0	25% (1)	75% (3)

CHD, congenital heart disease; Combined, sonographers made the diagnosis using both the 2D and 4D-2 data; DORV, double-outlet right ventricle; GW, gestational weeks; TCA, truncus arteriosus; TGA, transposition of the great arteries; TOF, tetralogy of Fallot; Compared with 2D method
[*]P < 0.05; [#]P < 0.01

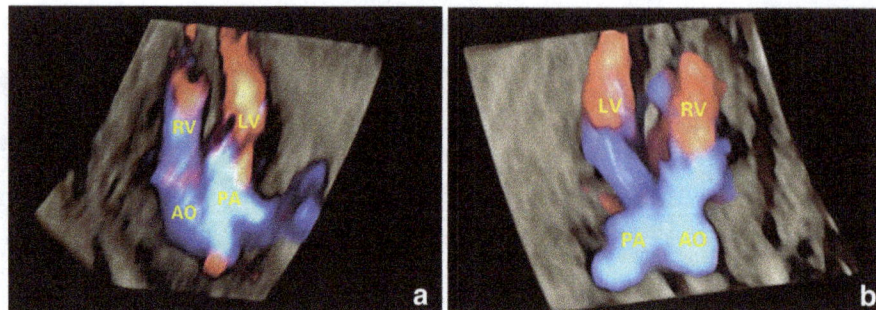

Fig. 6 Detection of great arteries alignment in TGA and normal fetuses using 4D volumes with color flow information. In a 24-gestational-week fetus with TGA (**a**), parallel great arteries were clearly identified by the 4D rendered image. The pulmonary artery was originated from the left ventricle while the right ventricle gave off the aorta. In a normal fetus (**b**) of similar gestational age, the 4D rendered image demonstrated that the two great arteries were orthogonal to each other originating from each ventricle. AO, aorta; LV, left ventricle; PA, pulmonary artery; RV, right ventricle; TGA, transposition of the great arteries

temporal domain. Dynamic image sequences are then extracted and displayed in a cine loop, which could be a multi-planar cross-sectional display and/or a surface-rendered display [16]. The examiner could then navigate within the volumes, re-slice, and get sufficient number of the standard planes for a comprehensive diagnosis [16].

Nowadays, 4D techniques are mainly used in fetal echocardiography but seldom used in prenatal screenings. We have used 4D STIC in fetal echocardiography since 2007 and the 4D technique has shown its value in helping diagnosis. We conducted this study with an aim to spur the use of 4D STIC in routine screenings. Uittenbogaard et al. [25] found that some key roles (i.e., fetal movement artifact, ROI setting, acquisition angle, fetal apex position, and fetal shadowing artifact) in volume acquisition may affect the volume quality, and thus proposed an acquisition condition scoring system. A study by Avnet et al. [26] demonstrated that trainees could get high quality volumes under the guidance of this condition scoring system. In fact, we have been performing volume acquisition in our obstetric screenings center since 2012. Screening sonographers were trained

in a short-term session to familiarize with the acquisition conditions similar to that proposed by Uittenbogaard et al. [25] and no additional time out of the scheduled 30-min slots was needed to perform volume acquisition for fetus in the second trimester, either for normal or CHD fetuses. A training session including these acquisition conditions may obviously improve over time for the incorporation of STIC in routine screenings. In our experience, a clear 4CV on 2D is essential before commencing acquisition, and a clear image without distortion and shadows in Panel B confirms the quality of the volumes, which is reasonable when the acquisition angel is set to (GW + 5)°. Longer acquisition times with smaller angles assure maximal information in a 4D volume, while the acquisition time must decrease when fetal movement is frequent. Parameter settings should be made according to actual situation. However, volumes obtained in late pregnancy were not satisfactory as more shadows may present or useful information may not be included due to the large size of the fetus.

In fact, the great impediment for the application of 4D STIC in prenatal screening is volume process, which consumes much time and expertise. If the sonographers

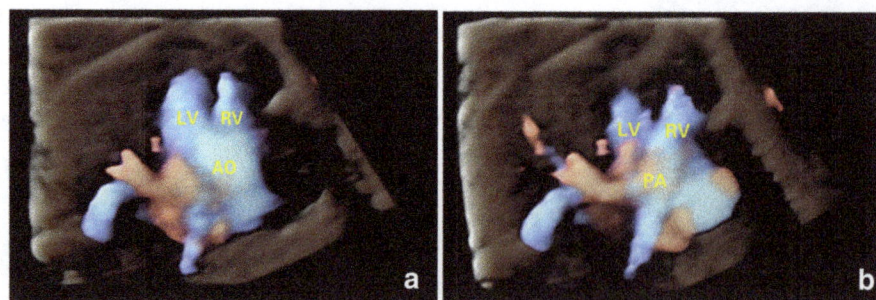

Fig. 7 Detection of TOF in a fetus of 24 gestational weeks using 4D volumes with color flow information. The 4D rendered image clearly showed that the large in sized aorta was connected to both ventricles (**a**). Another image showed the stenosis pulmonary artery was connected to the right ventricle (**b**). AO, aorta; LV, left ventricle; PA, pulmonary artery; RV, right ventricle; TOF, tetralogy of Fallot

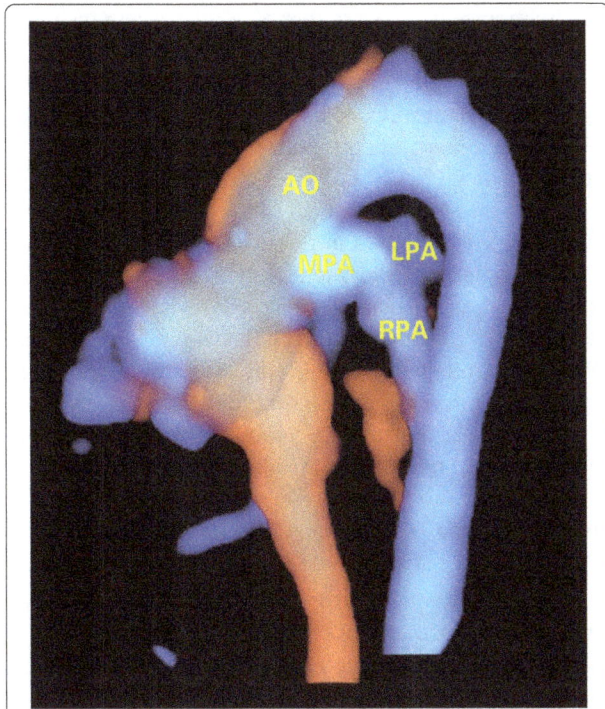

Fig. 8 Detection of TCA in a fetus of 28 gestational weeks using 4D volumes with color flow information. The 4D rendered image clearly showed that a large in sized great artery(aorta) was originated from both ventricles. The main pulmonary artery was connected to the root of aorta. AO, aorta; LPA, left pulmonary artery; MPA, main pulmonary artery; RPA, right pulmonary artery; TCA, truncus arteriosus

reformatting multi-planar volumes by rotating images in different panels with different angles do not have an effective algorithm, useful diagnostic views can still be retrieved but with much effort and difficulty. Our results showed an unsatisfactory detection rate and lower repeatability for 4D-1 modality, which suggested a limited value in routine screenings. Shih et al. [27] proposed

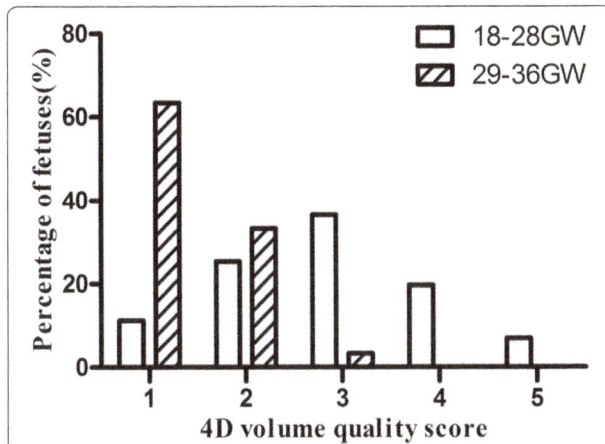

Fig. 9 Distribution of STIC volume quality for 101 CTA fetuses. 1, unacceptable; 2, marginal; 3, acceptable; 4, good; 5, excellent; GW, gestational weeks

a "Big-eyed frog" sign when they processed 4D volumes of fetal TGA and justified its value in improving diagnosis. However, the complex steps require higher experience and expertise and is better suitable for a specialist, and may be difficult to understand and manipulate by a screening sonographer.

In the current study, we proposed the protocol that could identify fetal ventriculoarterial connections by simply moving the reference point in three orthogonal planes without complex rotation of the images. When navigating the reference point, the great arteries were gradually revealed with its characteristics (i.e., the bifurcation of the pulmonary artery). For conventional 2D imaging, it is impossible for post-processing and only the original sonographic cuts were stored. If the characteristics of the great arteries are not well recorded, the screening sonographers are unable to make a correct diagnosis. It was also one of the reasons for the higher detection rate of 4D-2 modality in evaluating fetal TGA, when compared with the 2D method. In fact, screening sonographers can easily adapt to this protocol following a short few-days training session. This standardized method of processing 4D volumes is also more likely to be incorporated by beginners than acquiring many diagnostic views by the 2D method.

In the current study, we also included volumes of blood flow information to obtain the 4D–rendered images of the great arteries. The 4D–rendered images obtained from the 4D volumes obviously enhanced depth perception. These images reconstructed information and displayed a more complete and comprehensive picture. The data processing was very easy and the screening sonographers were apt to read the origin, course, and the spatial relationships of the great arteries. Therefore, inexperienced screening sonographers could be benefit from this technique given its ease. For cases of TGA, identification of the parallel great arteries when reviewing the 4D-rendered images was not challenging. Potential existing cardiac anomaly was then suspected. It is worth noting that the commitment of pulmonary arteries could be identified by the 4D–rendered images in some cases of TCA, while they could not be visualized by traditional 2D method. We must stress it is impossible to make a full diagnosis by just using a volume with blood flow information. Including a volume of gray-scale is necessary to evaluate cardiac anatomy in detail.

Usually, 4D STIC is not used alone in fetal echocardiography, but is considered a valuable method providing additional information during diagnosis. The echocardiographer or pediatrician reviews the 2D videos, and if needed, obtains the 4D images to help the diagnosis. In fact, accurate diagnosis cannot be made by just relying on a 4D volume without 2D images. Though standard cardiac views can be retrieved from volumes [28–31], the quality and resolution of these images were not as good as those from a 2D scan. Based on this point, we designed the combined method to test the feasibility of incorporating 4D volumes into routine screenings. After reviewing 2D images, the screening sonographers may have a preliminary judgement, thus could process the volumes more dedicatedly. At the same time, the sonographers may reevaluate the 2D images to determine whether there are some previously missed details after reviewing the 4D images. The results showed that the combined method could effectively improve the diagnostic accuracy in TGA, TOF, and TCA during the second trimester, when compared with using the 2D modality alone, which suggested the value for potential incorporation of the 4D STIC technique into routine screenings.

In the current study, our results suggested that 4D STIC did not help the diagnosis of fetal DORV. This may be due to the fact that DORV is a complex CHD with many classifications according to the spatial relationship of the great arteries. The ascending aorta and the pulmonary artery may lie side by side, or the aorta is on the right-anterior or left-anterior to the pulmonary artery, or the two great arteries are orthogonal to each other, similar to the situation of TOF. For the first three situations, the two great arteries were in parallel and were easy to distinguish from TOF. For the last situation, it was necessary to discern the sub-aortic conus. Our proposed protocol of volume analysis apparently could not provide an image of higher resolution than traditional 2D method and could not help the detection of the conus. Zidere et al. [32] published a report in which they demonstrated that the 4D−rendered images could provide more information and enhance prognostication with respect to the postnatal surgical approach. The authors made a detailed assessment of intracardiac anatomy, including the spatial relationship of the great arteries and the position of the VSD by post-processing the 4D STIC volumes. A pediatric cardiologist apparently could obtain more information from the 4D volumes than a screening sonographer.

The detection rate of the 4D modalities during late pregnancy was low. We evaluated the volume quality referenced in the scoring system by Goncalves et al. [20] and found that the mean score for the third trimester was significantly lower than the second trimester. The detection rate was likely correlated to volume quality, which was consistent with previous report [33]. As a retrospective study, we did not evaluate the acquisition quality as some factors (i.e., fetal movement) were not recorded. Furthermore, as the volumes used in the current study were acquired by an echocardiographer who was familiar with the acquisition conditions, it seemed that obtaining a valuable volume during late pregnancy was difficult, suggesting the limited value of 4D in late pregnancies.

It is important to stress that STIC has a few technical limitations. Volume quality apparently affects the diagnostic efficiency.Image distortion could be created by acoustic shadows, fetal movement artifact, and changes in heart rate. In our report, the poor quality of the 4D volumes in late pregnancy (29–36 GW) could have been caused by the increased acoustic shadows of the fetal ribs.

The study was limited in that we used the 4D volumes acquired by echocardiographers, not by screening sonographers. It might be impossible to observe large numbers of CHDs during routine screenings. As the largest fetal echocardiography center and consultation center in northeast China, we are able to obtain relatively large number of volumes of CTA fetuses. The current design, therefore, was intended to include more CHD fetuses to evaluate the utility of the proposed protocol in screening ventriculoarterial connections anomalies, which might compromise the study.

Conclusion

In conclusion, we have proposed a step-by-step technique, the "tracing" technique, which allowed the examiner to identify fetal ventriculoarterial connections by 4D volumes. The inclusion of blood flow information into the volumes also improved the diagnosis. The addition of 4D STIC into routine screenings could improve the detection for TGA, TOF, and TCA. A prospective study in a large population is further warranted.

Additional files

Additional file 1: Video. Multiplanar slicing of a fetus with normal cardiac structure of 19 gestational weeks. Panels A, B, and C represent three orthogonal planes (A, transverse; B, sagittal; and C, coronal). The cardiac apex in the 4CV was oriented upwards and the reference point was placed in the crux of the heart in Panel A. Move the reference point to the left ventricle in Panel A. By adjusting the position of the reference point in Panel A, near the position of the outflow tract (at the basal part of the left ventricle, near the crux of the heart), a great artery with clear course could be visualized in Panel B. Moving the reference point to this artery and then navigating along the course of the artery in Panel B, we could demonstrate a round (transverse) cross section of one great artery and a longitudinal section of the other great artery (characterized by the short trunk with bifurcation). They were aorta and the pulmonary artery. As the reference point was located at the aorta, it could be confirmed

Additional file 2: Video. Multiplanar slicing of a fetus with normal cardiac structure of 19 gestational weeks (the same fetus with Additional file 1). Panels A, B, and C represent three orthogonal planes (A, transverse; B, sagittal; and C, coronal). The cardiac apex in the 4CV was oriented upwards and the reference point was placed in the crux of the heart in Panel A. Move the reference point to the right ventricle in Panel A. By adjusting the position of the reference point in Panel A, near the position of the outflow tract (at the basal part of the right ventricle, near the crux of the heart), a great artery with its valve could be clearly visualized in Panel B. Moving the reference point to the valve in Panel B, two great arteries with cross section and longitudinal section respectively could be visualized in Panel A. As the reference point was located at the pulmonary artery, it could be confirmed that the pulmonary artery was

Additional file 3: Video. Multiplanar slicing of TGA in a fetus of 25 gestational weeks. Panels A, B, and C represent three orthogonal planes (A, transverse; B, sagittal; and C, coronal). The cardiac apex in the 4CV was oriented upwards and the reference point was placed in the crux of the heart in Panel A. Move the reference point to the right ventricle in Panel A. By adjusting the position of the reference point in Panel A, a great artery connecting to the right ventricle could be visualized in Panel B. Moving the reference point to the valve and then navigating along the artery in Panel B, we could then confirm that aorta was originated from the right ventricle and the pulmonary artery (characterized by the short trunk with bifurcation) from the left in Panel A. The parallel relationship

Additional file 4: Video. Multiplanar slicing of DORV in a fetus of 26 gestational weeks. Panels A, B, and C represent three orthogonal planes (A, transverse; B, sagittal; and C, coronal). The cardiac apex in the 4CV was oriented upwards and the reference point was placed in the crux of the heart in Panel A. Move the reference point to the right ventricle in Panel A. By adjusting the position of the reference point in Panel A, a great artery connecting to the right ventricle could be visualized in Panel B. Moving the reference point to the valve and then navigating along the artery in Panel B, we could then confirm that aorta and the pulmonary artery (characterized by the short trunk with bifurcation) were both originated from the right ventricle and were coursing in parallel in Panel A.

Additional file 5: Video. Multiplanar slicing of DORV in the fetus (the same with Additional file 4) using the "tracing" method in a different way. Panels A, B, and C represent three orthogonal planes (A, transverse; B, sagittal; and C, coronal). The cardiac apex in the 4CV was oriented upwards and the reference point was placed in the crux of the heart in Panel A. Moving the reference point to the right ventricle and navigating it to a certain point (close to the interventricularseptem, compared to the position mentioned in Additional file 4) in Panel A, a great artery connecting to the right ventricle could be visualized in Panel B. Moving the reference point to the valve and then navigating along the artery in Panel B, we could then confirm that aorta and the pulmonary artery (characterized by the short trunk with bifurcation) were both originated from the right ventricle and were coursing in parallel in Panel A. In this movie, the reference point was located at the pulmonary valve and the navigation was on the course of the main pulmonary artery. A subpulmoic ventricular septal defect could also be identified.

Additional file 6: Video. Multiplanar slicing of TOF in a fetus of 24 gestational weeks. Panels A, B, and C represent three orthogonal planes (A, transverse; B, sagittal; and C, coronal). The cardiac apex in the 4CV was oriented upwards and the reference point was placed in the crux of the heart in Panel A. Move the reference point to the position of the outflow tracts (at the basal part of the ventricles, near the crux of the heart) in Panel A. By adjusting the position of the reference point in Panel A, a great artery could be visualized in Panel B. Moving the reference point to the valve and then navigating along the artery in Panel B, we could then confirm that aorta was originated from both left and right ventricles in Panel A. Navigating the reference point further along aorta in Panel B, we could visualize that the pulmonary artery (characterized by the short trunk with bifurcation) was originated from the right ventricle with a thickened

Additional file 7: Video. Multiplanar slicing of TCA in a fetus of 28 gestational weeks. Panels A, B, and C represent three orthogonal planes (A, transverse; B, sagittal; and C, coronal). The cardiac apex in the 4CV was oriented upwards and the reference point was placed in the crux of the heart in Panel A. Move the reference point to the position of the outflow tracts (at the basal part of the ventricles, near the crux of the heart) in Panel A. By adjusting the position of the reference point in Panel A, a great artery could be visualized in Panel B. A VSD could also be identified. Moving the reference point to the valve and then navigating along the artery in Panel B, we could then confirm that only one great artery arising from both ventricles (mainly from the right ventricle) in Panel A. This great artery is aorta. The pulmonary artery was visualized

Acknowledgments
Not applicable.

Funding
This work was supported by grants from scientific research projects sponsored by the Science and Technology Agency of Liaoning province (NO. 2012225098), and sponsored by the Science and Technology Agency of Shenyang, China (NO. F16–206–9-11). M-lW was supported by grant from Natural Science Foundation of Liaoning Province (No. 2013021010). The funders had no role in study design, data collection and analysis, decision to publish, or preparation of the manuscript.

Authors' contributions
YZ and YW designed the whole study. YW, YZ, MF, WS, M-lW, and FAS drafted the manuscript. YZ performed some of the fetal echocardiography. XS and W-jL contributed to part of the analysis and interpretation of image data. M-lW made the data analysis. All authors read and approved the final manuscript.

Competing interests
The authors declare that they have no competing interests.

Consent for publication
Not applicable.

Author details
[1]Department of Sonography, Shengjing Hospital of China Medical University, Heping District, Shenyang, China. [2]Department of Radiology, The first Affiliated Hospital of Sun Yat-sen University, Guangzhou, China. [3]Department of Entomology, The Pennsylvania State University, University Park, PA 16802, USA. [4]Department of Microbiology and Parasitology, College of Basic Medical Sciences, China Medical University, Heping District, Shenyang, China.

References
1. Benjamin EJ, Blaha MJ, Chiuve SE, et al. Heart disease and stroke statistics-2017 update: a report from the American Heart Association. Circulation. 2017;135:e146–603.
2. Gillum RF. Epidemiology of congenital heart disease in the United States. Am Heart J. 1994;127(4 Pt 1):919–27.
3. Gembruch U. Prenatal diagnosis of congenital heart disease. Prenat Diagn. 1997;17:1283–98.
4. Hoffman JIE, Kaplan S. The incidence of congenital heart disease. J Am Coll Cardiol. 2002;39:1890–900.
5. Galindo A, Mendoza A, Arbues J, Grañeras A, Escribano D, Nieto O. Conotruncal anomalies in fetal life: accuracy of diagnosis, associated defects and outcome. Eur J Obstet Gynecol Reprod Biol. 2009;146:55–60.
6. Houston MR, Kirby ML. Neural crest and cardiovascular development: a 20-year perspective. Birth Defects Res Part C Embryo Today. 2003;60:2–13.
7. Rustico MA, Benettoni A, D'Ottavio G, Maieron A, Fischer-Tamaro I, Conoscenti G, et al. Fetal heart screening in low-risk pregnancies. Ultrasound Obstet Gynecol. 1995;6:313–9.
8. Allan L. Technique of fetal echocardiography. Pediatr Cardiol. 2004;25:223–33.
9. Goncalves LF, Espinoza J, Romero R, Lee W, Beyer B, Treadwell MC, et al. A systematic approach to prenatal diagnosis of transposition of the great arteries using 4-dimensional ultrasonography with spatiotemporal image correlation. J Ultrasound Med. 2004;23:1225–31.
10. Chaoui R. The four-chamber view: four reasons why it seems to fail in screening for cardiac abnormalities and suggestions to improve detection rate. Ultrasound Obstet Gynecol. 2003;22:3–10.
11. Huhta JC. Evaluating the fetus with transposition. Cardiol Young. 2005; 15(Suppl 1):88–92.
12. Zhang Y, Ding C, Fan M, Ren W, Guo Y, Sun W, et al. Evaluation of normal fetal pulmonary veins using B-flow imaging with spatiotemporal image correlation and by traditional color Doppler echocardiography. Prenat Diagn. 2012;32:1186–91.
13. Gindes L, Hegesh J, Weisz B, Gilboa Y, Achiron R. Three and four dimensional ultrasound: a novel method for evaluating fetal cardiac anomalies. Prenat Diagn. 2009;9:645–53.
14. Nelson TR, Pretorius DH, Sklansky M, Hagen-Ansert S. Three-dimensional echocardiographic evaluation of fetal heart anatomy and function:

acquisition, analysis, and display. J Ultrasound Med. 1996;15:1–9. quiz 11-2

15. Chaoui R, Heling KS. New developments in fetal heart scanning: three- and four-dimensional fetal echocardiography. Semin Fetal Neonatal Med. 2005;10:567–77.

16. DeVore GR, Falkensammer P, Sklansky MS, Platt LD. Spatio-temporal image correlation (STIC): new technology for evaluation of the fetal heart. Ultrasound Obstet Gynecol. 2003;22:380–7.

17. Viñals F, Poblete P, Giuliano A. Spatio-temporal image correlation (STIC): a new tool for the prenatal screening of congenital heart defects. Ultrasound Obstet Gynecol. 2003;22:388–94.

18. Zhang D, Zhang Y, Ren W, Sun F, Guo Y, Sun W, et al. Prenatal diagnosis of fetal interrupted aortic arch type A by two-dimensional echocardiography and four-dimensional echocardiography with B-flow imaging and spatiotemporal image correlation. Echocardiography. 2016;33:90–8.

19. Hu G, Zhang Y, Fan M, Wang M, Siddiqui FA, Wang Y, et al. Evaluation of fetal cardiac valve anomalies by four-dimensional echocardiography with spatiotemporal image correlation (4DSTIC). Echocardiography. 2016;33:1726–34.

20. Goncalves LF, Espinoza J, Romero R, Lee W, Treadwell MC, Huang R, et al. Four-dimensional fetal echocardiography with spatiotemporal image correlation (STIC): a systematic study of standard cardiac views assessed by different observers. J Matern Fetal Neonatal Med. 2005;17:323–31.

21. Paladini D, Rustico M, Todros T, Palmieri S, Gaglioti P, Benettoni A, et al. Conotruncal anomalies in prenatal life. Ultrasound Obstet Gynecol. 1996;8:241–6.

22. Sivanandam S, Glickstein JS, Printz BF, Allan LD, Altmann K, Solowiejczyk DE, et al. Prenatal diagnosis of conotruncal malformations: diagnostic accuracy, outcome, chromosomal abnormalities, and extracardiac anomalies. Am J Perinatol. 2006;23:241–5.

23. American Institute of Ultrasound in Medicine. AIUM practice guideline for the performance of fetal echocardiography. J Ultrasound Med. 2011;30:127–36.

24. Sun X, Zhang Y, Fan M, Wang Y, Wang M, Siddiqui FA, et al. Role of four-dimensional echocardiography with high definition flow imaging and spatiotemporal image correlation in detecting fetal pulmonary veins. Echocardiography. 2017; doi:10.1111/echo.13543.

25. Uittenbogaard LB, Haak MC, Spreeuwenberg MD, Van Vugt JMG. A systematic analysis of the feasibility of four-dimensional ultrasound imaging using spatiotemporal image correlation in routine fetal echocardiography. Ultrasound Obstet Gynecol. 2008;31:625–32.

26. Avnet H, Mazaaki E, Shen O, Cohen S, Yagel S. Evaluating spatiotemporal image correlation technology as a tool for training Nonexpert Sonographers to perform examination of the fetal heart. J Ultrasound Med. 2016;35:111–9.

27. Shih JC, Shyu MK, Su YN, Chiang YC, Lin CH, Lee CN. 'Big-eyed frog' sign on spatiotemporal image correlation (STIC) in the antenatal diagnosis of transposition of the great arteries. Ultrasound Obstet Gynecol. 2008;32:762–8.

28. DeVore GR, Polanco B, Sklansky MS, Platt LD. The 'spin' technique: a new method for examination of the fetal outflow tracts using three-dimensional ultrasound. Ultrasound Obstet Gynecol. 2004;24:72–82.

29. Abuhamad AZ. Standardization of 3-dimensional volumes in obstetric sonography: a required step for training and automation. J Ultrasound Med. 2005;24:397–401.

30. Gotsch F, Romero R, Espinoza J, Kusanovic JP, Erez O, Hassan S, et al. Prenatal diagnosis of truncus arteriosus using multiplanar display in 4D ultrasonography. J Matern Fetal Neonatal Med. 2010;23:297–307.

31. Yeo L, Romero R, Jodicke C, Oggè G, Lee W, Kusanovic JP, et al. Four-chamber view and 'swing technique' (FAST) echo: a novel and simple algorithm to visualize standard fetal echocardiographic planes. Ultrasound Obstet Gynecol. 2011;37:423–31.

32. Zidere V, Pushparajah K, Allan LD, Simpson JM. Three-dimensional fetal echocardiography for prediction of postnatal surgical approach in double outlet right ventricle: a pilot study. Ultrasound Obstet Gynecol. 2013;42:421–5.

33. Votino C, Cos T, Abu-Rustum R, Dahman Saidi S, Gallo V, Dobrescu O, et al. Use of spatiotemporal image correlation at 11-14 weeks' gestation. Ultrasound Obstet Gynecol. 2013;42:669–78.

5

Carotid plaque rather than intima-media thickness as a predictor of recurrent vascular events in patients with acute ischemic stroke

Hyun Ju Yoon[1,2], Kye Hun Kim[1,2]*, Hyukjin Park[1], Jae Yeong Cho[1,2], Young Joon Hong[1], Hyung Wook Park[1], Ju Han Kim[1], Youngkeun Ahn[1], Myung Ho Jeong[1], Jeong Gwan Cho[1,2] and Jong Chun Park[1,2]

Abstract

Background: To investigate the impacts of carotid plaque and intima-media thickness (IMT) on future vascular events (VEs) in the patients with acute ischemic stroke.

Methods: A total of 479 consecutive Korean patients with acute ischemic stroke were divided into 2 groups according to development of VEs; VE group (65.4 ± 10.9 years) vs no VE group (62.8 ± 13.2 years). VEs were defined as the development of recurrent stroke, coronary events, peripheral arterial disease, and death. Clinical, laboratory, and imaging findings were compared between the groups.

Results: During 105.5 ± 29.0 months of follow up, VEs were developed in 142 patients (29.6%). In univariate analysis, VEs were significantly associated with age, gender, diabetes, renal function, lipid levels, left ventricular function, carotid plaque or IMT. In multivariate analysis, the presence of carotid plaque, diabetes, renal function and male gender were independent predictors of future VEs in the patients with ischemic stroke, but carotid IMT was not a predictor of future VEs. Event free survival was significantly lower in patients with carotid plaque than without carotid plaque on Kaplan-Meier analysis (log rank $p < 0.001$).

Conclusion: The present study demonstrated that diabetes, impaired renal function, male gender, and the presence of carotid plaque rather than IMT were independent predictors of future VEs in Korean patients with acute ischemic stroke. Active medical management and careful monitoring for the development of recurrent VEs are strongly recommended in patients with acute ischemic stroke and carotid plaque.

Keywords: Carotid artery, Plaque, Intima-media thickness, Stroke

Background

Atherosclerotic cardiovascular disease (CVD) is a major cause of mortality and morbidity in worldwide. Carotid atherosclerosis is not only a marker of systemic atherosclerosis but also a predictor of ischemic cerebrovascular disease [1]. Carotid ultrasound is an efficient, relatively inexpensive, highly reproducible method to evaluate atherosclerotic change of the carotid artery by measuring the presence of plaques or intima-media thickness (IMT) of the carotid artery. The increased carotid IMT and the presence of carotid plaques are well established predictors of CVD and ischemic stroke [2–5]. Because intima-media thickening or plaques of the carotid artery may reflect different biological aspects of atherosclerotic process, the significance of carotid plaque or IMT in the prediction of atherosclerotic CVD or ischemic stroke may be different. According to the results of a recent meta-analysis, the measurement of carotid plaque seems to be a superior method than carotid IMT in predicting the development of CVD [6, 7]. In contrary to carotid plaque,

* Correspondence: cvkimkh@gmail.com
[1]Department of Cardiovascular Medicine, Chonnam National University Hospital, 42 Jaebong-ro, Donggu, Gwangju 501-757, South Korea
[2]Translational Research Center on Aging, Chonnam National University Hospital, 42 Jaebong-ro, Donggu, Gwangju 501-757, South Korea

furthermore, the association between carotid IMT and CVD has been questioned in some studies [8, 9].

After a first attack of stroke, secondary prevention for future vascular events (VEs) including recurrent stroke is very important. Major hemispheric stroke, ischemic stroke, and atrial fibrillation have been suggested as clinical predictors of recurrent stroke after an index stroke [10]. Recent studies have also suggested that carotid IMT or plaque can be a useful imaging marker for stroke recurrence [11–14]. However, the comparison between carotid IMT and plaque on future VEs including stroke recurrence after an index stroke has been poorly studied. We hypothesized that the significance of carotid IMT and plaque on future VEs would be different after a first attack of stroke of ischemic etiology. Therefore, the aim of this study was to investigate the impacts of carotid IMT and plaque on future VEs in the patients with acute ischemic stroke.

Methods
Study design and population
The present study is a single center, retrospective observational study, and the study protocol was approved by the Institutional Review Board of our institution (No = 2010–05-092).

From 2007 to 2008, a total of 2607 Korean patients were diagnosed as acute stroke. After excluding 2128 patients, a total of 479 patients with ischemic stroke who had baseline echocardiography and carotid ultrasound at admission were finally enrolled and divided into 2 groups according to the development of VE: VE group (n = 142, 65.42 ± 10.9 years, 99 males) vs no VE group (n = 337, 62.77 ± 13.2 years, 166 males). The reasons of exclusion were as follows; 1) no baseline echocardiography or carotid ultrasound study (n = 837), 2) previous history of stroke (n = 361), 3) cardio-embolic stroke including atrial fibrillation, mechanical valve, or mitral stenosis (n = 276), 4) transient ischemic attack (n = 269), 5) hemorrhagic stroke (n = 260), 6) cryptogenic stroke with confirmed patent foramen ovale (n = 125). After discharge from an index stroke, the study subjects underwent clinical follow up at out-patient clinic for 105.5 ± 29.0 months, and follow up information including VEs were obtained from medical records.

Definition of stroke and VEs
According to the updated definition of stroke of the current guideline, ischemic stroke was diagnosed by the combination of symptoms and/or signs of typical neurological dysfunction and imaging evidence of central nervous system infarction. Therefore, ischemic stroke was defined as an episode of neurological dysfunction caused by focal cerebral, spinal, or retinal infarction on imaging studies [15].

VEs were defined as the development of recurrent stroke, coronary events, peripheral arterial disease, and cardiovascular death during the study period in the present study. Recurrent stroke was defined as the development of a new focal neurologic deficit or new deterioration of a previous deficit accompanied by a de novo imaging evidence of brain infarction, but the development of transient ischemic attack or hemorrhagic transformation of the previous infarct lesion was excluded in the present study. Coronary event was defined as the development of obstructive atherosclerotic coronary artery disease (% diameter stenosis >70%) or myocardial infarction demonstrated by conventional coronary or cardiac CT angiography. Peripheral arterial disease was defined as the development of a narrowing of the arteries other than those that supply the heart or the brain with an ankle brachial index <0.9.

Laboratory tests
Routine laboratory study was performed as soon as possible after admission, and blood samples to assess the serum lipid profile and glucose were obtained in the next morning after fasting more than 9 h. C-reactive protein (CRP) was measured by the immunoturbidimetric CRP-Latex (II) assay using an Olympus 5431 auto analyzer (Olympus America Inc., Melville, NY, USA).

Carotid ultrasound examination
Carotid ultrasound examination was performed on both common carotid arteries (CCA) and internal carotid arteries (ICA) using a 10 MHz linear probe (Vivid 7, GE Vingmed Ultrasound, Horten, Norway) according to the current guideline [16, 17]. With the subject in the supine position and with slight hyperextension of the neck, the CCA and carotid bulb were identified.

Carotid arteries were examined bilaterally in the transversal and longitudinal planes. Following short-axis 2D image acquisition of the CCA, long-axis B-mode ultrasound images were acquired for the subsequent measurements. After placing a region of interest in the far wall of the CCA, the mean IMT was estimated in a region free of atherosclerotic plaques by using semi-automated vessel-wall detection software, AutoIMT® by GE Healthcare [18]. Averaged IMT values of the left and right CCAs were subsequently used in all analyses. Carotid IMT is defined as a double-line pattern visualized by echo 2D on both walls of the CCA in a longitudinal view. Two parallel lines (leading edges of two anatomical boundaries) form it. Mean IMT was computed from 80 to 120 measurements over a 10 mm span ending 5 mm proximal to the transition between the CCA and bulb regions. Intra- and inter-operator coefficients of variation were 2.8% and 3.0%, respectively, and intra- and inter-operator intra-class correlations were both 0.97. Plaque was defined as a protrusion of the vessel wall into the arterial lumen of at least 0.5 mm, with an IMT 50% that of the surrounding sites or an IMT > 1.5 mm as measured from the media-adventitia interface to the intima lumen interface. Regardless of locations, the presence of any plaque in CCA or bulb or ICA was considered as the presence of carotid plaque in the present study. First of all, the presence or absence of carotid plaques were evaluated and then texture were classified into soft, mixed, and calcified based on echogenicity. In the case of multiple plaques, we measured maximal protruding diameter from carotid wall. On a longitudinal two-dimensional ultrasound image of the carotid artery, the anterior (near) and posterior (far) walls of the carotid artery appear as two bright white lines separated by a hypoechogenic space. End-diastolic images were frozen, and the far wall IMT was identified as the region between the lumen-intima interface and the media-adventitia interface using semiautomatic method. It contained CCA, bulb and proximal ICA plaques. Peak systolic and end diastolic carotid flow velocity was measured by pulse wave Doppler on the CCA and the ICA [19].

Echocardiographic examination

Echocardiographic images from various echocardiographic windows were obtained by using a digital ultrasonographic equipment system (Vivid 7, GE Vingmed Ultrasound, Horten, Norway). Digital cine loops were obtained for subsequent offline analysis. All of the data were analyzed by using the computerized offline software package (Echo-PAC PC 6.0.0, GE Vingmed Ultrasound, Horten, Norway). Routine echocardiographic examinations were performed in accordance with the recommendation of the current guideline [20]. Ejection fraction were measured by using Simpson's biplane method. The intra-observer and inter-observer variabilities of Simpson's method were 4% ± 5% and 5% ± 4% (absolute difference divided by the mean measurement value). The early (E) and late diastolic velocities (A) of the mitral inflow were measured by using pulsed wave Doppler from the apical 4-chamber view, with the sample volume positioned at the tip of the mitral leaflets. The early (e′), late diastolic (a′), and systolic velocities of the mitral septal annulus were measured by using tissue Doppler imaging in the apical four chamber view.

Statistical analysis

The statistical Package for Social Sciences (SPSS) for Windows, version 18.0 (Chicago, Illinois, USA) was used for statistical analysis. Data are presented as percents or mean ± standard deviation. The differences of the categorical variables were evaluated by Chi-square test, and the continuous variables were compared using independent t test. The event-free survival rate was evaluated by using the Kaplan-Meier analysis, and the event rates were compared using the log-rank test. To identify the independent predictor of long term vascular events, multivariate logistic regression analysis was applied to the significant variables in univariate analysis. A p-value less than 0.05 was considered as statistically significant.

Results

Baseline characteristics

Baseline characteristics are summarized in the Table 1. Age was older and male gender was more prevalent in VE group than in no VE group. Diabetes mellitus and prior history of cerebrovascular accident were more frequent in VE group than in no VE group. Other baseline characteristics were not different between the groups.

Laboratory findings and discharge medication

Laboratory findings are summarized in the Table 2. The levels of serum glucose, hemoglobin A1c, and creatinine were significantly higher, whereas the levels of total and low density lipoprotein cholesterol were significantly lower in VE group than in no VE group. There was no significant difference in discharge medication between groups (Table 3).

Echocardiographic findings

Echocardiographic findings are summarized in the Table 4. Left ventricular end-systolic dimension was larger, whereas ejection fraction was decreased in VE group than in no VE group. Other echocardiographic findings were not different between the groups.

Table 1 Baseline clinical characteristics of the patients

	VE (n = 142)	No VE (n = 337)	P value
Age (years)	65.4 ± 10.9	62.7 ± 13.4	0.035
Male (%)	99 (70.2%)	166 (50%)	<0.001
Height (cm)	162.2 ± 9.1	161.5 ± 839	0.525
Weight (kg)	63.7 ± 9.6	63.4 ± 11.3	0.825
BMI (kg/m²)	25.5 ± 14	24.9 ± 9.1	0.655
Hypertension (%)	86 (61.8%)	159 (54.1%)	0.077
Diabetes (%)	53 (38.1%)	62 (21.0%)	<0.001
Dyslipidemia (%)	92 (67.1%)	202 (68.7%)	0.414
Smoking (%)	31 (22.3%)	59 (20.1%)	0.664
Territory infarction (%)	54 (38.8%)	127 (41.7%)	0.317
SBP (mmHg)	135.4 ± 22.7	133.1 ± 19.5	0.277
DBP (mmHg)	82.3 ± 14.6	81.9 ± 13.3	0.845
Pulse pressure (mmHg)	53.9 ± 16.7	51.5 ± 13.6	0.106

BMI body mass index, *CVA* cerebrovascular accident, *SBP* systolic blood pressure, *DBP* diastolic blood pressure

Table 2 Laboratory findings of the patients

	VE (*n* = 142)	No VE (*n* = 337)	P value
WBC (/mm^3)	7498 ± 4545	7383 ± 4746	0.814
Hb (g/dL)	13.0 ± 1.9	13.5 ± 2.7	0.095
TC (mg/dL)	179.1 ± 39.0	187.2 ± 37.1	0.044
TG (mg/dL)	129.2 ± 63.0	127.5 ± 70.9	0.819
LDL-C (mg/dL)	110.4 ± 35.1	124.2 ± 42.3	0.002
HDL-C (mg/dL)	45.7 ± 14.8	63.2 ± 26.3	0.456
LP(a) (mg/dL)	32.2 ± 30.4	38.2 ± 12.1	0.601
Glucose (g/dL)	146.1 ± 64.4	129.8 ± 55.8	0.011
HbA1c (%)	6.45 ± 1.1	6.27 ± 1.3	0.017
Creatinine (mg/dL)	1.10 ± 0.98	0.83 ± 0.363	0.001
CRP (mg/dL)	1.68 ± 3.5	1.04 ± 2.1	0.057
Homocystein (umol/L)	12.0 ± 5.2	12.0 ± 10.3	0.993

WBC white blood cell, *Hb* hemoglobin, *TC* total cholesterol, *TG* triglyceride, *LDL-C* low density lipoprotein-cholesterol, *HDL-C* high density lipoprotein-cholesterol, *LP* lipoprotein, *HbA1c* glycosylated hemoglobin, *CRP* C reactive protein

Carotid ultrasound findings

Carotid ultrasound findings are summarized in the Table 5. Carotid plaques were found in 181 cases (37.8%) out of 479 patients with stroke. Regardless of location, the presence of CCA, bulb, or ICA plaque was significantly frequent in VE group than in no VE group. Significant ICA stenosis (>50%) was not different between the groups. Carotid revascularization was performed only in 2 patients of VE group and 2 patients of no VE group. IMT of the left CCA and mean IMT of the both CCA were thicker in VE group than in no VE group, but IMT of the right CCA was not different between the groups. The size and types of carotid plaque and blood flow variables of the CCA were not different between the groups.

VEs and predictors of VEs during clinical follow up

During 105.5 ± 29 months of clinical follow up, VEs were developed in 142 patients (29.6%); recurrent stroke in 73 patients (15.2%), coronary events in 57 patients (11.9%), peripheral arterial disease in 16 patients (3.3%), and death in 9 patients (1.9%).

Table 3 Prescribed medications of the patients

	VE (*n* = 142)	No VE (*n* = 337)	P value
Aspirin (%)	50 (35.2)	107 (31.7)	0.416
Plavix (%)	49 (34.5)	106 (31.4)	0.161
Warfarin (%)	28 (19.7)	54 (16.0)	0.321
ACEI or ARB (%)	56 (39.4)	128 (37.9)	0.307
Beta blocker (%)	30 (21.1)	69 (20.4)	0.238
CCB (%)	53 (37.3)	102 (30.2)	0.064
Statin (%)	42 (29.5)	81 (24.0)	0.308

ACEI angiotensin converting enzyme, *ARB* aldosterone receptor blocker, *CCB* calcium channel blocker

Table 4 Baseline echocardiographic findings of the patients

	VE (*n* = 142)	No VE (*n* = 337)	P value
LVEDD (mm^2)	48.7 ± 5.3	48.1 ± 4.5	0.174
LVESD (mm^2)	31.8 ± 4.9	30.8 ± 4.2	0.046
IVS thickness (mm)	9.7 ± 1.7	9.7 ± 1.6	0.913
PW thickness (mm)	9.4 ± 1.3	9.4 ± 1.2	0.737
LA dimension (mm)	39.5 ± 7.6	38.4 ± 7.7	0.150
Aorta (mm)	32.5 ± 3.8	32.6 ± 7.5	0.917
EF (%)	63.4 ± 6.5	64.8 ± 6.	0.043
E (m/s)	0.62 ± 0.30	0.62 ± 0.63	0.974
A (m/s)	0.71 ± 0.16	0.70 ± 0.21	0.458
DT (msec)	213.5 ± 117	219.3 ± 88	0.607
E' (m/s)	0.06 ± 0.06	0.07 ± 0.06	0.572
S' (m/s)	0.09 ± 0.13	0.10 ± 0.52	0.814
E/E'	11.2 ± 7.8	10.4 ± 6.9	0.290

LVEDD left ventricle end diastolic dimension, *LVESD* left ventricle end systolic dimension, *LA* left atrium, *EF* ejection fraction, *E* early diastolic mitral inflow velocity, *A* late diastolic mitral inflow velocity, *DT* deceleration time, *E'*: early diastolic velocity of mitral septal annulus, *S'*: systolic velocity of mitral septal annulus

Multivariate analyses to identify independent predictors of VEs were performed, and the results are summarized in the Table 6. Diabetes, renal function, male gender, and the presence of carotid plaque in any site were independent predictors of future VEs in patients with acute ischemic

Table 5 Carotid ultrasound findings of the patients

	VE (*n* = 142)	No VE (*n* = 337)	P value
Plaque, CCA (%)	17 (11.9)	22 (6.5)	0.038
Plaque, bulb (%)	50 (35.2)	91 (27.0)	0.046
Plaque, ICA (%)	22 (15.4)	32 (9.5)	0.044
Plaque, any site (%)	66 (46.5)	114 (33.8)	0.006
Maximal plaque size (mm)	2.4 ± 0.6	2.5 ± 0.9	0.729
Types of plaque			
Soft (%)	31 (21.8)	57 (16.9)	0.121
Calcified (%)	10 (7.0)	13 (3.9)	0.098
Mixed (%)	25 (17.6)	44 (13.1)	0.454
RCCA IMT(mm)	0.82 ± 0.23	0.78 ± 0.22	0.061
LCCA IMT (mm)	0.86 ± 0.23	0.81 ± 0.22	0.043
Mean CCA IMT (mm)	0.84 ± 0.21	0.79 ± 0.20	0.022
RCCA PSV(cm/s)	47.9 ± 22.3	49.9 ± 22.3	0.373
LCCA PSV (cm/s)	51.4 ± 25.7	52.8 ± 25.3	0.609
RCCA EDV (cm/s)	13.4 ± 6.7	14.5 ± 7.5	0.958
LCCA EDV (cm/s)	13.6 ± 7.7	15.6 ± 8.1	0.124
ICA stenosis >50% (%)	9 (6.3)	11 (3.2)	0.102
Carotid revascularization (%)	2 (1.4)	2 (0.6)	0.343

RCCA right common carotid artery, *LCCA* left common carotid artery, *ICA* internal carotid artery, *Rt* right, *Lt* left, *CA* carotid artery, *IMT* intima-media thickness, *PSV* peak systolic velocity, *EDV* end diastolic velocity

Table 6 Predictors of vascular events by multivariate analysis

	RR	CI	P value
Age	1.018	1.000–1.036	0.051
Male	2.255	1.474–3.449	<0.001
DM	2.061	1.1311–3.239	0.002
Creatinine	1.969	1.205–3.217	0.007
LVESD	1.030	0.982–1.081	0.228
EF	0.983	0.952–1.015	0.290
Plaque, CCA	1.947	1.000–3.790	0.050
Plaque, bulb	1.469	0.965–2.236	0.073
Plaque, ICA	1.749	0.946–3.015	0.060
Plaque, any site	1.699	1.139–2.533	0.027
LCCA IMT	1.696	0.692–4.158	0.248
RCCA IMT	1.766	0.719–4.339	0.215
Mean CCA IMT	2.207	0.800–6.091	0.126
DM + plaque	3.779	2.101–6.796	<0.001

RR relation risk, *CI* confidence interval, *DM* diabetes mellitus, *LVESD* left ventricle end systolic dimension, *EF* ejection fraction, *CCA* right common carotid artery, *ICA* internal carotid artery, *Rt* right, *Lt* left, *CA* carotid artery, *IMT* intima-media thickness

stroke on multivariate analysis. However, carotid IMT was not an independent predictor of future VEs. The risk of future VEs was greatest in acute ischemic stroke patients with both carotid plaque and diabetes. In subgroup analysis, carotid IMT was not an independent predictor of future VEs in stroke patients without carotid plaque.

Carotid plaque and VEs

The presence of carotid plaque was significantly associated with recurrent stroke and total VEs, but it was not a predictor of coronary events, peripheral arterial disease and deaths (Fig. 1). On Kaplan-Meier analysis, event free survival for recurrent stroke and total VEs was significantly lower in acute ischemic stroke patients with carotid plaque than in without carotid plaque (log rank $p < 0.001$) (Fig. 2).

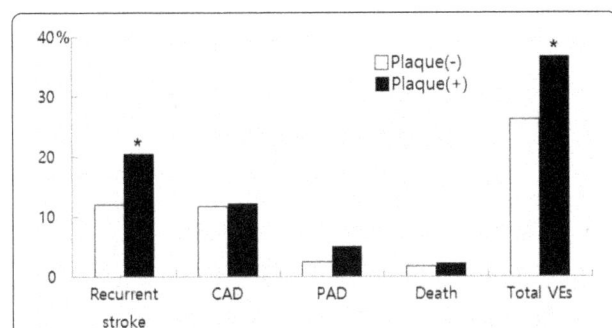

Fig. 1 Future vascular event according to the presence of carotid plaque (* means $p < 0.05$). CAD: coronary artery disease, PAD: peripheral vascular disease, VEs: vascular events

Discussion

In the present study, the authors want to compare the significance between carotid IMT and plaque on future VEs including stroke recurrence after an index stroke, and the results of the present study demonstrated several clinically important findings. First, recurrent VEs are not infrequent in Korean patients with ischemic stroke after an index event, and non-cerebral VEs including coronary and peripheral artery disease comprise about a half of VEs. Second, carotid plaque rather than carotid IMT is a useful prognostic marker for the development of future VEs in Korean patients with ischemic stroke. Therefore, careful search for non-cerebral vascular diseases and active medical management for preventing recurrent stroke are strongly recommended in acute ischemic stroke patients with carotid plaque. Thirdly, the presence of carotid plaque at any sites, as a whole, was an independent predictor of future VEs, whereas the presence of plaque at CCA or bulb or ICA showed marginal significance for predicting VEs. Therefore, the present study suggested that a thorough evaluation for the presence of plaques in whole carotid arterial trees including CCA, bulb, and ICA should be performed for risk stratification in patients with acute ischemic stroke.

The risk for the development of future stroke is significantly higher in survivors of first-ever stroke than in general population [21], the risk of stroke recurrence is known to be greatest during the first week after index stroke [22]. According to a current meta-analysis, the cumulative risk of stroke recurrence is gradually increased as time goes by and is 3.1% at 30 days, 11.1% at 1 year, 26.4% at 5 years, and 39.2% at 10 years after initial stroke [23]. In the present study, recurrent stroke was developed in 15.2% during 8.7 years of clinical follow up, and the rate of stroke recurrence seems to be lower than that of a current meta-analysis [23]. The rate of stroke recurrence was 18.4% at 5 years in the retrospective cohort study of Sun et al. [24] and 19.8% at years in the study of Lee et al. [25], and the recurrence rate of these studies were similar to that of our study. The differences of stroke recurrence might be explained by the differences in study population among the studies. In contrary to a current meta-analysis [23], the present study cannot reflect true incidence of stroke recurrence, because the present study only included stroke patients of ischemic etiology with carotid ultrasound and echocardiography studies.

Stroke recurrence is known to be associated with poor long-term clinical outcomes and quality of life [22, 26]. After a first attack of stroke, therefore, early identification of high risk group and secondary prevention for future vascular events (VEs) including recurrent stroke would be very important. Despite of high prevalence of classic risk factors such as hypertension and dyslipidemia in patients

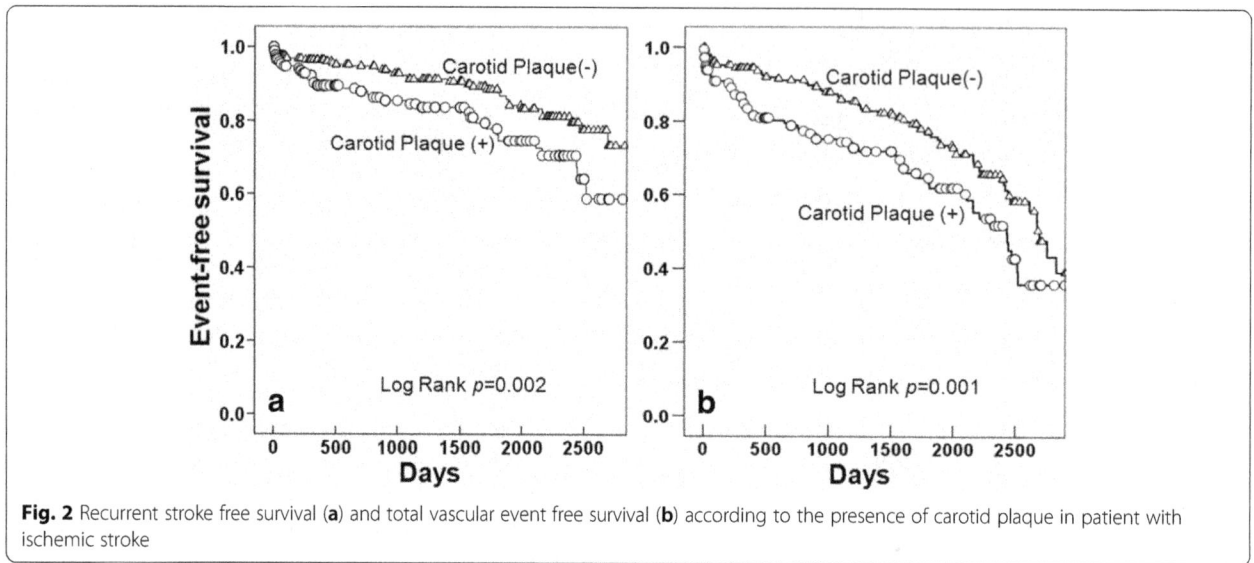

Fig. 2 Recurrent stroke free survival (**a**) and total vascular event free survival (**b**) according to the presence of carotid plaque in patient with ischemic stroke

with recurrent stroke as in the study of Leoo et al., hypertension and dyslipidemia were not predictors of stroke recurrence in the present study [27]. Rather, among classic risk factors for CVD, diabetes was the only significant predictor of stroke recurrence in the present study. In addition to classic risk factors, therefore, it is suggested that other risk factors or predictors for stroke recurrence should be identified to improve clinical outcomes. The previous studies have suggested several clinical predictors for stroke recurrence, and these include major hemispheric stroke, ischemic stroke, male gender, diabetes, advanced age, and atrial fibrillation [10, 23–25]. In the present study, diabetes, renal function, and male gender were significant clinical predictors of future VEs. History of coronary artery disease, severe stenosis or occlusion of large cerebral artery, and multiple acute cerebral infarcts suggested as independent predictors of recurrent ischemic stroke or TIA within one year [28]. Several studies have suggested that carotid plaque or IMT can be used as imaging marker not only in the prediction of development of first-ever stroke [2–5] but also in the prediction of stroke recurrence [11–14], even though the significance of carotid IMT or plaque may differ [6–9]. Our previous study also demonstrated that the significance of carotid IMT is different from carotid plaque on ischemic stroke [29]. Despite of these differences, the comparison between carotid IMT and plaque on future VEs after an index stroke has been poorly studied previously. And the results of the present study demonstrated that carotid plaque than carotid IMT is a significant imaging marker for stroke recurrence. The present study also suggested that a thorough evaluation for the presence of plaques in whole carotid arterial trees including CCA, bulb, and ICA should be performed for risk stratification in patients with acute ischemic stroke. In the present study, the presence of

both carotid plaque and diabetes was more strongly associated with stroke recurrence, and thus this subgroup of ischemic stroke patients should be more carefully monitored and actively managed for preventing VEs.

As a whole, the prevalence of carotid plaque was 37.8% in the present study population with ischemic stroke (8.1% in CCA, 29.4% in carotid bulb, 11.3% in ICA, respectively), and carotid bulb was also the most common site for plaque formation in this study as in previous studies [16]. In the previous studies involving Korean population, the prevalence of carotid plaque was 5.7% in general population [30] and 24.6 ~ 42.1% in patients with atherosclerotic CVD such as coronary artery disease [31], and the result of the present study also showed quite similar to those of the previous studies.

In addition to the presence of carotid plaque, the characteristics of plaques are also important for predicting stroke recurrence. The previous studies have shown that echolucent or large or mobile plaques are associated with stroke recurrence [13, 32, 33], but the echogenicity, size or mobility of carotid plaque was not associated with stroke recurrence in the present study. The reason why the characteristics of plaque were not associated with VEs in the present study is unclear, and selection bias from the retrospective nature of this study or ethnic differences might be possible explanations.

In population with ischemic stroke, future coronary or peripheral artery disease events and need for revascularization are not infrequent and the result of the present study was also demonstrated the association between stroke and systemic atherosclerotic vascular events [34, 35]. The development or identification of coronary or peripheral artery disease was also not infrequent in the present study and developed in 57 patients (11.9%) and in 16 patients (3.3%), respectively. Therefore, careful evaluation for coronary or peripheral artery disease should be performed by non-invasive coronary imaging or ankle-brachial index in patients with ischemic stroke. Although the presence of carotid plaque was a significant predictor of recurrent stroke, it was not an independent predictor of future coronary or peripheral vascular events in the present study. No association between carotid plaque and systemic vascular events might be explained by multi-factorial pathogenic mechanism of coronary or peripheral artery disease or small number of study population of the present study. Increased value of CCA IMT is known to be associated with a higher long-term risk of extracranial vascular events such as coronary or peripheral artery disease in a cohort study of Purroy et al. [36], it was not s predictor of future VEs in the present study.

Study limitations

The present study has several potential limitations. First, the present study has all limitations of a retrospective analysis including selection bias. As discussed already, the present study only included stroke patients of ischemic etiology with carotid ultrasound and echocardiography studies. Many of the patients with ischemic stroke were excluded because of the absence of ultrasound studies, and thus the result of the present study cannot be generalized. Second, the present study did not consider the impacts of interventional therapy or medications, and these also might influence on future VEs. Third, the incidence of coronary or peripheral vascular events might be underestimated because non-cerebral systemic vascular events were not evaluated routinely and usually evaluated in symptomatic patients.

Conclusion

In conclusion, despite these potential limitations, the results of the present study demonstrated that diabetes, impaired renal function, male gender, and the presence of carotid plaque rather than IMT were independent predictors of future VEs in Korean patients with acute ischemic stroke. Active medical management and careful monitoring for the development of recurrent VEs are strongly recommended in patients with acute ischemic stroke and carotid plaque.

Acknowledgements
Not applicable.

Funding
This research was supported by a grant (CRI 13904–21) of Chonnam National University Hospital Biomedical Research Institute.

Authors' contributions
HJY, KHK, HP, JYC, YJH, HWP and JHK made substantial contributions to patient inclusion, HJY and KHK to data analysis and YA, MHJ, JGC and JCP to data interpretation. All authors have contributed in writing and correcting the manuscript and approved the submission of the manuscript.

Consent for publication
Not applicable.

Competing interests
The authors declare that they have no competing interests.

References
1. Rothwell PM. Carotid artery disease and the risk of ischaemic stroke and coronary vascular events. Cerebrovasc Dis. 2000;10:21–33.
2. Ebrahim S, Papacosta O, Whincup P, Wannamethee G, Walker M, Nicolaides AN, et al. Carotid plaque, intima media thickness, cardiovascular risk factors, and prevalent cardiovascular disease in men and women: the British regional heart study. Stroke. 1999;30:841–50.
3. Polak JF, Pencina MJ, Pencina KM, O'Donnell CJ, Wolf PA, D'Agostino RB Sr. Carotid-wall intima-media thickness and cardiovascular events. N Engl J Med. 2011;365:213–21.
4. Lorenz MW, Polak JF, Kavousi M, Mathiesen EB, Volzke H, Tuomainen TP, et al. Carotid intima-media thickness progression to predict cardiovascular events in the general population (the PROG-IMT collaborative project): a meta-analysis of individual participant data. Lancet. 2012;379:2053–62.
5. Touboul PJ, Elbaz A, Koller C, Lucas C, Adraï V, Chédru F, et al. Common carotid artery intima-media thickness and brain infarction: the etude du Profil Genetique de l'Infarctus cerebral (GENIC) case-control study: the GENIC investigators. Circulation. 2000;102:313–8.
6. Inaba Y, Chen JA, Bergmann SR. Carotid plaque, compared with carotid intima-media thickness, more accurately predicts coronary artery disease events: a meta-analysis. Atherosclerosis. 2012;220:128–33.
7. Naqvi TZ, Lee MS. Carotid intima-media thickness and plaque in cardiovascular risk assessment. JACC Cardiovasc Imaging. 2014;7:1025–38.
8. del Sol AI, Moons KG, Hollander M, Hofman A, Koudstaal PJ, Grobbee DE, et al. Is carotid intima-media thickness useful in cardiovascular disease risk assessment? The Rotterdam study. Stroke. 2001;32:1532–8.
9. Johnsen SH, Mathiesen EB. Carotid plaque compared with intima-media thickness as a predictor of coronary and cerebrovascular disease. Curr Cardiol Rep. 2009;11:21–7.
10. Moroney JT, Bagiella E, Paik MC, Sacco RL, Desmond DW. Risk factors for early recurrence after ischemic stroke: the role of stroke syndrome and subtype. Stroke. 1998;29:2118–24.
11. Talelli P, Terzis G, Katsoulas G, Chrisanthopoulou A, Ellul J. Recurrent stroke: the role of common carotid artery intima-media thickness. J Clin Neurosci. 2007;14:1067–72.
12. Roquer J, Segura T, Serena J, Cuadrado-Godia E, Blanco M, García-García J, et al. Value of carotid intima-media thickness and significant carotid stenosis as markers of stroke recurrence. Stroke. 2011;42:3099–104.
13. Singh AS, Atam V, Jain N, Yathish BE, Patil MR, Das L. Association of carotid plaque echogenicity with recurrence of ischemic stroke. N Am J Med Sci. 2013;5:371–6.
14. Tadokoro Y, Sakaguchi M, Yamagami H, Okazaki S, Furukado S, Matsumoto M, et al. Echogenicity of medium-to-large carotid plaques predicts future vascular events. Cerebrovasc Dis. 2014;38:354–61.
15. Sacco RL, Kasner SE, Broderick JP, Caplan LR, Connors JJ, Culebras A, et al. An updated definition of stroke for the 21st century: a statement for healthcare professionals from the American Heart Association/American Stroke Association. Stroke. 2013;44:2064–89.
16. Stein JH, Korcarz CE, Hurst RT, Lonn E, Kendall CB, Mohler ER. Et al; American Society of Echocardiography carotid Intima-media thickness task force. Use of carotid ultrasound to identify subclinical vascular disease and evaluate cardiovascular disease risk: a consensus statement from the American Society of Echocardiography carotid Intima-media thickness task force. Endorsed by the Society for Vascular Medicine. J Am Soc Echocardiogr. 2008;21:93–111.
17. Roman MJ, Naqvi TZ, Gardin JM, Gerhard-Herman M, Jaff M, Mohler E. American Society of Echocardiography report. Clinical application of noninvasive vascular ultrasound in cardiovascular risk stratification: a report from the American society of echocardiography and the society for vascular medicine and biology. Vasc Med. 2006;11:201–11.

18. Vermeersch SJ, Rietzschel ER, De Buyzere ML, Van Bortel LM, D'Asseler Y, Gillebert TC, et al. Validation of a new automated IMT measurement algorithm. J Hum Hypertens. 2007;21:976–8.

19. Grant EG, Benson CB, Moneta GL, Alexandrov AV, Baker JD, Bluth EI, et al. Carotid artery stenosis: grayscale and Doppler ultrasound diagnosis-Society of Radiologists in ultrasound consensus conference. Ultrasound Q. 2003;19:190–8.

20. Lang RM, Badano LP, Mor-Avi V, Afilalo J, Armstrong A, Ernande L, et al. Recommendations for cardiac chamber quantification by echocardiography in adults: an update from the American Society of Echocardiography and the European Association of Cardiovascular Imaging. J Am Soc Echocardiogr. 2015;28:1–39.

21. Boysen G, Truelsen T. Prevention of recurrent stroke. Neurol Sci. 2000;21:67–72.

22. Furie KL, Kasner SE, Adams RJ, Albers GW, Bush RL, Fagan SC, et al. Guidelines for the prevention of stroke in patients with stroke or transient ischemic attack: a guideline for healthcare professionals from the American Heart Association/American Stroke Association. Stroke. 2011;42:227–76.

23. Mohan KM, Wolfe CD, Rudd AG, Heuschmann PU, Kolominsky-Rabas PL, Grieve AP. Risk and cumulative risk of stroke recurrence: a systematic review and meta-analysis. Stroke. 2011;42:1489–94.

24. Sun Y, Lee SH, Heng BH, Chin VS. 5-year survival and rehospitalization due to stroke recurrence among patients with hemorrhagic or ischemic strokes in Singapore. BMC Neurol. 2013;13:133.

25. Lee AH, Somerford PJ, Yau KK. Risk factors for ischaemic stroke recurrence after hospitalisation. Med J Aust. 2004;181:244–6.

26. Wang YL, Pan YS, Zhao XQ, Wang D, Johnston SC, Liu LP, et al. CHANCE investigators. Recurrent stroke was associated with poor quality of life in patients with transient ischemic attack or minor stroke: finding from the CHANCE trial. CNS Neurosci Ther. 2014;20:1029–35.

27. Leoo T, Lindgren A, Petersson J, von Arbin M. Risk factors and treatment at recurrent stroke onset: results from the recurrent stroke quality and epidemiology (RESQUE) study. Cerebrovasc Dis. 2008;25:254–60.

28. Zhang C, Zhao X, Wang C, Liu L, Ding Y, Akbary F, et al. Prediction factors of recurrent ischemic events in one year after minor stroke. PLoS One. 2015;10:1–12.

29. Yoon HJ, Jeong MH, Kim KH, Ahn Y, Cho JG, Park JC, et al. Carotid Intima-media thickness, not carotid plaque, is associated with large territory cerebral infarction in patients with ischemic stroke. Korean Circ J. 2010;40:272–6.

30. Kweon SS, Shin MH, Jeong SK, Nam HS, Lee YH, Park KS, et al. Cohort profile: the Namwon study and the dong-gu study. Int J Epidemiol. 2014;43:558–67.

31. Park HW, Kim KH, Song IG, Kwon TG, Kim WH, Bae JH. Body mass index, carotid plaque, and clinical outcomes in patients with coronary artery disease. Coron Artery Dis. 2017;28:278–86.

32. Lenzi GL, Vicenzini E. The ruler is dead: an analysis of carotid plaque motion. Cerebrovasc Dis. 2007;23:121–5.

33. Ogata T, Yasaka M, Wakugawa Y, Kitazono T, Okada Y. Morphological classification of mobile plaques and their association with early recurrence of stroke. Cerebrovasc Dis. 2010;30:606–11.

34. Calvet D, Touzé E, Varenne O, Sablayrolles J, Weber S, Mas J. Prevalence of asymptomatic coronary artery disease in ischemic stroke patients: the PRECORIS study. Circulation. 2010;121:1623–9.

35. Banerjee A, Fowkes FG, Rothwell PM. Associations between peripheral artery disease and ischemic stroke: implications for primary and secondary prevention. Stroke. 2010;41:2102–7.

36. Purroy F, Montserrat J, Begué R, Gil MI, Quílez A, Sanahuja J, et al. Higher carotid intima media thickness predicts extracranial vascular events and not stroke recurrence among transient ischemic attack patients. Int J Stroke. 2012;7:125–32.

6

Left ventricular diastolic function is strongly correlated with active emptying of the left atrium: a novel analysis using three-dimensional echocardiography

Johannes Scherr[1][*] ⓘ, Philip Jung[2], Tibor Schuster[3], Lars Pollmer[1], Gert Eisele[4], Franz Goss[4], Jens Schneider[5] and Martin Halle[1,6]

Abstract

Background: Increased left atrial (LA) dimensions are known to be a risk factor in predicting cardiovascular events and mortality and to be one key diagnostic tool to assess diastolic dysfunction. Currently, LA measurements are usually conducted using 2D-echocardiography, although there are well-known limitations. Real-time 3D-echocardiography is able to overcome these limitations, furthermore being a valid measurement tool compared to reference standards (e.g. cardiac magnetic resonance imaging).

We investigated LA function and volume and their association to left ventricular (LV) diastolic function, using newly designed and validated software for 3D-echocardiographic analysis. This software is the first to allow for a sophisticated analysis of both passive and active LA emptying.

Methods: We analyzed 2D- and 3D-echocardiographic measurements of LA volume and function in 56 subjects and compared the results between patients with normal LV diastolic function (NDF) ($n = 30$, 52 ± 15 years, BMI 24.7 ± 2.6 kg/m^2) and patients in which diastolic dysfunction (DDF) was suspected ($n = 26$, 65 ± 9 years, BMI 26.7 ± 3.7 kg/m^2).

Results: Volumes during LA active emptying were significantly smaller in DDF compared to NDF (active atrial stroke volume (ASV): 3.0 (0.1–4.5) vs. 5.5 (2.7–7.8) ml, $p = 0.005$; True-EF: 7.3(0.1–11.5) vs. 16.2 (8.1–25.4) %, $p = 0.002$). Furthermore, ASV showed a stronger association to E/e'_{mean} than all other measured LA volumes ($\beta = -0.35$, $p = 0.008$). Neither total stroke LA volume, nor maximum or minimum LA volume differed significantly between the groups.

Conclusions: Diastolic LV dysfunction results in a reduction in active LA emptying, which is more strongly associated with LV filling pressure than other previously investigated LA parameters.

Keywords: Three-dimensional echocardiography, Left atrium, Left ventricular diastolic function

Background

Heart failure (HF) with preserved ejection fraction (EF) (HFpEF) significantly contributes to morbidity, mortality and health care costs in both the U.S. and Europe [1]. Currently the best non-invasive diagnostic strategies and criteria to characterize HFpEF have yet to be determined, largely because opinions addressing diagnostic strategy differ substantially between cardiac associations [2, 3].

The left atrium (LA) seems to play a pivotal role in the development of HFpEF, as LA size is strongly associated with left ventricular (LV) diastolic function and is an independent predictor of heart failure hospitalization in subjects with preserved ejection fraction and coronary heart disease [4, 5]. Suggested mechanisms of ventricular filling modulation are strongly related to the reservoir, conduit, and pump functions of the LA [6, 7].

As a potential tool in the measurement of LV diastolic function, LA volume is considered to reflect the

---
* Correspondence: scherr@sport.med.tum.de
[1]Department of Prevention and Sports Medicine, Klinikum rechts der Isar, Technische Universitaet Muenchen, Georg-Brauchle-Ring 56, D-80992 Munich, Germany
Full list of author information is available at the end of the article

cumulative effects of filling pressure over time in terms of atrial remodeling. This would be superior to the currently used technique of measuring left ventricular inflow, which only reflect the filling pressure at the time of measurement [3]. Therefore, LA volume seems to be a good surrogate parameter for cardiovascular risk, as well as a powerful predictor of cardiovascular outcomes [4, 8].

Left atrial size is clinically assessed by linear 2-dimensional (2D) echocardiographic (2DE) measurements in 2- and 4-chamber views, which provides a fairly good estimation of the true dimension [9]. Although this measurement has been accepted as having sufficient clinical feasibility and reliability, in recent years 3-dimensional (3D) echocardiography (3DE) assessment has become increasingly available.

The 3D-echocardiographic measurements for chamber quantifications have shown high correlations with the gold standard of cardiac magnetic resonance imaging (cMRI) and computed tomography (CT) [10–12]. In contrast to cMRI and CT, which is costly both in terms of time and money, 3DE is a relatively fast and economical bedside method to assess LA size and function [13]. Furthermore, other LA parameters such as the left atrial function – generated by both the passive early filling of the left ventricle (LV) caused by the movement of the valvular plane and the active atrial contraction – were rarely analyzed until the introduction of 3DE.

In a recent study, it was shown that a decreased contribution of active left atrial emptying to ventricular filling during diastole was strongly predictive of adverse cardiac events and death [14].

Therefore, we performed the first evaluation of passive and active left atrial function and size using newly designed, already validated software for 3D-echocardiographic analysis and its correlation with left ventricular diastolic function [11, 12].

Methods
Study population
Sixty consecutive, randomly assigned subjects (14 women, 46 men) who underwent echocardiography with a commercially available ultrasound system (iE33, Philips Healthcare, Hamburg, Germany) were recruited from 1) the out-patient clinic for Prevention and Sports Medicine, Klinikum rechts der Isar, Technische Universitaet Muenchen or 2) the Division of Cardiology, Department of Medicine, Medizinische Klinik und Poliklinik, Ludwig-Maximilians-Universität, Campus Innenstadt.

The study protocol was approved by the university's ethical board (Klinikum rechts der Isar der Technischen Universitat Munchen) and the investigation conforms to the principles outlined in the Declaration of Helsinki. All participants gave written informed consent.

Inclusion criteria were age ≥18 years and written informed consent. Exclusion criteria were significant cardiac valvular disease (at least moderate (2nd degree) mitral or aortic regurgitation or mitral stenosis), cardiac arrhythmias or conduction abnormalities (e.g. (intermittent) atrial fibrillation or flutter, left or right bundle branch block (QRS duration >120 ms), pacemaker rhythm, frequent premature beats), previous cardiac surgery, reduced left ventricular ejection fraction (EF <55 %), previous transcoronary ablation of septal hypertrophy (TASH), acute coronary syndrome (ACS) within four weeks or myocardial infarction within 2 months, or severe pulmonary hypertension with clinical relevant right ventricular impairment.

The participants were divided into the following groups: (1) a control group consisting of subjects with an $E/e'_{mean} < 8$; and (2) subjects with an $E/e'_{mean} \geq 8$ and also maximal LA volume (LAV_{max}) ≥ 34 mL*m^{-2} and therefore meeting criteria for diastolic LV dysfunction according to current guidelines using 2DE [2, 3]. Study design aimed to include 30 subjects in each group. Four participants were excluded because of very poor image quality (as recommended by the current guidelines [15]). In the group with normal diastolic function (control group), mainly leisure time athletes (all performance category ranging from hobby sportspeople to former elite athletes, all being free of any cardiovascular diseases) were examined who presented within the Department of Prevention and Sports Medicine for primary prevention purposes. In the group with evidence of diastolic LV dysfunction, mainly patients with heart failure with preserved ejection fraction (HFpEF) were included (recruited both in the Department of Prevention and Sports Medicine and Division of Cardiology).

Hypertension was defined as previously described [16]. Hyperlipidemia was defined as a total fasting cholesterol level of more than 6.21 mmol/L or use of lipid-lowering medication.

Echocardiography
Transthoracic echocardiographic investigations (standard 2D parasternal short- and long-axis images and apical 2-, 3- and 4-chamber views, and 3-dimensional echocardiography) were conducted during end-expiratory apnea in a left lateral decubitus position by experienced echocardiographers in accordance to current recommendations [17]. Echocardiographic images were collected at all sites and analyses were performed at the core laboratory at the Department of Prevention and Sports Medicine. Indexes of LA volumes for body surface area were calculated as previously described with a variation of the formula from DuBois [18]:

$$BSA \left[m^2 = 0.007184 \times Heightcm^{0.725} \times Weightkg \right]^{0.425}.$$

2D echocardiography (2DE)

For 2D-echocardiography, a transthoracic broadband S5-1 transducer (frequency transmitted 1.7 MHz, received 3.4 MHz, Philips Medical Imaging, Hamburg, Germany) was used.

2D atrial size was assessed with the biplane method of discs (modified Simpson's rule) and the area-length method from apical two- and four-chamber views as recommended by the American Society of Echocardiography [9]. The maximal length of the LA was measured at ventricular end-systole in an apical-four chamber view. Maximal left atrial volume (LAV_{max}) was measured at the ventricle end-systole just before opening of the mitral valve. Minimal left atrial volume (LAV_{min}) was measured at the end-diastole on ECG just before closure of the mitral valve [9].

Peak velocities of trans-mitral inflow during early filling (E), atrial contraction (A), and the deceleration time of the E-wave velocity (DT) were measured in apical four-chamber view using pulsed Doppler echocardiography with positioning of the Doppler sample volume perpendicular to the flow jet at the tips of the mitral valve leaflets; E/A ratio was subsequently calculated. The early diastolic mitral annular velocity (e') was measured at the septal side as well as the free LV wall of the mitral annulus using tissue Doppler imaging on the longitudinal axis in the apical 4-chamber view. E/e'_{med} and E/e'_{lat} as well as E/e'_{mean} (calculated as $E/mean(e'_{med}$ and e'_{lat})) were subsequently calculated.

Diastolic function was graded as "normal" when E/e'_{mean} was <8 and "at least suggestive of diastolic dysfunction" when E/e'_{mean} was ≥8 and LAV_{max} was ≥34 mL*m^{-2} [2, 3, 19]. The latter one with evidence of diastolic dysfunction was subdivided into the three stages of diastolic dysfunction in accordance to the classification of Khouri [20]. Also in the current guidelines, consistency between at least two indices is required to make the diagnosis of a diastolic dysfunction [15]. We chose E/e'_{mean} and LAV_{max} because these indices seem to be feasible and reproducible [15]. Furthermore, LAV_{max} represents a marker of chronicity of elevated LA pressure [15]. Additionally, E/e'_{mean} ratio seems to be less age dependent than other indices and therefore also suitable to compare groups with different mean ages [15]. An E/e'_{mean} ratio <8 usually indicates normal LV filling pressure [15].

Real-time 3D-echocardiography (RT3DE)

For each patient, RT3DE was performed directly after 2DE with a 3 to 1 MHz transthoracic matrix array transducer (X3-1) in the harmonic mode from an apical window to acquire full-volume 3D images in accordance to the current recommendations [17]. To encompass the entire left heart into the real-time 3-dimensional echocardiographic data set, a full volume up to 92° × 84° scan was acquired from seven R-wave-triggered sub-volumes during an end-expiratory breath-hold. The depth and angle of the ultrasound scan sector were adjusted to the minimal level still encompassing the entire left ventricle and atrium. The temporal resolution of the data sets ranged from 25 to 34 ms.

Analysis of systolic function of the left ventricle ($3D-EF_{LV}$) and left ventricular volumes (LV stroke volume [LV-SV]) was performed as previously described [21].

3D LA volume (3D-LAV) was analyzed with RT3DE software (4D LA Function, TomTec Imaging Systems, Munich, Germany) as previously described (see Fig. 1) [11, 12]. 3-dimensionally measured maximum left atrial volume (LAV_{max3D}) was assessed at ventricular end systole right before opening of the mitral valve by semiautomatic tracing of the LA endocardial surface. Minimal 3-dimensionally measured volume (LAV_{min3D}) was measured at ventricular end-diastole just after closure of the mitral valve. Total stroke volume of the left atrium (Total SV) was calculated as the difference between the minimum and maximum left atrial volumes.

After manual setting of five to seven tracing points in each view, the endocardial border was automatically delineated, and the LAV was obtained automatically throughout the heart cycle, resulting in LA volume-time curves. LA appendages and the confluence of the pulmonary veins were excluded from the tracing. Manual corrections were made to modify the automatic tracings in some subjects where necessary (inaccuracy of endocardial automated detection). To differentiate between early diastolic filling (E = LA passive emptying) and atrial contraction (A = LA active emptying) a marker (preA) was set at the moment of the second opening component of the biphasic opening movement of the mitral valve. Corresponding volume was defined as pre-atrial contraction volume (V_{preA}). For LA, atrial stroke volume (ASV) was calculated as $LAV_{preA} - LAV_{min3D}$. Total-EF was calculated as $(LAV_{max3D} - LAV_{min3D})/LAV_{max3D} \times 100\%$. True-EF was calculated as $ASV/LAV_{max3D} \times 100\%$. Left atrial conduit volume (LA-CV) was calculated as followed: LA-CV = LV-SV – Total SV. Additionally, LA-CV was expressed as percentage of LV stroke volume ($LA-CV_{rel}$) to present the magnitude of LA-CV on LV systolic function.

3D LA size and function were interpreted blinded to the 2D measurements of diastolic function.

Statistics

Data analysis was performed using PASW Statistics 22.0 (SPSS Inc., Chicago IL, USA). For quantitative data, the

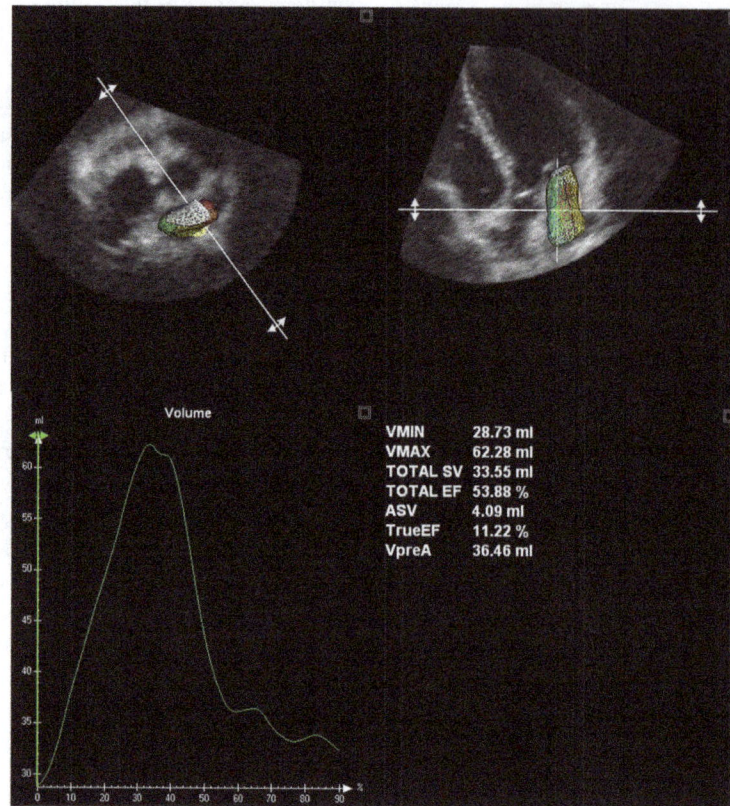

Fig. 1 3D image analysis (4D LA Function, TomTec Imaging Systems) depicting the performed measurements

mean, standard deviation and range or if more appropriate (non-normally distributed data) the median and interquartile range (IQR: 25th/75th percentile) were reported for descriptive purpose. Assumption of normal distribution of data was verified by using descriptive methods (skewness, outliers and distribution plots) and inferential statistics (Shapiro–Wilk test).

Non-normally distributed main outcome parameters were logarithmically transformed prior to parametric data analysis. Thus, relative effects of potential explanatory variables were modeled. Back-transformation was performed using simple exponential functions. Thus back-transformation of regression coefficients gives an estimate for the median relative change of outcome measure by a one-unit increment of the corresponding explanatory variable.

For correlation analyses of left ventricular inflow parameters and parameters of left atrial function, Spearman correlation coefficients (ρ) were calculated. Agreements between 2D- and 3D-methods were assessed by the Bland–Altman analysis.

We performed a receiver operating characteristics (ROC) analysis with participants meeting criteria for diastolic LV dysfunction (E/e'$_{mean} \geq 8$ and also maximal LA volume (LAV$_{max}$) ≥ 34 mL*m^{-2}) as event of interest and

various quantities of the 3D assessment as potential predictors. Areas under the ROC curve (AUCs) and corresponding 95 % confidence intervals are presented. For the most important measures (True-EF, Total-EF, and ASV) the ROC curves are shown.

For analysis of the interobserver variability, measurements were performed by two blinded observers. To assess intraobserver variability, measurements were repeated 2 weeks later by an observer blinded to the previous measurements. Inter- and intraobserver variabilities were calculated as the difference between the two measurements in terms of the percentage of their mean.

A p-value <0.05 was considered to indicate statistical significance. Testing was performed two-sided.

Results
Participants' characteristics
Baseline characteristics and 2-dimensional echocardiographic data are presented in Table 1.

In the group with evidence of diastolic dysfunction ($n = 26$), 14 (54 %) had impaired relaxation (stage I diastolic dysfunction), 7 (27 %) had pseudonormal function (stage II diastolic dysfunction) and 5 (19 %) had a reversible restriction (stage III diastolic dysfunction).

Table 1 Baseline characteristics of participants

	Normal diastolic function (E/e'$_{mean}$ < 8) n = 30	With evidence of diastolic LV dysfunction (E/e'$_{mean}$ ≥ 8 & LAV$_{max}$ ≥ 34 mL/m^2) n = 26	p-value
Anthropometry			
Women [%]	4 (13 %)	10 (38 %)	0.07
Age [yrs]	52.3 ± 15.1	64.8 ± 9.3	0.001
Weight [kg]	76.5 ± 9.7	78.3 ± 12.8	0.63
Height [m]	1.76 ± 0.07	1.71 ± 0.08	0.02
Body mass index [kg/m^2]	24.7 ± 2.6	26.7 ± 3.7	0.01
Fat Free Mass [kg]	63.0 ± 9.5	57.2 ± 6.8	0.09
Body surface area [m^2]	1.92 ± 0.14	1.90 ± 0.18	0.55
Cardiovascular Risk Factors			
Hypercholesterolemia (total cholesterol ≥6.21 mmol/L)	5 (17 %)	7 (27 %)	0.61
RR$_{sys}$/RR$_{dia}$	128 ± 16/83 ± 10	144 ± 22/85 ± 9	0.01/0.25
Hypertension (RR$_{sys}$ > 140 mmHg or RR$_{dia}$ > 90 mmHg)	9 (30 %)	16 (62 %)	0.07
Echocardiography			
Heart rate [bpm]	59 ± 11	68 ± 10	0.001
3D-EF$_{LV}$ [%]	59.7 ± 5.2	60.6 ± 12.0	0.14
LV mass [g/m^2]	86.6 ± 16.0	96.9 ± 30.4	0.35
E [cm/s]	68.4 ± 18.1	79.6 ± 16.4	0.02
Left ventricle internal diameter, diastole [mm]	47 ± 6	39 ± 11	0.002
Posterior wall thickness, diastole [mm]	11 ± 2	13 ± 3	<0.001
Septum wall thickness, diastole [mm]	11 ± 2	14 ± 3	<0.001
A [cm/s]	60.6 ± 14.5	79.2 ± 20.0	0.001
E/A ratio	1.20 ± 0.44	1.05 ± 0.35	0.10
Dct [ms]	218 ± 8	262 ± 6	0.004
e'$_{lat}$ [cm/s]	14.0 ± 3.6	8.9 ± 2.7	<0.001
E/e'$_{lat}$	5.01 ± 1.12	9.9 ± 4.6	<0.001
e'$_{med}$ [cm/s]	9.3 ± 2.8	6.4 ± 1.5	0.001
E/e'$_{med}$	7.42 ± 1.57	13.01 ± 3.46	<0.001
E/e'$_{mean}$	5.55 ± 1.33	11.30 ± 2.92	<0.001
E/e'$_{mean}$ [range]	2.9–7.9	8.0–20.0	<0.001

Mean ± SD or median (IQR)
(*RR$_{sys}$/RR$_{dia}$* systolic and diastolic blood pressure, *E* early diastolic filling peak velocity, *A* peak velocity during atrial contraction, *Dct* Deceleration time of the E-wave velocity, *e'$_{lat}$* early diastolic mitral annular velocity free LV wall, *e'$_{med}$* early diastolic mitral annular velocity septal)

3-dimensional echocardiographic parameters

No significant between-group differences were observed in left atrial dimensions (both minimal and maximal volume and total stroke volume) when measured with 2DE and 3DE. However, there were significant differences in volumes caused by active left atrial emptying, like ASV and true atrial ejection fraction (see Table 2 and Fig. 2). In these investigations, the group with suspected diastolic dysfunction had decreased atrial stroke volume (median [IQR]: 3.0 [0.1–4.5] ml vs. 5.5 [2.7–7.8] ml, p = 0.005), also when corrected for BSA and BMI, respectively. Furthermore, the true ejection fraction was significantly lower in the group with diastolic impairment (7.3 vs. 16.2 %, p = 0.002).

These significant associations between E/e'$_{mean}$ and LA volumes were also supported in univariate and multivariate linear regression models. In the correlation analysis there were highly significant inverse associations between E/e'$_{mean}$ and parameters of active left atrial emptying (correlation coefficients: ASV: ρ = –0.472; True EF ρ = –0.488, all p < 0.001). In contrast, total left atrial function (represented by Total SV and Total-EF) was not different between the groups (all p > 0.05). There were no significant associations between 2-dimensionally measured (such as A or a' wave) and 3-dimensionally assessed (e.g. ASV) parameters of active LA emptying (all p > 0.05).

In ROC analyses, True-EF showed the highest AUC (0.753 (0.623–0.883)), followed by ASV (0.731 (0.598–

Table 2 3D-echocardiographic characteristics (volumetric and functional) of the left atrium

	Normal diastolic function (E/e'$_{mean}$ < 8) n = 30	With evidence of diastolic LV dysfunction (E/e'$_{mean}$ ≥ 8 & LAV$_{max}$ ≥ 34 mL/m^2) n = 26	p-value
2DE			
LAV$_{Simpson}$ (ml)	65.4 ± 20.2	69.8 ± 30.0	0.71
LAV$_{area-length\ method}$ (ml)	55.3 ± 21.3	56.2 ± 10.1	0.27
3DE			
LAV$_{max3D}$ (ml)	54.5 ± 13.2	57.1 ± 21.3	0.87
LAV$_{max3D}$/BSA (ml/m^2)	28.5 ± 7.2	30.3 ± 12.6	0.88
LAV$_{max3D}$/BMI (ml × m^2 × kg^{-1})	2.2 ± 0.5	2.2 ± 1.2	0.21
LAV$_{min3D}$ (ml)	23.6 ± 7.4	28.4 ± 15.8	0.38
LAV$_{min3D}$/BSA (ml/m^2)	12.3 ± 4.0	15.1 ± 8.5	0.44
LAV$_{min3D}$/BMI (ml × m^2 × kg^{-1})	0.96 ± 0.31	1.10 ± 0.71	0.85
Total SV (ml)	30.7 (26.7–34.8)	27.1 (22.1–32.3)	0.13
Total SV/BSA (ml/m^2)	15.4 (13.3–18.5)	14.1 (12.0–16.6)	0.16
Total SV/BMI (ml × m^2 × kg-1)	1.24 (1.02–1.44)	1.03 (0.86–1.17)	0.009
ASV (ml)	5.5 (2.7–7.8)	3.0 (0.1–4.5)	0.005
ASV/BSA (ml/m^2)	2.8 (1.3–4.3)	1.5 (0.0–2.4)	0.007
ASV/BMI (ml × m^2 × kg-1)	0.21 (0.11–0.35)	0.10 (0.00–0.16)	0.002
V$_{preA}$ (ml)	34.5 (27.3–42.2)	38.1 (28.0–51.4)	0.31
Total-EF (%)	57.0 ± 7.3	52.2 ± 11.9	0.09
True-EF (%)	16.2 (8.1–25.4)	7.3 (0.1–11.5)	0.002
LA-CV (ml)	31.6 (18.7–44.0)	29.9 (17.0–32.9)	0.27
LA-CV$_{rel}$ (%)	52.3 ± 15.2	44.9 ± 17.9	0.11

Mean ± SD or median (IQR)

(*LAV* left atrial volume, *LAV$_{max3D}$* 3d-measured maximal left atrial volume, *LAV$_{min3D}$* 3d-measured minimal left atrial volume, *SV* stroke volume, *V$_{preA}$* pre-atrial contraction volume, *ASV* atrial stroke volume, *LA-CV* left atrial conduit volume, *LA-CV$_{rel}$* LA-CV expressed as percentage of LV stroke volume, *BSA* body surface area, *BMI* body mass index)

0.865)) and Total-EF (0.605 (0.452–0.758)). These AUCs were not significantly different between the examined parameters (p-value ranging from 0.114 to 0.409). ROC curves are presented in Fig. 3.

In regression analyses, total SV (β = –0.024, p = 0.862) and LAV$_{max3D}$ (β = 0.125, p = 0.357) showed weak associations to E/e'$_{mean}$, whereas LAV$_{min3D}$ showed a modest association (β = 0.196, p = 0.148). ASV showed the strongest association (β = –0.421, p = 0.001). Also after adjustment for age, blood pressure, heart rate and LV mass, active atrial emptying (ASV) remained strongly associated with E/e'$_{mean}$ in a linear regression model including all LA volumes (see Table 3).

Reproducibility

The correlation coefficients ranged from 0.90 (ASV) to 0.99 (LAV$_{min3D}$ and LAV$_{max3D}$) between measurements (performed by one observer, intra-observer variability) and from 0.90 (ASV) to 0.99 (LAV$_{min3D}$) between observers (inter-observer variability). Cronbach's Alpha ranged from 0.90 (ASV) to 0.99 (LAV$_{min3D}$).

Agreement of 2D- and 3D- determined left atrial volumes

Agreement of 2-dimensionally and 3-dimensionally measured left atrial volumes are presented within Bland-Altman correlation (see Fig. 4). The left atrial volume measured 2-dimensionally using the Simpson method seems to overestimate the volume compared to the 3-dimensionally measurement. In contrast, LA volume analyzed with the area-length technique resulted in smaller sizes when compared to 3D measurements.

Discussion

Our study is the first to analyze both active and passive LA emptying components with regard to diastolic function.

We were able to detect differences between a group with normal diastolic function compared to a group with participants representing with diastolic dysfunction with regard to active LA emptying. In contrast, all other parameters of LA volume showed no significant differences. Therefore, it can be assumed that using 3DE with special focus on active LA emptying might result in

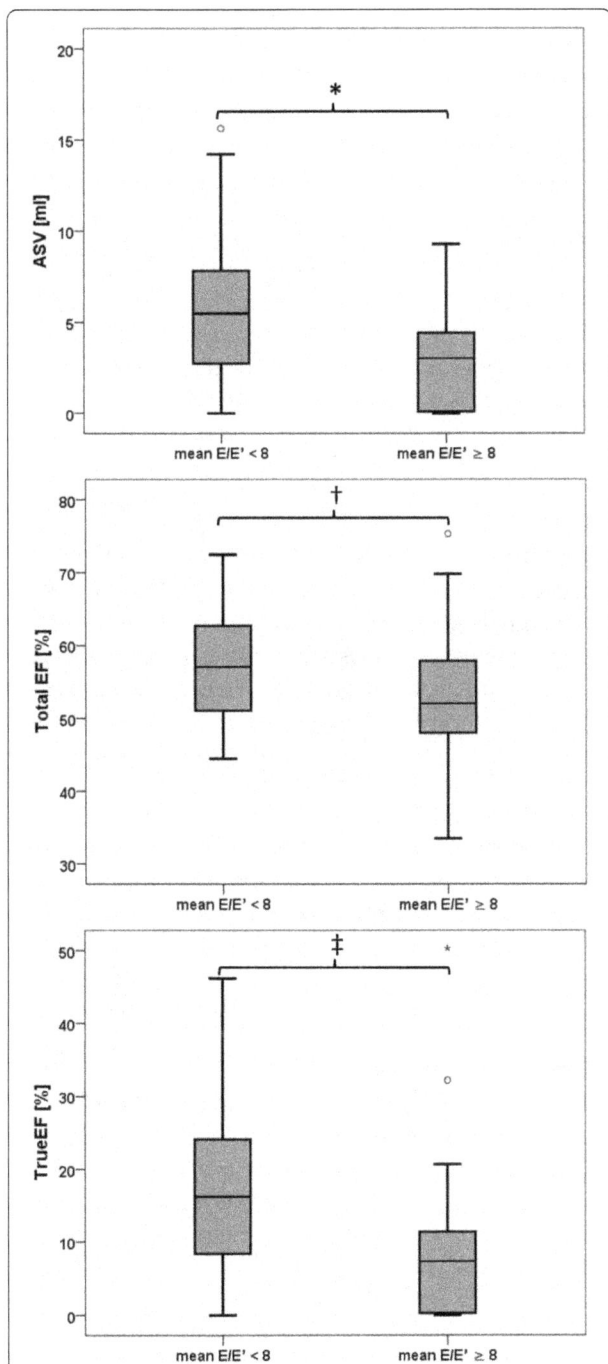

Fig. 2 LA volumes and function in the investigated groups.
* indicating $p = 0.005$, †indicating $p = 0.09$, ‡ indicating $p = 0.002$

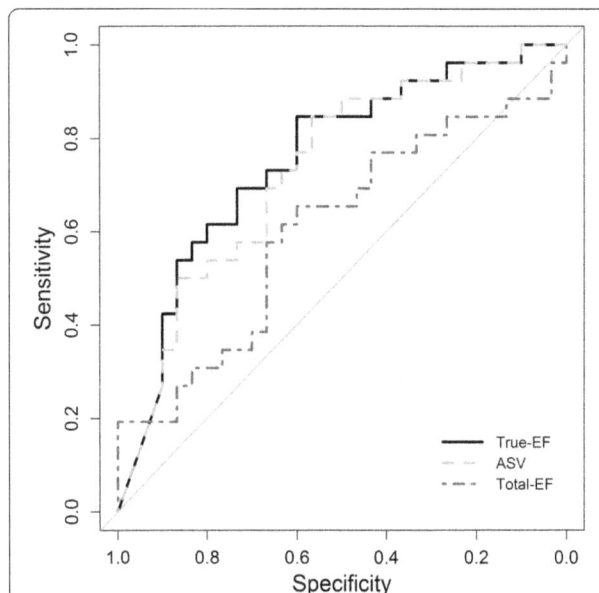

Fig. 3 ROC curves for True-EF, ASV and Total-EF with respect to participants meeting criteria for diastolic LV dysfunction (E/e'$_{mean} \geq 8$ and also maximal LA volume (LAV$_{max} \geq 34$ mL*m^{-2}) as event of interest

we also found LAV$_{min3D}$ to better correlate with LV diastolic function than LAV$_{max3D}$. However, the newly investigated parameters of LA function (True-EF and ASV) showed even stronger associations and seem therefore to be a more sensitive instrument to measure small but meaningful alterations of diastolic function. One reason for this reduction during active LA emptying might be the decreasing compliance of the left ventricle with progressive filling at end-diastole in patients with impaired diastolic LV function [3].

Regarding another three-dimensionally assessed parameter (relative LA conduit volume) which was prior linked to diastolic dysfunction [23], we were not able to demonstrate an association between increased LA-CV$_{rel}$ and impaired diastolic LV function. However, the populations between our study and the cohort of Nappo et al. differ significantly (e.g. LV-EF: 60.1 ± 9.3 % vs. 37.1 ± 11.3 %) and LV stroke volume and EF play a decisive role in the calculation of LA-CV$_{rel}$ and determination of impaired diastolic LV function [15], the results of these two studies cannot be compared. Therefore, further studies are needed with

earlier and more sensitive diagnosis of diastolic dysfunction compared to conventional approaches.

New parameters and left ventricular diastolic function

In a recent study, Russo et al. observed that minimum LA volume was closer correlated to LV diastolic function than maximum LA volume [22]. This is in accordance with our results. In the multivariate regression analysis,

Table 3 Linear regression of left atrial volumes with E/e'$_{mean}$

	Unadjusted			Adjusted[a]		
	B (SE)	β	p-value	B (SE)	β	p-value
ASV	−0.41 (0.13)	−0.40	0.002	−0.35 (0.13)	−0.35	0.008
Total SV	−0.03 (0.05)	−0.08	0.55	−0.07 (0.05)	−0.19	0.19
LAV$_{min3D}$	0.05 (0.047)	0.17	0.20	−0.02 (0.05)	−0.08	0.64

Values represent parameter estimates (B), standard errors (SE), and standardized parameter estimates (β)
[a]Adjusted for age, heart rate, hypertension and left ventricular mass

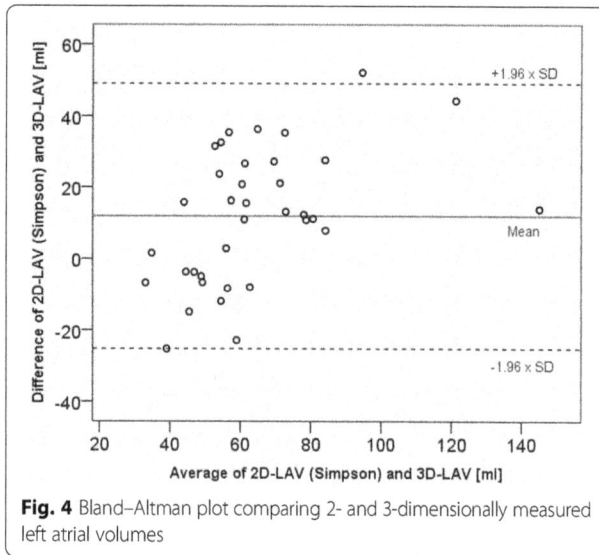

Fig. 4 Bland–Altman plot comparing 2- and 3-dimensionally measured left atrial volumes

larger numbers of participants to be able to calculate reference values which can be generalized.

In another recent study on 2-dimensional evaluation of LA volumes and function, Teo et al. observed that in subjects in the initial stages of diastolic dysfunction, the active emptying volume is increased compared to subjects with normal diastolic function [24]. However, as the grade of LV diastolic dysfunction increases, this compensatory mechanism reduces and is eventually lost as mechanical atrial dysfunction sets in, resulting in a lower total LA emptying volume. Similar results were observed by Prioli et al., while investigating left atrial volumes and function with 2D-echocardiography and left ventricular catheterization [7]. This is consistent with the current study in which nearly half of the participants had higher stages of diastolic dysfunction; however, we were able to observe decreases in active LA emptying even at the very early stages of diastolic dysfunction. The reason behind this might be due to the fact that the analyses of the LA volumes in both of the aforementioned studies were conducted with conventional 2D methods, which are known to be less precise then CMR imaging or 3D echo [12]. Furthermore, in the study of Prioli et al., left atrial volume and function were estimated based on 2D-measured ventricular filling volumes and mitral flow patterns.

Similar results to those of Teo and Prioli were demonstrated in a study of Murata et al., who were able to show in cases of impaired relaxation, an initial increase in active LA emptying followed by a decrease of active LA emptying in the stages of pseudonormalisation and restriction (and vice versa regarding passive LA emptying) [25].

However, in studies assessing left atrial volumes 3-dimensionally, the software application tool (QLAB,

Philips Medical System, Andover, Massachusetts) used was originally designed for analysis of LV volumes. Therefore, the analysis of these studies might be less precise compared to the software we used and which was specifically designed for volumetric analysis of the left atrium [26].

Clinical implications of new LA parameters

Studies investigating the impact of left atrium as a prognostic marker concentrate mainly on maximum LA volume [6, 27, 28]. This parameter can be assessed easily with 2D-echocardiography, and therefore there is a large amount of data available.

However, newer studies suggest that other measures of left atrium dimensions and function (e.g. minimum LA volume or ejection fraction) have higher prognostic impact and a closer correlation to left ventricular diastolic function than maximum LA volume [5, 14, 22, 29]. Especially LA function has attracted scientific attention recently. Epidemiologically, left atrial function seems to play an important role as a risk factor in all-cause mortality. In particular, LA True-EF seems to be superior to LAVI with respect to cardiovascular death but also all-cause mortality even after adjustment for traditional cardiovascular risk factors and LV parameters [29].

Therefore, future studies investigating the impact of left atrial volumes and function should focus on novel and easily accessible LA markers such as total left atrial function and active left atrial emptying. These markers can be determined validly with the new method including the software used in the current study and correlate well with conventional markers of diastolic function.

Limitations and strengths

It can certainly be argued that our study included a relatively small number of participants and data should be validated by larger patient cohorts. However, the sample was heterogeneous (both randomly selected healthy subjects referred to the out-patient clinic and seriously ill patients consulted in by cardiologists in a University Hospital were included) and therefore representative. Therefore, the findings of our study can be generalized.

Secondly, we did not perform direct measurements of LV end-diastolic pressure because this requires invasive procedures. However, we used Doppler-derived E/e' ratio as a surrogate parameter of LV end-diastolic pressure. This method is routinely used in clinical settings and studies and has been clinically validated [30, 31]. Additionally, we refrained from strain or speckle LA analyses, which are parameters investigated in the context of diastolic function most recently [32, 33]. However, these investigations would go beyond the scope of the current paper and might reduce the clarity. Therefore, this might be a topic of future analyses.

Furthermore, recording of the total duration of the diastole was not possible due to the modality of acquisition which required a record of seven subsamples to attain a sufficient resolution. Therefore, LAV_{min} could not be measured with complete assuredness. However, there are two studies demonstrating that the measurement of minimum LA volume assessed by the new software correlated excellently with the gold standard measurements (cardiac magnetic resonance imaging and computed tomography) [11, 12]. Especially in the study of Mor-Avi et al. cMRI and 3D-echocardiography showed identical results regarding LAV_{min} (bias: 0 ml, $r = 0.88$) [12]. In the study of Rohner et al., LA_{min} measured by RT3DE was even lower than measured by CT [11]. Therefore, we are confident that the data for LA_{min} measured with RT3DE are valid. Furthermore, this limitation would be relevant for both the NDF and DDF groups, leaving the results based on group differences unbiased in this aspect. Nevertheless, future studies should examine whether a significant difference between the left atrial volumes analyzed in loops covering the whole diastole also exists.

However, there are several strengths of the current study. First of all, state-of-the-art techniques (e.g. 3D-echocardiography and tissue Doppler imaging) were used. The 3-dimensional examination procedure of left cardiac dimensions and function has been demonstrated to be superior to 2-dimensional investigations [12, 21].

Another strength of our study is the use of a novel, yet validated software tool which was specifically designed for detailed assessment of both left atrial volumes and dimensions. This software allows sophisticated analyses of both passive and active emptying of the left atrium, which allowed for the new results of the present study.

Lastly, our study was conducted with a multi-centre setting and therefore has greater general applicability than single-centre studies.

Conclusion

Diastolic dysfunction causes a reduction in active left atrial emptying which is more strongly associated to left ventricular filling pressure than maximum or minimum left atrial volume.

Acknowledgments
The investigational software package used in this study was provided free of charge by TomTec Imaging Systems, Unterschleissheim, Germany.

Funding sources
No funding was received for this study.

Authors' contributions
The study was primarily designed by JSche. JSche, MH and PJ represent the principal investigators. All other authors contributed to the design of the study and supervised the trial. Data acquisition was conducted by JSche, PJ, GE, FG and JSchn. The statistical analysis plan and statistical analysis of the data were made by TS, JSche and LP. The first author (JSche) wrote the first draft of the manuscript, which was next revised in detail by MH. Subsequent drafts were prepared by all authors. JSche has the primary responsibility for the final content of the manuscript. All authors read and approved the final manuscript.

Competing interests
There are neither financial relationship with the organization that sponsored the research nor any other financial interests. The authors had full control of all primary data and they agree to allow the journal to review their data if requested.

Disclosures
None.

Author details
[1]Department of Prevention and Sports Medicine, Klinikum rechts der Isar, Technische Universitaet Muenchen, Georg-Brauchle-Ring 56, D-80992 Munich, Germany. [2]Medizinische Klinik und Poliklinik I, Klinikum der Universität München, Munich, Germany. [3]Department for Medical Statistics and Epidemiology, Klinikum rechts der Isar, Technische Universitaet Muenchen, Munich, Germany. [4]Heart Center "Alter Hof", Munich, Germany. [5]Universitäts Herz-Zentrum Freiburg - Bad Krozingen, Klinik für Kardiologie und Angiologie II, Bad Krozingen, Germany. [6]Munich Heart Alliance, Munich, Germany.

References
1. Liao L, Anstrom KJ, Gottdiener JS, Pappas PA, Whellan DJ, Kitzman DW, Aurigemma GP, Mark DB, Schulman KA, Jollis JG. Long-term costs and resource use in elderly participants with congestive heart failure in the Cardiovascular Health Study. Am Heart J. 2007;153(2):245–52.
2. Paulus WJ, Tschope C, Sanderson JE, Rusconi C, Flachskampf FA, Rademakers FE, Marino P, Smiseth OA, De KG, Leite-Moreira AF, Borbely A, Edes I, Handoko ML, Heymans S, Pezzali N, Pieske B, Dickstein K, Fraser AG, Brutsaert DL. How to diagnose diastolic heart failure: a consensus statement on the diagnosis of heart failure with normal left ventricular ejection fraction by the Heart Failure and Echocardiography Associations of the European Society of Cardiology. Eur Heart J. 2007;28(20):2539–50.
3. Nagueh SF, Appleton CP, Gillebert TC, Marino PN, Oh JK, Smiseth OA, Waggoner AD, Flachskampf FA, Pellikka PA, Evangelista A. Recommendations for the evaluation of left ventricular diastolic function by echocardiography. J Am Soc Echocardiogr. 2009;22(2):107–33.
4. Tsang TS, Barnes ME, Gersh BJ, Bailey KR, Seward JB. Left atrial volume as a morphophysiologic expression of left ventricular diastolic dysfunction and relation to cardiovascular risk burden. Am J Cardiol. 2002;90(12):1284–9.
5. Welles CC, Ku IA, Kwan DM, Whooley MA, Schiller NB, Turakhia MP. Left atrial function predicts heart failure hospitalization in subjects with preserved ejection fraction and coronary heart disease longitudinal data from the heart and soul study. J Am Coll Cardiol. 2012;59(7):673–80.
6. Abhayaratna WP, Seward JB, Appleton CP, Douglas PS, Oh JK, Tajik AJ, Tsang TS. Left atrial size: physiologic determinants and clinical applications. J Am Coll Cardiol. 2006;47(12):2357–63.
7. Prioli A, Marino P, Lanzoni L, Zardini P. Increasing degrees of left ventricular filling impairment modulate left atrial function in humans. Am J Cardiol. 1998;82(6):756–61.
8. Suh IW, Song JM, Lee EY, Kang SH, Kim MJ, Kim JJ, Kang DH, Song JK. Left atrial volume measured by real-time 3-dimensional echocardiography predicts clinical outcomes in patients with severe left ventricular dysfunction and in sinus rhythm. J Am Soc Echocardiogr. 2008;21(5):439–45.
9. Lang RM, Bierig M, Devereux RB, Flachskampf FA, Foster E, Pellikka PA, Picard MH, Roman MJ, Seward J, Shanewise JS, Solomon SD, Spencer KT, Sutton MS, Stewart WJ. Recommendations for chamber quantification: a report from the American Society of Echocardiography's Guidelines and Standards Committee and the Chamber Quantification Writing Group, developed in conjunction with the European Association of Echocardiography, a branch of the European Society of Cardiology. J Am Soc Echocardiogr. 2005;18(12):1440–63.
10. Artang R, Migrino RQ, Harmann L, Bowers M, Woods TD. Left atrial volume measurement with automated border detection by 3-dimensional echocardiography: comparison with Magnetic Resonance Imaging. Cardiovasc Ultrasound. 2009;7:16.

11. Rohner A, Brinkert M, Kawel N, Buechel RR, Leibundgut G, Grize L, Kuhne M, Bremerich J, Kaufmann BA, Zellweger MJ, Buser P, Osswald S, Handke M. Functional assessment of the left atrium by real-time three-dimensional echocardiography using a novel dedicated analysis tool: initial validation studies in comparison with computed tomography. Eur J Echocardiogr. 2011;12(7):497–505.

12. Mor-Avi V, Yodwut C, Jenkins C, Kuhl H, Nesser HJ, Marwick TH, Franke A, Weinert L, Niel J, Steringer-Mascherbauer R, Freed BH, Sugeng L, Lang RM. Real-time 3D echocardiographic quantification of left atrial volume: multicenter study for validation with CMR. JACC Cardiovasc Imaging. 2012; 5(8):769–77.

13. Shimada YJ, Shiota T. A meta-analysis and investigation for the source of bias of left ventricular volumes and function by three-dimensional echocardiography in comparison with magnetic resonance imaging. Am J Cardiol. 2011;107(1):126–38.

14. Kaminski M, Steel K, Jerosch-Herold M, Khin M, Tsang S, Hauser T, Kwong RY. Strong cardiovascular prognostic implication of quantitative left atrial contractile function assessed by cardiac magnetic resonance imaging in patients with chronic hypertension. J Cardiovasc Magn Reson. 2011;13:42.

15. Nagueh SF, Smiseth OA, Appleton CP, Byrd 3rd BF, Dokainish H, Edvardsen T, Flachskampf FA, Gillebert TC, Klein AL, Lancellotti P, Marino P, Oh JK, Popescu BA, Waggoner AD. Recommendations for the evaluation of left ventricular diastolic function by echocardiography: an update from the American Society of Echocardiography and the European Association of Cardiovascular Imaging. J Am Soc Echocardiogr. 2016;29(4):277–314. doi:10.1016/j.echo.2016.01.011.

16. Chobanian AV, Bakris GL, Black HR, Cushman WC, Green LA, Izzo Jr JL, Jones DW, Materson BJ, Oparil S, Wright Jr JT, Roccella EJ. Seventh report of the Joint National Committee on Prevention, Detection, Evaluation, and Treatment of High Blood Pressure. Hypertension. 2003;42(6):1206–52.

17. Lang RM, Badano LP, Tsang W, Adams DH, Agricola E, Buck T, Faletra FF, Franke A, Hung J, de Isla LP, Kamp O, Kasprzak JD, Lancellotti P, Marwick TH, McCulloch ML, Monaghan MJ, Nihoyannopoulos P, Pandian NG, Pellikka PA, Pepi M, Roberson DA, Shernan SK, Shirali GS, Sugeng L, Ten Cate FJ, Vannan MA, Zamorano JL, Zoghbi WA. EAE/ASE recommendations for image acquisition and display using three-dimensional echocardiography. J Am Soc Echocardiogr. 2012;25(1):3–46.

18. Wang Y, Moss J, Thisted R. Predictors of body surface area. J Clin Anesth. 1992;4(1):4–10.

19. Chahal NS, Lim TK, Jain P, Chambers JC, Kooner JS, Senior R. Normative reference values for the tissue Doppler imaging parameters of left ventricular function: a population-based study. Eur J Echocardiogr. 2010;11(1):51–6.

20. Khouri SJ, Maly GT, Suh DD, Walsh TE. A practical approach to the echocardiographic evaluation of diastolic function. J Am Soc Echocardiogr. 2004;17(3):290–7.

21. Soliman OI, Kirschbaum SW, van Dalen BM, van der Zwaan HB, Mahdavian DB, Vletter WB, van Geuns RJ, Ten Cate FJ, Geleijnse ML. Accuracy and reproducibility of quantitation of left ventricular function by real-time three-dimensional echocardiography versus cardiac magnetic resonance. Am J Cardiol. 2008;102(6):778–83.

22. Russo C, Jin Z, Homma S, Rundek T, Elkind MS, Sacco RL, Di Tullio MR. Left atrial minimum volume and reservoir function as correlates of left ventricular diastolic function: impact of left ventricular systolic function. Heart. 2012;98(10):813–20.

23. Nappo R, Degiovanni A, Bolzani V, Sartori C, Di Giovine G, Cerini P, Fossaceca R, Kovacs SJ, Marino PN. Quantitative assessment of atrial conduit function: a new index of diastolic dysfunction. Clin Res Cardiol. 2016;105(1): 17–28. doi:10.1007/s00392-015-0882-8.

24. Teo SG, Yang H, Chai P, Yeo TC. Impact of left ventricular diastolic dysfunction on left atrial volume and function: a volumetric analysis. Eur J Echocardiogr. 2010;11(1):38–43. doi:10.1093/ejechocard/jep153.

25. Murata M, Iwanaga S, Tamura Y, Kondo M, Kouyama K, Murata M, Ogawa S. A real-time three-dimensional echocardiographic quantitative analysis of left atrial function in left ventricular diastolic dysfunction. Am J Cardiol. 2008; 102(8):1097–102.

26. Hoit BD. Assessment of echocardiographic left atrial size: how accurate do we need to be? JACC Cardiovasc Imaging. 2012;5(8):778–80.

27. Zile MR, Gottdiener JS, Hetzel SJ, McMurray JJ, Komajda M, McKelvie R, Baicu CF, Massie BM, Carson PE. Prevalence and significance of alterations in cardiac structure and function in patients with heart failure and a preserved ejection fraction. Circulation. 2011;124(23):2491–501.

28. Pritchett AM, Mahoney DW, Jacobsen SJ, Rodeheffer RJ, Karon BL, Redfield MM. Diastolic dysfunction and left atrial volume: a population-based study. J Am Coll Cardiol. 2005;45(1):87–92.

29. Gupta S, Matulevicius SA, Ayers CR, Berry JD, Patel PC, Markham DW, Levine BD, Chin KM, de Lemos JA, Peshock RM, Drazner MH. Left atrial structure and function and clinical outcomes in the general population. Eur Heart J. 2013;34(4):278–85. doi:10.1093/eurheartj/ehs188.

30. Nagueh SF, Middleton KJ, Kopelen HA, Zoghbi WA, Quinones MA. Doppler tissue imaging: a noninvasive technique for evaluation of left ventricular relaxation and estimation of filling pressures. J Am Coll Cardiol. 1997;30(6): 1527–33.

31. Garcia MJ, Ares MA, Asher C, Rodriguez L, Vandervoort P, Thomas JD. An index of early left ventricular filling that combined with pulsed Doppler peak E velocity may estimate capillary wedge pressure. J Am Coll Cardiol. 1997;29(2):448–54.

32. Freed BH, Daruwalla V, Cheng JY, Aguilar FG, Beussink L, Choi A, Klein DA, Dixon D, Baldridge A, Rasmussen-Torvik LJ, Maganti K, Shah SJ. Prognostic utility and clinical significance of cardiac mechanics in heart failure with preserved ejection fraction: importance of left atrial strain. Circ Cardiovasc Imaging. 2016;9(3). doi:10.1161/CIRCIMAGING.115.003754

33. Hoit BD. Left atrial size and function: role in prognosis. J Am Coll Cardiol. 2014;63(6):493–505. doi:10.1016/j.jacc.2013.10.055.

7

Preoperative single ventricle function determines early outcome after second-stage palliation of single ventricle heart

Jacek Pająk[1*] (iD), Michał Buczyński[1], Piotr Stanek[2], Grzegorz Zalewski[2], Marek Wites[2], Lesław Szydłowski[3], Bogusław Mazurek[3] and Lidia Tomkiewicz-Pająk[4]

Abstract

Background: Second-stage palliation with hemi-Fontan or bidirectional Glenn procedures has improved the outcomes of patients treated for single-ventricle heart disease. The aim of this study was to retrospectively analyze risk factors for death after second-stage palliation of single-ventricle heart and to compare therapeutic results achieved with the hemi-Fontan and bidirectional Glenn procedures.

Material and methods: We analyzed 60 patients who had undergone second-stage palliation for single-ventricle heart. Group HF consisted of 23 (38.3%) children who had been operated with the hemi-Fontan method; Group BDG consisted of 37 (61.7%) who had been operated with the bidirectional Glenn method. The analysis focused on 30-day postoperative mortality rates, clinical and echocardiographic data, and early complications.

Results: The patients' ages at the time of repair was 33 ± 11.2 weeks; weight was 6.7 ± 1.2 kg. The most common anatomic subtype was hypoplastic left heart syndrome, in 36 (60%) patients. The early mortality rate was 13.3%. Significant preoperative atrioventricular valve regurgitation, single-ventricle heart dysfunction, pneumonia/sepsis, and arrhythmias were associated with higher mortality rates after second-stage palliation. Multivariate analysis identified significant preoperative single-ventricle heart dysfunction as an independent predictor of early death after second-stage palliation. No differences were found in the analyzed variables after bidirectional Glenn compared with hemi-Fontan procedures.

Conclusion: Significant preoperative atrioventricular valve regurgitation, arrhythmias and pneumonia/sepsis are closely correlated with mortality in patients with single-ventricle heart after second-stage palliation. Preoperative significant single-ventricle heart dysfunction is an independent mortality predictor in this group of patients. There are no differences in clinical, echocardiographic data, or outcomes in patients treated with the hemi-Fontan compared with bidirectional Glenn procedures.

Keywords: Second-stage single-ventricle palliation, Single-ventricle heart, Hemi-Fontan, bidirectional Glenn procedure, Hypoplastic left heart syndrome, Extracellular matrix, CorMatrix

* Correspondence: jacekpajak@poczta.onet.pl
[1]Pediatric Heart Surgery and General Pediatric Surgery Department, Medical University of Warsaw, ul. Żwirki i Wigury 63A, 02-091 Warszawa, Poland
Full list of author information is available at the end of the article

Background

Second-stage palliation, using the hemi-Fontan or bidirectional Glenn procedures in the surgical treatment of single-ventricle heart has reduced the complication rate and improved outcomes after the final stage, i.e. the Fontan operation. Anatomically, second-stage palliation for single-ventricle heart represents one-half of systemic venous-to-pulmonary arterial anastomosis, while hemodynamically it leads to normalization of the volume load of the single ventricle [1–3]. Such an intermittent stage promotes better tolerance and gradual transition to the hemodynamic model after the Fontan operation. Second-stage palliation of single-ventricle heart performed with the hemi-Fontan method consists of anastomosing the superior vena cava (SVC) with the pulmonary arteries close to the SVC insertion to the right atrium, while the SVC insertion is separated from the right atrial cavity by means of a transverse patch sutured to the right atrial walls. Such a location of the incision line, anastomosis and patch suturing lines, and future scar formation in this region, pose a risk of damaging the sinus node and/or impulse conduction pathways from the sinus node. These issues may lead to arrhythmias, a severe complication, given the post-Fontan operation circulation physiology [4]. Performing hemi-Fontan as second-stage palliation necessitates performing the Fontan operation, using the "lateral tunnel" technique, which consists of suturing a patch inside the right atrium that directs flow from the vena cava to the pulmonary arteries. Thus, hemi-Fontan does not allow for a selection of the Fontan operation technique to match the anatomy of a defect [5].

In 2011, we decided to switch our second-stage palliation surgical technique from the hemi-Fontan to the bidirectional Glenn. In bidirectional Glenn, the SVC is anastomosed with the pulmonary arteries at a distance from the sinus node region and conduction pathways, an arrangement that would seem to decrease the risk of arrhythmias developing. However, no reports have been published that unambiguously favor either of the methods. Hence, we are our attempting to evaluate hemi-Fontan and bidirectional Glenn based on our clinical outcomes. Both in the hemi-Fontan and bidirectional Glenn technique, achieving a wide anastomosis between the SVC and the pulmonary arteries may require using a biological or artificial patch to enlarge the anastomosed site. Since the beginning of 2013, we have placed an extracellular matrix (ECM) patch, derived from porcine small intestinal submucosa [6, 7], in all children with single-ventricle heart operated for enlargement of pulmonary artery anastomoses.

The aim of the present study was to retrospectively analyze risk factors of mortality after second-stage palliation of single-ventricle heart, and to compare the therapeutic results achieved with hemi-Fontan and bidirectional Glenn procedures.

Methods

We conducted a retrospective review of all the patients who had undergone second-stage palliation for single-ventricle heart in the Pediatric Heart Surgery Department (University School of Medicine in Katowice, Poland) between 2003 and 2015. The study protocol was approved by the local ethics committee. Depending on the method of surgical treatment, the patients were assigned to one of two groups. Group HF consisted of 23 (38.3%) children, in whom second-stage palliation had been performed using the hemi-Fontan method in the years 2003–2011. Group BDG consisted of 37 (61.7%) children who had been treated in the years 2011–2015, with the bidirectional Glenn procedure. In this group, 15 (40.5%) patients had a direct end-to-side anastomosis made between the SVC and the right pulmonary artery, while the remaining 22 (59.5%) patients had the SVC and right pulmonary artery anastomosis extended by use of an ECM patch (CorMatrix®; Cardiovascular, Inc., Roswell GA, USA).

Patient demographics, clinical characteristics, imaging, operative reports, hospital records, and clinical reports were collected, and a retrospective analysis of the data was performed.

In all the patients, anatomical details were determined, and the children were deemed qualified for surgical treatment based on echocardiographic findings. Echocardiograms were interpreted by two readers, who assessed the single-ventricle morphology and function and atrioventricular valve function. The single-ventricle function was assessed semi-quantitatively according to the following scale: 1, good; 2, fair; 3, decreased, and 4, poor [8, 9]. Significant impairment of the single-ventricle heart function was defined as a score of more than fair. Semi-quantitative assessment was also used in evaluating valvular competence, the scale being 0, none; 1, mild; 2, moderate; 3, severe [8–10]. Significant regurgitation was defined as a score more than mild. The examinations were performed before operation and on day 2 postoperatively.

The analyses performed in the two groups included postoperative 30-day mortality rates and these variables: anatomy of the defect; age; body mass; aortic clamp time; oxygen arterial blood saturation (Sat O_2) on day 1, 3 and 5 postoperatively; pneumonia or sepsis; atrioventricular valve regurgitation (AVVR); single-ventricle function; arrhythmias; intubation time; duration of hospitalization; and relations between these variables and their effect on the outcomes.

The diagnosis of a clinically significant arrhythmia in the perioperative period was based on the Cardiosurgical Postoperative Intensive Care Unit monitoring system and a review of all available electrocardiograms. "Arrhythmia" was defined as a rhythm requiring treatment with an antiarrhythmic medication or pacing, or led to cardiopulmonary resuscitation.

Statistical methods

To assess differences between the groups in qualitative data, we employed the chi-square test or the Fisher's exact test, whereas quantitative data were evaluated with the t-Student test or Mann-Whitney test. Correlation of quantitative data was analyzed by the Spearman's correlation coefficient (r_s); for qualitative data, we employed the chi-square or the Fisher's exact test. The stepwise logistic regression was used to determine factors affecting postoperative mortality rates.

Surgical technique

In all patients in both groups, the procedure was performed through a median sternotomy. The ascending aorta was cannulated. In 10 (27.0%) patients in Group BDG, two venous cannulas were inserted, one into the right atrium and another high in the SVC. In these patients, a direct SVC-right pulmonary artery anastomosis was performed with the patient in moderate hypothermia (approximately 32° C). In the remaining children from both groups, a single venous cannula was inserted into the right atrium, and the procedure was performed in deep hypothermia (approximately 18° C) with low flow (cardiac output approx. 50 ml/kg) or with cardiac arrest; crystalline cardioplegia was administered.

In Group HF, all children had a hemi-Fontan anastomosis constructed between the SVC and the pulmonary arteries, and an oval polytetrafluoroethylene patch was sutured below the SVC outlet to the right atrium, which separated the SVC outlet from the remaining RA. The anterior part of the SVC-PAs anastomosis was enlarged by use of a homogenous pulmonary artery patch.

In Group BDG, 5 (13.5%) children had a direct bidirectional Glenn anastomosis performed in deep hypothermia with low flow. The remaining 22 patients (59.5%) had a modified Norwood I procedure (aortic arch ECM patch reconstruction and bilateral pulmonary artery banding), in which the pulmonary arteries were dissected from the main pulmonary artery trunk, the stumps were proximally closed with sutures, and the junction between the pulmonary arteries and SVC was reconstructed with an ECM (CorMatrix®) tube larger in diameter than the pulmonary artery diameter (Fig. 1). No patient had a surgical correction because of insufficient tricuspid valve.

Postoperatively, all the patients were hospitalized in the Cardiosurgical Postoperative Intensive Care Unit. All patients received heparin in the early postoperative period, then antiplatelet medication until the Fontan operation was performed.

Results

Patients characteristics are reported in Tables 1 and 2. All children with HLHS operated on in the years

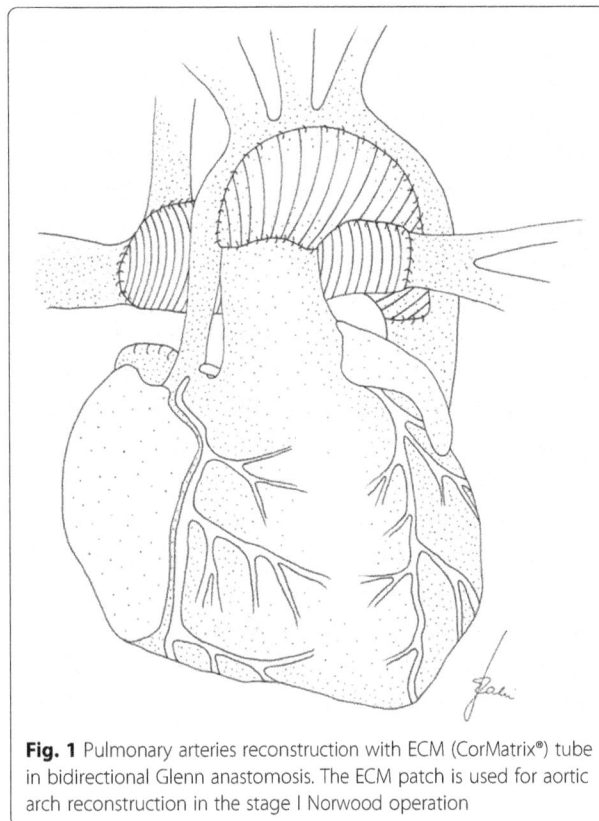

Fig. 1 Pulmonary arteries reconstruction with ECM (CorMatrix®) tube in bidirectional Glenn anastomosis. The ECM patch is used for aortic arch reconstruction in the stage I Norwood operation

2003–2013 received the Norwood I procedure as modified by Sano et al. [11] as the first-stage operation (part of Group HF). Since 2013, we have routinely used our modification of the Norwood procedure in the first-stage of HLHS treatment; the modification consists of reconstructing the aortic arch with an ECM patch and in bilateral pulmonary arteries banding (part of Group BDG). Patients with diagnoses other than HLHS had made earlier main pulmonary artery banding or systemic – pulmonary anastomosis as a first stage operation or they required no operation.

Table 1 illustrates that Group BDG patients were significantly older than Group HF patients at the time of operation [36 weeks (range 19–72) vs. 28 weeks (range 10–42); p = 0.03]. Otherwise, no significant differences were noted in body mass, intubation time, aortic clamp time, arterial blood saturation, duration of hospitalization, arrhythmias, pneumonia/sepsis, mortality rate, AVVR, or systemic ventricular function.

Risk factors and mortality (Table 2)
Postoperative arrhythmias

Postoperative arrhythmias were recorded in 9 of the 60 (15%) children, 5 (22%) in Group HF; 3 (13.0%) of these children had slow sinus rhythm, and 2 (9%) had sinus bradycardia. Among the 4 (11%) in Group BDG, 1 (3%)

Table 1 Comparison of patients with single-ventricle heart operated on with the hemi-Fontan (Group HF) or bidirectional Glenn (Group BDG) procedure

		Group HF (n = 23) m (min-max, %)	Group BDG (n = 37) m (min/max, %)	p value
Age 33 ± 11.2 (weeks)		28 (10–42)	36 (19–72)	0.03
Body mass 6.7 ± 1.2 (kg)		6 (4–9)	7 (4–10)	0.19
Mechanical ventilation (days)		4 (2–25)	4 (1–20)	0.46
Type of single-ventricle	HLHS	13 (56.5%)	23 (62,2%)	0,66
	TA	2 (8,7%)	4 (10,8%)	0,99
	Unbalanced A-V canal	2 (8,7%)	3 (8,1%)	0,99
	DILV	1 (4,3%)	3 (8,1%)	0,99
	Other	5 (21,7%)	4 (10,8%)	0,28
Aortic clamping time (min)		39 (27–58)	39 (21–61)	0.62
Mechanical ventilation (days)		4 (2–25)	4 (1–20)	0.46
SatO$_2$ (%) - 1 postoperative day		75 (40–86)	77 (61–92)	0.96
SatO$_2$ (%) - 3 postoperative day		78 (63–85)	80 (65–92)	0.64
SatO$_2$ (%) - 5 postoperative day		78 (70–87)	81 (60–91)	0.642
Length of stay (days)		11 (5–19)	10 (7–18)	0.42

M median, *SatO2* oxygen arterial blood saturation, *HLHS* hypoplastic left heart syndrome, *TA* tricuspid atresia, *DILV* double inlet left ventricle

had slow sinus rhythm, 1 (3%) had sinus bradycardia, and 2 (5%) had tachyarrhytmias with a moderate reaction to pharmacotherapy.

Pneumonia/sepsis

Pneumonia/sepsis developed in 9 of the 60 children (15.0%), 5 of 23 (22%) in Group HF and 4 of 37 (11%) in Group BDG, a statistically insignificant difference. The children who developed postoperative pneumonia/sepsis

Table 2 Echocardiographic data, complication and outcome in patients with SV operated on employing the hemi-Fontan and bidirectional Glenn procedures

	Group HF (n = 23) n (%)	Group BDG (n = 37) n (%)	Total (n = 60) n (%)	p value
Postoperative Arrhythmias	5 (22)	4 (11)	9 (15.0)	0.28
Postoperative Sepsis	2 (9)	4 (11)	6 (10)	0.99
Preoperative AVVR (0 + 1)	18 (78)	30 (81)	48 (80)	0.89
Preoperative AVVR (2 + 3)	5 (22)	7 (19)	12 (20)	
Postoperative AVVR (0 + 1)	20 (87)	33 (89)	53 (88)	0.79
Postoperative AVVR (2 + 3)	3 (13)	4 (11)	7 (12)	
Preoperative SV function (1 + 2)	19 (83)	31 (84)	50 (83)	0.99
Preoperative SV function (3 + 4)	4 (17)	6 (16)	10 (17)	
Postoperative SV function (1 + 2)	20 (87)	33 (89)	53 (88)	0.99
Postoperative SV function (3 + 4)	3 (13)	4 (11)	7 (12)	
Death	4 (17,4)	4 (10,8)	8 (13,3)	0,464

AVVR atrioventricular valve regurgitation, *SV* single ventricle

were intubated significantly longer than those who did not develop postoperative pneumonia/sepsis, both in Group HF ($p = 0.025$) and in Group BDG ($p = 0.009$).

Pre-and postoperative A-V valve regurgitation and single-ventricle heart function

Significant preoperative AVVR (Grade 2 or 3) was present in 12 (20%) of the 60 investigated patients, and postoperative AVVR was present in 7 (12%).

In Group HF, significant preoperative AVVR was present in 5 of 23 (22%) patients, of whom 4 (80%) had significant single-ventricle dysfunction. AVVR developed in 3 (13%) children with HLHS and 2 (8%) patients with unbalanced atrioventricular septal defect (UAVSD). Two (9%) children with HLHS had postoperative improvement of atrioventricular valve function, whereas 3 (13%) with this defect had no improvement (and died) - 2 (9%) of them developed arrhythmias, and 1 (4%) had fatal pneumonia/sepsis.

In Group BDG, 7 of 37 (19%) children had significant AVVR, shown in preoperative echocardiography; 5 (14%) had HLHS and 2 (5%) had UAVSD. Six (86%) patients with significant AVVR also had significant single-ventricle dysfunction. After bidirectional Glenn, echocardiography in 3 (8%) patients with HLHS revealed improvement in tricuspid valve competence, whereas no improvement was seen in the other 4 (11%); 2 (5%) of these patients developed arrhythmias, and 2 (5%) developed pneumonia/sepsis; these four children died.

The rates of postoperative single-ventricle heart function of grades 1–2 and 3–4 were similar in the two groups.

Mortality

Four of 23 (17.4%) children in Group HF died. Three (75%) had significant atrioventricular valve regurgitation before and after operation. Postoperatively, 2 of the patients (50%) developed arrhythmias – sinus bradycardia in 1 (25%) and slow sinus heart rhythm in the other (25%). None of the deceased children presented with tachyarrhythmia. One (25%) deceased child, with significant atrioventricular valve regurgitation, developed sepsis. In 1 (25%) child, sinus bradycardia occurred, and the patient died due to low cardiac output despite effective atrial pacing. The deceased patients in Group HF had significantly more frequent arrhythmias (75% vs. 11%; p = 0.02) and AVVR (75% vs. 11%; p = 0.02) than did the survivors.

Four for 37 (10.8%) children from Group BDG died. All had significant atrioventricular valve regurgitation. Two (50%) of the children also developed supraventricular tachyarrhythmia, and 2 (50%) had pneumonia/sepsis. The deceased patients In Group BDG had significantly more frequent arrhythmias (50% vs. 6%; p = 0.05), more frequent significant AVVR (100% vs. 9%; p < 0.001) and more frequent pneumonia/sepsis (50% vs. 6%; p = 0.05) than did the survivors.

Univariate and multivariate analysis of risk factors and death

Univariate analysis was performed to identify risk factors for death by patient characteristics and clinical and echocardiographic data (Table 3). Preoperative single-ventricle heart dysfunction (grade 3–4; significant impairment); preoperative clinically significant AVVR (grade 2–3; worse than mild); arrhythmias; and sepsis were associated with death. Multivariate analysis then was performed, with logistic regression in a model that took statistically significant preoperative variables from the univariate analysis. In the multivariate analysis, significant preoperative single-ventricle heart dysfunction was the only independent prognostic risk factor for

death in second-stage palliation of single-ventricle heart anatomy (odds ratio 4.7; p < 0.001) (Fig. 2).

Discussion

Our study showed that clinically significant preoperative AVVR, preoperative single-ventricle dysfunction, pneumonia/sepsis, and arrhythmias were associated with increased mortality in patients with single-ventricle heart disease who underwent second-stage palliation. Only significant preoperative single-ventricle dysfunction was an independent prognostic risk factor. We did not find significant differences in clinical data, echocardiographic findings, or outcomes of patients treated with the hemi-Fontan compared with the bi-directional Glenn technique.

The mortality rate in our patients was higher than rates reported by centers treating larger numbers of patients [10]. This difference might be due to greater patient complexity in our population, as we aggressively accept high-risk patients. In recent years, the mortality rate in our patients from Group BDG has decreased compared with the rate in Group HF, even though Group BDG included older children with more complex defects than did Group I. A high percentage of our patients (20%) had significant AVVR, which has been reported to have a high perioperative risk [10, 12]. We emphasize that, except for one patient with complex heterotaxy syndrome, all children in our study who died had significant AVVR preoperatively; the significant AVVR persisted after operation, and the children also developed arrhythmias and/or pneumonia/sepsis.

Significant AVVR in our patients was due to dysfunction of the very valve and/or dysfunction of the single-ventricle. Disturbances of the structure/competence of the valve are most commonly associated with the anatomical background of the single ventricle heart and usually appear as unbalanced forms of common atrioventricular canal, as well as in heterotaxy syndrome. A study [10] has shown that even in the absence of associated defects and physiologic derangements, UAVSD confers risk on patients with single-ventricle heart. Mortality rates in these patients are high, regardless of whether valvuloplasty is performed in parallel with the second-stage palliation of single-ventricle heart [13]. In view of problems inherent in A-V valvuloplasty and the unimpressive results, we have not attempted this procedure. In cases of AVVR combined with ventricular dysfunction, we tried to perform stage II palliation at an earlier age (about 4 months of life), so the volume load of the single-ventricle could normalize earlier [1, 3]; with earlier operation, AVV competence was improved in children with HLHS but not in those with UAVSD, a result that is concordant with those of others [10].

Table 3 Univariate analysis of risk factors for second-stage palliation of single-ventricle heart

Variables		Survived		Deaths		Total		p value
		n	%	n	%	n	%	
Preoperative SV function (0 = 1 + 2,1 = 3 + 4)	0	49	94.2	1	12.5	50	83.3	<0.001
	1	3	5.8	7	87.5	10	16.7	
Preoperative AVVR (0 = 0 + 1,1 = 2 + 3)	0	31	59.6	1	12.5	32	53.3	0.020
	1	21	40.0	7	87.5	28	46.7	
Arrhythmias	0	48	92.3	3	37.5	51	85.0	0.001
	1	4	7.7	5	62.5	9	15.0	
Postoperative sepsis	0	49	94.2	5	62.5	54	90.0	0.027
	1	3	5.8	3	37.5	6	10.0	
Total		52	100	8	100	60	100	–

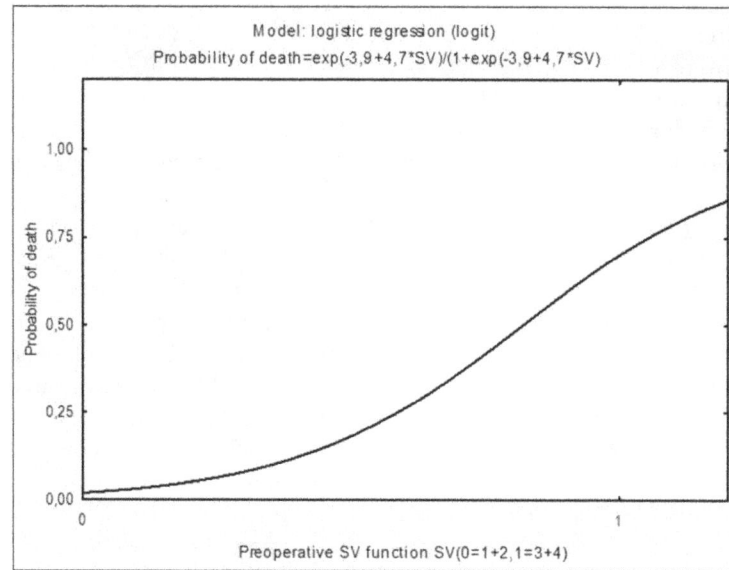

Fig. 2 Following the stepwise elimination of the least significant factor in each step, SV (single ventricle) dysfunction was found to significantly affect mortality rates ($p < 0.001$)

In this study, significant single-ventricle dysfunction was an independent prognostic risk factor in patients with single-ventricle heart after second-stage palliation. Dysfunction of the single ventricle determines the occurrence of other complications that increase the risk of death in the early postoperative period. Bharucha et al. [14] demonstrated that right ventricular mechanical dyssynchrony and inhomogeneous contraction were worse in patients with clinically important tricuspid regurgitation and HLHS. Ventricular dysfunction leads to atrioventricular regurgitation, which in time results in progressive circulatory insufficiency. Patients with this insufficiency are susceptible to infections and often are operated on after numerous infectious episodes, when they are colonized by pathological bacterial and fungal flora.

Changing the surgical technique from the hemi-Fontan to bidirectional Glenn procedure did not significantly affect the prevalence of postoperative arrhythmias in our cohort. Similarly, as in other reports [15, 16], sinus bradycardia and slow sinus rhythm were the predominant postoperative cardiac rhythm abnormalities after second-stage palliation of single-ventricle heart. In 2 patients, supraventricular tachyarrhythmia developed after the bidirectional Glenn procedure, a complication that we believe has not been described. In each case of second-stage single-ventricle palliation, interatrial communication was enlarged surgically. On the one hand, such management allows for achieving wide interatrial communication, whereas on the other, it poses a threat of damaging the impulse conduction pathways between the sinus node and the sinoatrial node. Love et al. [17]

showed that the atriotomy, right atrial free-wall scars, and atrial septal scars were predictors of tachyarrhythmias in patients after congenital heart diseases operations. Our patients with tachyarrhythmias had both atriotomy and atrioseptostomy, which we feel may have triggered arrhythmias.

For reconstruction of the pulmonary arteries and widening the SVC-pulmonary arteries anastomoses we have used an ECM (CorMatrix®) patch. This material has proven safe in reconstruction of low-pressure vessels. However, Hibino et al. [18] observed that at a mean follow-up of 9.7 months, 8 of 10 patients who underwent central pulmonary artery reconstruction with CorMatrix® tube had progressive significant stenosis. To avoid this complication, we used oversized anastomoses between the pulmonary arteries and the SVC.

There are limitations of this study. First, the number of the patients was small, although the study does have the advantage of uniform management in a single center. Second, the retrospective nature of the study could have introduced bias that affected comparisons between treatment groups. A prospective, randomized study of second-stage palliation (hemi-Fontan vs bidirectional Glenn procedure) of single-ventricle heart disease is needed. Third, in all patients, the ventricular function was evaluated semi-quantitatively. All patients were qualified to stage II on the base of echocardiographic examination; in some examinations it was impossible to visualize the size of all pulmonary arteries; thus, unfortunately, we could not include this important measurement in our analysis.

Conclusions

Significant preoperative atrioventricular valve regurgitation, arrhythmias and sepsis are closely correlated with mortality in patients with single-ventricle heart disease after second-stage surgical palliation. Preoperative significant single-ventricle dysfunction is an important problem that has not been overcome by staged repair and has the highest impact on the mortality rate after second-stage surgical palliation. The bidirectional Glenn technique in surgical treatment of single-ventricle heart does not have a lower the incidence of early complications than does the hemi-Fontan operation.

Abbreviations

AVVR: Atrioventricular valve regurgitation; DILV: Double inlet left ventricle; ECM: Extracellular matrix; HLHS: Hypoplastic left heart syndrome; SatO2: Oxygen arterial blood saturation; SVC: Superior vena cava; TA: Tricuspid atresia; UAVSD: Unbalanced atrioventricular septal defect

Acknowledgments

We thank to Dr. H. Stanuch for statistical analysis.

Funding

Not applicable.

Authors' contributions

JP contributed to study conception and design, acquisition of data, analysis and interpretation of data, drafting and critical revision of the manuscript. MB participated in the design of the study, collection of data, and drafting of the manuscript. PS participated in analysis and interpretation of data and drafting the manuscript. GZ participated in collection and interpretation of the data. MW contributed to study conception, design and to acquisition of data. LS contributed to study conception and design, critical revision for important intellectual content, and final approval of the version to be published. BM collected data, analyzed and interpreted data, and critically revised the manuscript. LT-P contributed to acquisition of data, analysis and interpretation of data, and critical revision of the manuscript. All authors read and approved the final manuscript.

Consent for publication

All authors read and approved the final manuscript.

Competing interests

The authors declare that they have no competing interests.

Author details

[1]Pediatric Heart Surgery and General Pediatric Surgery Department, Medical University of Warsaw, ul. Żwirki i Wigury 63A, 02-091 Warszawa, Poland. [2]Pediatric Heart Surgery Department, The Independent Public Clinical Hospital no. 6 of the Medical University of Silesia, Katowice, Poland. [3]Department of Pediatric Cardiology, Medical University of Silesia, Katowice, Poland. [4]Institute of Cardiology, Jagiellonian University, Medical College and John Paul II Hospital, Krakow, Poland.

References

1. Seliem MA, Baffa JM, Vetter JM, Chen SL, Chin AJ, Norwood WI Jr. Changes in right ventricular geometry and heart rate early after hemi-Fontan procedure. Ann Thorac Surg. 1993;55:1508–12.
2. Fogel MA, Weinberg PM, Chin AJ, Fellows KE, Hoffman EA. Late ventricular geometry and performance changes of functional single-ventricle throughout staged Fontan reconstruction assessed by magnetic resonance imaging. J Am Coll Cardiol. 1996;28:212–21.
3. Jacobs ML, Rychik J, Rome JJ, Apoustopoulou S, Pizarro C, Murphy ID, et al. Early reduction of the volume work of the single-ventricle: the hemi fontan operation. Ann Thorac Surg. 1996;62:456–62.
4. Deal BJ, Mavroudis C, Backer CL. Arrhythmia Management in the Fontan Patient. Pediatric Cardiology November. 2007;28:448–56.
5. Pekkan K, Dasi LP, de Zélicourt D, Sundareswaran KS, Fogel MA, Kanter KR, Yoganathan AP. Hemodynamic performance of stage-2 univentricular reconstruction: Glenn vs. hemi-Fontan templates. Ann Biomed Eng. 2009;37:50–63.
6. Scholl FG, Boucek MM, Chan KC, Valdes-Cruz L, Perryman R. Preliminary experience with cardiac reconstruction using decellularized porcine extracellular matrix scaffold: human applications in congenital heart disease. World J Pediatr Congenit Heart Surg. 2010;1:132–6.
7. Quarti A, Nardone S, Colaneri M, Santoro G, Pozzi M. Preliminary experience in the use of an extracellular matrix to repair congenital heart diseases. Interact Cardiovasc Thorac Surg. 2011;13:569–72.
8. Wong DJ, Iyengar AJ, Wheaton GR, Ramsay JM, Grigg LE, Horton S, Konstantinov IE, Brizard CP, d'Udekem Y. Long-term outcomes after atrioventricular valve operations in patients undergoing single-ventricle palliation. Ann Thorac Surg. 2012;94:606–13.
9. Tomkiewicz-Pająk L, Hoffman P, Trojnarska O, Bednarek J, Płazak W, Pająk JW, Olszowska M, Komar M, Podolec PS. Long-term follow-up in adult patients after Fontan operation. Polish Journal of Thoracic and Cardiovascular Surgery. 2013;10:357–63.
10. Lee TM, Aiyagari R, Hirsch JC, Ohye RG, Bove EL, Devaney EJ. Risk factor analysis for second-stage palliation of single-ventricle anatomy. Ann Thorac Surg. 2012;93:614–8.
11. Sano S, Ishino K, Kawada M, Arai S, Kasahara S, Asai T, Masuda Z, Takeuchi M, Ohtsuki S. Right ventricle-pulmonary artery shunt in first-stage palliation of hypoplastic left heart syndrome. J Thorac Cardiovasc Surg. 2003;126:504–9.
12. Scheurer MA, Hill EG, Vasuki N, Maurer S, Graham EM, Bandisode V, Shirali GS, Atz AM, Bradley SM. Survival after bidirectional cavopulmonary anastomosis: analysis of preoperative risk factors. J Thorac Cardiovasc Surg. 2007;134:82–9.
13. Owens GE, Gomez-Fifer C, Gelehrter S, Owens ST. Outcomes for patients with unbalanced atrioventricular septal defects. Pediatr Cardiol. 2009;30:431–5.
14. Bharucha T, Khan R, Mertens L, Friedberg MK. Right ventricular mechanical dyssynchrony and asymmetric contraction in hypoplastic heart syndrome are associated with tricuspid regurgitation. J Am Soc Echocardiogr. 2013;2610:1214–20.
15. Reichlin A, Prêtre R, Dave H, Hug MI, Gass M. Balmer C postoperative arrhythmia in patients with bidirectional cavopulmonary anastomosis. Eur J Cardiothorac Surg. 2014;45:620–4.
16. Trivedi B, Smith PB, Barker PC, Jaggers J, Lodge AJ, Kanter RJ. Arrhythmias in patients with hypoplastic left heart syndrome. Am Heart J. 2011;161:138–44.
17. Love BA, Collins KK, Walsh EP, Triedman JK. Electroanatomic characterization of conduction barriers in sinus/atrially paced rhythm and association with intra-atrial reentrant tachycardia circuits following congenital heart disease surgery. J Cardiovasc Electrophysiol. 2001;12:17–25.
18. Hibino N, McConnell P, Shinoka T, Malik M, Galantowicz M. Preliminary experience in the use of an extracellular matrix (CorMatrix) as a tube graft: word of caution. Semin Thorac Cardiovasc Surg. 2015;27:288–95.

8

Left ventricular outflow tract velocity time integral outperforms ejection fraction and Doppler-derived cardiac output for predicting outcomes in a select advanced heart failure cohort

Christina Tan, David Rubenson, Ajay Srivastava, Rajeev Mohan, Michael R. Smith, Kristen Billick, Samuel Bardarian and J. Thomas Heywood[*]

Abstract

Background: Left ventricular outflow tract velocity time integral (LVOT VTI) is a measure of cardiac systolic function and cardiac output. Heart failure patients with low cardiac output are known to have poor cardiovascular outcomes. Thus, extremely low LVOT VTI may predict heart failure patients at highest risk for mortality.

Methods: Patients with heart failure and extremely low LVOT VTI were identified from a single-center database. Baseline characteristics and heart failure related clinical outcomes (death, LVAD) were obtained at 12 months. Correlation between clinical endpoints and the following variables were analyzed: ejection fraction (EF), pulmonary artery systolic pressure (PASP), NYHA class, renal function, Doppler cardiac output (CO), and LVOT VTI.

Results: Study cohort consisted of 100 patients. At the 12-month follow up period, 30 events (28 deaths, 2 LVADs) were identified. Occurrence of death and LVAD implantation was statistically associated with a lower LVOT VTI ($p = 0.039$) but not EF ($p = 0.169$) or CO ($p = 0.217$). In multivariate analysis, LVOT VTI ($p = 0.003$) remained statistically significant, other significant variables were age ($p = 0.033$) and PASP ($p = 0.022$). Survival analysis by LVOT VTI tertile demonstrated an unadjusted hazard ratio of 4.755 (CI 1.576-14.348, $p = 0.006$) for combined LVAD and mortality at one year.

Conclusions: Extremely low LVOT VTI strongly predicts adverse outcomes and identifies patients who may benefit most from advanced heart failure therapies.

Keywords: Congestive heart failure, Velocity time integral, Time velocity integral, Echocardiography

Background

Congestive heart failure is persistently growing health care dilemma in the United States, resulting in more than 50,000 deaths annually and more than 2 million yearly hospitalizations [1, 2]. The clinical assessment of patients with heart failure has been shown to be a valuable tool in guiding therapy and predicting prognosis, with the presence or absence of congestion and hypoperfusion dividing heart failure patients into one of four

* Correspondence: Heywood.james@scrippshealth.org
Fellow, Scripps Clinic Cardiology, 10666 N. Torrey Pines Road, La Jolla, CA 92037, USA

hemodynamic profiles [3]. Patients with both congestion and low cardiac output have been shown to have more than twice the mortality and cardiac transplantation rates of those without hypoperfusion and congestion [3]. Thus, accurate and timely identification of high risk profiles is crucial. Due to the burden of disease, as more patients with heart failure are cared for by clinicians without expertise in advanced heart failure, an easily utilized screening tool for identifying such patients would be helpful to facilitate timely assessment for advanced therapies such as left ventricular assist device and cardiac transplantation [4].

Echocardiography has emerged as an invaluable tool in the diagnosis and management of congestive heart failure (CHF) and is routinely performed in patients with CHF [5]. Measurements of left and right ventricular dysfunction, presence of valvular disease, Doppler derived cardiac output, and estimates of intracardiac pressures are frequently obtained metrics [6]. Multiple studies have demonstrated a close correlation between cardiac output calculated by Doppler echocardiography and invasive thermodilution and Fick methods [7, 8]. Doppler derived cardiac output is typically obtained by measuring flow across the left ventricular outflow tract (LVOT) which is determined by the velocity time integral of the Doppler signal directed across the LVOT (LVOT velocity time integral or LVOT VTI), multiplied by the cross sectional area of the LVOT and heart rate. LVOT VTI has been shown to be a reproducible measurement even in the context of severe chronic heart failure [8, 9] and is superior to flow measured at other locations, including the right ventricle, pulmonary artery, mitral valve, and aortic arch [10] due to multiple factors: ability to obtain insonation parallel to blood flow and a relatively flat profile of blood velocity distribution [11].

Because estimation of the area of LVOT represents the major source of error in deriving cardiac output due to the elliptoid shape of the LVOT and squaring of the measured radius (πr^2) [12, 13], using LVOT VTI alone rather than Doppler derived cardiac output has been suggested as a reliable surrogate for cardiac output in the absence of left ventricular outflow tract abnormalities [9]. Prior studies have evaluated LVOT VTI in acute myocardial infarction, demonstrating 100% one-month survival for subjects with LVOT VTI greater than 100% predicted for age and greater than 80% survival at 5 years. In contrast, mortality rate at one month and five years were 18% and 43% respectively when LVOT VTI was less than 65% predicted [14]. More recently, a study of 990 patients with stable

coronary artery disease demonstrated increased rates of heart failure hospitalization for subjects within the lowest VTI quartile [15]. Our study was designed to test the following concept: for those within the lowest VTI quartile, is extremely low VTI a marker for patients at highest risk of death and who will go on to need advanced therapies such as transplant or LVAD? We hypothesized that because extremely low LVOT VTI is an accurate marker of the low output state, LVOT VTI may be used to discriminate between early stage heart failure versus advanced heart failure with low cardiac output, thus providing clinicians with a readily obtainable noninvasive tool to identify patients who may benefit most from advanced heart failure interventions such as LVAD and heart transplantation.

Methods

LVOT VTI is used to estimate stroke volume since it reflects the column of blood which moves through the LV outflow tract during each systole, per the following equation [16]:

$$\text{Stroke Volume} = \text{LVOT VTI} \times \text{Cross Sectional Area}$$
$$\text{of the Left Ventricular Outflow Tract.}$$

LVOT VTI is calculated by placing the pulsed Doppler sample volume in the outflow tract below the aortic valve and recording the velocity (cm/s). When the velocity signal is integrated with respect to time, the distance blood moves with each systole is calculated in cm/systole (Fig. 1). Assuming laminar flow through the LVOT, this has been shown to correlate well with cardiac output, which is equivalent to stroke volume x heart rate [16].

The study protocol was approved by the Institutional Review Board of Scripps Health, La Jolla, CA. Subject selection: The transthoracic echocardiogram (TTE) database at our institution was queried for studies performed between June 2009 and May 2011 for patients with heart

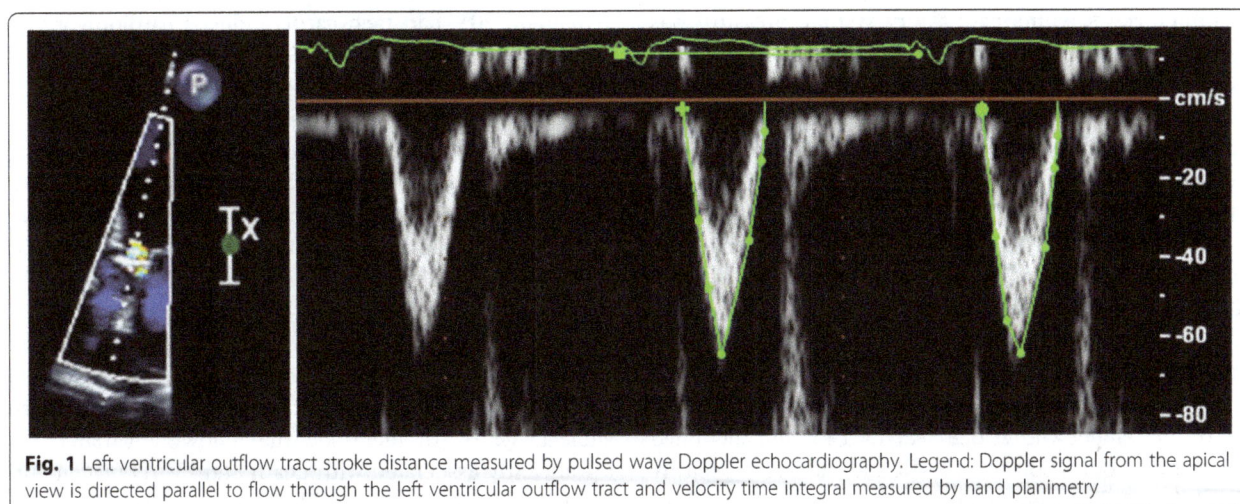

Fig. 1 Left ventricular outflow tract stroke distance measured by pulsed wave Doppler echocardiography. Legend: Doppler signal from the apical view is directed parallel to flow through the left ventricular outflow tract and velocity time integral measured by hand planimetry

failure. As over 20,000 echocardiograms per year are performed at our institution, in order to identify subjects with extremely low LVOT VTI, a cutoff LVOT VTI of no more than 10 cm was applied in order to limit the number of included studies.

Exclusion criteria included any one of the following: alternative causes for shock (including hypovolemia and sepsis), acute myocardial infarction, significant valvular disease affecting accurate estimation of forward cardiac output by LVOT VTI (i.e, severe aortic regurgitation) [5], significant tachycardia (defined as >120 beats per minute), and pulmonary arterial hypertension. Subjects with multiple TTEs were reviewed at time of earliest study and subsequent studies were excluded. Valvular disease was characterized according to guidelines from the American College of Cardiology [17]. Diagnosis of heart failure was established by review of the electronic medical record (EMR): clinical documentation of heart failure in an admission history and physical, discharge summary, or cardiologist's note and/or referral to a dedicated heart failure clinic.

Echocardiographic measurements
LVOT VTI was measured from an anteriorly angled apical four-chamber view using pulsed wave Doppler with the interrogation beam directed across the LVOT. The pulsed wave Doppler sample volume was placed in the left ventricular outflow tract just proximal to the aortic valve and thin spectral envelopes were obtained using very low gain. In patients with atrial fibrillation, LVOT VTI was averaged over three to five consecutive beats. In cases of aortic stenosis, the pulsed Doppler sample volume was placed far enough from the stenotic valve to avoid falsely elevated readings. Inter- and intra-observer variability testing for LVOT VTI was performed and validated (intra-class correlation coefficient 0.989-0.997). Ejection fraction (EF) was calculated using bi-plane method of disks from apical two and four chamber views. Pulmonary artery systolic pressure was calculated from Doppler derived tricuspid regurgitation velocity using the simplified Bernoulli equation ($\triangle P = 4v^2$). Doppler derived cardiac output was calculated using the previously described equation for Doppler derived stroke volume, followed by multiplication by heart rate (i.e. CO = SV x HR).

Data collection: Baseline demographic information and laboratory data at time of TTE were obtained from the EMR via retrospective chart review.

Statistical analysis:
The primary endpoint was defined as death, transplant or LVAD placement within one year of TTE and identified by review of our institution's EMR and the Social Security Death Index. The study population was analyzed in cohort design based on subjects meeting the primary endpoint versus event-free subjects. Differences in categorical and continuous variables were analyzed by chi-squared and independent t-test analyses respectively.

Survival analysis
The prognostic ability of various factors including LVOT VTI to predict the primary endpoint over 12 months following TTE was tested by Cox regression analysis. Univariate Cox regression was performed using a set of predefined variables: age, gender, presence of renal dysfunction, hemoglobin, NYHA class, diabetes, ejection fraction, echo-derived pulmonary artery systolic pressure and Doppler derived cardiac output. Variables from the univariate analysis found to be significant at $p \leq 0.1$ were combined in the multiple variable analysis. The study population was divided into tertiles based on LVOT VTI and survival was compared between groups using Kaplan Meier and Cox regression analysis. Study data was analyzed using IBM SPSS software (IBM SPSS, version 21.0, IBM, Rochester, Minnesota).

Results
Study sample
Twenty-six thousand one hundred thirty-five TTE studies were performed during the selected time period; of these, 265 studies were identified with LVOT VTI < 10 cm; duplicate studies from the same subject (n = 125), subjects without at least a year of follow up (n = 22), heart rate > 120 beats per minute (n = 7), acute myocardial infarction at time of TTE (n = 6), pulmonary arterial hypertension (n = 1) and alternative causes for shock (n = 4) were excluded. The study sample consisted of 100 subjects; all subjects carried a diagnosis of heart failure (age 73.5 ± 14.7 years, 72% male, mean ejection fraction 28.9%). More than 60% of the study population had ischemic cardiomyopathy as the cause of their heart failure, 18% had dilated, non-ischemic cardiomyopathy, and the remaining 20% had tachycardia-induced cardiomyopathy (10%), viral myocarditis (5%), drugs/toxins (4%) and postpartum cardiomyopathy (1%). Other baseline subject characteristics are described in Table 1. A total of thirty events occurred (28 deaths and 2 LVADs) over 1 year of follow up from TTE study. No cardiac transplants were identified. When divided into LVOT VTI tertiles, ejection fraction demonstrated statistical significant across tertiles, (p = 0.024).

Outcome group analysis
Comparison of subjects meeting primary endpoints (death or LVAD or transplant, n = 30) versus event-free subjects (n = 70) identified the following variables as significantly associated with death and LVAD placement: LVOT VTI (p = 0.039), older age (p = 0.001), higher

Table 1 Baseline characteristics

	Total study population (n = 100)	LVOT VTI < 8.1 cm, lowest tertile (n = 34)	LVOT VTI 8.1-9.0 cm, median tertile (n = 33)	LVOT VTI > 9.0 cm, highest tertile (n = 33)	P-value
Clinical characteristics					
Age (years)	73.53 ± 14.7	71.26 ± 15.3	74.82 ± 15.1	74.58 ± 13.8	0.547
Gender (% male)	72	79.4	75.8	60.6	0.194
Diabetes	27%	29.4%	24.2%	27.3%	0.892
Hypertension	57%	52.9%	51.5%	66.7%	0.388
Atrial Fibrillation	68%	77%	62%	67%	0.485
Prior revascularization	50%	56%	49%	45%	0.679
NYHA Class					0.643
I	1.1%	3.1%	0%	0%	
II	41.5%	40.6%	33.3%	51.7%	
III	45.7%	43.8%	54.5%	37.9%	
IV	11.7%	12.5%	12.1%	10.3%	
Smoking	14%	11.8%	10%	21.2%	0.328
Alcohol	17%	15%	24%	12%	0.385
Illicit drugs	4%	6%	3%	3%	0.797
Medical Therapy					
Diuretics	68.7%	72.7%	72.7%	60.6%	0.472
ACE/ARB	57.6%	64.7%	51.5%	56.3%	0.541
Beta blocker	84%	82.4%	84.8%	84.8%	0.949
Digoxin	28.3%	27.3%	30.3%	27.3%	0.951
Spironolactone	32%	35.3%	39.4%	21.2%	0.251
Statin	45.4%	41.2%	51.6%	43.8%	0.683
CRT	31.6%	31.3%	43.3%	21.2%	0.169
ICD	42.9%	51.5%	50.0%	27.3%	0.084
Objective Parameters					
SBP (mmHg)	114.57 ± 16.8	111 ± 17	113 ± 16	119 ± 17	0.128
DBP (mmHg)	72.00 ± 14.4	70 ± 16	71 ± 14	74 ± 13	0.581
HR (beats per minute)	82.93 ± 16.3	85.6 ± 18	80.9 ± 15	82.1 ± 16	0.481
Weight (kg)	76.6 ± 19.2	77.2 ± 16	80 ± 24	73.1 ± 17	0.391
Body mass index	25.8 ± 5	25.8 ± 5	26.4 ± 6	25.2 ± 5	0.657
Hgb (g/dL)	13.28 ± 2.0	13.7 ± 1.7	12.9 ± 1.7	13.2 ± 2.5	0.205
Creatinine (mg/dL)	1.40 ± 0.6	1.51 ± 0.8	1.46 ± 0.6	1.21 ± 0.4	0.101
Blood urea nitrogen (mg/dL)	27.0 ± 14	25.8 ± 10	30.5 ± 18	24.9 ± 13	0.221
Glomerular filtration rate < 60 ml/min	60.2%	67.7%	51.5%	62.1%	0.403
Sodium (mEq/L)	137 ± 4	137 ± 4	137 ± 3	138 ± 3	0.270
Cholesterol, total (mg/dL)	149 ± 41	142 ± 35	147 ± 41	158 ± 46	0.286
QRS > 120 msec	51.2%	61.3%	46.2%	44.4%	0.364
Ejection fraction (%)	28.9 ± 17	25.1 ± 17	26.4 ± 11	35 ± 19	0.024
Mean PA pressure (mmHg)	47.7 ± 15	47.8 ± 16	48.2 ± 13	47.1 ± 15	0.961
LV end diastolic dimension (cm)	5.81 ± 1.3	6.06 ± 1.2	5.94 ± 1.1	5.42 ± 1.5	0.092
Aortic Stenosis	11.1%	15.2%	10.0%	10.0%	0.900

Table 1 Baseline characteristics *(Continued)*

Aortic Insufficiency	16.2%	24.2%	21.2%	3.0%	0.060
Tricuspid Regurgitation*	51.5%	54.5%	51.5%	48.4%	0.738
Mitral Regurgitation*	61%	55.9%	75.8%	51.5%	0.302

Legend: *SD* standard deviation, *NYHA* New York Heart Association; Diuretics furosemide, toresmide, bumetanide, *ACE* angiotensin converting enzyme, *ARB* angiotensin receptor blocker, *CRT* cardiac resynchronization therapy, *ICD* implantable cardiac defibrillator, *SBP* systolic blood pressure, *DBP* diastolic blood pressure, *bpm* beats per minute, *GFR* glomerular filtration rate, *PA* pulmonary artery, *LV* left ventricle
*denotes meaningful valve disease classified as greater than mild

NYHA class (p = 0.014), higher pulmonary artery systolic pressure (53.0 ± 16.9 vs. 45.3 ± 12.6 mmHg; p = 0.019), higher blood urea nitrogen (33.8 ± 15.4 vs 24.1 ± 12.5, p = 0.001), lower hemoglobin (12.7 ± 1.4 vs. 13.5 ± 2.2 g/dL; p = 0.030), and glomerular filtration rate < 60 ml/min (75.9% vs 53.1%, p = 0.038), results summarized in Table 2.

Univariate outcomes prediction analysis

A set of predefined variables including age, gender, presence of diabetes, NYHA class, hemoglobin, blood urea nitrogen, glomerular filtration rate < 60 ml/min, pulmonary artery systolic pressure, ejection fraction, LVOT VTI, and Doppler derived cardiac output were assessed (Table 3). Significant variables that were associated with death and LVAD implatation included LVOT VTI, hazard ratio (HR) of 0.729 (95% confidence interval [CI] 0.55 - 0.96, p = 0.024), age (HR 1.05, CI 1.02 - 1.09, p = 0.001), NYHA class (HR 2.13, CI 1.26 - 3.60, p = 0.005), blood urea nitrogen (HR 1.03, CI1.01 - 1.05, p = 0.005), and glomerular filtration rate (HR 2.437, CI 1.04 - 5.71, p = 0.029).

Multivariate analysis

In the multivariate model, all variables in the univariate analysis with p value ≤0.1 and the prespecified addition of ejection fraction were included (Table 3). In model 1 LVOT VTI was adjusted by age; model 2 consisted of all variables in model 1 with the addition of echocardiographic

factors including ejection fraction and echo derived pulmonary artery systolic pressure. Model 3 consisted of all variables in model 2 with the addition of NYHA class, glomerular filtration rate < 60 ml/min and blood urea nitrogen. In all models, lower LVOT VTI remained significantly associated with death and LVAD implantation (Table 3).

Survival analysis

Subjects were divided into three groups based on LVOT VTI tertile: lowest tertile (LVOT VTI < 8.1 cm, n = 34), median tertile (LVOT VTI 8.1-9.0 cm, n = 33), and upper tertile (LVOT VTI > 9.0 cm, n = 33). Event free survival rates were 55.9% for the lowest LVOT VTI tertile, 66.7% for the median tertile, and 87.9% for the upper tertile, p = 0.008 (Fig. 2. Kaplan Meier Survival analysis by LVOT VTI Tertile). The hazard ratio for death and LVAD placement for the lowest tertile (LVOT VTI > 8.1 cm, n = 34) in comparison to the upper two tertiles (LVOT VTI > 8.1 cm, n = 66) was 4.755 (CI 1.576-14.348, p = 0.006), and the HR was 12.680 (CI 2.638 – 60.949, p = 0.002) when adjusted for age, creatinine, ejection fraction, pulmonary artery systolic pressure and NYHA class (Table 4).

Discussion

Because extremely low LVOT VTI was the focus of our investigation, a cut off of <10 cm was used for subject inclusion. Similar to previously described heart failure

Table 2 Comparison of baseline variables by outcome group: Primary outcome vs Event free subgroups

Variable	Primary outcome group (n = 30)	Event-free group (n = 70)	p-value
LVOT VTI	8.0	8.5	0.039
Ejection fraction (%)	32.3	27.4	0.169
Doppler derived cardiac output (L/min)	2.29	2.44	0.217
Age, years	80.1 ± 11.3	70.7 ± 15.1	0.003
NYHA class (% in stage III or IV)	80%	48.60%	0.014
Hemoglobin, g/dL	12.7 ± 1.4	13.5 ± 2.2	0.030
Blood urea nitrogen, g/dL	33.8 ± 15.4	24.1 ± 12.5	0.001
GFR <60 ml/min	75.90%	53.10%	0.038
Pulmonary artery pressure, mmHg	53.0 ± 16.9	45.3 ± 12.6	0.019

Primary outcome was met in 30 subjects (28 death and 2 LVADs); Event free subjects were those alive at one year of follow up from TTE and without requirement for mechanical circulatory support
Abbrev: *GFR* glomerular filtration rate, *LVOT VTI* Left ventricular outflow tract velocity time integral, *NYHA* New York Heart Association

Table 3 Univariate and multiple variable analyses of factors related to death or LVAD placement

	Hazard ratio (95% CI)	P-value
Univariate analysis		
LVOT VTI, cm	0.729 (0.55 - 0.96)	0.024
Age, years	1.05 (1.02 - 1.09)	0.001
Male gender	1.66 (0.678 - 4.058)	0.245
Diabetes	1.38 (0.65 - 2.95)	0.416
NYHA class	2.13 (1.26 - 3.60)	0.005
Hemoglobin, g/dL	0.876 (0.74 - 1.04)	0.107
Blood urea nitrogen, g/dL	1.03 (1.01 - 1.05)	0.005
Glomerular filtration rate < 60 ml/min	2.437 (1.04 - 5.71)	0.029
Pulmonary artery pressure, mmHg	1.03 (1.01 - 1.06)	0.010
Ejection fraction	1.01 (0.99 - 1.03)	0.179
Doppler derived cardiac output, L/min	0.677 (0.378-1.213)	0.190
Multivariate analysis		
Model 1: LVOT VTI + age	0.661 (0.502 – 0.871)	0.003
Model 2: Model 1 + Pulmonary artery pressure and Ejection fraction	0.619 (0.452 – 0.849)	0.003
Model 3: Model 2 + Blood urea nitrogen, glomerular filtration rate < 60 ml/min and NYHA class	0.590 (0.415 – 0.838)	0.003

Legend: *HR* hazard ratio, *CI* confidence interval, *LVAD* left ventricular assist device, *LVOT VTI* left ventricular outflow tract velocity time integral; other abbreviations described in Table 1

Table 4 Cox proportional hazard analysis by LVOT VTI tertile

	Lowest tertile (LVOT VTI < 8.1, n = 34) vs Upper 2/3 s study population (n = 66)	P-value
Unadjusted analysis	4.755 (CI 1.576 - 14.348)	0.006
Adjusted analysis*	12.680 (CI 2.638 – 60.949)	0.002

*Adjusted for Age, Creatinine, Ejection fraction, Pulmonary artery systolic pressure and NYHA class

cohorts, our study population was predominantly male (72 out of 100), elderly (mean age, 73.5 years) with systolic CHF due to ischemic cardiomyopathy (mean EF, 28%). Our findings demonstrate that extremely diminished LVOT VTI was robustly associated with the combination of 12-month death and LVAD implantation. In the multivariate analysis, LVOT VTI was most predictive of adverse outcomes [HR 0.589 (95% CI 0.41 - 0.83), $p = 0.003$], hazard ratio of less than one indicating that higher LVOT VTI correlates with better outcomes, other significant variables being older age [HR 1.04 (95% CI 1.004 - 1.095, $p = 0.033$] and higher echo-derived systolic pulmonary artery pressure [HR 1.03 (95% CI 1.005 - 1.065, $p = 0.022$].

When comparing cohort tertiles, the unadjusted and adjusted hazard ratios for LVOT VTI were even more predictive, with an unadjusted mortality and LVAD likelihood ratio of 4.755 (95% CI 1.576 - 14.348) in the lowest LVOT VTI tertile compared with the rest of the

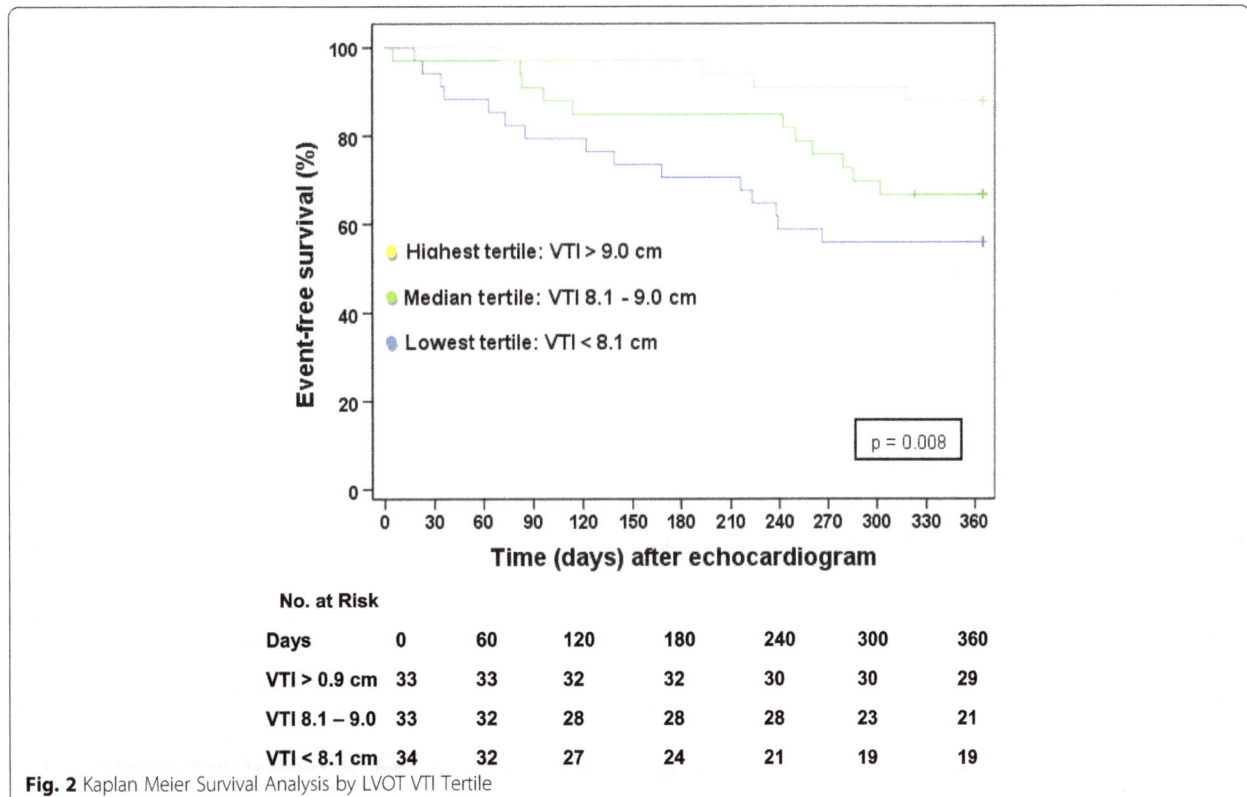
Fig. 2 Kaplan Meier Survival Analysis by LVOT VTI Tertile

study group and an adjusted likelihood ratio of 12.680 (95% CI 2.638 – 60.949).

Several reasons may explain why low LVOT VTI correlates closely with adverse clinical outcomes. LVOT VTI provides enhanced prognostic information over ejection fraction, as it focuses on forward cardiac output which at times maybe normal even in compensated heart failure patients with low ejection fraction. Low cardiac output is a known precursor to overt cardiogenic shock, multi-organ dysfunction and death [18]. Whereas the accuracy of Doppler derived cardiac output is primarily limited by errors in determining the cross sectional area of the LVOT, as defined by the formula πr^2, utilizing LVOT VTI alone rather than Doppler derived cardiac output eliminates this source of error. In patients who are tachycardic due to cardiogenic shock and poor LV function, rapid heart rate partially offsets the decline LV function, allowing for maintenance of cardiac output in the setting of a sick ventricle, however LVOT VTI remains depressed. Thus, in cases of low cardiac output with compensatory tachycardia, LVOT VTI may be a very sensitive predictor of cardiogenic shock and impaired ability to meet systemic tissue perfusion and metabolic demands. Because LVOT VTI is an easily obtainable and reproducible measurement, we propose that LVOT VTI may be a useful and accessible tool to identify heart failure patients with very low cardiac output and who may benefit from advanced heart failure therapies appropriate for end-stage HF.

Conclusions

As numerous therapies emerge that increase cardiac output for patients with advanced heart failure [19], there is an ever greater need to identify those who stand to benefit most from such therapies [4]. LVOT VTI is an easily available non-invasive tool that identifies patients at highest risk for decreased survival at one year, thus allowing for earlier identification and advanced treatment.

Study limitations and future directions

Accurate determination of LVOT VTI assumes laminar flow and is affected by LVOT abnormalities such as severe aortic regurgitation, hypertrophic obstructive cardiomyopathy, systolic anterior motion of the anterior mitral leaflet, and subaortic stenosis; subjects with these diagnoses were excluded in our study as LVOT VTI is not an accurate predictor of forward cardiac flow in these settings [5].

Our study was designed as a novel proof-of-concept study, no prior study to our knowledge at the time of this writing has examined the relationship between extremely low LVOT VTI and outcomes in advanced heart failure. Given the retrospective nature of this study, findings should be confirmed a larger, prospective cohort.

Abbreviations
CI: 95% confidence interval; CO: Doppler derived cardiac output; EF: Ejection fraction; EMR: Electronic medical record; GFR: Glomerular filtration rate; HR: Hazard ratio; HR: Heart rate; LVAD: Left ventricular assist device; LVOT VTI: Left ventricular outflow tract velocity time integral; NYHA class: New York Heart Association class; PASP: Pulmonary artery systolic pressure,; SV: Stroke volume; TTE: Transthoracic echocardiogram

Acknowledgements
The authors would like to acknowledge Dr. Jill Waalen for her assistance with the statistical analyses performed.

Funding
No funding was received for this study.

Authors' contributions
The study was designed by JTH. KB assisted with data acquisition. CWT was the major contributor in writing the manuscript. The manuscript was edited by AS and RM. All authors read and approved the final article.

Competing interests
Dr. Heywood serves as a speaker for Thoratec®. The remaining authors have no disclosures or competing interests.

Consent for publication
No patient identifying information is used in this article.

References
1. Go AS, Mozaffarian D, Roger VL, Benjamin EJ, Berry JD, Borden WB, et al. Heart disease and stroke statistics—2013 update: a report from the American Heart Association. Circulation. 2013;127:e6–e245.
2. Adams KF, Fonarow GC, Emerman CL, LeJemtel TH, Costanzo RM, Abraham WT, et al. Characteristics and outcomes of patients hospitalized for heart failure in the United States: rationale, design, and preliminary observations from the first 100,000 cases in the acute Decompensated heart failure National Registry. Am Heart J. 2005;149:209–16.
3. Noria A, Tsang SW, Fang JC, Lewis EF, Jarcho JA, Mudge GH, et al. Clinical assessment identifies hemodynamic profiles that predict outcomes in patients admitted with heart failure. J Am Coll Cardiol. 2003;21:1797–804.
4. Miller LW, Guglin M. Patient selection for ventricular assist devices. J Am Coll Cardiol. 2013;61:1209–21.
5. Beigel R, Cercek B, Siegel RJ, Hamilton MA. Echo-Doppler Hemodynamics: an important management tool for Today's heart failure care. Circulation. 2015 Mar 17;131(11):1031–4. doi:10.1161/CIRCULATIONAHA.114.011424.
6. Hunt SA, Abraham WT, Chin MH, et al. 2009 focused update incorporated into the ACC/AHA 2005 guidelines for the diagnosis and Management of Heart Failure in adults: a report of the American College of Cardiology Foundation/American Heart Association task force on practice guidelines: developed in collaboration with the International Society for Heart and Lung Transplantation. Circulation. 2009;119:e391–479.
7. Gola A, Pozzoli M, Capomolla S, Traversi E, Sanarico M, Cobelli F, et al. Comparison of Doppler echocardiography with thermodilution for assessing cardiac output in advanced congestive heart failure. Am J Cardiol. 1996 Sep 15;78:708–12.
8. Pozzoli M, Capomolla S, Cobelli F, Tavazzi L. Reproducibility of Doppler indices of left ventricular systolic and diastolic function in patients with severe chronic heart failure. Eur Heart J. 1995;16:194–200.
9. Mowat DH, Haites NE, Rawles JM. Aortic blood velocity measurement in healthy adults using a simple ultrasound technique. Cardiovasc Res. 1983;17:75–80.
10. Labovitz AJ, Buckingham TA, Habermehl K, Nelson J, Kennedy HL, Williams GA. The effects of sampling site on the two-dimensional echo-Doppler determination of cardiac output. Am Heart J. 1985 Feb;109:327–32.
11. Coats AJ. Doppler ultrasonic measurement of cardiac output: reproducibility and validation. Eur Heart J. 1990;11(Suppl I):49–61.
12. Dittmann H, Voelker W, Karsch KR, Seipel L. Influence of sampling site and flow area on cardiac output measurements by Doppler echocardiography. J Am Coll Cardiol. 1987;10:818–23.
13. Evangelista A, Garcia-Dorado D, Garcia del Castillo H, Gonzalez-Alujas T, Soler-Soler J. Cardiac index quantification by Doppler ultrasound in patients without left ventricular outflow tract abnormalities. J Am Coll Cardiol. 1995; 25:710–6.

14. Trent RJ, Rawles JM. Risk stratification after acute myocardial infarction by Doppler stroke distance measurement. Heart. 1999;82:187–91.

15. Ristow B, Na B, Ali S, Whooley MA, Schiller NB. Left ventricular outflow tract and pulmonary artery stroke distances independently predict heart failure hospitalization and mortality: the heart and soul study. J Am Soc Echocardiogr. 2011;24:565–72.

16. Huntsman LL, Stewart DK, Barnes SR, Franklin SB, Colocousis JS, Hessel EA. Noninvasive Doppler estimation of cardiac output in man, clinical validation. Circulation. 1983;67:593–602.

17. Nishimura RA, et al. 2014 American Heart Association/American College of Cardiology Guideline for the Management of Patients with Valvular heart disease. Circulation. 2014;129:000.

18. Abraham WT, Adams KF, Fonarow GC, Costanzo MR, Berkowitz RL, LeJemtel TH, et al. In-hospital mortality in patients with acute decompensated heart failure requiring intravenous vasoactive medications: an analysis from the acute Decompensated heart failure National Registry. J Am Coll Cardiol. 2005;46(1):57.

19. Stewart GC, Givertz M. Advances in mechanical circulatory support: mechanical circulatory support for advanced heart failure: patients and Technology in Evolution. Circulation. 2012;125:1304–15. doi:10.1161

9

Comparison of strain parameters in dyssynchronous heart failure between speckle tracking echocardiography vendor systems

Wouter M. van Everdingen[1][*], Alexander H. Maass[2], Kevin Vernooy[3], Mathias Meine[1], Cornelis P. Allaart[4], Frederik J. De Lange[5], Arco J. Teske[1], Bastiaan Geelhoed[2], Michiel Rienstra[2], Isabelle C. Van Gelder[2], Marc A. Vos[6] and Maarten J. Cramer[1]

Abstract

Background: Although mechanical dyssynchrony parameters derived by speckle tracking echocardiography (STE) may predict response to cardiac resynchronization therapy (CRT), comparability of parameters derived with different STE vendors is unknown.

Methods: In the MARC study, echocardiographic images of heart failure patients obtained before CRT implantation were prospectively analysed with vendor specific STE software (GE EchoPac and Philips QLAB) and vendor-independent software (TomTec 2DCPA). Response was defined as change in left ventricular (LV) end-systolic volume between examination before and six-months after CRT implantation. Basic longitudinal strain and mechanical dyssynchrony parameters (septal to lateral wall delay (SL-delay), septal systolic rebound stretch (SRSsept), and systolic stretch index (SSI)) were obtained from either separate septal and lateral walls, or total LV apical four chamber. Septal strain patterns were categorized in three types. The coefficient of variation and intra-class correlation coefficient (ICC) were analysed. Dyssynchrony parameters were associated with CRT response using univariate regression analysis and C-statistics.

Results: Two-hundred eleven patients were analysed. GE-cohort (n = 123): age 68 years (interquartile range (IQR): 61–73), 67% male, QRS-duration 177 ms (IQR: 160–192), LV ejection fraction: 26 ± 7%. Philips-cohort (n = 88): age 67 years (IQR: 59–74), 60% male, QRS-duration: 179 ms (IQR: 166–193), LV ejection fraction: 27 ± 8. LV derived peak strain was comparable in the GE- (GE: -7.3 ± 3.1%, TomTec: −6.4 ± 2.8%, ICC: 0.723) and Philips-cohort (Philips: −7.7 ± 2.7%, TomTec: −7.7 ± 3.3%, ICC: 0.749). SL-delay showed low ICC values (GE vs. TomTec: 0.078 and Philips vs. TomTec: 0.025). ICC's of SRSsept and SSI were higher but only weak (GE vs. TomTec: SRSsept: 0.470, SSI: 0.467) (Philips vs. QLAB: SRSsept: 0.419, SSI: 0.421). Comparability of septal strain patterns was low (Cohen's kappa, GE vs. TomTec: 0.221 and Philips vs. TomTec: 0.279). Septal strain patterns, SRSsept and SSI were associated with changes in LV end-systolic volume for all vendors. SRSsept and SSI had relative varying C-statistic values (range: 0.530–0.705) and different cut-off values between vendors.

Conclusions: Although global longitudinal strain analysis showed fair comparability, assessment of dyssynchrony parameters was vendor specific and not applicable outside the context of the implemented platform. While the standardization taskforce took an important step for global peak strain, further standardization of STE is still warranted.

Keywords: Speckle tracking echocardiography, Cardiac resynchronization therapy, Strain, Dyssynchrony, Heart failure, Vendor comparison, Response

* Correspondence: w.m.vaneverdingen@umcutrecht.nl
[1]Department of Cardiology, University Medical Centre Utrecht, P.O. Box 855500, 3508, GA, Utrecht, The Netherlands
Full list of author information is available at the end of the article

Background

Speckle tracking echocardiography (STE) is used to assess myocardial deformation and strain in research setting as well as in clinical practice [1, 2]. The use of STE in cardiac resynchronization therapy (CRT) has received increasing interest the past years, with respect to multiple aspects: optimization of left ventricular (LV) lead positioning, myocardial viability, optimization of CRT device configuration, determining mechanical dyssynchrony, and predicting volumetric response and outcome [3–7]. Response prediction is an important aspect of clinical decision making, since 20–50% of patients are still non-responders to CRT despite meeting internationally acknowledged selection criteria [8]. Prediction of volumetric response and outcome to CRT has been approached using several STE derived parameters for mechanical dyssynchrony [3, 7, 9, 10]. Publications on these parameters mainly use STE software of General Electric EchoPac (Chicago, Illinois, United States) [9, 11, 12]. However, several other commercially available vendor dependent and independent software platforms have been developed for STE [9, 10, 13]. Between these platforms, differences in derived results are known, complicating the interpretation of specific study results and restricting their use in clinical practice [14, 15]. A taskforce of the European Association of Cardiovascular Imaging and American Society of Echocardiography (EACVI/ASE) was appointed to standardize longitudinal strain results and specifically global values [16]. However, inter vendor comparability of results obtained in patients with LV dyssynchrony is unknown. It was the aim of this study to compare strain parameters and more specifically dyssynchrony parameters derived from longitudinal strain analysis of different vendors of STE software, implemented specifically in CRT patients, as well as the association of derived dyssynchrony parameters with volumetric response to CRT. STE software of two commonly used vendors was used (i.e. GE EchoPac and Philips QLAB (Philips Medical Systems, Best, The Netherlands)), and the vendor-independent system of TomTec 2DCPA (TomTec Imaging Systems GmbH, Unterschleissheim, Germany). The hypothesis of this study is that vendors may have good agreement on global parameters and timing indices in patients eligible for CRT, while agreement on more detailed parameters and dyssynchrony parameters may be poor.

Methods

Study design

The Markers and Response to CRT (MARC) study was designed to investigate predictors for response on CRT, including several echocardiographic parameters [17]. The study was initiated and coordinated by the six centres within the framework of the Centre for Translational Molecular Medicine (CTMM), project

COHFAR (grant 01C-203), and additionally supported by Medtronic (Fridley, Minnesota, USA). Study monitoring was done by Medtronic, data management and validation by the investigators (MR, BG) in collaboration with Medtronic. The study was approved by the institutional review boards of all participating centres. All patients gave written informed consent. The trial was registered at clinicaltrials.gov: NCT01519908.

Study participants

Two hundred forty patients eligible for CRT according to the most recent international guidelines were included in the MARC study [18, 19]. In short, MARC study inclusion criteria were: sinus rhythm and optimal pharmacological heart failure therapy, QRS-duration ≥130 ms in patients with left bundle branch block (LBBB) and QRS-duration of ≥150 ms in non-LBBB patients with NYHA class II and QRS-duration ≥120 ms in LBBB patients with NYHA class III. Exclusion criteria were severe renal insufficiency, an upgrade from a bradycardia pacemaker or CRT-P to CRT-D, permanent atrial fibrillation, flutter or tachycardia, right bundle branch block, and permanent 2nd or 3rd degree atrioventricular block. Before and 6 months after CRT implantation, data were recorded at the outpatient department, including electrocardiographic and echocardiographic examination. Patients were excluded for this sub-analysis if frame rate of the apical four chamber (4CH) view was below 35 Hz, in case of irregular heart rhythm, unanalysable images due to technical errors or if image quality was very poor.

Echocardiographic examination

Echocardiographic examinations were performed by participating centres and analysed at the echocardiographic core lab situated in the UMC Utrecht (Utrecht, the Netherlands). Echocardiographic examinations made in this study were performed on either GE Vivid7, GE Vivid9, or Philips iE33 ultrasound machines. Standard images included a 4CH view, zoomed and focused on the LV. Of these images both image quality and frame rate were optimized for offline analysis. Analysis of apical rocking and interventricular mechanical delay (IVMD) are described in earlier work [17]. Pulsed-wave Doppler images of the LV outflow tract were obtained for definition of aortic valve closure time. QRS-onset and aortic valve closure time were used to define systole.

Volumetric response

LV ejection fraction, LV end-diastolic and end-systolic (LVESV) volumes were measured by biplane Simpson's method [20]. Volumetric response to CRT was defined as the percentage of change in LVESV between echocardiographic examination before and 6 months after CRT implantation. Patients were classified as responder in case of ≥15% reduction in LVESV.

Speckle tracking echocardiography

Echocardiographic 4CH images were subjected to offline speckle tracking analysis (WE, MC). The optimal images for speckle tracking were selected and used for the vendor dependent and independent platform (Additional file 1: Figure S1). All images were scored for quality (poor, average, or high) by two experienced observers. Image quality was categorized as high if the total LV myocardium was visible during the entire cardiac cycle, average if one or two segments were not clearly visible and poor in all other cases. Images were exported to vendor specific software (GE EchoPac 11.3 and Philips QLAB 10.0) in standard formats and exported as DICOM-files for vendor independent software (TomTec 2D Cardiac Performance Analysis (2DCPA) version 1.2.1.2). Speckle tracking was performed with standard settings for all vendors. For each platform, a region of interest (ROI) was placed by user defined markers to incorporate the entire myocardial wall. Repeat adjustments of the ROI were done if tracking quality was insufficient. The myocardial wall was separated into six segments by all platforms (i.e. basal and mid inferoseptal, apical septal, apical lateral and basal and mid anterolateral). Philips QLAB analyses an additional true apical segment (i.e. 17 segment model of the AHA), which was excluded for the septal and lateral wall strain curves, as it was part of both walls [21]. Segments were also excluded if adequate tracking was not achievable. The basal inferoseptal, mid inferoseptal and apical septal segment were averaged into a global septal wall strain curve. The apical lateral, basal anterolateral and mid anterolateral segment were averaged into a global lateral wall strain curve. Results from a single wall were excluded if tracking of more than one segment was unachievable. The entire myocardial wall was used for both Philips and GE analysis. TomTec analysis resulted in separate datasets for the endocardial and epicardial border. The epicardial border at the apical and mid ventricular lateral wall was often outside the echocardiographic window, and was therefore excluded in TomTec analysis. This was done even though differences between endo- and epicardial layers are known [22]. The marker for reference length (L_0) was placed at onset of QRS-complex for GE derived images, both for GE EchoPac and TomTec 2DCPA. L_0 of Philips derived images could not be altered in QLAB and was automatically placed in the QRS-complex. L_0 was manually placed at a similar position for Philips derived images analysed with TomTec 2DCPA. Therefore,

both direct comparisons (GE vs. TomTec and Philips vs. TomTec) had similar L_0 positions.

Offline analysis

Results of speckle tracking analysis were stored and exported for offline analysis with Matlab 2014b (Mathworks, Natick, MA, USA). Author written Matlab scripts allowed for input of valve closure times and semi-automatic calculation of strain parameters. Results of strain parameters were based on global strain curves. Global strain curves were averages of the segments representing the global LV or the separate septal or lateral wall.

Parameters

Basic strain parameters Five basic strain parameters were obtained for global LV, septal wall and lateral wall strain curves. 1) Pre-stretch was defined as maximal positive peak strain, occurring after QRS onset and before shortening (Fig. 1). 2) Peak strain was the maximal negative peak strain during the entire cardiac cycle. 3) Systolic strain was the maximal negative strain during systole. 4) Time to maximal peak (TTP_{max}) was the time difference from L_0 to most negative peak strain. 5) Time to first peak (TTP_{first}) was the time difference from L_0 to first negative peak.

Dyssynchrony parameters Four dyssynchrony parameters were compared. a) Septal to lateral wall delay (SL-delay) was calculated as the difference in TTP_{max} of the septal and lateral walls. b) Septal systolic rebound stretch (SRSsept) was defined as the cumulative amount of stretch after initial shortening of the septum, occurring during systole (Fig. 1) [3]. c) Systolic stretch index (SSI) was defined as the sum of SRSsept and lateral wall pre-stretch [9]. d) Septal strain curves were categorized in three LBBB pattern types, determined by their shape, based on earlier work of our group [23]. LBBB-1: double-peaked systolic stretch, LBBB-2: early pre-ejection shortening peak followed by prominent systolic stretching and LBBB-3: pseudo normal shortening with a late-systolic shortening peak followed by less pronounced end-systolic stretch (Fig. 2).

Cross-correlation The similarity of strain curves between vendor dependent and independent software was analysed by cross correlation of strain signals obtained from the same patient and image. Strain data of the vendor dependent analysis was interpolated and plotted on the horizontal axis, while data of the vendor independent analysis was plotted on the vertical axis. Least squares fitting ($y = a*x$) of this data was used to calculate the coefficient of determination (R^2). Strain

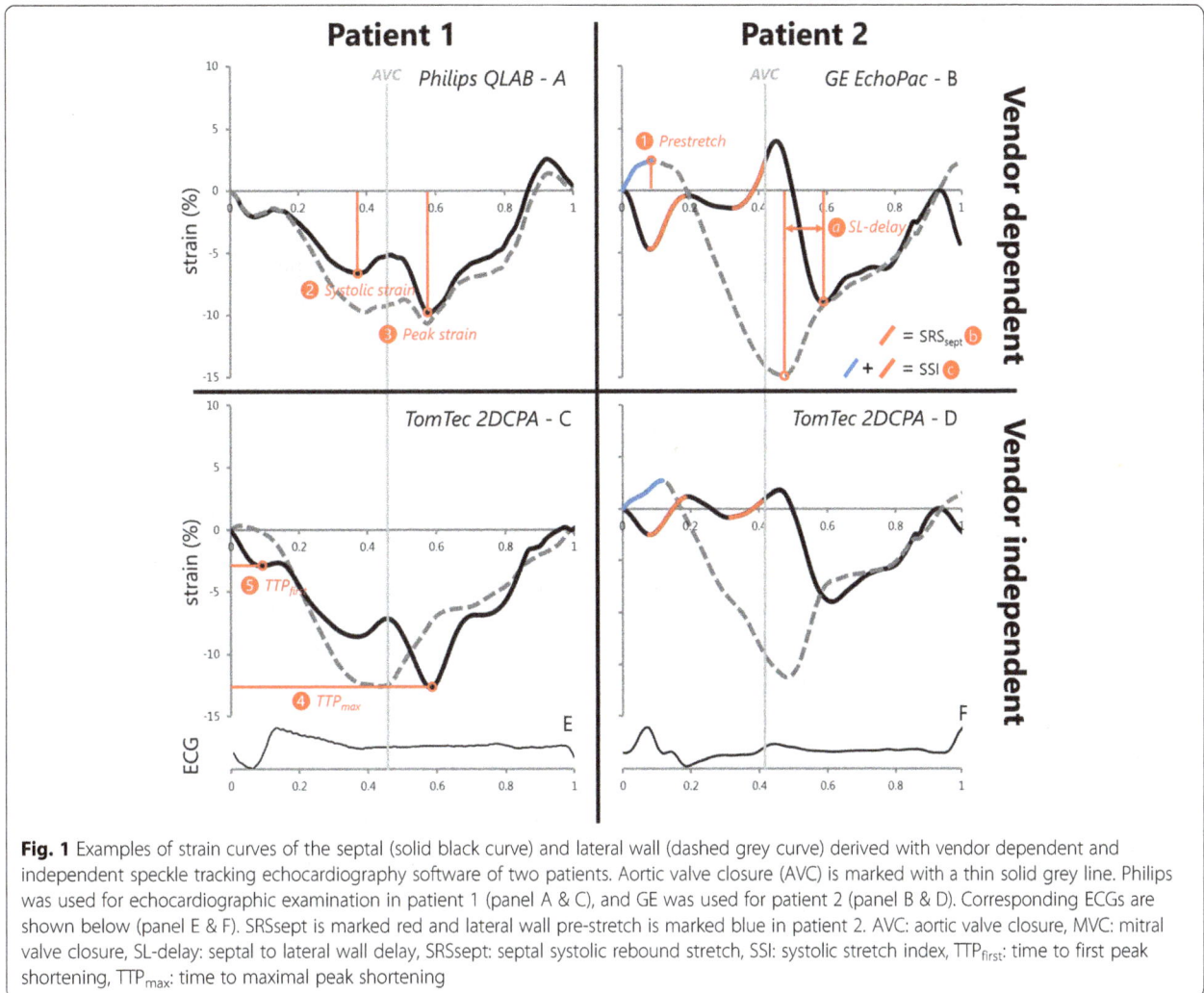

Fig. 1 Examples of strain curves of the septal (solid black curve) and lateral wall (dashed grey curve) derived with vendor dependent and independent speckle tracking echocardiography software of two patients. Aortic valve closure (AVC) is marked with a thin solid grey line. Philips was used for echocardiographic examination in patient 1 (panel A & C), and GE was used for patient 2 (panel B & D). Corresponding ECGs are shown below (panel E & F). SRSsept is marked red and lateral wall pre-stretch is marked blue in patient 2. AVC: aortic valve closure, MVC: mitral valve closure, SL-delay: septal to lateral wall delay, SRSsept: septal systolic rebound stretch, SSI: systolic stretch index, TTP$_{first}$: time to first peak shortening, TTP$_{max}$: time to maximal peak shortening

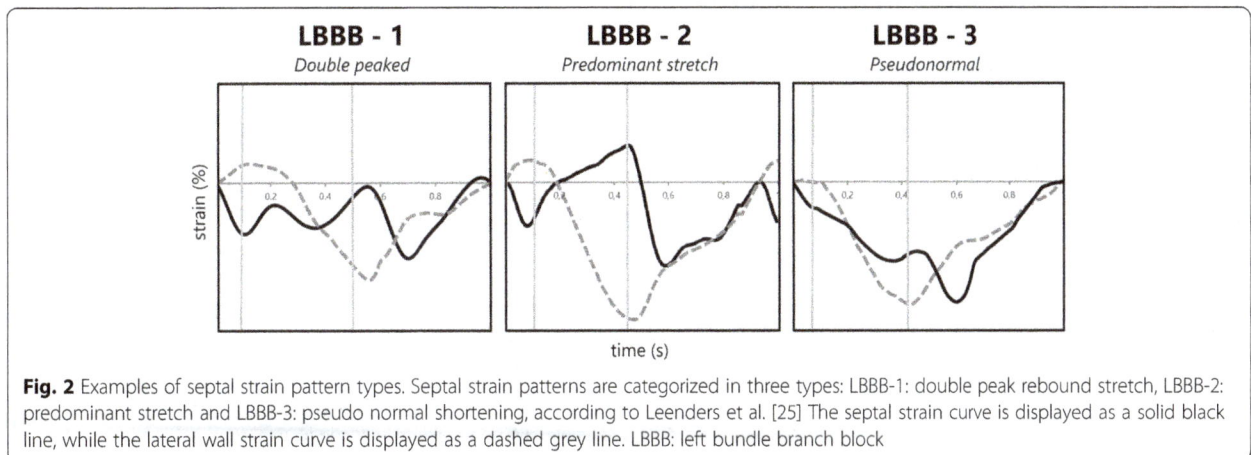

Fig. 2 Examples of septal strain pattern types. Septal strain patterns are categorized in three types: LBBB-1: double peak rebound stretch, LBBB-2: predominant stretch and LBBB-3: pseudo normal shortening, according to Leenders et al. [25] The septal strain curve is displayed as a solid black line, while the lateral wall strain curve is displayed as a dashed grey line. LBBB: left bundle branch block

data of the vendor dependent analysis was shifted by steps of 1 ms and R^2 was calculated for each step. After a total shift of 100 ms, the highest value was used as the optimal correlation coefficient.

Intra-observer agreement

Categorization of septal strain curves of all patients were analysed a second time with vendor-specific and vendor independent software for intra-observer agreement. There was an interval of at least 20 weeks between the data-analyses.

Statistical analysis

Statistical analysis was performed (BG and MR) using R version 3.2.4 (The R foundation for Statistical Computing), SAS software version 9.4 (SAS Institute, Cary, NC, USA) and the R-packages psych version 1.5.8 (for calculation of Cohen's kappa coefficients, ICCs and their associated p-values). Comparison of subgroups on baseline characteristics and strain parameters of GE and Philips was performed using a student t-test or Wilcoxon test, dependent on normality of data. Categorical data was compared using a Fisher exact test or Chi-Square tests if more than two categories were present. To compare vendor dependent to vendor independent data, strain parameters were compared by a paired t-test or Wilcoxon test, dependent on normality of data. The coefficient of variation (COV), intra-class correlation coefficient (ICC), and Bland-Altman plots were also used for comparison between vendors. For Bland-Altman plots, the mean, standard deviation and 95% confidence interval (i.e. limits of agreement) were calculated. Cross-correlation results were compared using a pairwise t-test with Bonferroni correction. Agreement of LBBB pattern categorization was assessed using Cohen's kappa coefficient. ICC and Cohen's kappa results were classified as follows; ≥0.75: excellent, 0.60–0.74: good, 0.40–0.59: weak, and <0.40: poor. Univariate regression analysis with change in LVESV as a continuous variable was used to test dyssynchrony parameters as predictors for response to CRT. The C-statistic and cut-off value were calculated for each dyssynchrony parameter, with volumetric response (LVESV reduction ≥15%) as a dichotomous parameter. A p-value <0.05 was considered significant for all tests.

Results

Study population

Two-hundred-eleven of 240 MARC study patients were included in this sub-analysis, 123 in the GE-cohort and 88 in the Philips-cohort. Nineteen patients were excluded for GE analysis, of which five were excluded from the main study, two had irregular heart rhythm, four had a frame rate below 35 Hz, four had overall low

image quality and two had only one analysable segment for the lateral wall. Ten patients were excluded for Philips analysis, of which four were already excluded from the main study, five were stored in a datafile not analysable for STE and one had a frame rate below 35 Hz. There were no significant differences in baseline characteristics between cohorts (Table 1), except for frame rate. Frame rate was higher in the GE-cohort (61 ± 12 Hz) compared to the (Philips-cohort 55 ± 7 Hz, p < 0.001). LV end-diastolic and end-systolic volumes tended to be lower in the Philips-cohort compared to the GE-cohort. LV ejection fraction was comparable, as were conventional electrical dyssynchrony (i.e. QRS duration and morphology) and mechanical dyssynchrony parameters (i.e. IVMD, apical rocking and septal flash). IVMD was above the cut-off value of 40 ms in both groups, septal flash was seen in approximately half of all patients, while apical rocking was observed in around 60%

Table 1 Baseline characteristics

	GE-cohort (n = 123)	Philips-cohort (n = 88)	p-value
Age (years)	68.3 (61.3–73.4)	67.2 (59.0–73.9)	0.450
Gender (n, % male)	82 (66.7%)	53 (60.2%)	0.384
BMI (kg/m²)	26.5 (23.8–29.6)	26.2 (23.6–29.3)	0.813
NYHA Class (n, %)			
I	1 (0.8%)	0 (0.0%)	0.869
II	77 (62.6%)	53 (60.2%)	
III	45 (36.6%)	35 (39.8%)	
QRS duration (ms)	177 (160–192)	179 (166–193)	0.293
QRS morphology (n, %)			
LBBB	68 (56.7%)	55 (64.7%)	0.311
IVCD	52 (43.3%)	30 (35.3%)	
LVEDV (ml)	183.3 (148.8–247.7)	168.0 (132.0–211.8)	0.051
LVESV (ml)	135.3 (100.7–194.7)	130.3 (92.8–167.3)	0.087
LVEF (%)	25.6 ± 7.3	26.5 ± 7.9	0.406
LVEDD (cm)	6.3 ± 0.8	6.2 ± 0.8	0.591
IVMD (ms)	47.1 ± 28.8	46.3 ± 30.2	0.855
Apical rocking (n, %)	71 (58.2%)	56 (63.6%)	0.476
Septal flash (n, %)	56 (47.5%)	42 (48.8%)	0.888
Frame rate (Hz)	61 ± 12	55 ± 7	<.001
Image quality (n, %)			
Poor	31 (25.2%)	8 (9.1%)	0.011
Average	54 (43.9%)	50 (56.8%)	
High	38 (31.0%)	30 (34.1%)	
ESV reduction	20.4 ± 22.9	24.9 ± 25.7	0.208
Responders (n, %)	65 (58.6%)	54 (65.1%)	0.375

Standard deviations are given with ± symbol, for non-normal distributed data, the median is given with the interquartile range between brackets
BMI body mass index, *NYHA* New York Heart Association, *LBBB* left bundle branch block, *LV* left ventricular, *LVEDV* LV end-diastolic volume, *LVESV* LV end-systolic volume, *LVEF* LV ejection fraction, *LVEDD* LV end-diastolic diameter, *IVCD* intra-ventricular conduction delay, *IVMD* interventricular mechanical delay

of patients. CRT response rate was non-significantly different in the two cohorts (GE-cohort: 59% vs. Philips-cohort: 65%), with non-significantly differences in ESV reduction (GE-cohort: 20 ± 23% vs. Philips-cohort: 25 ± 26, $p = 0.208$).

GE echocardiographic images
GE basic strain parameters
Comparison of strain results obtained with vendor dependent and independent STE software resulted in a good to excellent ICC for peak strain and systolic strain for global LV and septal wall (Table 2). COV was relatively low, as was the mean difference in Bland-Altman plots (Fig. 3). Nevertheless, the standard deviations of the Bland-Altman plots were relatively large, ranging from 2.2 to 2.8%. The ICC of peak and systolic strain of the lateral wall were weak (0.595 and 0.565 respectively),

with an even larger standard deviation in Bland-Altman plots (3.6 and 3.7%, respectively). The ICC of TTP_{first} and TTP_{max} of both walls and the global LV were poor to weak, with relatively large COV and large standard deviations in Bland-Altman plots.

GE dyssynchrony parameters
Dyssynchrony indices derived from GE images showed varied results. SL-delay showed a poor ICC (0.078) and high COV (−14.4) and wide limits of agreement in the Bland-Altman plots (mean difference: 2 ± 226 ms). The ICC of SRSsept was weak (0.470), COV was relatively high (0.937) and the Bland-Altman plots showed relative wide limits of agreement (1.0 ± 2.0%, Fig. 4). SSI showed similar results, ICC was also weak (0.467), COV was relatively high (0.720) and Bland-Altman plots showed a difference between vendors with

Table 2 Strain parameters derived from GE echocardiographic images

	GE EchoPac ($n = 123$)	TomTec 2DCPA ($n = 123$)	COV	ICC (p-value)	Bland-Altman (mean diff ±SD)
LV					
1) Pre-stretch (%)	0.4 (0.0–1.4)	0.7 (0.1–1.7)	1.218	0.631 (<0.001)	−0.3 ± 1.0
2) Peak strain (%)	−7.3 ± 3.1	−6.4 ± 2.8	−0.424	0.723 (<0.001)	−0.8 ± 2.2
3) Systolic strain (%)	−6.4 ± 3.2	−5.6 ± 3.2	−0.504	0.752 (<0.001)	−0.8 ± 2.2
4) TTP_{max} (ms)	511 (426–587)	488 (429–593)	0.201	0.676 (<0.001)	−2 ± 86
5) TTP_{first} (ms)	400 (158–458)	421 (316–471)	0.480	0.195 (0.015)	−34 ± 205
Septum					
1) Pre-stretch (%)	0.3 (0.0–1.0)	0.7 (0.0–1.5)	1.337	0.470 (<0.001)	−0.4 ± 1.1
2) Peak strain (%)	−8.0 ± 3.1	−7.2 ± 3.2	−0.392	0.707 (<0.001)	−0.8 ± 2.4
3) Systolic strain (%)	−6.7 ± 3.5	−6.0 ± 3.5	−0.517	0.667 (<0.001)	−0.7 ± 2.8
4) TTP_{max} (ms)	531 (378–626)	520 (414–606)	0.336	0.261 (0.002)	−9 ± 189
5) TTP_{first} (ms)	208 (135–376)	311 (151–420)	0.521	0.486 (<0.001)	−39 ± 142
Lateral wall					
1) Pre-stretch (%)	1.6 (0.5–3.1)	1.2 (0.2–2.4)	0.951	0.524 (<0.001)	0.3 ± 1.9
2) Peak strain (%)	−8.5 (−11.4- -5.8)	−6.5 (−10.2- -4.3)	−0.462	0.595 (<0.001)	−1.4 ± 3.6
3) Systolic strain (%)	−6.6 (−10.8- -4.2)	−5.5 (−9.0- -3.0)	−0.532	0.565 (<0.001)	−1.2 ± 3.7
4) TTP_{max} (ms)	500 (456–541)	514 (445–556)	0.149	0.444 (<0.001)	−7 ± 101
5) TTP_{first} (ms)	475 (419–520)	431 (300–522)	0.302	0.136 (0.066)	47 ± 206
Dyssynchrony					
a) SL-delay (ms)	25 (−132–110)	−13 (−121–101)	−14.440	0.078 (0.194)	−2 ± 226
b) SRSsept (%)	1.7 (0.8–3.4)	1.1 (0.1–1.9)	0.937	0.470 (<0.001)	1.0 ± 2.0
c) SSI (%)	3.8 (2.1–5.9)	2.6 (1.3–3.8)	0.720	0.467 (<0.001)	1.3 ± 3.0
d) LBBB type (n, %)					
LBBB-1	46 (37.4%)	36 (29.3%)			
LBBB-2	17 (13.8%)	10 (8.1%)			
LBBB-3	60 (48.8%)	77 (62.6%)			

Means and standard deviations are given with ± symbol. For non-normal distributed data, the median is given with the interquartile range between brackets
COV coefficient of variation, *ICC* intra-class correlation coefficient, *diff* difference, *SD* standard deviation, *LV* strain derived from global LV in apical four chamber view, TTP_{max} time to maximal peak shortening, TTP_{first} time to first peak shortening, *SL-delay* time delay between septal and lateral peak shortening, *SSI* systolic stretch index, *SRSsept* septal systolic rebound stretch, *LBBB type* type of LBBB strain patterns, based on definition by Leenders et al. [23]

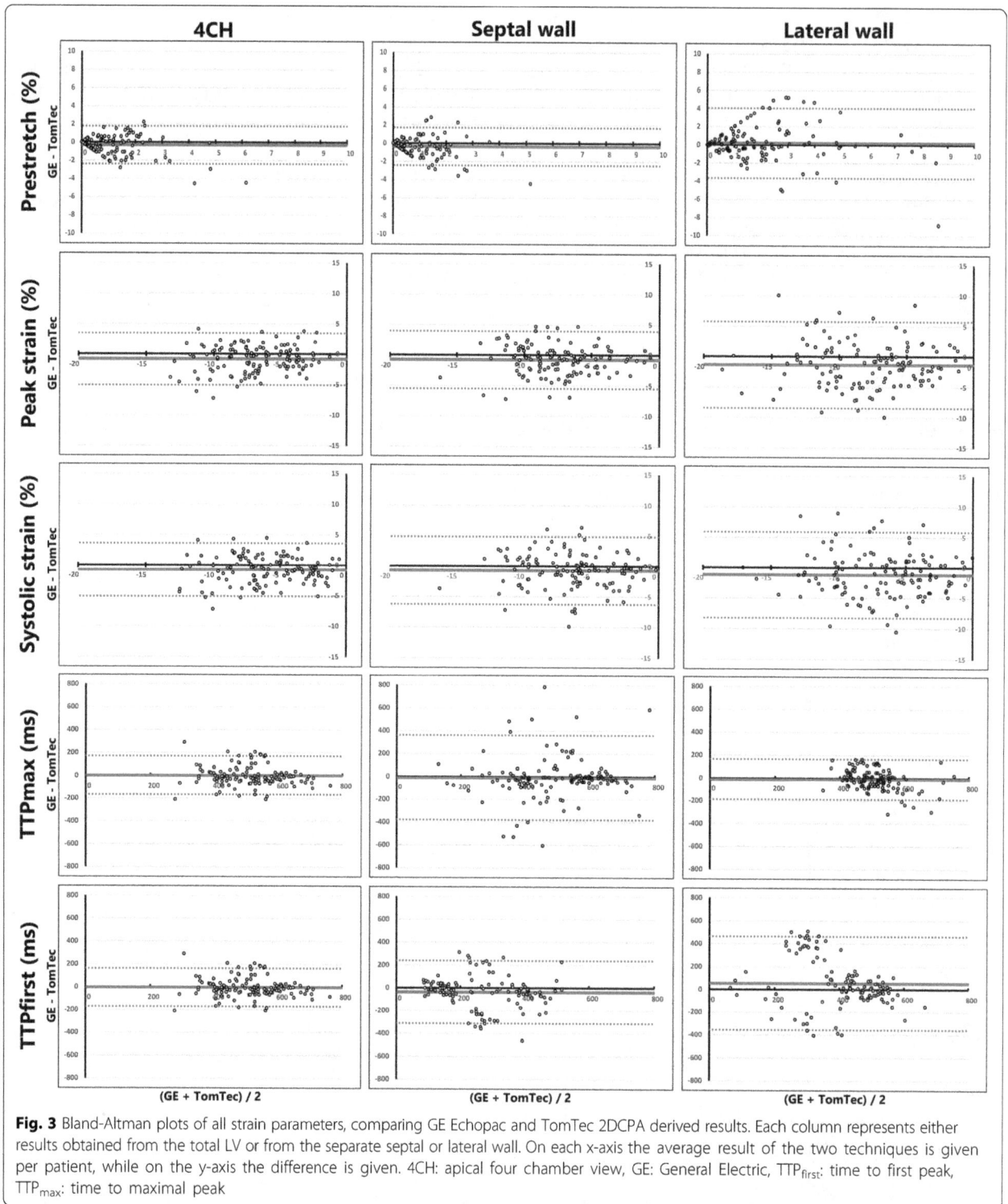

Fig. 3 Bland-Altman plots of all strain parameters, comparing GE Echopac and TomTec 2DCPA derived results. Each column represents either results obtained from the total LV or from the separate septal or lateral wall. On each x-axis the average result of the two techniques is given per patient, while on the y-axis the difference is given. 4CH: apical four chamber view, GE: General Electric, TTP$_{first}$: time to first peak, TTP$_{max}$: time to maximal peak

relative wide limits of agreement (1.3 ± 3.0%, Fig. 4). Cohen's kappa coefficient of agreement on LBBB pattern categorization was low (0.221). Cohen's kappa coefficient of intra-observer agreement was good for GE EchoPac (0.685) and weak for TomTec 2DCPA analysis (0.493) (Fig. 5).

Philips echocardiographic images
Philips basic strain parameters
Comparison of vendor dependent and independent STE results derived from Philips echocardiographic images showed a similar pattern in results to GE (Table 3). Namely, peak and systolic strain showed a

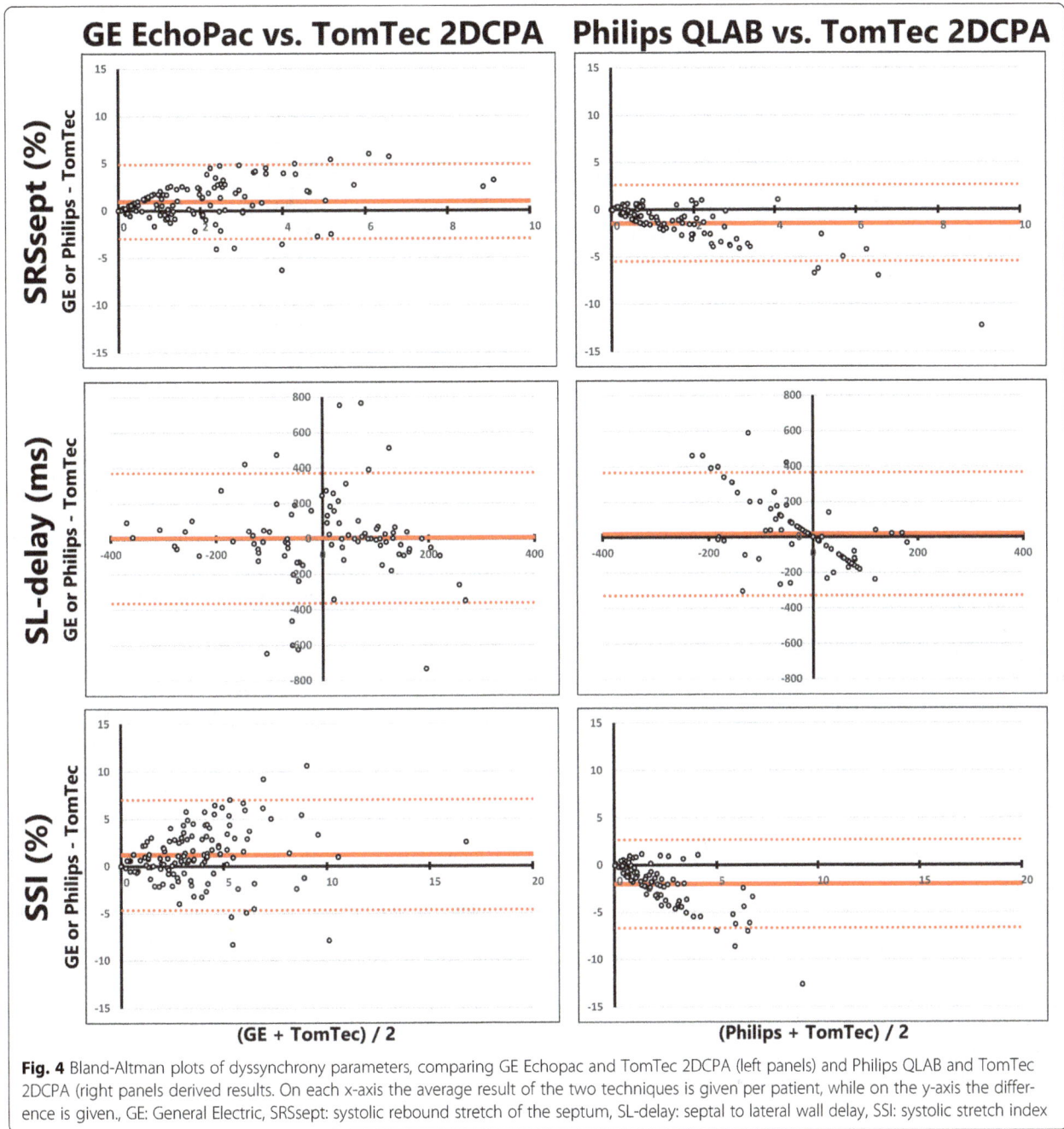

GE EchoPac vs. TomTec 2DCPA

Philips QLAB vs. TomTec 2DCPA

Fig. 4 Bland-Altman plots of dyssynchrony parameters, comparing GE Echopac and TomTec 2DCPA (left panels) and Philips QLAB and TomTec 2DCPA (right panels derived results. On each x-axis the average result of the two techniques is given per patient, while on the y-axis the difference is given., GE: General Electric, SRSsept: systolic rebound stretch of the septum, SL-delay: septal to lateral wall delay, SSI: systolic stretch index

smaller bias and COV than pre-stretch, timing parameters (i.e. TTP$_{max}$ and TTP$_{first}$) and dyssynchrony indices. ICCs were overall lower than GE derived results. Peak strain and systolic strain of the global LV showed an excellent ICC (0.749 and 0.802 respectively), with a relatively low COV and low mean difference in Bland-Altman plots (Table 3 and Fig. 6). The ICC of peak and systolic strain of the septal and lateral wall were good (ranging from 0.626 to 0.680). Results on pre-stretch showed a high COV, poor ICC

and wide limits of agreement in Bland-Altman results for all three comparisons (i.e. global LV, septal and lateral wall).

Philips dyssynchrony parameters

For Philips vs. TomTec, results on comparison of dyssynchrony parameters were lower for SL-delay (ICC: 0.025, COV: -10.7, Bland-Altman mean difference: 24 ± 180 ms) compared to SRSsept (ICC: 0.419, COV: 1.03, Bland-Altman mean difference: −1.5 ± 2.1%, Fig. 4)

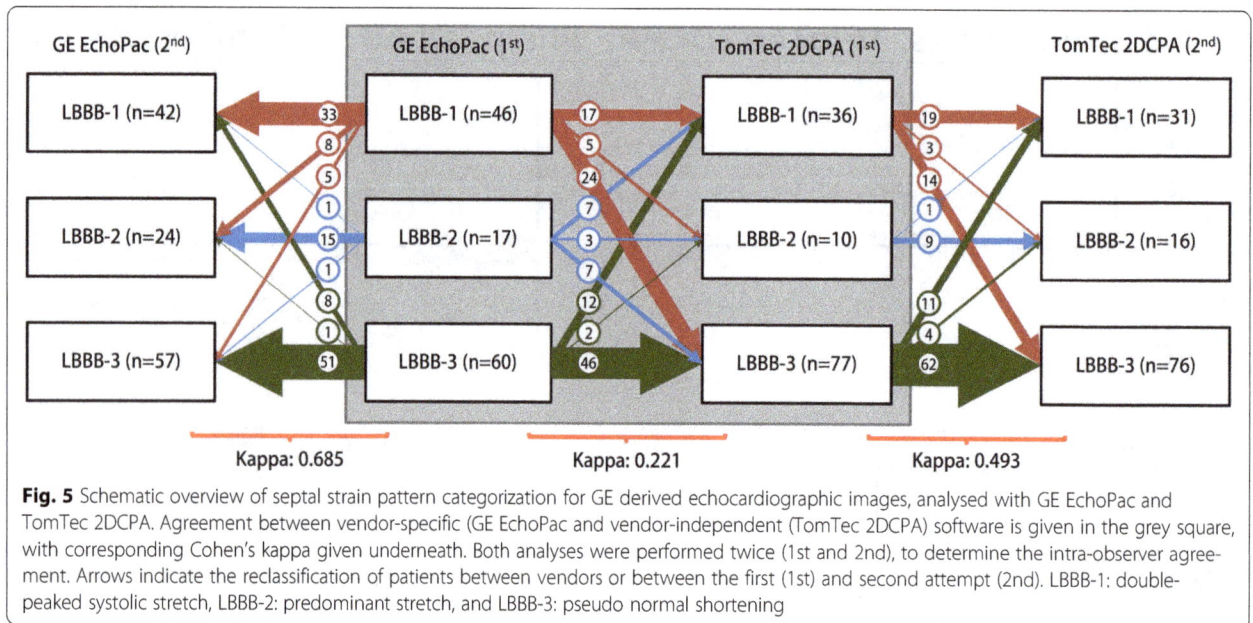

Fig. 5 Schematic overview of septal strain pattern categorization for GE derived echocardiographic images, analysed with GE EchoPac and TomTec 2DCPA. Agreement between vendor-specific (GE EchoPac and vendor-independent (TomTec 2DCPA) software is given in the grey square, with corresponding Cohen's kappa given underneath. Both analyses were performed twice (1st and 2nd), to determine the intra-observer agreement. Arrows indicate the reclassification of patients between vendors or between the first (1st) and second attempt (2nd). LBBB-1: double-peaked systolic stretch, LBBB-2: predominant stretch, and LBBB-3: pseudo normal shortening

and SSI (ICC: 0.421, COV: 1.024, Bland-Altman mean difference: −2.0 ± 2.4%, Fig. 4). Cohen's kappa coefficient of agreement on LBBB pattern categorization was poor (0.279). The Cohen's kappa coefficient of intra-observer agreement was good for both QLAB (0.612) and TomTec 2DCPA analysis (0.683) (Fig. 7).

Cross-correlation

Septal wall cross correlation was significantly lower compared to the LV and lateral wall for GE vs. TomTec (septum: 0.682 ± 0.290, LV: 0.835 ± 0.213, lateral wall: 0.800 ± 0.244, $p < 0.05$) and for Philips vs. TomTec ((septum: 0.712 ± 0.293, global LV: 0.898 ± 0.156, lateral wall: 0.827 ± 0.226, $p < 0.05$). There was no apparent statistical difference between the three subgroups based on image quality (Additional file 2: Table S1). Only for the lateral wall in GE vs. TomTec did the high-quality images (0.892 ± 0.123) have significantly higher R^2 compared to the poor-quality images (0.713 ± 0.312, $p < 0.05$).

Prediction of volumetric response
GE echocardiographic images

For GE derived images, GE EchoPac derived SRSsept, SSI, and LBBB pattern categorization showed a significant association with volumetric response to CRT in univariate analysis, while TomTec 2DCPA derived parameters did not (Table 4). The SL-delay showed no significant association with volumetric response. C-statistic values were comparable between GE EchoPac and TomTec 2DCPA Except for SSI, cut-off values for response prediction were higher for GE EchoPac (SL-delay: 144 ms,

SRSsept: 1.61% and SSI: 2.98%) compared to TomTec 2DCPA (SL-delay: -101 ms, SRSsept 0.46%, SSI: 3.72%).

Philips echocardiographic images

For Philips derived images, both Philips QLAB and TomTec 2DCPA showed a significant association with volumetric response to CRT for SRSsept, SSI and LBBB pattern categorization (Table 5). Only the SL-delay showed no significant association with volumetric response. The C-statistic values were overall reasonable (i.e. ranging from 0.564 to 0.705) and comparable between vendor dependent and independent analysis. The cut-off values for response prediction were apparently different, with lower values for Philips QLAB (SL-delay: 0 ms, SRSsept: 0.79% and SSI: 0.83%) compared to TomTec 2DCPA (SL-delay: -80 ms, SRSsept: 1.18% and SSI: 2.35%).

Discussion

Comparability of speckle tracking echocardiography platforms on apical four chamber LV peak and systolic strain is fair in patients with heart failure and dyssynchrony. We observed relevant differences in more specific strain parameters (i.e. pre-stretch, TTP_{max} and TTP_{first}) and indices representing dyssynchrony (i.e. SRSsept, SSI and SL-delay). Results on strain pattern categorization (i.e. LBBB patterns) were disappointing as agreement between vendors was low. However, the inter-observer agreement, using the same STE software twice, on strain pattern categorization was better. Although most dyssynchrony parameters showed a weak but significant association with changes in LV end-

Table 3 Strain parameters derived from Philips echocardiographic images

	Philips QLAB (n = 88)	TomTec 2DCPA (n = 88)	COV	ICC (p-value)	Bland-Altman (mean diff ±SD)
LV					
1) Pre-stretch (%)	0.0 (0.0–0.0)	0.0 (0.0–0.2)	4.125	−0.052 (0.684)	−0.1 ± 0.6
2) Peak strain (%)	−7.7 ± 2.7	−7.7 ± 3.3	−0.350	0.749 (<0.001)	0.0 ± 2.1
3) Systolic strain (%)	−6.8 ± 3.0	−7.0 ± 3.5	−0.435	0.802 (<0.001)	0.2 ± 2.0
4) TTP_{max} (ms)	527 (444–592)	492 (396–559)	0.185	0.376 (<0.001)	34 ± 113
5) TTP_{first} (ms)	361 (112–438)	361 (118–413)	0.567	0.165 (0.061)	2 ± 213
Septum					
1) Pre-stretch (%)	0.0 (0.0–0.0)	0.0 (0.0–0.4)	3.990	−0.035 (0.627)	−0.3 ± 0.9
2) Peak strain (%)	−7.6 ± 2.7	−8.0 ± 3.7	−0.363	0.626 (<0.001)	0.5 ± 2.8
3) Systolic strain (%)	−6.5 ± 3.0	−7.0 ± 3.9	−0.468	0.667 (<0.001)	0.5 ± 2.9
4) TTP_{max} (ms)	541 (442–598)	477 (346–575)	0.202	0.109 (0.155)	61 ± 179
5) TTP_{first} (ms)	361 (118–426)	161 (114–342)	0.534	0.232 (0.014)	84 ± 185
Lateral wall					
1) Pre-stretch (%)	0.0 (0.0–0.1)	0.3 (0.0–0.8)	2.728	0.324 (<0.001)	−0.5 ± 1.0
2) Peak strain (%)	−8.0 (−9.4 - -6.1)	−9.0 (−11.1 - -6.3)	−0.345	0.631 (<0.001)	1.3 ± 3.0
3) Systolic strain (%)	−6.4 (−9.0 - -5.2)	−8.0 (−11.1 - -4.9)	−0.436	0.680 (<0.001)	1.5 ± 3.0
4) TTP_{max} (ms)	542 (454–597)	476 (434–538)	0.175	0.531 (<0.001)	36 ± 87
5) TTP_{first} (ms)	376 (107–461)	433 (216–481)	0.550	0.060 (0.290)	−41 ± 239
Dyssynchrony					
a) SL-delay (ms)	0 (0–0)	−20 (−121–120)	−10.694	0.025 (0.409)	24 ± 180
b) SRSsept (%)	0.7 (0.3–1.2)	1.7 (0.6–3.3)	1.030	0.419 (<0.001)	−1.5 ± 2.1
c) SSI (%)	0.8 (0.4–1.5)	2.3 (1.1–4.2)	1.024	0.421 (<0.001)	−2.0 ± 2.4
d) LBBB type (n, %)					
LBBB-1	33 (38.4%)	33 (37.5%)			
LBBB-2	3 (3.5%)	11 (12.5%)			
LBBB-3	50 (58.1%)	44 (50.0%)			

Means and standard deviations are given with ± symbol, for non-normal distributed data, the median is given with the interquartile range between brackets
COV coefficient of variation, ICC intra-class correlation coefficient, diff: difference, SD standard deviation, LV strain derived from global LV in apical four chamber view, TTP_{max} time to maximal peak shortening, TTP_{first} time to first peak shortening, SL-delay time delay between septal and lateral peak shortening, SSI systolic stretch index, SRSsept septal systolic rebound stretch, LBBB type type of LBBB strain patterns, based on definition by Leenders et al. [23]

systolic volume, the cut-off values were apparently different. STE software of different vendors can therefore not be used interchangeably for more specific purposes than peak strain.

Vendor variability
To the best of our knowledge, this is the first study to compare results of different STE software packages, specifically for mechanical dyssynchrony in CRT-candidates. The average differences of peak strain and systolic strain were small and non-significant between vendor dependent and vendor independent STE packages. Nevertheless, TomTec had lower values compared to GE EchoPac and higher values compared to Philips QLAB. Unfortunately, we cannot define the source of discordance, as a gold-standard for deformation imaging (i.e. sonomicrometry) was not available in our study.

The relative high correlation for global longitudinal strain between STE platforms is in accordance with earlier publications [16]. There are currently no publications on vendor comparison studies on STE in patients with heart failure and dyssynchrony, besides a small comparative study by our own group [24]. Moreover, comparison to earlier publications on peak strain and timing values is difficult as previous studies implemented older versions of STE software, while we used the most recent versions. STE software is constantly under development, partly due to the STE standardization taskforce of the EACVI/ASE. This task force includes among its members representatives of several vendors. Their efforts resulted in small and acceptable differences between vendors for global longitudinal strain [16, 25]. However, the variability among vendors in more specific longitudinal strain features is not yet elucidated, nor is the exact

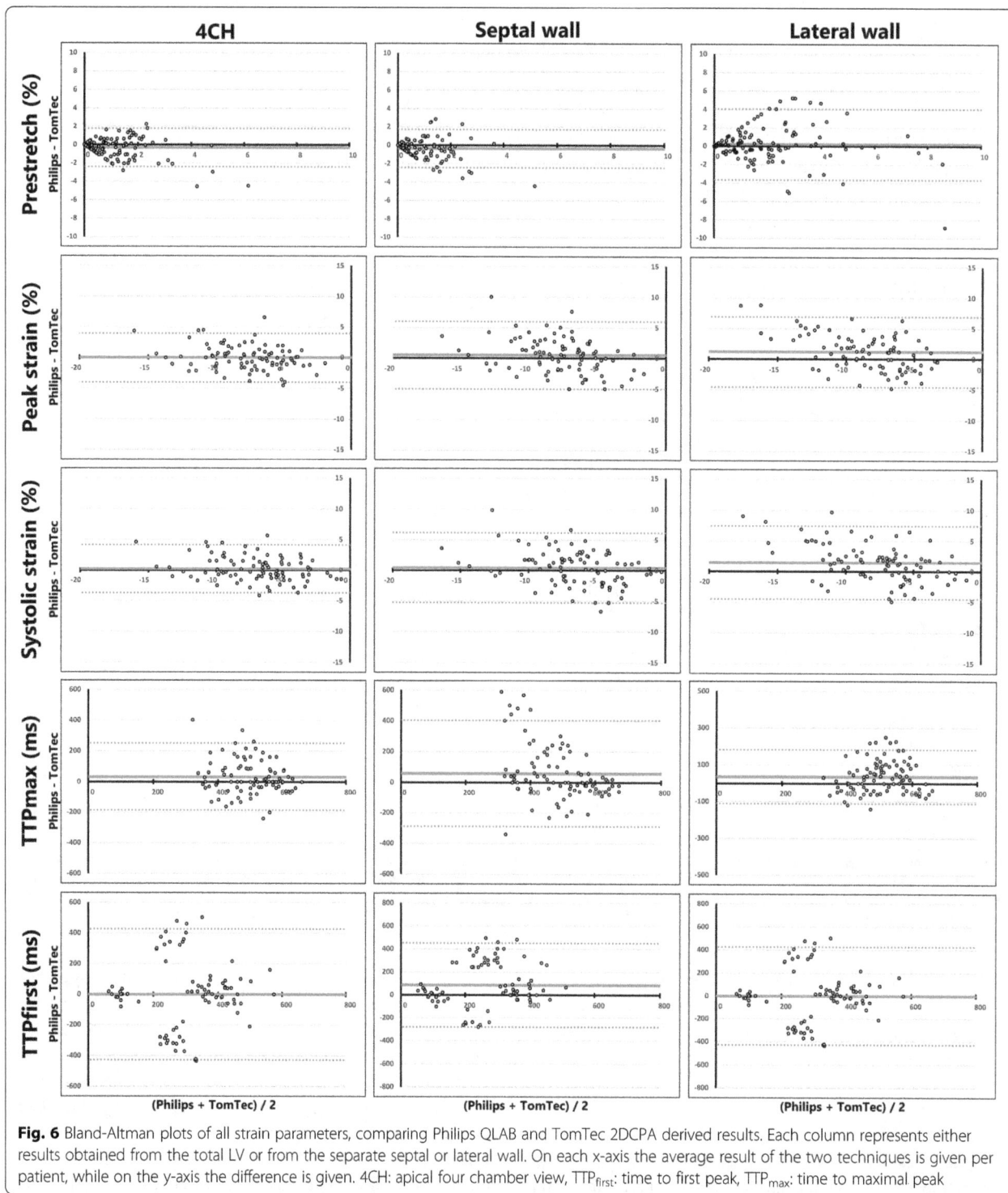

Fig. 6 Bland-Altman plots of all strain parameters, comparing Philips QLAB and TomTec 2DCPA derived results. Each column represents either results obtained from the total LV or from the separate septal or lateral wall. On each x-axis the average result of the two techniques is given per patient, while on the y-axis the difference is given. 4CH: apical four chamber view, TTP$_{first}$: time to first peak, TTP$_{max}$: time to maximal peak

bias between vendors with respect to regional strain assessment. Furthermore, the cohort studied for standardization consisted of a wide range of subjects (mean LVEF 60%, global longitudinal strain −19.2%) and is therefore not representative for CRT patients with dilated hearts, reduced LV function, and complex deformation characteristics [23]. Moreover, CRT patients can have suboptimal acoustic windows which affects image quality and reliability of strain analysis. In the current study, comparable 4CH peak longitudinal strain values were found in CRT patients, although the limits of agreement of Bland-Altman plots were relatively wide, and results for

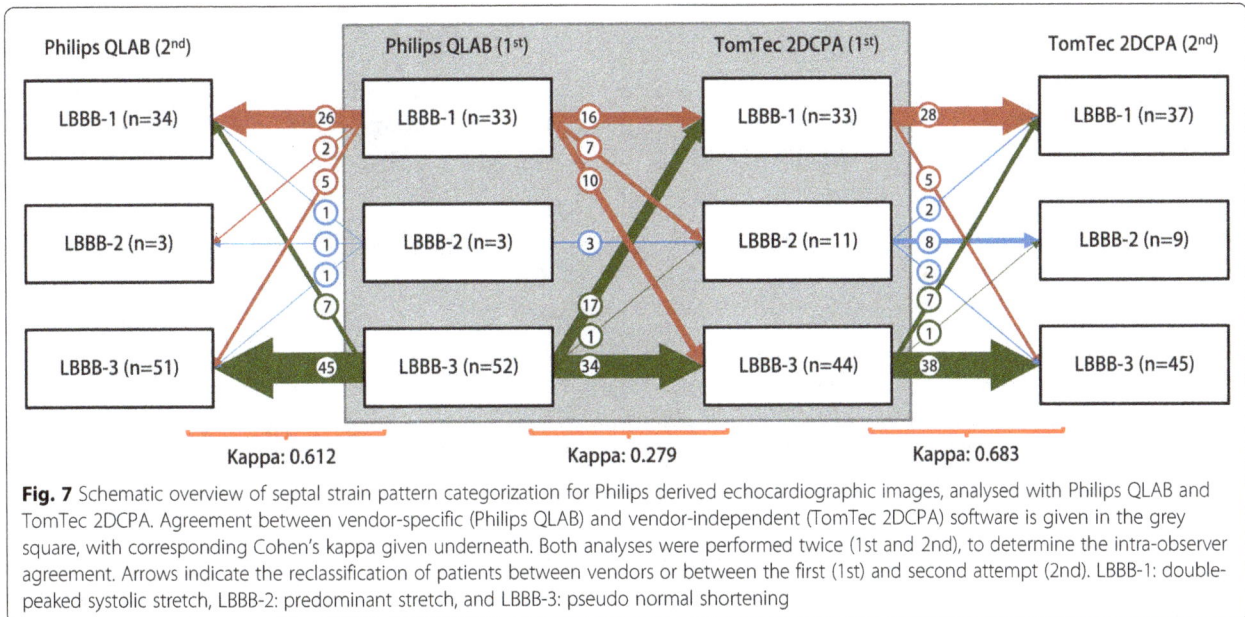

Fig. 7 Schematic overview of septal strain pattern categorization for Philips derived echocardiographic images, analysed with Philips QLAB and TomTec 2DCPA. Agreement between vendor-specific (Philips QLAB) and vendor-independent (TomTec 2DCPA) software is given in the grey square, with corresponding Cohen's kappa given underneath. Both analyses were performed twice (1st and 2nd), to determine the intra-observer agreement. Arrows indicate the reclassification of patients between vendors or between the first (1st) and second attempt (2nd). LBBB-1: double-peaked systolic stretch, LBBB-2: predominant stretch, and LBBB-3: pseudo normal shortening

individual patients varied significantly. The discrepancies between the current study and the publications by Farsalinos et al.. and Yang et al. may therefore be ascribed to the examined populations [16, 26]. A mechanistic modelling study showed higher variability in peak strain among vendors and a higher inter-observer variability in a dilated thin-walled LV [27]. This modelling study suggests a lower level of agreement among vendors in heart failure patients, which might explain the findings in our current observations.

Echocardiographic images and speckle tracking algorithms

Differences between manufacturers are largely attributed to discrepancies in STE algorithms. Albeit recently

thoroughly investigated, [16] the algorithms of the majority of commercially available speckle tracking software have lacked published validation [27]. They are furthermore not open-source. TomTec 2DCPA uses DICOM images and thereby imports images with lower frame rate and lower image quality compared to the raw image files used by the vendor dependent platforms. Lower frame rates influence temporal resolution, which hampers reliable assessment of both strain values and timing indices. The image quality directly influences spatial resolution, decreasing reliable tracking of speckles. TomTec also displays separate endo- and epicardial strain curves for each segment, and mean myocardial wall strain results are not given. The use of endocardial strain data might have caused a slight overestimation of peak strain values

Table 4 Prediction of volumetric response to CRT with GE derived echocardiographic images

Parameter	Univariate analysis ($n = 123$)			Receiver operating characteristics ($n = 123$)	
	B	SD	p-value	C-statistic	Cut-off value
GE SL-delay	0.820	12.997	0.950	0.512	0.144
TomTec SL-delay	22.334	13.081	0.091	0.573	−0.101
GE SRSsept	3.146	0.911	<0.001	0.599	1.614
TomTec SRSsept	0.503	1.362	0.713	0.544	0.455
GE SSI	2.296	0.653	<0.001	0.619	2.980
TomTec SSI	1.250	0.818	0.129	0.530	3.715
GE LBBB-type (type 1 or 2 vs. 3)	18.536	4.003	<0.001		
TomTec LBBB-type (type 1 or 2 vs. 3)	8.151	4.464	0.071		

Prediction of volumetric response to CRT, with results of univariate regression analysis (B, SD and *p*-value) and receiver operating characteristics (C-statistic, R^2 and cut-off). Univariate analyses are based on a change in LVESV on a continuous scale, while receiver operating characteristics are based on a cut-off of ≥15% reduction in LVESV

GE General Electric EchoPac, *TomTec* TomTec 2DCPA, *B* beta coefficient, *SD* standard deviation, *SL-delay* septal-to-lateral wall delay, *SRSsept* septal systolic rebound stretch, *SSI* systolic stretch index, *LBBB-type* septal strain pattern categorization according to Leenders et al

Table 5 Prediction of volumetric response to CRT with Philips derived echocardiographic images

Parameter	Univariate analysis (n = 88)			Receiver operating characteristics (n = 88)	
	B	SD	p-value	C-statistic	Cut-off value
Philips SL-delay	58.897	38.368	0.129	0.564	0.000
TomTec SL-delay	−23.910	16.952	0.162	0.569	−0.080
Philips SRSsept	10.072	2.653	<0.001	0.697	0.790
TomTec SRSsept	3.842	0.997	<0.001	0.686	1.180
Philips SSI	7.346	2.257	0.002	0.661	0.830
TomTec SSI	3.860	0.863	<0.001	0.705	2.345
Philips LBBB-type (type 1 or 2 vs. 3)	20.091	5.418	<0.001		
TomTec LBBB-type (type 1 or 2 vs. 3)	22.069	5.122	<0.001		

Prediction of volumetric response to CRT, with results of univariate regression analysis (B, SD and *p*-value) and receiver operating characteristics (C-statistic, R^2 and cut-off). Univariate analyses are based on a change in LVESV on a continuous scale, while receiver operating characteristics are based on a cut-off of ≥15% reduction in LVESV

Philips Philips QLAB, *TomTec* TomTec 2DCPA, *B* beta coefficient, *SD* standard deviation, *SL-delay* septal-to-lateral wall delay, *SRSsept* septal systolic rebound stretch, *SSI* systolic stretch index, *LBBB-type* septal strain pattern categorization according to Leenders et al

[22]. GE EchoPac uses 'global' wall myocardial strain by default, although users can choose between endocardial, epicardial or mid myocardial layers. Lastly, the method used by Philips QLAB is unknown, although a global myocardial based approach is likely. Timing of the reference length is also of importance for standardization, as differences in the onset of strain curves directly influences absolute strain values as wells as timing indices. As mentioned, timing of reference length was uniformed for TomTec analysis compared to both vendor dependent platforms.

Mechanical dyssynchrony indices

Absolute values of mechanical dyssynchrony indices were significantly lower for Philips, compared to TomTec. Whereas the results on dyssynchrony parameters obtained from GE images displayed higher values for GE compared to TomTec. Although the source of discordance is unknown, dyssynchrony seems underestimated by Philips QLAB speckle tracking algorithms. Underestimation of dyssynchrony is exemplified by results for the SL-delay obtained by Philips QLAB (median 0 ms, interquartile range 0 – 0 ms). The discrepancies of Philips QLAB with both other vendors are remarkable, as both GE EchoPac and TomTec 2DCPA displayed large variation for SL-delay. Moreover, as the Bland-Altman plot of SL-delay in Fig. 4 shows, the discrepancy between Philips QLAB and TomTec 2DCPA, a large number of results are on a line (y = −0.5*x), indicating a large variation in SL-delay for TomTec, while Philips values were mainly close to zero. Philips' derived septal and lateral wall strain curves were often quite similar, as can be appreciated in the example in Fig. 1. It seems that segmental strain curves are more smoothened by Philips QLAB. While no gold-standard for deformation imaging was applied, the relative absence of dyssynchrony obtained with Philips STE software is striking.

Although intra-observer agreement of strain pattern categorization is relatively good, strain pattern categorization showed apparent variations among vendors. Strain patterns were earlier found to be more robust between vendors [24]. This discrepancy could be attributed to changes in STE algorithms, as there were almost no LBBB type 2 patterns found by Philips. LBBB type 2 is the most distinctive septal deformation pattern, with predominant stretch almost in completely opposite direction to the lateral wall. Higher percentages of LBBB type 2 were observed in the same (i.e. Philips imaged) patient with TomTec. The cohorts of GE and Philips were not significantly different, and conventional dyssynchrony parameters such as apical rocking, septal flash and IVMD were comparable. Therefore, the relative absence of LBBB type 2 patterns is likely caused by the inability to detect dyssynchrony using QLAB. Given the above-mentioned differences in both continuous and categorical dyssynchrony parameters, one might postulate that STE with Philips QLAB is less suitable for detection of dyssynchrony in a CRT population. However, despite the lower values, the predictive value of Philips QLAB derived dyssynchrony parameters is at least comparable to the vendor independent analysis of TomTec 2DCPA. Although Philips QLAB and TomTec 2DCPA were able to predict volumetric response to CRT with the implemented dyssynchrony parameter, the cut-off values were different. Even though cut-off values for GE EchoPac derived parameters were higher, the values are different from earlier published values [3, 9]. These differences may be ascribed to the used software versions or the examined populations. Vendor specific cut-off values should therefore be used for each STE platform.

Echocardiographic image quality

Echocardiographic analysis in the current study was restricted to 4CH images, as speckle tracking analysis of these images is relevant for dyssynchrony in patients with left bundle branch block and has higher reproducibility [15]. However, echocardiographic 4CH images with adequate image quality can be difficult in patients with dilated hearts. Patient anatomy and cardiac size both complicate echocardiographic acquisition, as can be observed from the number of echocardiograms with poor image quality. Although this is not reflected in our results, lateral wall acquisition can be difficult in heart failure patients. It was surprising that lateral wall cross-correlation values were significantly higher compared to septal wall values for all vendors. Lower septal wall cross-correlation values can be explained by the higher complexity of septal strain patterns (i.e. LBBB type 1 and 2, Fig. 2). This in contrast to strain patterns of the lateral wall, which often had a similar shape between patients, also seen in the agreement on TTP_{max} for lateral wall strain. Complex septal deformation pattern can more easily be misinterpreted, resulting in lower correlations and wider limits of agreement in Bland-Altman plots. The poor agreement in septal strain analysis was also seen in the low Cohen's kappa values of septal strain pattern categorization.

Limitations

Although this study consists of relatively large subgroups, it is a sub-analysis with inherent limitations. However, images were prospectively collected for analysis with STE software. Nonetheless, patients underwent echocardiographic examination by a single vendor, which was assigned dependent of the centre of implantation and therefore non-randomized. Ideally patients would undergo echocardiographic examination by both vendors, making a direct comparison between GE and Philips possible. Moreover, there was no gold-standard used in this study, making it impossible to determine the source of variability. Test-retest variability was not part of the imaging protocol, although consecutive measurements are subject to variation [16]. Nevertheless, the large and comparable subgroups permitted a reliable comparison of vendors, and large differences were seen. This is in contrast to previous studies, in which most echocardiographic dyssynchrony parameters (i.e. SRSsept, SSI, and SL-delay) were tested solely on one vendor (i.e. GE EchoPac).

Clinical implications

Although global LV peak strain correlates reasonable between vendor systems, the results of individual patients between vendors may vary, as indicated by the wide limits of agreement in Bland-Altman plots. This variation hampers translation of deformation parameters obtained by STE to clinical practice. All three STE vendors were capable to predict response to CRT, using

the implemented dyssynchrony parameters. Although the diagnostic value of GE EchoPac derived parameters is well validated in prior studies, [10, 28] further work is needed to confirm the predictive value of these parameters in clinical practice. Differences between vendors can be large, hampering direct translation from pre-clinical work to the clinical implementation of speckle tracking derived dyssynchrony parameters and patterns in all echo laboratories, with a myriad of echo-machines. We recommend that in patients eligible for CRT, clinicians should use reference and cut-off values specific to the STE vendor.

Conclusions

This study proves the general fair comparability of longitudinal peak strain, although results for individual cases and more complex strain parameters can differ significantly. Moreover, we have demonstrated that dyssynchrony parameters derived with different vendors are associated with volumetric response to CRT, but that cut-off values do not correlate well between vendors. While the standardization taskforce took an important first step for global peak strain, further standardization of STE in patients eligible for CRT is still warranted.

Abbreviations

4CH: Apical four chamber view; ASE: American Society of Echocardiography; COV: Coefficient of variation; CRT: Cardiac resynchronization therapy; EACVI: European Association of Cardiovascular Imaging; ESV: End-systolic volume; GE: General Electric; ICC: Intra-class correlation coefficient; IVMD: Interventricular mechanical dyssynchrony; LBBB: Left bundle branch block; LV: Left ventricular; MARC: Markers and Response to Cardiac Resynchronization Therapy; R^2: Coefficient of determination; ROI: Region of interest; SL-delay: Septal to lateral wall delay; SRSsept: Systolic rebound stretch of the septum; SSI: Systolic stretch index; STE: Speckle tracking echocardiography; TTP_{first}: Time to first peak; TTP_{max}: Time to maximal peak

Acknowledgements

The authors would like to acknowledge Diana J.Z. Dalemans for her contribution to this study, by importing a considerable proportion of echocardiograms.

Funding

This research was performed within the framework of CTMM, the Centre for Translational Molecular Medicine (www.ctmm.nl), project COHFAR (grant 01C-203), and supported by the Dutch Heart Foundation.

Authors' contributions

WE and MC analyzed and interpreted the patient data regarding the echocardiograms and speckle tracking analysis. AM, KV, MM, FL and CA were local principal investigators. IG and MV were central principal investigators. BG and MR performed the statistical analyses. WE, MC, and AT were a major contributor in writing the manuscript. All authors read and approved the final manuscript.

Consent for publication
Not applicable.

Competing interests
Dr. Vernooy reports consultancy for Medtronic; research grants from Medtronic; speaker fees from St. Jude Medical. Dr. Maass reports lecture fees from Medtronic and LivaNova. Dr. Vos reports funding from CTMM COHFAR, CVON Predict, EU TrigTreat, EU CERT-ICD and GiLead to perform (pre)clinical studies. All other authors declare that they have no conflict of interests.

Author details
[1]Department of Cardiology, University Medical Centre Utrecht, P.O. Box 855500, 3508, GA, Utrecht, The Netherlands. [2]Department of Cardiology, Thoraxcenter, University of Groningen, University Medical Centre Groningen, Groningen, The Netherlands. [3]Department of Cardiology, Maastricht University Medical Centre, Maastricht, The Netherlands. [4]Department of Cardiology, VU University Medical Centre, Amsterdam, The Netherlands. [5]Department of Cardiology, Academic Medical Centre, Amsterdam, The Netherlands. [6]Department of Medical Physiology, University of Utrecht, Utrecht, The Netherlands.

References
1. Teske AJ, De Boeck BW, Melman PG, Sieswerda GT, Doevendans PA, Cramer MJ. Echocardiographic quantification of myocardial function using tissue deformation imaging, a guide to image acquisition and analysis using tissue Doppler and speckle tracking. Cardiovasc Ultrasound. 2007;5:27.
2. Schroeder J, Hamada S, Grundlinger N, Rubeau T, Altiok E, Ulbrich K, Keszei A, Marx N, Becker M. Myocardial deformation by strain echocardiography identifies patients with acute coronary syndrome and non-diagnostic ECG presenting in a chest pain unit: a prospective study of diagnostic accuracy. Clin Res Cardiol. 2016;105(3):248–56.
3. De Boeck BW, Teske AJ, Meine M, Leenders GE, Cramer MJ, Prinzen FW, Doevendans PA. Septal rebound stretch reflects the functional substrate to cardiac resynchronization therapy and predicts volumetric and neurohormonal response. Eur J Heart Fail. 2009;11(9):863–71.
4. Khan FZ, Virdee MS, Palmer CR, Pugh PJ, O'Halloran D, Elsik M, Read PA, Begley D, Fynn SP, Dutka DP. Targeted left ventricular lead placement to guide cardiac resynchronization therapy: the TARGET study: a randomized, controlled trial. J Am Coll Cardiol. 2012;59(17):1509–18.
5. van Deursen CJ, Wecke L, van Everdingen WM, Stahlberg M, Janssen MH, Braunschweig F, Bergfeldt L, Crijns HJ, Vernooy K, Prinzen FW. Vectorcardiography for optimization of stimulation intervals in cardiac resynchronization therapy. J Cardiovasc Transl Res. 2015;8(2):128–37.
6. Leenders GE, Cramer MJ, Bogaard MD, Meine M, Doevendans PA, De Boeck BW. Echocardiographic prediction of outcome after cardiac resynchronization therapy: conventional methods and recent developments. Heart Fail Rev. 2011;16(3):235–50.
7. van Everdingen WM, Schipper JC, van 't Sant J, Ramdat Misier K, Meine M, Cramer MJ. Echocardiography and cardiac resynchronisation therapy, friends or foes? Neth Hear J. 2016;24(1):25–38.
8. Daubert JC, Saxon L, Adamson PB, Auricchio A, Berger RD, Beshai JF, Breithard O, Brignole M, Cleland J, DeLurgio DB, et al. 2012 EHRA/HRS expert consensus statement on cardiac resynchronization therapy in heart failure: implant and follow-up recommendations and management. Europace. 2012;14(9):1236–86.
9. Lumens J, Tayal B, Walmsley J, Delgado-Montero A, Huntjens PR, Schwartzman D, Althouse AD, Delhaas T, Prinzen FW, Gorcsan J 3rd. Differentiating electromechanical from non-electrical substrates of mechanical Discoordination to identify responders to cardiac resynchronization therapy. Circ Cardiovasc Imaging. 2015;8(9):e003744.
10. Leenders GE, De Boeck BW, Teske AJ, Meine M, Bogaard MD, Prinzen FW, Doevendans PA, Cramer MJ. Septal rebound stretch is a strong predictor of outcome after cardiac resynchronization therapy. J Card Fail. 2012;18(5):404–12
11. Marechaux S, Guiot A, Castel AL, Guyomar Y, Semichon M, Delelis F, Heuls S, Ennezat PV, Graux P, Tribouilloy C. Relationship between two-dimensional speckle-tracking septal strain and response to cardiac resynchronization therapy in patients with left ventricular dysfunction and left bundle branch block: a prospective pilot study. J Am Soc Echocardiogr. 2014;27(5):501 11.
12. Risum N, Tayal B, Hansen TF, Bruun NE, Jensen MT, Lauridsen TK, Saba S, Kisslo J, Gorcsan J 3rd, Sogaard P. Identification of typical left bundle branch block contraction by strain echocardiography is additive to electrocardiography in prediction of long-term outcome after cardiac resynchronization therapy. J Am Coll Cardiol. 2015;66(6):631–41.
13. Riffel JH, Keller MG, Aurich M, Sander Y, Andre F, Giusca S, Aus dem siepen F, Seitz S, Galuschky C, Korosoglou G, et al. Assessment of global longitudinal strain using standardized myocardial deformation imaging: a modality independent software approach. Clin Res Cardiol. 2015;104(7):591–602.
14. Koopman LP, Slorach C, Hui W, Manlhiot C, McCrindle BW, Friedberg MK, Jaeggi ET, Mertens L. Comparison between different speckle tracking and color tissue Doppler techniques to measure global and regional myocardial deformation in children. J Am Soc Echocardiogr. 2010;23(9):919–28.
15. Negishi K, Lucas S, Negishi T, Hamilton J, Marwick TH. What is the primary source of discordance in strain measurement between vendors: imaging or analysis? Ultrasound Med Biol. 2013;39(4):714–20.
16. Farsalinos KE, Daraban AM, Unlu S, Thomas JD, Badano LP, Voigt JU. Head-to-head comparison of global longitudinal strain measurements among nine different vendors: the EACVI/ASE inter-vendor comparison study. J Am Soc Echocardiogr. 2015;28(10):1171–81. e1172
17. Maass AH, Vernooy K, Wijers SC, van 't Sant J, Cramer MJ, Meine M, Allaart CP, De Lange FJ, Prinzen FW, Gerritse B, et al. Refining success of cardiac resynchronization therapy using a simple score predicting the amount of reverse ventricular remodelling: results from the markers and response to CRT (MARC) study. Europace. 2017. doi:10.1093/europace/euw445. (Epub ahead of print)
18. Brignole M, Auricchio A, Baron-Esquivias G, Bordachar P, Boriani G, Breithardt OA, Cleland J, Deharo JC, Delgado V, Elliott PM, et al. 2013 ESC guidelines on cardiac pacing and cardiac resynchronization therapy. Eur Heart J. 2013;34(29):2281–329.
19. Russo AM, Stainback RF, Bailey SR, Epstein AE, Heidenreich PA, Jessup M, Kapa S, Kremers MS, Lindsay BD, Stevenson LW. ACCF/HRS/AHA/ASE/HFSA/SCAI/SCCT/SCMR 2013 appropriate use criteria for implantable cardioverter-defibrillators and cardiac resynchronization therapy: a report of the American College of Cardiology Foundation appropriate use criteria task force, Heart Rhythm Society, American Heart Association, American Society of Echocardiography, Heart Failure Society of America, Society for Cardiovascular Angiography and Interventions, Society of Cardiovascular Computed Tomography, and Society for Cardiovascular Magnetic Resonance. J Am Coll Cardiol. 2013;61(12):1318–68.
20. Lang RM, Badano LP, Mor-Avi V, Afilalo J, Armstrong A, Ernande L, Flachskampf FA, Foster E, Goldstein SA, Kuznetsova T, et al. Recommendations for cardiac chamber quantification by echocardiography in adults: an update from the American Society of Echocardiography and the European Association of Cardiovascular Imaging. Eur Heart J Cardiovasc Imaging. 2015;16(3):233–70.
21. Cerqueira MD, Weissman NJ, Dilsizian V, Jacobs AK, Kaul S, Laskey WK, Pennell DJ, Rumberger JA, Ryan T, Verani MS. Standardized myocardial segmentation and nomenclature for tomographic imaging of the heart: a statement for healthcare professionals from the cardiac imaging Committee of the Council on clinical cardiology of the American Heart Association. Circulation. 2002;105(4):539–42.
22. Leitman M, Lysiansky M, Lysyansky P, Friedman Z, Tyomkin V, Fuchs T, Adam D, Krakover R, Vered Z. Circumferential and longitudinal strain in 3 myocardial layers in normal subjects and in patients with regional left ventricular dysfunction. J Am Soc Echocardiogr. 2010;23(1):64–70.
23. Leenders GE, Lumens J, Cramer MJ, De Boeck BW, Doevendans PA, Delhaas T, Prinzen FW. Septal deformation patterns delineate mechanical dyssynchrony and regional differences in contractility: analysis of patient data using a computer model. Circulation Heart failure. 2012;5(1):87–96.
24. van Everdingen WM, Paiman ML, van Deursen CJ, Cramer MJ, Vernooy K, Delhaas T, Prinzen FW. Comparison of septal strain patterns in dyssynchronous heart failure between speckle tracking echocardiography vendor systems. J Electrocardiol. 2015;48(4):609–16.
25. Voigt JU, Pedrizzetti G, Lysyansky P, Marwick TH, Houle H, Baumann R, Pedri S, Ito Y, Abe Y, Metz S, et al. Definitions for a common standard for 2D speckle tracking echocardiography: consensus document of the EACVI/ASE/industry task force to standardize deformation imaging. J Am Soc Echocardiogr. 2015;28(2):183–93.
26. Yang H, Marwick TH, Fukuda N, Oe H, Saito M, Thomas JD, Negishi K. Improvement in strain concordance between two major vendors after the strain standardization initiative. J Am Soc Echocardiogr. 2015;28(6):642–8. e647

10

Different determinants of exercise capacity in HFpEF compared to HFrEF

Arlind Batalli[1,2], Pranvera Ibrahimi[1,3], Ibadete Bytyçi[1], Artan Ahmeti[1,2], Edmond Haliti[1,2], Shpend Elezi[2], Michael Y. Henein[3,4] and Gani Bajraktari[1,2,3]*

Abstract

Background: Quality of life is as important as survival in heart failure (HF) patients. Controversies exist with regards to echocardiographic determinants of exercise capacity in HF, particularly in patients with preserved ejection fraction (HFpEF). The aim of this study was to prospectively examine echocardiographic parameters that correlate and predict functional exercise capacity assessed by 6 min walk test (6-MWT) in patients with HFpEF.

Methods: In 111 HF patients (mean age 63 ± 10 years, 47% female), an echo-Doppler study and a 6-MWT were performed in the same day. Patients were divided into two groups based on the 6-MWT distance (Group I: ≤ 300 m and Group II: >300 m).

Results: Group I were older ($p = 0.008$), had higher prevalence of diabetes ($p = 0.027$), higher baseline heart rate ($p = 0.004$), larger left atrium - LA ($p = 0.001$), longer LV filling time - FT ($p = 0.019$), shorter isovolumic relaxation time ($p = 0.037$), shorter pulmonary artery acceleration time - PA acceleration time ($p = 0.006$), lower left atrial lateral wall myocardial velocity (a') ($p = 0.018$) and lower septal systolic myocardial velocity (s') ($p = 0.023$), compared with Group II. Patients with HF and reduced EF (HFrEF) had lower hemoglobin ($p = 0.007$), higher baseline heart rate ($p = 0.005$), higher NT-ProBNP ($p = 0.001$), larger LA ($p = 0.004$), lower septal s', e', a' waves, and septal mitral annular plane systolic excursion (MAPSE), shorter PA acceleration time ($p < 0.001$ for all), lower lateral MAPSE, higher E/A & E/e', and shorter LVFT ($p = 0.001$ for all), lower lateral e' ($p = 0.009$), s' ($p = 0.006$), right ventricular e' and LA emptying fraction ($p = 0.012$ for both), compared with HFpEF patients.

In multivariate analysis, only LA diameter [2.676 (1.242–5.766), $p = 0.012$], and diabetes [0.274 (0.084–0.898), $p = 0.033$] independently predicted poor 6-MWT performance in the group as a whole. In HFrEF, age [1.073 (1.012–1.137), $p = 0.018$] and LA diameter [3.685 (1.348–10.071), $p = 0.011$], but in HFpEF, lateral s' [0.295 (0.099–0.882), $p = 0.029$], and hemoglobin level [0.497 (0.248–0.998), $p = 0.049$] independently predicted poor 6-MWT performance.

Conclusions: In HF patients determinants of exercise capacity differ according to severity of overall LV systolic function, with left atrial enlargement in HFrEF and longitudinal systolic shortening in HFpEF as the the main determinants.

Keywords: Six-minute walk test, Doppler echocardiography, Heart failure, HFpEF, Exercise capacity

Background

Despite advances in the diagnosis and treatment of heart failure (HF), it still presents a major public health problem [1], with increased incidence [2, 3] and poor prognosis [4–6]. In patients with HF and reduced left ventricular (LV) ejection fraction (HFrEF) several echo parameters correlated with functional capacity [7–16]. In contrast, in patients with HF and preserved LV EF (HFpEF), determinants of functional capacity are not well investigated [15–18]. Exercise capacity has been objectively assessed in the setting of HF using the six-min walk test (6-MWT) [19]. While several echocardiographic markers at rest predicted limited exercise capacity in patients with HFrEF [7–16], none of them correlate with functional capacity in those with HFpEF [15, 17]. The aim of this study was to prospectively examine whether 6-MWT results correlate with

* Correspondence: gani.bajraktari@umu.se; ganibajraktari@yahoo.co.uk
[1]Clinic of Cardiology, University Clinical Centre of Kosova, "Rrethi i Spitalit", p.n., Prishtina, Kosovo
[2]Medical Faculty, University of Prishtina, Prishtina, Kosovo
Full list of author information is available at the end of the article

Table 1 Patients with limited exercise vs. good exercise capacity (6-MWT distance)

Variable	All patients (n = 111)	6MWT > 300 m (n = 70)	6MWT ≤ 300 m (n = 41)	P value
Clinical and biochemical data				
Age (years)	63 ± 10	61 ± 10	66 ± 9	0.008
Female (%)	47	41	56	0.135
Smoking (%)	31.5	30	34	0.676
Diabetes (%)	28	20	41	0.027
Arterial hypertension (%)	69.4	68.6	70.7	0.835
Waist/hips ratio	0.97 ± 0.06	0.96 ± 0.06	0.98 ± 0.05	0.064
BMI (kg/m²)	28.6 ± 4.1	28.7 ± 4.2	28.4 ± 3.8	0.764
BSA (m²)	1.13 ± 0.2	1.15 ± 0.1	1.08 ± 0.1	0.067
Fasting glucose (mmol/L)	6.8 ± 2.8	6.4 ± 2.4	7.9 ± 2.9	0.009
Total cholesterol (mmol/L)	4.9 ± 1.2	4.9 ± 1.1	4.8 ± 1.2	0.439
Triglycerides (mmol/L)	1.7 ± 0.7	1.7 ± 0.7	1.6 ± 0.8	0.747
Creatinine (µmol/L)	96 ± 46	98 ± 56	93 ± 21	0.527
Hemoglobin (g/dl)	12.7 ± 1.8	12.8 ± 1.6	12.3 ± 2.0	0.166
NT-ProBNP (pg/mL)	1178 ± 1635	970 ± 1286	1534 ± 2072	0.124
Baseline heart rate (beats/min)	74 ± 16	71 ± 15	80 ± 13	0.004
Echocardiographic data				
Ejection fraction (%)	47 ± 15	48 ± 14	45 ± 15	0.409
IVSd (cm)	1.1 ± 0.2	1.1 ± 0.2	1.11 ± 0.1	0.923
Left atrium (cm)	4.4 ± 0.8	4.2 ± 0.7	4.8 ± 0.9	0.001
LV EDD (cm)	5.8 ± 1.0	5.7 ± 0.8	5.9 ± 1.1	0.319
LV ESD (cm)	4.4 ± 1.2	4.2 ± 1.1	4.5 ± 1.3	0.281
Lateral MAPSE (cm)	1.15 ± 0.4	1.2 ± 0.4	1.05 ± 0.3	0.051
Septal MAPSE (cm)	1.0 ± 0.3	1.0 ± 0.3	0.9 ± 0.2	0.054
TAPSE (cm)	2.15 ± 0.5	2.2 ± 0.4	2.1 ± 0.5	0.466
LVPWd (cm)	1.05 ± 0.15	1.05 ± 0.2	1.05 ± 0.1	0.960
LVM (g)	266 ± 85	260 ± 75	279 ± 101	0.324
LVMI (g/m²·⁷)	58 ± 21	53 ± 16	67 ± 26	0.006
E/A ratio	1.05 ± 0.7	1.0 ± 0.7	1.1 ± 0.8	0.414
E wave DT	174 ± 49	178 ± 50	167 ± 44	0.228
Filling time (ms)	414 ± 132	434 ± 141	376 ± 104	0.019
IVRT (ms)	126 ± 41	131 ± 42	110 ± 34	0.037
PA acceleration time (ms)	110 ± 24	114 ± 23	100 ± 21	0.006
E/e' ratio	11 ± 5.9	10 ± 4.1	13 ± 8.0	0.053
Lateral e' (cm/s)	6.1 ± 2.1	6.1 ± 2.4	6.0 ± 2.6	0.817
Lateral a'(cm/s)	7.9 ± 3.6	8.1 ± 3.7	7.5 ± 3.5	0.461
Lateral s' (cm/s)	5.3 ± 1.6	5.5 ± 1.5	4.9 ± 1.6	0.101
Septal e' (cm/s)	4.9 ± 2.2	5.1 ± 2.2	4.6 ± 2.1	0.312
Septal a' (cm/s)	7.15 ± 2.3	7.5 ± 2.4	6.4 ± 1.8	0.018
Septal s' (cm/s)	4.4 ± 1.5	4.6 ± 1.6	4.0 ± 1.0	0.023
Right e' (cm/s)	8.7 ± 3.0	8.9 ± 3.1	8.3 ± 2.7	0.305
Right a' (cm/s)	12.5 ± 4.4	12.7 ± 4.3	11.8 ± 4.3	0.333
Right s' (cm/s)	8.8 ± 3.0	9.8 ± 2.8	8.0 ± 3.2	0.086
LAV max (ml)	73 ± 35	68 ± 26	80 ± 47	0.218
LAV min (ml)	40 ± 29	35 ± 20	49 ± 38	0.067
LA EF (%)	47 ± 18	49 ± 17	45 ± 16	0.314

LV left ventricle, *EDD* end-diastolic dimension, *ESD* end-systolic dimension, *DT* deceleration time, *FT* filling time, *ET* Ejection time, *HR* heart rate, *IVSd* interventricular septum in diastole, *LVPWd* left ventricular posterior wall in diastole, *MAPSE* mitral annular plane systolic excursion, *TAPSE* tricuspid annular plane systolic excursion, *PA* pulmonary artery, *A* atrial diastolic velocity, *E* early diastolic filling velocity, *e'* early diastolic myocardial velocity, *s'* systolic myocardial velocity, *LA* left atrium, *LAV max* left atrial maximal volume, *LAV min* left atrial minimal volume, *LA EF* left atrial emptying fraction, *LVM* left ventricular mass, *LVMI* left ventricular mass index

Table 2 Comparison of patients' data between patients HFpEF and HFrEF

Variable	HFpEF (n = 55)	HFrEF (n = 56)	P value
Clinical and biochemical data			
Age (years)	63 ± 6.8	62 ± 12	0.767
Body-mass index (kg/m²)	29 ± 4	28 ± 3.6	0.130
Waist/hips ratio	0.96 ± 0.06	0.96 ± 0.06	0.996
Fasting glucose (mmol/L)	7.1 ± 3.1	6.7 ± 2.3	0.462
Total cholesterol (mmol/L)	5.1 ± 1.1	4.7 ± 1.1	0.054
Triglycerides (mmol/L)	1.8 ± 0.7	1.5 ± 0.7	0.137
Creatinine (μmol/L)	87 ± 16	105 ± 63	0.052
Hemoglobin (g/dL)	12.8 ± 1.9	12.4 ± 1.5	0.078
Baseline heart rate (beats/min)	70 ± 15	79 ± 15	0.005
NT-ProBNP (pg/mL)	681 ± 1280	1665 ± 1801	0.001
6-min walk distance (m)	339 ± 106	282 ± 119	0.010
PPV of 6-min walk distance (%)	56 ± 19	45 ± 20	0.004
Echocardiographic data			
IVSd (cm)	1.1 ± 0.1	1.1 ± 0.2	0.666
Left atrium (cm)	4.2 ± 0.8	4.6 ± 0.7	0.004
LV EDD (cm)	5.2 ± 0.7	6.3 ± 0.9	<0.001
LV ESD (cm)	3.5 ± 0.7	5.1 ± 1	<0.001
EDV (ml)	135 ± 44	213 ± 67	<0.001
ESV (ml)	56 ± 8.7	140 ± 52	<0.001
LV EF (%)	59.6 ± 8.7	35 ± 7.5	<0.001
Lateral MAPSE (cm)	1.27 ± 0.3	1.02 ± 0.4	0.001
Septal MAPSE (cm)	1.14 ± 0.2	0.85 ± 0.2	<0.001
TAPSE (cm)	2.3 ± 0.4	2.1 ± 0.5	0.062
LVPWd (cm)	1.05 ± 0.2	1.06 ± 0.2	0.688
E/A ratio	0.81 ± 0.3	1.3 ± 0.9	0.001
LVM (g)	224 ± 69	310 ± 77	<0.001
LVMI (g/m²·⁷)	50 ± 16	67 ± 23	<0.001
E wave DT	189 ± 44	159 ± 49	0.002
Filling time (ms)	454 ± 147	372 ± 99	0.001
IVRT (ms)	122 ± 39	130 ± 43	0.407
PA acceleration time (ms)	118 ± 20	101 ± 23	<0.001
E/e' ratio	9.4 ± 4.7	13.5 ± 6.4	0.001
Lateral e' (cm/s)	6.7 ± 2.6	5.3 ± 2.2	0.009
Lateral a' (cm/s)	8.6 ± 3.3	7.1 ± 3.8	0.051
Lateral s' (cm/s)	5.7 ± 1.3	4.8 ± 1.7	0.006
Septal e' (cm/s)	5.7 ± 2.5	4.0 ± 1.1	<0.001
Septal a' (cm/s)	7.9 ± 2.1	6.2 ± 2.0	<0.001
Septal s' (cm/s)	4.9 ± 1.6	3.8 ± 0.9	<0.001
Right e' (cm/s)	9.4 ± 3.2	7.9 ± 2.4	0.012
Right a' (cm/s)	12.7 ± 4.5	12.2 ± 4.2	0.593
Right s' (cm/s)	9.1 ± 3.1	8.3 ± 2.7	0.187
LAV max	62 ± 23	83 ± 57	0.005
LAV min	29 ± 18	51 ± 34	<0.001
LA EF (%)	53 ± 15	43 ± 18	0.012

LV left ventricle, EDD end-diastolic dimension, ESD end-systolic dimension, DT deceleration time, FT filling time, ET Ejection time, HR heart rate, IVSd interventricular septum in diastole, LVPWd left ventricular posterior wall in diastole, MAPSE mitral annular plane systolic excursion, TAPSE tricuspid annular plane systolic excursion, PA pulmonary artery, A atrial diastolic velocity, E early diastolic filling velocity, e' early diastolic myocardial velocity, s' systolic myocardial velocity, LA left atrial, LAV max left atrial maximal volume, LAV min left atrial minimal volume, LA EF left atrial eemptying fraction, LVM left ventricular mass, LVMI left ventricular mass index, PPV percentage of the predicted value

cardiac function parameters in a consecutive group of patients with HF and to identify possible determinants of exercise capacity in those with HFpEF.

Methods

Study population

We studied 111 patients (mean age 63 ± 10 years, 47% female), with clinical diagnosis of HF, and New York Heart Association (NYHA) functional class I-III, secondary to ischemic or non-ischemic etiology. Patients were referred to the Clinic of Cardiology, University Clinical Centre of Kosova, between May 2013 and June 2016. At the time of the study all patients were on optimum HF medications, optimized at least 2 weeks prior to enrollment, based on patient's symptoms and renal function: 82% were receiving ACE inhibitors or ARB, 78% beta-blockers, 12% calcium-blockers, 10% digoxin, 52% spironolactone, 62% diuretics. Patients with HFrEF had ischemic aetiology in 45%, hypertensive in 38%, and unknown aetiology in 17%. Patients with HFpEF had ischemic aetiology in 41% and hypertensive in 59%. All patients were in sinus rhythm. Patients with clinical evidence for cardiac decompensation, limited physical activity due to factors other than cardiac symptoms (e.g. arthritis), more than moderate mitral regurgitation, more than mild renal failure, chronic obstructive pulmonary disease or those with recent acute coronary syndrome, stroke or anemia were excluded. Patients gave a written informed consent to participate in the study, which was approved by the local Ethics Committee.

Data collection

Detailed history and clinical assessment were obtained in all patients, in whom routine biochemical tests were also performed including hemoglobin, lipid profile, blood glucose level, and kidney function tests. Estimated body mass index (BMI) was calculated from weight and height measurements. Waist, hip measurements were also made and waist/hip ratio was calculated.

Echocardiographic examination

A single operator performed all echocardiographic examinations using a Philips Intelligent E-33 system with a multifrequency transducer, and harmonic imaging as appropriate. Images were obtained with the patient in the left lateral decubitus position and during quiet expiration. Measurements of interventricular septal thickness, posterior wall thickness, and LV dimensions were made at end-diastole and end-systole, as recommended by the American Society of Echocardiography [19]. LV mass (LVM) was calculated

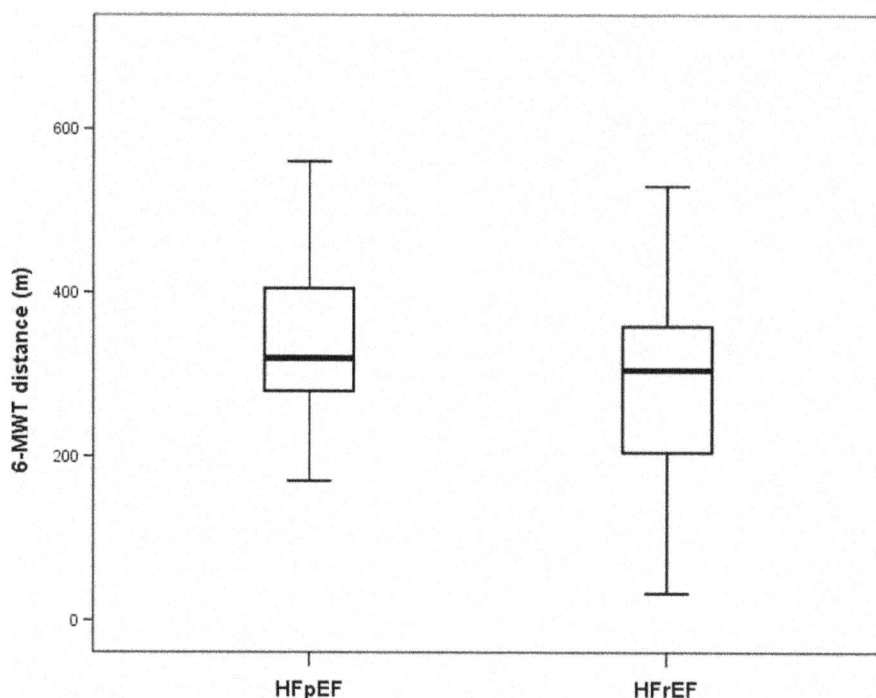

Fig. 1 Six-minute walk test (6-MWT) distance in patients with heart failure and preserved ejection fraction (HFpEF) and in patients with heart failure and reduced ejection fraction (HFrEF)

using the Devereux formula [20] and normalized to body surface area (LV mass index [LVMI]).

LV volumes and EF were calculated from the apical 2 and 4 chamber views using the modified Simpson's method. Ventricular long axis motion was studied by placing the M-mode cursor at the lateral and septal angles of the mitral ring and the lateral angle of the tricuspid ring. Total amplitude of long axis motion was measured as previously described [21] from peak inward to peak outward points. LV and right ventricular (RV) long axis myocardial velocities were also studied using Doppler myocardial imaging technique. From the apical 4-chamber view, longitudinal velocities were recorded with the sample volume placed at the basal part of LV lateral and septal segments as well as RV free wall. Systolic (s'), as well as early and late (e' and a') diastolic myocardial velocities were measured with the gain optimally adjusted. Mean value of lateral and septal LV velocities were calculated.

Left atrial diameter was measured from aortic root recordings with the M-mode cursor positioned at the level of the aortic valve leaflets. LA volumes were measured using area-length method from the apical four chamber views, according to the guidelines of the American Society of Echocardiography and European Association of Echocardiography [22]. Left atrial maximal volume (LAV max) was measured at the end of LV systole, just before the opening of the mitral valve, LA minimal volume (LAV

min) was measured at end diastole, right after mitral valve closure. LA emptying fraction (LA EF) was calculated with the formula [22, 23]:

$$LA\ total\ emptying\ fraction$$
$$= LAV\ max - LAV\ min/LAV\ max \times 100$$

Diastolic LV and RV function was assessed from filling velocities using spectral pulsed wave Doppler with the sample volume positioned at the tips of the mitral and tricuspid valve leaflets, respectively, during a brief apnea. Peak LV and RV early (E wave) and late (A wave) diastolic velocities were measured and E/A ratios were calculated. E wave deceleration time (DT) was also measured from peak E wave to the end of its deceleration in all study patients. The E/e' ratio was calculated from the transmitral E wave and the mean lateral and septal segments e' wave velocities. The isovolumic relaxation time was also measured from aortic valve closure to mitral valve opening, on the pulsed wave Doppler recording. LV filling pattern was considered 'restrictive' when E/A ratio was >2.0, E wave deceleration time < 140 ms and the left atrium dilated of more than 40 mm in transverse diameter [24]. Total LV filling time was measured from the onset of the E wave to the end of the A wave and ejection time from the onset to the end of the aortic Doppler flow velocity.

Table 3 Determinants of limited exercise in HF patients

Variable	OR	(CI 95%)	P value
Determinants of all HF study patients			
Univariate determinants			
Age	1.062	(1.014–1.112)	0.011
Diabetes mellitus	0.353	(0.150–0.892)	0.017
NYHA class >1	0.290	(0.108–0.783)	0.015
LVMI	1.035	(1.011–1.060)	0.004
Left atrium	2.410	(1.404–4.137)	0.001
E wave	1.023	(1.004–1.043)	0.019
FT	0.996	(0.993–1.000)	0.036
Heart rate	1.039	(1.010–1.069)	0.008
PAAC	0.972	(0.952–0.993)	0.010
E/e′	1.092	(1.009–1.181)	0.028
Septal a′	0.786	(0.631–0.979)	0.032
Septal s′	0.661	(0.444–0.984)	0.041
Multivariate determinants			
Left atrium diameter	2.676	(1.242–5.766)	0.012
Diabetes mellitus	0.274	(0.084–0.898)	0.033
Age	1.067	(0.999–1.140)	0.052
NYHA class >1	2.068	(0.859–4.978)	0.105
Gender	0.406	(0.122–1.350)	0.141
E/e′	1.043	(0.943–1.153)	0.415
FT	0.997	(0.989–1.005)	0.463
Septal s′	0.854	(0.512–1.422)	0.543
Heart rate	1.011	(0.940–1.088)	0.764
Determinants in HFpEF patients			
Univariate determinants			
Diabetes mellitus	0.276	(0.082–0.926)	0.037
Haemoglobin	0.697	(0.502–0.968)	0.031
NYHA class >1	0.206	(0.043–0.993)	0.049
BSA	0.005	(0.000–0.308)	0.012
LVMI	1.049	(1.006–1.094)	0.025
Lateral a′	0.772	(0.603–0.987)	0.039
Lateral s′	0.489	(0.270–0.886)	0.018
Multivariate determinants			
Lateral s′	0.295	(0.099–0.882)	0.029
Haemoglobin	0.497	(0.248–0.998)	0.049
NYHA class >1	0.051	(0.003–1.034)	0.053
BSA	0.081	(0.000–6.016)	0.463
Lateral a′	1.049	(0.734–1.500)	0.793
Age	0.988	(0.827–1.179)	0.891
Diabetes	0.860	(0.109–6.786)	0.886
Determinants in HFrEF patients			
Univariate determinants			
Age	1.067	(1.010–1.127)	0.020

Table 3 Determinants of limited exercise in HF patients *(Continued)*

Left atrium	3.236	(1.333–7.856)	0.009
LAV max	1.021	(1.001–1.042)	0.045
LAV min	1.029	(1.003–1.055)	0.032
Multivariate determinants			
Age	1.073	(1.012–1.137)	0.018
Left atrium diameter	3.685	(1.348–10.071)	0.011
Gender	2.147	(0.556–8.288)	0.268

BMI body mass index, *BSA* body surface area, *NYHA* New York Heart Association, *LV* left ventricle, *EDD* end-diastolic dimension, *ESD* end-systolic dimension, *FT* filling time, *ET* ejection time, *PA* pulmonary artery, *A* atrial diastolic velocity, *E* early diastolic filling velocity, *e′* early diastolic myocardial velocity, *s′* systolic myocardial velocity, *LVMI* left ventricular mass index

Mitral regurgitation severity was assessed by colour and continuous wave Doppler and was graded as mild, moderate, or severe according to the relative jet area to that of the left atrium as well as the flow velocity profile, in line with the recommendations of the American and European Society of Echocardiography [25, 26]. Likewise, tricuspid regurgitation was assessed by colour Doppler and continuous-wave Doppler. Retrograde trans-tricuspid pressure drop > 35 mmHg was taken as an evidence for pulmonary hypertension [26, 27]. All M-mode and Doppler recordings were made at a fast speed of 100 mm/s with a superimposed ECG (lead II).

Measurement of amino-terminal pro BNP
Fasting venous blood was collected from study participants after they had rested in a supine position for 20 min. Samples were placed in disposable EDTA containers (1 g/L of plasma), and N-terminal proBNP was measured by a Cobas Elecsys E 411 analyzer (measuring range 5–35000 pg/mL) using a chemiluminescent immunoassay kit (Roche Diagnostics, Grenach-Wyhlen, Germany).

Six minute walk test
Within 24 h of the echocardiographic examination a 6-MWT was performed on a level hallway surface, administered by a specialized nurse who was blinded to the results of the echocardiogram. According to the method of Gyatt et al. [28] patients were informed of the purpose and protocol of the 6 MWT which was conducted in a standardized fashion while patients on their regular medications [29, 30]. A 15 m flat, obstacle-free corridor was used and patients were instructed to walk as far as they can, turning 180° after they have reached the end of the corridor, during the allocated time of 6 min. Patients walked unaccompanied so not to influence walking speed. At the end of the 6 min the supervising nurse measured the total distance walked by the patient.

Using the norm-reference equation developed by Troosters [31] for the prediction of 6MWT distance

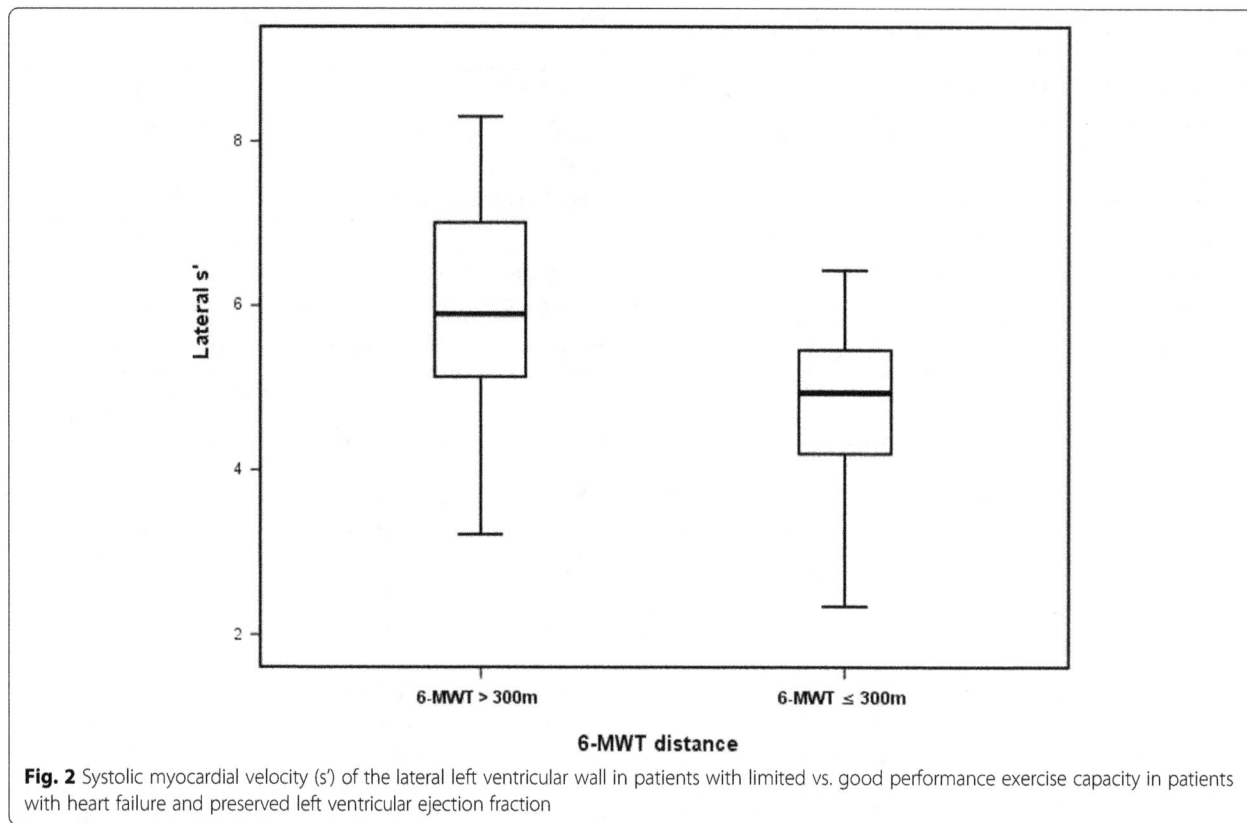

Fig. 2 Systolic myocardial velocity (s') of the lateral left ventricular wall in patients with limited vs. good performance exercise capacity in patients with heart failure and preserved left ventricular ejection fraction

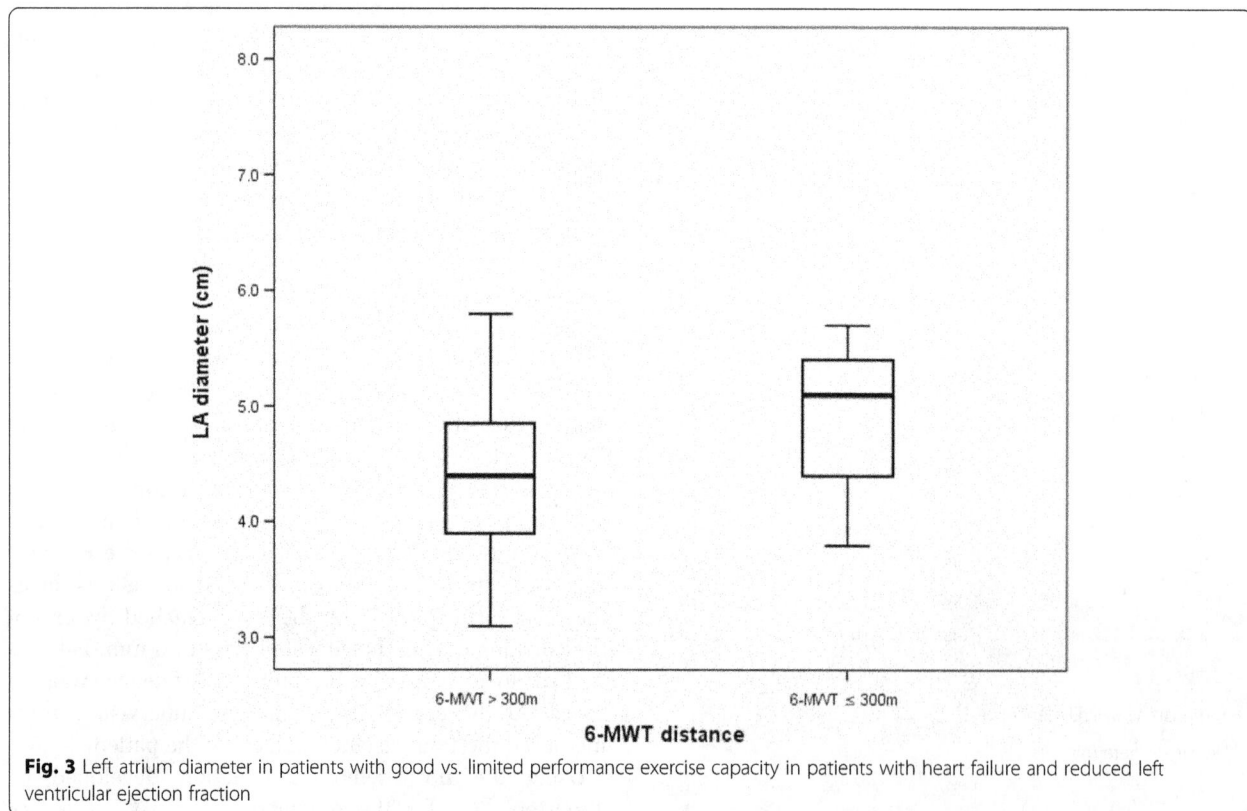

Fig. 3 Left atrium diameter in patients with good vs. limited performance exercise capacity in patients with heart failure and reduced left ventricular ejection fraction

according to age, height, weight, and gender that has been proposed for healthy patients, we derived the percentage of the predicted value (PPV). PPV is computed by dividing the actual 6MWT distance by the expected value of 6MWT distance and then multiplying by 100. Troosters' equation is as follows: Predicted 6MWT distance = 218 + 5.14 height (cm) – 5.32 age (years) –1.8 weight (kg) + 51.31 sex (1–male, 0–female).

Statistical analysis

Data are presented as mean ± SD or proportions (% of patients). Continuous data was compared with two-tailed unpaired Student's t test and discrete data with Chi-square test. Correlations were tested with Pearson coefficients. Determinants of 6 MWT distance were identified with univariate analysis and multivariate logistic regression was performed using the step-wise method. A significant difference was defined as $p < 0.05$ (2-tailed). Patients were divided according to their ability to walk >300 m into good and limited exercise performance groups [30], and were compared using unpaired Student t-test. Also, patients with HFpEF (>45%) were compared with those with HFrEF (<45%) using unpaired t-test.

Results

Patients with Limited vs. Good 6 MWT performance (Table 1)

Patients with limited exercise capacity were older ($p = 0.008$) and had higher prevalence of diabetes ($p = 0.027$) compared with those with good exercise capacity. Patients with limited 6-MWT had larger left atrium ($p = 0.001$), increased LVMI ($p = 0.006$), shorter LV filling time ($p = 0.019$), shorter isovolumic relaxation time ($p = 0.037$) and shorter PA acceleration time ($p = 0.006$), lower septal a' ($p = 0.018$) and s' ($p = 0.023$), compared to those with good 6-MWT performance. The rest of the clinical and echocardiographic indices were not different between groups.

Patients with HFpEF vs. HFrEF (Table 2)

The whole group of study patients walked a distance of 310 ± 116 m during 6-MWT. Patients with HFrEF walked significantly shorter distance compared those with HFpEF ($p = 0.01$, Fig. 1).

Mean PPV of 6-MWT distance for the whole group was 50 ± 20%, and was lower in HFrEF compared to HFpEF patients ($p = 0.004$). Patients with HFrEF had lower hemoglobin ($p = 0.007$), higher baseline heart rate ($p = 0.005$), higher NT-ProBNP ($p = 0.001$), larger LAV max ($p = 0.005$), larger LAV min ($p < 0.001$), larger LA ($p = 0.004$), increased LVM and LVMI ($p < 0.001$, for both), shorter pulmonary acceleration time, lower septal s', e' and a' velocities, and lower septal and lateral mitral annular plane systolic excursion (MAPSE) ($p < 0.001$ for

all), higher E/A, shorter LVFT and higher E/e' ($p = 0.001$ for all), shorter E wave DT ($p = 0.002$), lower lateral e' ($p = 0.009$) and s' ($p = 0.006$), RV e' and LA EF ($p = 0.012$ for both) compared to HFpEF patients. Eleven of the 55 HFpEF patients and 23 of 56 HFrEF patients had mild-moderate mitral regurgitation. Seven of the 55 HFpEF patients and 17 of 56 HFrEF patients had mild or more tricuspid regurgitation.

Determinants of limited 6 MWT distance (Table 3)

Determinants of limited 6 MWT distance in all HF patients

High baseline heart rate ($p = 0.008$), age ($p = 0.011$), diabetes ($p = 0.017$) and NYHA class ($p = 0.015$) predicted limited 6-MWT distance. Also, enlarged LA ($p = 0.001$), increased LVMI ($p = 0.004$), increased E wave velocity ($p = 0.019$), short LV filling time ($p = 0.036$) and pulmonary artery acceleration time ($p = 0.01$), raised E/e' ($p = 0.028$), low septal a' and s' ($p = 0.032$ and $p = 0.041$, respectively), predicted limited 6 MWT distance. In multivariate analysis [odds ratio 95% confidence interval], only enlarged LA diameter [2.676 (1.242–5.766), $p = 0.012$], and diabetes [0.274 (0.084–0.898), $p = 0.033$], independently predicted the limited 6-MWT distance.

Determinants of limited 6 MWT distance in HFpEF patients

In univariate analysis, body surface area - BSA ($p = 0.012$), low hemoglobin level ($p = 0.031$), diabetes ($p = 0.037$), and NYHA class > 1 ($p = 0.049$), increased LVMI ($p = 0.025$), low lateral s' ($p = 0.018$) and a' ($p = 0.039$) predicted limited 6-MWT distance. In multivariate analysis, lateral s' [0.295 (0.099–0.882), $p = 0.029$, Fig. 2], and hemoglobin level [0.497 (0.248–0.998), $p = 0.049$], independently predicted the limited 6-MWT distance.

Determinants of limited 6 MWT distance in HFrEF patients

In univariate analysis, age ($p = 0.02$) and enlarged LA ($p = 0.009$) predicted limited exercise distance, which also remained as independent determinants in multivariate analysis: age [1.073 (1.012–1.137), $p = 0.018$] and LA diameter [3.685 (1.348–10.071), $p = 0.011$, Fig. 3].

Discussion

Findings

The results of this study show that in general HF patients with limited exercise capacity are older and have worse left ventricular function and raised filling pressures than those with satisfactory exercise performance. However, determinants of exercise capacity differed significantly according to ejection fraction. While patients with reduced ejection fraction have the enlarged left atrium and advanced age as the independent determinants of exercise capacity, it was the low hemoglobin and reduced lateral s' the respective determinants in those with preserved ejection fraction.

Data interpretation

Patients with heart failure due to reduced ejection fraction are known to have worse segmental and overall ventricular function, with additional signs of myocardial stiffness and raised filling pressures in many of them [32]. These perpetual changes result in left atrial enlargement due to the raised pressure, either because of venous hypertension, additional mitral regurgitation or the combination of both [33]. Indeed left atrial enlargement has previously been shown to be the most important prognostic marker in heart failure patients, irrespective of the development of atrial fibrillation [34]. It has also been taken as a reflection of the severity of LV myocardial stiffness, which is an end-stage dysfunction, thus an irreversible damage. On the other hand, many factors contribute to the pathophysiology of heart failure with preserved ejection fraction [35], including atrial fibrillation, hypertension and kidney disease. Although none of our patients was in atrial fibrillation, the low hemoglobin levels were the main determinant of compromised exercise capacity. This reflects the need for acknowledging differences in the strategic management of these patients when compared with those of HFrEF. Finally, our findings discard ejection fraction, as the commonest marker of ventricular function as a determinant of exercise capacity.

Limitations

The main limitation of our study is that we did not investigate the response of echocardiographic measurements to exercise, at the time of symptoms development. However the objective of this study was to determine determinants of ordinary walking exercise limitation rather than heavy exercise in HF patients. The other limitation was the lack of invasive measurements of left atrial pressures, but the study was based on Doppler measurements which have been shown to be reproducible and correlate closely with invasive pressure measurements [36]. The small sample size was another limitation, but we believe that future studies with larger sample size should strength our findings.

Clinical implications

Patients with HF have significantly limited exercise tolerance. Although ejection fraction is considered as the most useful index of LV function and the corner stone for recruiting patients for various treatment modalities, the other echo parameters should be considered as part of the conventional protocol of the follow-up of such patients, depending on overall LV systolic function: enlarged left atrium in HFrEF and impaired longitudinal systolic shortening and reduced hemoglobin in those

with HFpEF. While management of patients with HFrEF could be standardized, and follow one protocol, that of patients with HFpEF is likely to be individualized.

Conclusions

In HF patients determinants of exercise capacity differ according to severity of overall LV systolic function, with left atrial enlargement in HFrEF and longitudinal systolic shortening and low hemoglobin in HFpEF as the the main determinants.

Abbreviations

6-MWT: Minute walk test; A: Atrial diastolic velovity; a': Atrial myocardial velocity; BMI: Body mass index; BSA: Body surface area; DT: Deceleration time; e': Early diastolic myocardial velocity; E: Early diastolic velocity; EF: Ejection fraction; FT: Filling time; HF: Heart failure; HFpEF: Heart failure with preserved ejection fraction; HFrEF: Heart failure with reduced ejection fraction; LA EF: Left atrial emptying fraction; LA: Left atrium; LAV max: Left atrial maximal volume; LAV min: Left atrial minimal volume; LV: Left ventricle; LVM: Left ventricular mass; LVMI: Left ventricular mass index; LVPWd: Left ventricular posterior wall in diastole; MAPSE: Mitral annular plane systolic excursion; NYHA: New York Heart Association; PA: Pulmonary artery; PPV: Percentage of the predicted value; RV: Right ventricle; s': Systolic myocardial velocity; TAPSE: Tricuspidal annular plane systolic excursion

Acknowledgements
Not applicable.

Authors' contributions
All authors have contributed (AB, GB, PI, and MH designed the manuscript; PI, IB and GB analyzed and interpreted the data; AB, PI, AA and EH drafted the manuscript; MH, GB and SE revised critically), read and approved the manuscript.

Competing interests
The authors declare that they have no competing interests.

Consent for publication
Not applicable.

Statement on ethics approval
Nr.3729, date 22.10.2010.

Name of the ethics committee
Ethics Committee of Medical Faculty, University of Prishtina.

Author details
¹Clinic of Cardiology, University Clinical Centre of Kosova, "Rrethi i Spitalit p.n., Prishtina, Kosovo. ²Medical Faculty, University of Prishtina, Prishtina, Kosovo. ³Department of Public Health and Clinical Medicine, Umeå University and Heart Centre, Umeå, Sweden. ⁴Molecular and Clinical Sciences Research Institute, St George University London, London, United Kingdom.

References
1. Mozaffarian D, Benjamin EJ, Go AS, Arnett DK, Blaha MJ, Cushman M, et al. Heart Disease and Stroke Statistics-2016 Update: A Report From the American Heart Association. Circulation. 2016;133(4):e38–360.

2.   Bui AL, Horwich TB, Fonarow GC. Epidemiology and risk profile of heart failure. Nat Rev Cardiol. 2011;8:30–41.

3.   Roger VL. Epidemiology of heart failure. Circ Res. 2013;113:646–59.

4.   Ho KK, Anderson KM, Kannel WB, Grossman W, Levy D. Survival after onset of congestive heart failure in Framingham Heart Study subjects. Circulation. 1993;88:107–15.

5.   Davies M, Hobbs F, Davis R, Kenkre J, Roalfe AK, Hare R, Wosornu D, Lancashire RJ. Prevalence of left-ventricular systolic dysfunction and heart failure in the Echocardiographic Heart of England Screening study: a population based study. Lancet. 2001;358:439–45.

6.   Bytyçi I, Bajraktari G. Mortality in heart failure patients. Anatol J Cardiol. 2015;15(1):63–8. doi:10.5152/akd.2014.5731.

7.   Ciampi Q, Pratali L, Porta MD, Petruzziello B, Manganiello V, Villari B, Picano E, Sicari R. Tissue Doppler systolic velocity change during dobutamine stress echocardiography predicts contractile reserve and exercise tolerance in patients with heart failure. Eur Heart J Cardiovasc Imaging. 2013;14(2):102–9.

8.   Gardin JM, Leifer ES, Fleg JL, Whellan D, Kokkinos P, Leblanc MH, Wolfel E, Kitzman DW, HF-ACTION Investigators. Relationship of Doppler-Echocardiographic left ventricular diastolic function to exercise performance in systolic heart failure: the HF-ACTION study. Am Heart J. 2009;158:S45–52.

9.   Chattopadhyay S, Alamgir MF, Nikitin NP, Rigby AS, Clark AL, Cleland JG. Lack of diastolic reserve in patients with heart failure and normal ejection fraction. Circ Heart Fail. 2010;3:35–43.

10. Berisha V, Bajraktari G, Dobra D, Haliti E, Bajrami R, Elezi S. Echocardiography and 6-minute walk test in left ventricular systolic dysfunction. Arq Bras Cardiol. 2009;92(2):121–34.

11. Leong DP, Grover S, Molaee P, Chakrabarty A, Shirazi M, Cheng YH, Penhall A, Perry R, Greville H, Joseph MX, Selvanayagam JB. Nonvolumetric echocardiographic indices of right ventricular systolic function: validation with cardiovascular magnetic resonance and relationship with functional capacity. Echocardiography. 2012;29:455–63.

12. Bajraktari G, Elezi S, Berisha V, Lindqvist P, Rexhepaj N, Henein MY. Left ventricular asynchrony and raised filling pressure predict limited exercise performance assessed by 6 minute walk test. Int J Cardiol. 2011;146(3):385–9. doi:10.1016/j.ijcard.2009.07.018.

13. Rubis P, Podolec P, Tomkiewicz-Pajak L, Kopec G, Olszowska M, Tracz W. Usefulness of the evaluation of isovolumic and ejection phase myocardial signals during stress echocardiography in predicting exercise capacity in heart failure patients. Echocardiography. 2009;26:1050–9.

14. Ohara T, Iwano H, Thohan V, Kitzman DW, Upadhya B, Pu M, Little WC. Role of Diastolic Function in Preserved Exercise Capacity in Patients with Reduced Ejection Fractions. J Am Soc Echocardiogr. 2015;28(10):1184–93.

15. Bajraktari G, Batalli A, Poniku A, Ahmeti A, Olloni R, Hyseni V, et al. Left ventricular markers of global dyssynchrony predict limited exercise capacity in heart failure, but not in patients with preserved ejection fraction. Cardiovasc Ultrasound. 2012;10(1):36. doi:10.1186/1476-7120-10-36.

16. Hasselberg NE, Haugaa KH, Sarvari SI, Gullestad L, Andreassen AK, Smiseth OA, Edvardsen T. Left ventricular global longitudinal strain is associated with exercise capacity in failing hearts with preserved and reduced ejection fraction. Eur Heart J Cardiovasc Imaging. 2015;16(2):217–24.

17. Mohammed SF, Borlaug BA, McNulty S, Lewis GD, Lin G, Zakeri R, et al. Resting ventricular-vascular function and exercise capacity in heart failure with preserved ejection fraction: a RELAX trial ancillary study. Circ Heart Fail. 2014;7(4):580–9.

18. Kosmala W, Rojek A, Przewlocka-Kosmala M, Mysiak A, Karolko B, Marwick TH. Contributions of Nondiastolic Factors to Exercise Intolerance in Heart Failure With Preserved Ejection Fraction. J Am Coll Cardiol. 2016;67(6):659–70.

19. Cheitlin MD, Armstrong WF, Aurigemma GP, Beller GA, Bierman FZ, et al. a report of the American College of Cardiology/American Heart Association Task Force on PracticeGuidelines (ACC/AHA/ASE Committee to Update the 1997 Guidelines for the Clinical Application of Echocardiography). Circulation. 2003;108(9):1146–62.

20. Devereux RB, Alonso DR, Lutas EM, Gottlieb GJ, Campo E, Sachs I, Reichek N. Echocardiographic assessment of left ventricular hypertrophy: comparison to necropsy findings. Am J Cardiol. 1986;57(6):450–8.

21. Höglund C, Alam M, Thorstrand C. Atrioventricular valve plane displacement in healthy persons. An echocardiographic study. Acta Med Scand. 1988;224:557–62.

22. Lang RM, Badano LP, Mor-Avi V, Afilalo J, Armstrong A, Ernande L, et al. Recommendations for cardiac chamber quantification by echocardiography in adults: an update from the American Society of Echocardiography and the European Association of Cardiovascular Imaging. Eur Heart J Cardiovasc Imaging. 2015;16(3):233–70. doi:10.1093/ehjci/jev014.

23. Wakatsuki Y, Funabashi N, Mikami Y, Shiina Y, Kawakubo M, Takahashi M, et al. Left atrial compensatory function in subjects with early stage primary hypertension assessed by using left atrial volumetric emptying fraction acquired by transthoracic echocardiography. Int J Cardiol. 2009;136(3):363–7.

24. Appleton CP, Hatle LK, Popp RL. Relation of transmitral flow velocity patterns to left ventricular diastolic function: new insights from a combined hemodynamic and Doppler echocardiographic study. J Am Coll Cardiol. 1988;12:426–40.

25. Zoghbi WA, Enriquez-Sarano M, Foster E, Grayburn PA, Kraft CD, Levine RA, Nihoyannopoulos P, Otto CM, Quinones MA, Rakowski H, Stewart WJ, Waggoner A, Weissman NJ, American Society of Echocardiography. Recommendations for evaluation of the severity of native valvular regurgitation with two-dimensional and Doppler echocardiography. J Am Soc Echocardiogr. 2003;16:777–802.

26. Galderisi M, Henein MY, D'hooge J, Sicari R, Badano LP, Zamorano JL, Roelandt JR, European Association of Echocardiography. Recommendations of the European Association of Echocardiography: how to use echo-Doppler in clinical trials: different modalities for different purposes. Eur J Echocardiogr. 2011;12(5):339–53. doi:10.1093/ejechocard/jer051.

27. Gardin JM, Adams DB, Douglas PS, Feigenbaum H, Forst DH, Fraser AG, Grayburn PA, Katz AS, Keller AM, Kerber RE, Khandheria BK, Klein AL, Lang RM, Pierard LA, Quinones MA, Schnittger I, American Society of Echocardiography. Recommendations for a standardized report for adult transthoracic echocardiography: a report from the American Society of Echocardiography's Nomenclature and Standards Committee and Task Force for a Standardized Echocardiography Report. J Am Soc Echocardiogr. 2002;15:275–90.

28. Guyatt GH, Sullivan MJ, Thompson PJ, Fallen EL, Pugsley SO, Taylor DW, Berman LB. The 6-minute walk test: a new measure of exercise capacity in patients with chronic heart failure. Can Med Assoc J. 1985;132:919–23.

29. Guyatt GH, Thompson PJ, Berman LB, Sullivan MJ, Townsend M, Jones NL, Pugsley SO. How should we measyre function in patients with chronic heart and lung disease? J Chronic Dis. 1985;28:517–24.

30. Ingle L, Rigby AS, Nabb S, Jones PK, Clark AL, Cleland JG. Clinical determinants of poor six-minute walk test performance in patients with left ventricular systolic dysfunction and no major structural heart disease. Eur J Heart Fail. 2006;8(3):321–5.

31. Troosters T, Gosselink R, Decramer M. Six minute walking distance in healthy elderly subjects. Eur Respir J. 1999;14:270–4.

32. Nagueh SF, Shah G, Wu Y, Torre-Amione G, King NM, Lahmers S, et al. Altered titin expression, myocardial stiffness, and left ventricular function in patients with dilated cardiomyopathy. Circulation. 2004;110(2):155–62.

33. Cioffi G, Gerdts E, Cramariuc D, Tarantini L, Di Lenarda A, Pulignano G, et al. Left atrial size and force in patients with systolic chronic heart failure: Comparison with healthy controls and different cardiac diseases. Exp Clin Cardiol. 2010;15(3):e45–51.

34. Rossi A, Temporelli PL, Quintana M, Dini FL, Ghio S, Hillis GS, et al. Independent relationship of left atrial size and mortality in patients with heart failure: an individual patient meta-analysis of longitudinal data (MeRGE Heart Failure). Eur J Heart Fail. 2009;11(10):929–36. doi:10.1093/eurjhf/hfp112.

35. Redfield MM. Heart Failure with Preserved Ejection Fraction. N Engl J Med. 2016;375(19):1868–77.

36. Kuppahally SS, Michaels AD, Tandar A, Gilbert EM, Litwin SE, Bader FM. Can echocardiographic evaluation of cardiopulmonary hemodynamics decrease right heart catheterizations in end-stage heart failure patients awaiting transplantation? Am J Cardiol. 2010;106:1657–62.

11

Does the internal jugular vein affect the elasticity of the common carotid artery?

Michał Podgórski[1*], Monika Winnicka[2], Michał Polguj[2], Piotr Grzelak[1], Maciej Łukaszewski[3] and Ludomir Stefańczyk[1]

Abstract

Background: Arterial stiffness is an early marker of atherosclerosis. The carotid arteries are easily accessible by ultrasound and are commonly used for the evaluation of atherosclerosis development. However, this stiffness assessment is based on the elastic properties of the artery, which may be influenced by the adjacent internal jugular vein (IJV).
The aim of the present study is to evaluate the influence of internal jugular vein morphology on the stiffness of the common carotid artery.

Methods: Bilateral carotid ultrasound was performed in 248 individuals. When no carotid plaque was detected (90.9 % cases), the distensibility coefficient and β - stiffness index were calculated. The global and segmental circumferential strain parameters of the carotid wall were evaluated with 2D-Speckle Tracking. The cross-sectional area of the IJV and degree of its adherence to the carotid wall (angle of adherence) were measured.

Results: The morphology of the IJV did not influence the standard stiffness parameters nor the global circumferential strain. However, segmental analysis found the sector adjacent to the IJV to have significantly higher strain parameters than its opposite counterpart. In addition, the strain correlated significantly and positively with IJV cross-sectional area and angle of adherence.

Conclusions: The movement of the carotid artery wall caused by the passage of the pulse wave is not homogeneous. The greatest strain is observed in a segment adjacent to the IJV, and the degree of wall deformation is associated with the size of the vein and the degree of its adherence.

Keywords: Atherosclerosis, Arterial stiffness, 2D-Speckle tracking, β-Stiffness index, Carotid artery

Background

Although loss of arterial elasticity naturally occurs with ageing, it is also an early marker of atherosclerosis. The pathomechanism of arterial stiffening is associated mostly with the exchange of elastin for collagen in the extracellular matrix of the arterial wall [1, 2]. Such structural changes have a strong impact on the generation, propagation and reflection of pressure waves in the arterial tree, resulting in an increased aortic systolic pressure, a greater burden on the left ventricle and increased risk of cardiovascular mortality [2, 3].

Arterial stiffness may be assessed through such systemic markers as pulse wave velocity or augmentation index, or locally in parts of the cardiovascular system most prone to development of atherosclerosis [4, 5].

Commonly-used markers of local arterial stiffness are distensibility coefficient, elastic modulus and β-stiffness index [2, 4–6]. A newly-developed method derived from echocardiography which can be employed in the evaluation of local arterial stiffness is 2D-Speckle Tracking [3]. This tool offers the advantage of a more detailed, segment-base analysis of arterial wall mechanics than standard stiffness parameters [3, 7]. Moreover, unlike tissue Doppler imaging and IMT measurements, it is angle independent [8]. It is also more sensitive than β-stiffness index in the detection of age-related changes in the arterial wall elasticity [5]. 2D-Speckle Tracking might therefore be useful in determining whether local conditions may influence the elastic properties of the arterial wall and bias any stiffness assessment.

The internal jugular vein (IJV) travels adjacent to the internal carotid and common carotid arteries (CCA) within the carotid sheath. Its size and course are highly

* Correspondence: michal.podgorski@umed.lodz.pl
[1]Department of Radiology and Diagnostic Imaging, Medical University of Lodz, 22, Kopcińskiego St., Barlicki Hospital, Lodz, Poland
Full list of author information is available at the end of the article

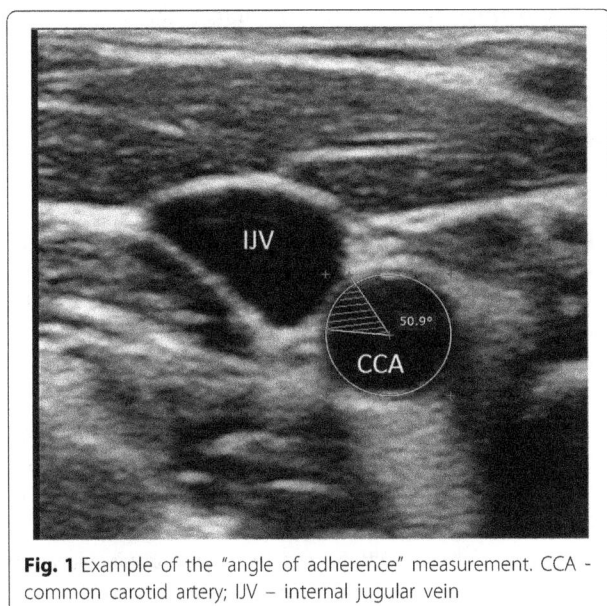

Fig. 1 Example of the "angle of adherence" measurement. CCA - common carotid artery; IJV – internal jugular vein

variable, nevertheless it is easily compressible due to its thin wall and low blood pressure [9, 10]. Hence, it is reasonable to assume that the elasticity of the common carotid artery may be affected by the size and alignment of the IJV.

Hence, the aim of the study was to evaluate the influence of IJV morphology on stiffness markers evaluated in the CCA.

Methods

Carotid ultrasound was performed in 248 participants of the "Diamentowy Grant" study (No DI2012 007742), the aim of which was to assess the relationship between asthma and risk of atherosclerosis. All participants gave their informed consent to take part in the study, and the study protocol was approved by the Local Bioethics Committee (RNN/41/13/KB).

Patients were recruited from the Pulmonology and Allergology Outpatient Clinics and through an internet advertisement. The only inclusion criterion was that the participant must be aged over 30 years old. The exclusion criteria were as follows: the presence of atrial fibrillation, which impair the evaluation of strain parameters, the presence of goitre or lymphadenopathy adjacent to CCA or IJV, or previous surgeries in the neck region.

When the atherosclerotic plaque was present in the CCA or its bifurcation, this side was excused from the analysis.

Examination

Carotid ultrasound was performed with a GE Vivid 7 ultrasound apparatus (GE Medical System, Milwaukee, WI, USA) with a high-resolution linear transducer (14 MHz).

The patient lay in the supine position. After 5 min rest under semi-dark, quiet conditions, brachial blood pressure was measured, an ECG trace was obtained and carotid ultrasound was performed. The patient's head was turned 45° opposite to the side of examination. The carotid arteries were evaluated for the presence of atherosclerotic changes. If no changes were noted, the short axis of the CCA was obtained one centimetre below the carotid bulb. Any movement between the two most distant points on the near and far walls of CCA was assessed using M-mode during three consecutive heart cycles. Afterwards, the short axis of the CCA was visualised in standard B-mode and a cine loop taken during another three consecutive heart cycles was saved. If the entire IJV did not fit within the field of view, another three consecutive heart cycle cine loop was recorded to see a complete cross-section of the IJV.

To minimize respiration-related motion artefacts, all acquisitions were performed during a short breath-hold at the end of expiration. The probe was placed with the least possible pressure to avoid compressing the IJV and to allow expansion of the CCA. All images were recorded with a high frame rate (>90 frames s^{-1}; mean frame rate: 112 ± 20 frames s^{-1}).

Further analysis was performed offline on a workstation equipped with EchoPac software (EchoPac PC, GE Medical System). The measurements from three cardiac cycles were averaged and used for further analysis. Based on the M-mode presentation, the classical arterial stiffness parameters were calculated according to the following formulas:

1. Distensibility coefficient (DC)

$$DC\left[Pa^{-1}\right] = \frac{\left(D_{max}^2 - D_{min}^2\right)}{D_{min}2} \times \Delta P$$

ΔP difference between systolic and diastolic blood pressure value; D_{max} and D_{min} are respectively the

Table 1 Measurements of common carotid arteries and internal jugular veins. Data presented as mean and (SD)

	RCCA	LCCA	p	RIJV	LIJV	p
AP diameter [mm]	7.6 (1.0)	7.4 (0.8)	**0.0001**	5.2 (3.1)	4.6 (2.6)	**0.0036**
ML diameter [mm]	7.7 (1.0)	7.5 (0.9)	**0.0001**	11.0 (3.9)	9.8 (3.9)	**0.0001**
Area [mm²]	47.0 (1.0)	44.1 (1.1)	**0.0001**	55.9 (5.8)	41.2 (3.8)	**0.0001**

RCCA right common carotid artery, LCCA left common carotid artery, RIJV right internal jugular vein, LIJV left internal jugular vein, AP antero-posterior diameter, ML medio-lateral diameter
p-value presented in bold style is significant (<0.05)

Table 2 Strain parameters for carotid arteries

	RCCA	LCCA	p
β - stiffness index	9.7 (4.6)	9.9 (5.1)	0.6028
Distensibility coefficient	0.06 (0.08)	0.07 (0.03)	0.2099
CS [%]	3.32 (1.34)	3.21 (1.21)	0.8319
CSR [1/s]	0.63 (0.22)	0.61 (0.21)	0.3952

RCCA right common carotid artery, *LCCA* left common carotid artery, β β-stiffness index, *DC* distensibility coefficient, *CS* circumferential strain, *CSr* circumferential strain rate

largest and the smallest distances between the intima media thickness on the near and far wall of the CCA.

2. β-stiffness index (β)

$$\beta = \frac{\ln\left(\frac{SBP}{DBP}\right) \times D}{\Delta D}$$

SBP - systolic blood pressure, DBP - diastolic blood pressure, D - mean value of D_{max} and D_{min}, ΔD - difference between D_{max} and D_{min}

Circumferential strain (CS) and strain rate (CSR) were evaluated using 2D-Speckle Tracking. The region of interest (ROI) was placed over the arterial wall along the border between the intima-media and the vessel lumen. The width of the ROI was narrower to cover the smallest possible portion of tissues adjacent to the arterial wall. The ROI segments were manually adjusted so that one of them covered the whole part of the CCA wall adherent to the IJV wall (venous segment). A mirror segment of the same length was placed against the opposite site (opposite segment). The parts of the wall between these segments were covered with remaining two parts of the ROI – the posterior and anterior segments. "Global" and "segmental" values of CS and CSR were calculated as the mean amplitudes between minimal and maximal measurements during the three heart beats of the cine loop.

The cross-sectional area of the CCA and the IJV were measured with a tracking-measuring tool. If the CCA and IJV were not in contact, the distance between them

was measured. If they were in contact, the segment including CCA and IJV adjacent to each other was measured as a portion of the complete circumference of the CCA in degrees and this was determined the "angle of adherence" (Fig. 1).

Statistical analysis

The statistical analysis was performed using Statistica 12 software (StatSoft Polska, Cracow, Poland). A *p*-value lower than 0.05 was considered significant. The results are presented as mean and standard deviation unless otherwise stated.

The normality of the continuous data distribution was checked with the Shapiro-Wilk test. The χ2 test was used for comparisons of nominal variables. Comparisons of continuous variables between different groups (e.g. men vs women) were performed with the Student *t*-test for independent variables. Differences in continuous variables between body sides was performed with the paired Student *t*-test. To evaluate the determinants of stiffness, multiple regression analysis was performed with age, BMI, systolic blood pressure, angle of adherence and cross-sectional area of the IJV, as potential explanatory variables. The correlation of continuous variables was assessed with the Persons correlation coefficient. Our previous studies have confirmed the reliability of strain measurements to be 84.83 % for interclass and 94.42 % for intraclass agreement [11].

Results

A carotid plaque was found on 25 left CCA and 20 right CCA. In five individuals, it was present bilaterally. Hence, 223 left CCA and 228 right CCA were included into the analysis: 90.9 % from all arteries. In the study group there were 66 (27 %) men and 177 (73 %) women, in the mean age of 57.2 (SD = 9.3) and 56.4 (SD = 9.4), respectively. The age difference was not significant (*p* = 0.5562).

The wall of the IJV was in contact with the wall of the CCA in 212 cases on the right side (93 %) and in 213 on the left side (96 %). In remaining cases, the vessels were separated by a mean distance of 6.2 mm (SD = 5.4) on the right side and 5.9 (SD = 4.8) on the left side. The difference was not significant (*p* = 0.81).

Table 3 Correlation between arterial stiffness parameters and vein related variables

		RIJV						LIJV			
		Angle		Area				Angle		Area	
		R^2	p	R^2	p			R^2	p	R^2	p
RCCA	β	0.04	0.6760	0.14	0.0770	LCCA	β	−0.10	0.2824	−0.01	0.8750
	DC	−0.02	0.8593	−0.15	0.0686		DC	0.07	0.4096	−0.03	0.6854
	CS [%]	0.01	0.9482	−0.10	0.1831		CS [%]	0.10	0.2180	−0.06	0.4054
	CSR [1/s]	−0.13	0.1005	**−0.21**	**0.0050**		CSR [1/s]	0.05	0.5061	−0.14	0.0634

RCCA right common carotid artery, *LCCA* left common carotid artery, *RIJV* right internal jugular vein, *LIJV* left internal jugular vein, β β-stiffness index, *DC* distensibility coefficient, *CS* circumferential strain, *CSr* circumferential strain rate, R^2 correlation coefficient, *p* value
p-value presented in bold style is significant (<0.05)

Table 4 Multiple regression analysis for arterial stiffness parameters (pooled data for right and left CCA)

	β $R^2 = 0.1054$ $p = 0.005$		DC $R^2 = 0.0855$ $p = 0.005$		CS [%] $R^2 = 0.1196$ $p = 0.002$		CSR [1/s] $R^2 = 0.2445$ $p < 0.001$	
	Beta	p	Beta	p	Beta	p	Beta	p
Age [years]	**0.154**	**0.0006**	**−0.001**	**0.0008**	**−0.053**	**0.0000**	**−0.011**	**0.0000**
BMI [kg/m²]	0.137	0.0903	−0.001	0.1793	−0.036	0.0934	**−0.007**	**0.0487**
SBP	−0.002	0.9170	0.000	0.0897	**0.009**	**0.0455**	**0.002**	**0.0213**
Angle of adherence	−0.012	0.2695	0.000	0.1775	0.004	0.2177	0.000	0.7683
Area of the RIJV	0.004	0.6777	0.000	0.2857	0.001	0.6520	0.000	0.7618

RCCA right common carotid artery, *LCCA* left common carotid artery, *RIJV* right internal jugular vein, *LIJV* left internal jugular vein, β β-stiffness index, *DC* distensibility coefficient, *CS* circumferential strain, *CSr* circumferential strain rate, *BMI* body mass index, *SBP* systolic blood pressure, *Beta* regression coefficient, *p* – value
p-value presented in bold style is significant (<0.05)

The diameters of the vessels are presented in Table 1. Both CCA and IJV were significantly larger on the right side. The mean angle of adherence was 69.9° (SD = 36.8°) on the right side and 74.8° (SD = 34.7°) on the left side. The difference was not significant ($p = 0.5821$).

Global stiffness analysis

Arterial stiffness parameters are presented in Table 2. The global CSR of the right CCA correlated significantly with the area of the right IJV. The remaining parameters did not significantly correlate with the angle of adherence nor with the area of the vein (Table 3). Furthermore, multiple regression analysis found all of the arterial stiffness parameters to be independent of vein area and adherence angle (Table 4).

Segment specific analysis

Both CS and CSR differed significantly between the analysed segments (Table 5). For the LCCA, the CS and CSR of the venous segment were significantly higher than of the opposite and posterior segments. These parameters were also significantly higher in the anterior segment than in the opposite segment (Fig 2.).

The CS and CSR of the RCCA were significantly higher only when the venous segment was compared with the opposite one (Fig 2.).

Table 5 Differences in circumferential strain and circumferential strain rate according to the analysed segment of the common carotid artery

Segment	LCCA		RCCA	
	CS [%] mean (SD)	CSr [1/s] mean (SD)	CS [%] mean (SD)	CSr [1/s] mean (SD)
Opposite	2.88 (1.25)	0.54 (0.24)	2.98 (1.32)	0.64 (0.26)
Posterior	3.10 (1.26)	0.59 (0.24)	3.23 (1.39)	0.58 (0.23)
Anterior	3.38 (1.43)	0.63 (0.27)	3.36 (1.48)	0.63 (0.25)
Venous	3.73 (1.57)	0.69 (0.29)	3.59 (1.56)	0.69 (0.28)
p	**<0.0001**	**<0.0001**	**0.0012**	**0.0017**

RCCA right common carotid artery, *LCCA* left common carotid artery, *CS* circumferential strain, *CSr* circumferential strain rate, *p* – value
p-value presented in bold style is significant (<0.05)

The CS and CSR of the venous segment correlated significantly with the area of the IJV cross-section (LCCA: strain - $R^2 = 0.51$, $p = 0.0031$; strain rate - $R^2 = 0.48$, $p = 0.0075$. RCCA: strain - $R^2 = 0.53$, $p = 0.0021$; strain rate - $R^2 = 0.50$, $p = 0.0125$) and angle of its adherence (LCCA: strain - $R^2 = 0.43$, $p = 0.0078$; strain rate - $R^2 = 0.40$, $p = 0.0097$. RCCA: strain - $R^2 = 0.49$, $p = 0.0010$; strain rate - $R^2 = 0.47$, $p = 0.0202$). The later correlation was not as tight.

Discussion

Our findings indicate that the local elasticity of the CCA is affected by the adherence of the IJV. Although it does not seem to affect the global elastic properties of the artery, it may bias one-dimensional measurement of elastic properties of the CCA.

It has been known for 50 years that the rigidity of the capillary vessel is largely affected by surrounding tissue according to the "tunnel-in-gel" concept [12]. This theory has also been confirmed in a pig animal model for carotid and femoral arteries. Liu [13] notes that the CSR was found to be 15 to 25 % less when subjected to radial constraint at physiological pressure. In addition, mean circumferential wall stress only constituted a maximum of 30 % of the untethered stress. Asymmetrical expansion of the carotid artery has also been reported in a rat model based on longitudinal sections of the CCA and external carotid artery [14]. However, no detailed analysis of neighbouring structures was included in any of the aforementioned experiments.

The local measurement of arterial stiffness reveals the relationship between changes in the arterial volume and distending pressure [2]. The calculation assumes that the luminal cross-sectional area changes linearly with pressure and that the length of the artery remains constant during contraction [2]. However, as luminal distensibility of the arterial wall is not representative of whole arterial wall stress, calculation of the β-stiffness index and distensibility coefficient produces inaccurate results [15], as demonstrated by the significant differences found in segmental strain parameters in the present study. The non-homogeneous pattern of arterial stiffening is reflected in the local formation of

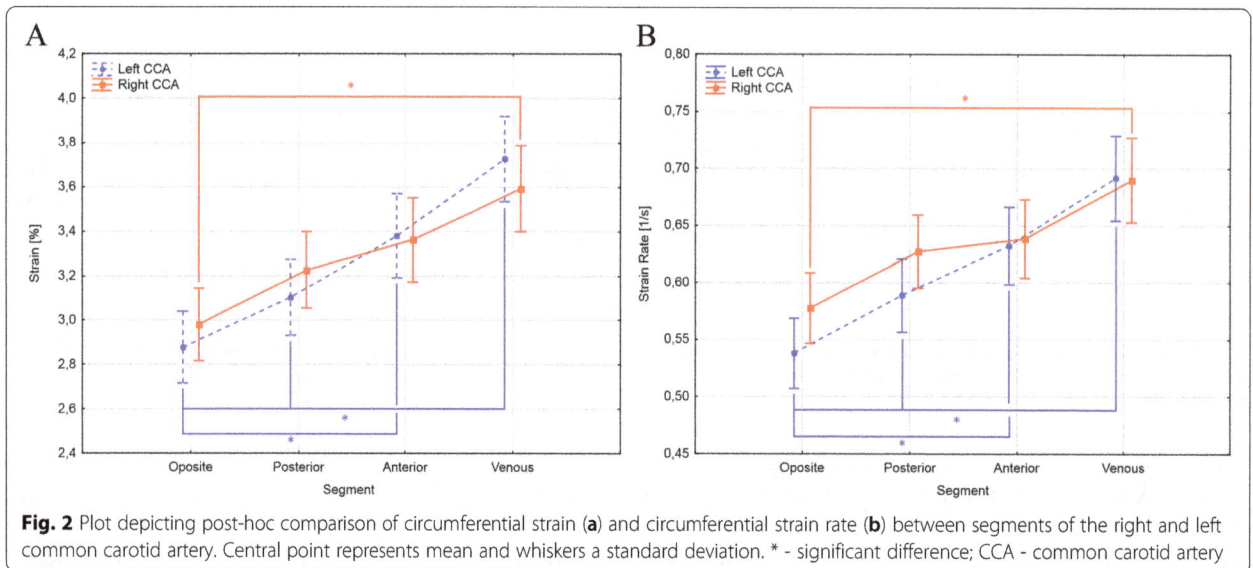

Fig. 2 Plot depicting post-hoc comparison of circumferential strain (**a**) and circumferential strain rate (**b**) between segments of the right and left common carotid artery. Central point represents mean and whiskers a standard deviation. * - significant difference; CCA - common carotid artery

atherosclerotic plaques which favours the posterior wall of the internal carotid artery [14]. This is in line with our results, because the opposite segment, usually comprising the posterior wall, was characterised by the least local elasticity, and so would be the most prone to plaque formation due to greater shearing stress.

2D-Speckle Tracking has been reported to offer excellent reproducibility when evaluating patients with subclinical atherosclerosis [3, 5, 15]. It gives better reproducibility when assessing arterial stiffness based on classical parameters [3, 7, 8]. This technique enables angle-independent calculations to be performed, which is especially important for operator-dependant ultrasound examination [4, 5, 7]. In addition, it has been found to be more sensitive than elastic modulus and β-stiffness index in detecting age-related differences in the elastic properties of CCA [5, 7]. In majority of studies, the global or far wall segment CS parameters were calculated because they offer better reproducibility than an analysis of each particular segment separately [2, 7]. Although one previous study, including 51 healthy subjects [8], has used bilateral segment-based analysis, it only reported significant variation in the anterior and inferior segments of the left CCA, the segments were determined automatically and their alignment was not adjusted for the neighbouring IJV.

Our findings indicate that movement of the carotid artery wall due to the passage of the pulse wave is non-homogeneous. Therefore, the evaluation of CCA diameter in a fixed manner, as the distance between a near and far wall, may not be as accurate as using 2D-Speckle Tracking to evaluate changes in diameter. Hence, standard stiffness parameters calculated based on routine measurements might be biased by the cross-sectional area of the IJV and the angle of its adherence to the CCA.

The potential limitation of this study is that it focuses only on the immediate neighbourhood of the IJV and not all surrounding tissues: It is possible that changes in the composition of loose connective tissue within the carotid sheath might also affect strain parameters. However, the aim of this research was to evaluate local (segmental) differences, and not the influence of homogeneous surroundings. The IJV was the most significant "soft point" adjacent to the CCA wall, which may increase its local elasticity. Secondly, assessment of brachial pressure instead of carotid pressure might have biased evaluation of stiffness parameters [6]. However, this effect is particularly pronounced in young subjects, when in our study the mean age of participants was 56 years. Furthermore, application of brachial pressure may lead to overestimation of stiffness parameters. Nevertheless, it might have increased the chance of significant relations between these parameters and internal jugular vein morphology but the results were not significant. Finally,, the study does not evaluate the actual error of standard measurements due to variations in IJV morphology. However, as it is now known that the IJV does play a role, this factor should be taken into account when planning further studies incorporating more advanced techniques, such as MRI.

Conclusion

This is the first report to indicate that IJV morphology has a direct influence on strain parameters of the CCA. Due to increasing role of stiffness parameters as markers of atherosclerosis and surrogates of cardiovascular events, their evaluation should be accurate. 2D-Speckle Tracking is a sensitive and reliable method that allows for evaluation of the complete circumference of the

CCA including the influence of IJV position. Hence, it offers the potential to become a superior tool for conventional stiffness measurements.

Abbreviations

2D: Two-dimensional; CCA: Common carotid artery; CS: Circumferential strain; CSr: Circumferential strain rate; D: Mean value of D_{max} and D_{min}; DBP: Diastolic blood pressure; DC: Distensibility coefficient; D_{max}: The largest distances between the intima media thickness on the near and far wall of the CCA; D_{min}: The smallest distances between the intima media thickness on the near and far wall of the CCA; IJV: Internal jugular vein; MRI: Magnetic resonance imaging; ROI: Region of interest; SBP: Systolic blood pressure; SD: Standard deviation; ΔD: Difference between D_{max} and D_{min}

Funding

This work was supported by the Polish Ministry of Science and Higher Education, as a research project within the "Diamentowy Grant" programme. Research number: DI2012 007742.
Role of the Funding Source: the Polish Ministry of Science and Higher Education covered costs of diagnostic and laboratory examinations, salary of the main researcher and costs of results publication.

Authors' contributions

Podgórski M and SL designed a study. WM recruited patients. GP and Polguj M performed the carotid ultrasound. Podgórski M and ŁM performed calculations. WM and SL conducted the statistical analysis. All the authors were involved in drafting and revising the manuscript and gafe final approval of the version to be published.

Competing interests

The authors declare that they have no competing interests.

Consent for publication

Not applicable.

Author details

[1]Department of Radiology and Diagnostic Imaging, Medical University of Lodz, 22, Kopcińskiego St., Barlicki Hospital, Lodz, Poland. [2]Department of Angiology, Chair of Anatomy, Medical University of Lodz, 60, Narutowicza St, Lodz, Poland. [3]Department of Diagnostic Imaging, Polish Mother's Memorial Hospital Research Institute, 281/289, Rzgowska St, Lodz, Poland.

References

1. Sehgel NL, Vatner SF, Meininger GA. "Smooth muscle cell stiffness syndrome"-revisiting the structural basis of arterial stiffness. Front Physiol. 2015;18(6):335.
2. Rhee MY, Lee HY, Bae PJ. Measurements of arterial stiffness: methodological aspects. Korean Circ J. 2008;38:343–50.
3. Catalano M, Lamberti-Castronuovo A, Catalano A, Filocamo D, Zimbalatti C. Two-dimensional speckle-tracking strain imaging in the assessment of mechanical properties of carotid arteries: feasibility and comparison with conventional markers of subclinical atherosclerosis. Eur J Echocardiogr. 2011;12:528–35.
4. Oliver JJ. Noninvasive assessment of arterial stiffness and risk of atherosclerotic events. Arterioscler Thromb Vasc Biol. 2003;23:554–66.
5. Bjällmark A, Lind B, Peolsson M, Shahgaldi K, Brodin L-A, Nowak J. Ultrasonographic strain imaging is superior to conventional non-invasive measures of vascular stiffness in the detection of age-dependent differences in the mechanical properties of the common carotid artery. Eur J Echocardiog. 2010;11:630–6.
6. Laurent S, Cockcroft J, Bortel L Van, Boutouyrie P, Giannattasio C, Hayoz D, et al. Expert consensus document on arterial stiffness: methodological issues and clinical applications. Eur Heart J. 2006;27:2588-605.
7. Saito M, Okayama H, Inoue K, Yoshii T, Hiasa G, Sumimoto T, et al. Carotid arterial circumferential strain by two-dimensional speckle tracking: a novel parameter of arterial elasticity. Hypertens Res. 2012;35:897–902.
8. Yuda S, Kaneko R, Muranaka A, Hashimoto A, Tsuchihashi K, Miura T, et al. Quantitative measurement of circumferential carotid arterial strain by two-dimensional speckle tracking imaging in healthy subjects. Echocardiography. 2011;28:899–906.
9. Qin X-H, Zhang H, Mi W-D. Anatomic relationship of the internal jugular vein and the common carotid artery in Chinese people. Chin Med J (Engl). 2010;123:3226–30.
10. Shoja MM, Ardalan MR, Tubbs RS, Loukas M, Vahedinia S, Jabbary R, et al. The relationship between the internal jugular vein and common carotid artery in the carotid sheath: the effects of age, gender and side. Ann Anat. 2008;190:339–43.
11. Podgórski M, Grzelak P, Szymczyk K, Szymczyk E, Drożdż J, Stefańczyk L. Peripheral vascular stiffness, assessed with two-dimensional speckle tracking versus the degree of coronary artery calcification, evaluated by tomographic coronary artery calcification index. Arch Med Sci. 2015;11:122–9.
12. Fung YC, Zweifach BW, Intaglietta M. Elastic environment of the capillary bed. Circ Res. 1966;19:441–61.
13. Liu Y, Dang C, Garcia M, Gregersen H, Kassab GS. Surrounding tissues affect the passive mechanics of the vessel wall: theory and experiment. Am J Physiol Heart Circ Physiol. 2007;293:H3290–300.
14. Nam K-H, Bok T-H, Jin C, Paeng D-G. Asymmetric radial expansion and contraction of rat carotid artery observed using a high-resolution ultrasound imaging system. Ultrasonics. 2014;54:233–40.
15. Park HE, Cho G-Y, Kim H-K, Kim Y-J, Sohn D-W. Validation of circumferential carotid artery strain as a screening tool for subclinical atherosclerosis. J Atheroscler Thromb. 2012;19:349–56.

12

Increased aortic intima-media thickness may be used to detect macrovascular complications in adult type II diabetes mellitus patients

Ayse Selcan Koc[1][*] and Hilmi Erdem Sumbul[2]

Abstract

Background: Carotid intima media thickness (C-IMT) and aortic IMT (A-IMT) increase in adult and pediatric patients with diabetes mellitus (DM), respectively. In both age groups IMT is used for early detection of macrovascular complications. In adult DM patients, A-IMT is still not a routine examination and is not used frequently. We aimed to determine whether there is an increase in A-IMT values measured from abdominal aorta besides traditional C-IMT in patients with type II DM and to determine parameters closely related to A-IMT in the same patient group.

Methods: We included 114 type II DM patients and 100 healthy control subjects similar in age and sex in our study. Bilateral C-IMT and A-IMT values were measured by B-mode ultrasonography (USG) in addition to anamnesis, physical examination and routine examinations of all patients.

Results: When the clinical, demographic and laboratory data of patients with and without DM were compared, there was a high level of glucose and HbA1c and low hemoglobin levels in the DM patient group. All other parameters were found to be similar between the two groups. When the B-mode USG findings were examined, it was found that C-IMT and A-IMT were increased in patients with DM, with the A-IMT increase being more prominent. A-IMT values were found to be strongly and positively correlated with age, systolic blood pressure, blood urea nitrogen, DM onset time and HbA1c levels, and a negatively and significantly correlated with hemoglobin levels ($p < 0.05$, for each). In the regression model, the parameters correlating most closely with A-IMT were DM diagnosis onset time, HbA1c and hemoglobin levels ($p = 0.001$ and $\beta = 0.353$, $p = 0.014$ and $\beta = 0.247$ and $p < 0.001$ and $\beta = -0.406$).

Conclusions: As in pediatric DM patients also in adult DM patients A-IMT can easily be measured with new model USG devices. A-IMT must be measured during abdominal USG which is routine in adult DM patients. A-IMT is an easy, reproducible and non-invasive parameter that may be used in the diagnosis of macrovascular complications of adult type II DM.

Keywords: Aortic intima-media thickness, Macrovascular complication, Type II diabetes mellitus

* Correspondence: drayseselcankoc@gmail.com
[1]Department of Radiology, University of Health Sciences - Adana Health Practices and Research Center, Adana, Turkey
Full list of author information is available at the end of the article

Background

Type II diabetes mellitus (DM) is a common metabolic disease, causing macrovascular and microvascular complications. DM is a major and known risk factor for atherosclerosis development. The most important macrovascular involvement in DM is coronary artery disease (CAD). Increased carotid intima-media thickness (C-IMT) in DM patients is closely related to asymptomatic or subclinical atherosclerosis and is recommended as a routine examination [1, 2].

The artery wall contains three layers; tunica intima, tunica media and tunica adventitia. The atherosclerotic process occurs in the first two walls, resulting in a structural change in the early period as an increase in IMT thickness. IMT on the posterior wall is clearly distinguishable with ultrasonography (USG). C-IMT and aortic IMT (A-IMT) increase in adult and pediatric patients with DM, respectively [1, 2]. IMT is used in early detection of macrovascular complications in both groups. Studies about the A-IMT evaluation obtained from abdominal aorta in adult DM patients are limited in the literature [3, 4]. For this reason, the importance of A-IMT in adult DM patients is unknown, it is not a routine examination and is not used.

A-IMT measurement can be used to detect the development of early atherosclerosis, since atherosclerosis is first started in the distal abdominal aorta [5–7]. Therefore, we hypothesize that A-IMT obtained with new model high-resolution USG devices may be more useful for early detection of macrovascular complications in adult DM patients than C-IMT. In our study, we aimed to determine whether there was an increase in A-IMT values measured from the abdominal aorta in addition to C-IMT, which became a routine for type II DM patients, and to identify parameters closely related to A-IMT in the same patient group.

Methods

Study population

We included 114 type II DM patients (mean age: 46.3 ± 12.8 years, male / female: 52/62) and 100 healthy control subjects similar in age and sex (mean age: 47.1 ± 12.3 years, male / female: 48/52) in our study. When we looked in terms of the control group, subjects that have major risk factors that may lead to an increase in IMT as smoking habits, hypertension (HT), hyperlipidemia and obesity were excluded from study. Those with secondary or malignant HT, calcific plaques, abdominal aneurysm or dissection, congestive heart failure, cerebrovascular disease, severe heart valve disease, inflammatory diseases, hematologic diseases, cancer, pregnancy and renal failure were also excluded from both groups. The Local Ethics Committee approved the study protocol and each participant gave written informed consent.

After a detailed medical history and a complete physical examination, basic characteristics of patients such as age, gender, HT, current smoking status, family history, and hyperlipidemia, presence of CAD and body mass index (BMI) were recorded.

Plasma glucose, HbA1c, triglyceride, low-density lipoprotein, high-density lipoprotein, hs-CRP, uric acid, creatinine, hemoglobin and white blood cell concentrations were measured using an automated chemistry analyzer using commercial kits.

Main carotid and abdominal aortic B-mode ultrasonography evaluation

The left and right main carotid artery and abdominal aorta were examined with a high resolution Doppler ultrasound system (Philips EPIQ 7) equipped with a 12 and 5 MHz high resolution linear and convex converter (Philips Health Care, Bothell, WA, USA) respectively. Ultrasound scanner setting was made to be useful for every patient for all B-mode USG examination (gain [55–75 dB]; penetration depth [2.5–16 cm]; dynamics range [50–60] and zoom range [0.8–2.0]). Arteries were examined both longitudinally and transversely. All arteries were scanned longitudinally to visualize the IMT on the posterior or distal artery wall. All measurements were made on frozen images. Two frozen images that the highest quality for the operator opinion's were selected for analysis in each study. The IMT is defined as the distance from the anterior edge of the first echogenic line to the anterior edge of the second echogenic line. The first line represents the intima-lumen interface and the second line represents the collagen-containing top layer of adventitia. Vascular IMT was measured using ultrasonic calipers in the presence of two independent and blind observers. All IMT values were calculated as averages of six measurements. Patients were examined in supine position. While studying carotid artery patients rotated their heads by 45 °counter from scanned area. IMT, which was measured from the distal wall of the right and left main carotid artery in the 10–20 mm proximal segment before bifurcation, was accepted as C-IMT. Abdominal A-IMT was examined in the 10–15 mm segment through from the level of renal artery bifurcation to iliac artery bifurcation. IMT measured from the posterior wall of the abdominal artery was accepted as A-IMT (Fig. 1). Increased A-IMT and C-IMT accepted as > 2.90 mm and > 0.90 mm respectively [8–10].

Statistical analysis

All analyzes were performed using SPSS 20.0 (SPSS for Windows 20.0, Chicago, IL, USA). Data are expressed as mean ± SD for continuous variables and as percent for categorical variables. Continuous variables with normal distribution were compared with Student t test, while

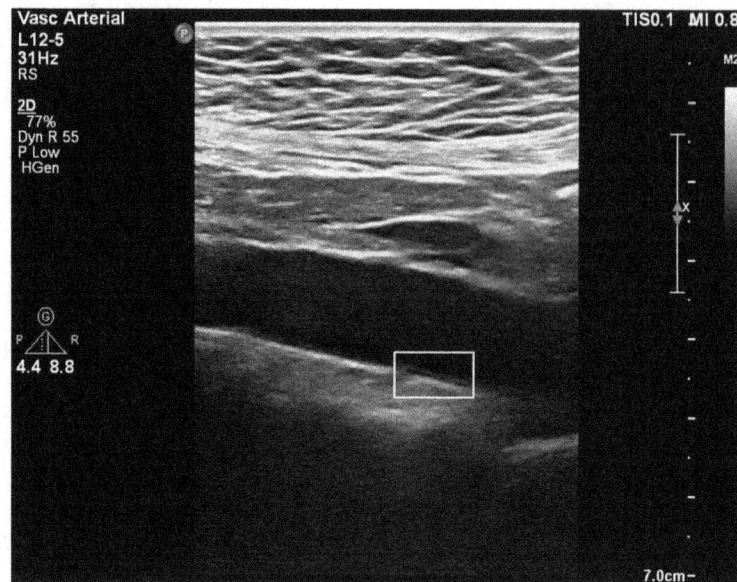

Fig. 1 Aortic IMT measurements with B-mode ultrasound from the level of renal artery bifurcation to iliac artery bifurcation

Mann-Whitney U test was used for not normally distributed samples. Categorical variables and frequencies were compared with chi-square (χ2) test. Statistical significance was defined as $p < 0.05$ for all comparisons. Pearson and Spearman correlations were used to examine the relationship between continuous variables. A multivariate, step-by-step forward conditional linear regression analysis was used to determine parameters much closer to the A-IMT. In the correlation analysis, the important parameters related to A-IMT were selected in the multivariate model. A receiver operator characteristic (ROC) curve analysis was carried out to identify the optimal cut-off point of A-IMT and C-IMT to detect presence of DM.

Results
Baseline characteristics
When the clinical, demographic and laboratory data of patients with and without DM were compared, there was a high level of glucose and HbA1c and a low hemoglobin level in the DM patient group. All other parameters were found to be similar between the two groups (Table 1). The incidence of smoking, HT and hypercholesterolemia in DM patients was 41.2, 57.9 and 51.8%, respectively. Patients were followed up for DM for an average of 4.8 ± 2.5 years, and the frequency of oral anti-diabetic and insulin treatment was 70.2 and 39.5%, respectively.

Vascular ultrasonography findings
A-IMT and C-IMT measurements were successfully performed in all patients who were included in the study. When the B-mode USG findings are examined we found

Table 1 Baseline characteristics and laboratory parameters in patients with type II DM and controls

	Type II DM $n = 114$	Controls $n = 100$	p
Age (year)	46.3 ± 12.8	47.1 ± 12.3	0.666
Gender (male)	62	58	0.435
Heart rate (beat/min)	84.9 ± 15.8	82.8 ± 16.1	0.331
Office systolic BP (mmHg)	132.9 ± 17.7	128.3 ± 8.1	0.069
Office diastolic BP (mmHg)	77.9 ± 8.3	75.9 ± 7.7	0.085
Body mass index (kg/m^2)	23.5 ± 4.1	23.2 ± 3.7	0.755
White blood cell (µL)	10.1 ± 3.4	9.8 ± 3.8	0.680
Hemoglobin (mg/dL)	12.8 ± 2.1	13.6 ± 2.8	0.045
Glukoz (mg/dL)	189.1 ± 86.2	91.2 ± 14.3	< 0.001
BUN (mg/dL)	38.9 ± 17.9	35.7 ± 16.6	0.178
Creatinine (mg/dL)	0.99 ± 0.86	1.01 ± 0.75	0.834
Total Cholesterol (mg/dL)	176 ± 44	183 ± 54	0.415
LDL Cholesterol (mg/dL)	103 ± 35	113 ± 44	0.080
HDL Cholesterol (mg/dL)	40.7 ± 13.9	41.9 ± 9.8	0.490
Triglyceride (mg/dL)	173 ± 108	150 ± 101	0.130
HbA1c (%)	8.3 ± 1.9	6.0 ± 0.9	< 0.001
hs-CRP (mg/L)	0.37 ± 0.29	0.42 ± 0.61	0.647
Uric acid (mg/dL)	5.68 ± 1.90	5.55 ± 1.68	0.656

BUN Blood urea nitrogen, *DM* Diabetes mellitus, *HDL* high density lipoprotein, *hs-CRP* high sensitive C reactive protein, *LDL* low density lipoprotein

that both IMT values were significantly higher in type II DM patients, with A-IMT being more prominent (Table 2). In DM patients, the frequency of increased A-IMT was significantly and 2 times higher than the control group (Table 2). However, although the increased C-IMT frequency was greater in the DM patient group, this difference was not statistically significant (Table 2).

Parameters associated with aortic intima-media thickness

Aortic IMT values were found to be strongly and positively correlated with age, systolic blood pressure, blood urea nitrogen, DM diagnosis time and HbA1c levels, and a negatively and significantly correlated with hemoglobin levels (Table 3). Patients with or without oral antidiabetic drug or insulin had similar A- IMT values ($p > 0.05$ both of them). In the linear regression model, the parameters correlating most closely with A-IMT were DM diagnosis time, HbA1c and hemoglobin levels (Table 3).

ROC analysis for A-IMT and C-IMT to detect patients with diabetes mellitus

In the ROC analysis, the area under the curve was 0.718 and 0.602 respectively for A-IMT and C-IMT ($p < 0.05$, Table 4). İf A-IMT and C-IMT cut-off values were taken as 1.5 mm and 0.9 mm, respectively, these values detect the patient with DM with a sensitivity of 70.3% and specificity of 63.0%, sensitivity of 60.5% and specificity of 55.8%, respectively (Table 4).

Discussion

The main result of this study is that A-IMT is found to be significantly increased in adult DM patients. Another striking finding is that the A-IMT increase in DM patients is greater than the C-IMT increase. In addition, the parameters most closely associated with A-IMT in our study were found to be DM diagnosis time, serum hemoglobin and HbA1c levels. In addition, as in pediatric DM patients, the A-IMT can easily be measured with new model USG devices in adult DM patients.

Diabetes mellitus causes an increase in smooth muscle cell proliferation in vessel walls, worsens oxidative stress exposure and leads to production of free oxygen radicals [2]. This entire process leads to extensive thickening of the arterial walls. Increased C-IMT is closely associated

Table 2 Vascular ultrasound finding in patients with type II DM and controls

	Type II DM $n = 114$	Controls $n = 100$	p
Common carotid IMT (mm)	0.82 ± 0.18	0.76 ± 0.17	0.023
Abdominal aort IMT (mm)	1.84 ± 0.77	1.49 ± 0.75	0.001
Increased common carotid IMT, n (%)	31 (27.2)	22 (22.0)	0.236
Increased abdominal aort IMT, n (%)	26 (22.8)	11 (11.0)	0.017

IMT Intima-media thickness

with asymptomatic atherosclerosis in DM patients and has been proposed as a routine examination [1, 2]. It is a known fact that the B-mode USG evaluation of C-IMT is a reproducible and useful method in the detection of asymptomatic atherosclerosis in DM patients [1, 2]. C-IMT is also associated with CAD, myocardial infarction, and stroke. [11–14]. For these reasons, C-IMT is the preferred method of vascular assessment. C-IMT is also preferred because it is superficially located in neck, easy to visualize, easy to examine, and has many C-IMT documents in the literature.

Aortic IMT is not routinely used in DM patients. The main reasons for this are: (i) There is limited data on the association of A-IMT with macrovascular organ involvement in DM patients [3, 4], (ii) A-IMT assessment is more difficult than C-IMT,(iii) It is not preferred as a routine method in DM disease, (iiii) especially abdominal fat tissue is thought to prevent A-IMT measurement [3]. Atherosclerosis begins to develop as fatty streaks in childhood and can be diagnosed early by sensitive visualization methods [15, 16]. Because atherosclerosis first occurs in the distal abdominal aorta, A-IMT measurement with new USG devices can be used to detect early atherosclerosis development [5–7]. Therefore, we hypothesize that A-IMT obtained with new model high-resolution USG devices may be more useful for early detection of macrovascular complications in adult DM patients than C-IMT. For this reason, we received A-IMT measurements of the abdominal aorta from our patients. Aortic IMT is preferred in pediatric and adolescent groups because tissue penetration is good; target organ damage begins here and is more susceptible to the risk of cardiovascular events. Aortic IMT is thought to be an early indicator of atherosclerosis in this age group. In high-risk children with hypercholesterolemia, DM and inflammatory bowel disease [7, 17–19]. A-IMT is more potent than C-IMT and can detect atherosclerosis earlier. There is no study showing that A-IMT is superior to C-IMT in predicting pre-clinical atherosclerosis, target organ damage, and cardiovascular event risk in adults and most USG devices do not have adequate tissue penetration in adult DM patients. For this reason, A-IMT measurement in adults is not a routine assessment. Diabetes mellitus is the equivalent of CAD and is one of the major risk factors for atherosclerosis. In our study, histopathologic vascular tissue examination was not performed but an explanatory result was obtained for the pathogenesis of macrovascular involvement in DM patients. In our study, the increase of A-IMT in patients with DM is more pronounced and significant than C-IMT. When performing ROC analyses for A-IMT and C-IMT measurements with DM presence, the limit values for A-IMT and C-IMT with DM presence were 1.5 mm and 0.9 mm respectively. The A-IMT increase was thought to be more prominent

Table 3 The parameters associated with A-IMT and linear regression analysis for parameters significantly correlated with A-IMT

A-IMT	Correlation analyze		Regression analyses	
	p	r	p	β
C-IMT (mm)	< 0.001	0.896	–	–
Age (year)	< 0.001	0.237	0.081	0.216
Office systolic blood pressure (mmHg)	0.044	0.177	0.201	0.106
DM diagnosis time (years)	< 0.001	0.450	0.001	0.353
Hemoglobin (mg/dL)	0.018	- 0.167	< 0.001	- 0.406
Glukoz (mg/dL)	0.012	0.174	0.756	0.064
HbA1c (%)	0.003	0.202	0.014	0.247
Blood urea nitrogen (mg/dL)	0.003	0.205	0.209	0.141

DM Diabetes mellitus, *IMT* Intima-media thickness * $R^2_{Adjusted}$ = 0.382 and C-IMT was excluded in linear regression analyses

than the C-IMT because the atherosclerosis was first detected at the beginning of the distal abdominal aorta, the abdominal aortic vessel diameter and thickness were larger than the carotid artery and C-IMT was affected after A-IMT. According to our evaluation, studies comparing abdominal A-IMT values in adult DM patients are limited in the literature [3, 4]. In a study conducted in adult type 1 DM patients a decade ago, A-IMT evaluations was performed and a lower mean A-IMT value was obtained than our study [3]. However, in this study, it was reported that A-IMT measurement was a difficult challenge and therefore only 69% of the patients had A-IMT measurements. Although there is no clear information on the measurement problem in this study, increased intraabdominal fat tissue, especially in DM patients, is thought to prevent A-IMT measurement. In a recent study of middle-aged sporadic idiopathic hypo parathyroid patients, just like our findings there was a strong correlation between A-IMT and C-IMT [20]. There is a serious difference in the A-IMT measurements obtained in these two studies and there is a reference value problem to standardize the A-IMT. In two small studies including 39 adult DM and 10 congenital adrenal hyperplasia patients, A-IMT measurement was evaluated and the A-IMT value was found to be 0.89 ± 0.17 mm and 1.84 ± 0.68 mm, respectively [3, 21]. Our study was performed with a 5 MHz high-resolution probe and the mean A-IMT value of DM patients was 1.84 ± 0.75 mm. In our study, the A-IMT value obtained in DM patients was very close to Sartorato et al. study [21] but our findings were obtained with more patients than previous study.

Table 4 ROC analysis for A-IMT and C-IMT to detect patients with diabetes mellitus

Variable	AUROC Curve	p	Cut-off	Sensitivity	Specificity
A-IMT	0.718 (0.542–0.790)	0.002	1.5 mm	70.3%	63.0%
C-IMT	0.602 (0.506–0.699)	0.012	0.9 mm	60.5%	55.8%

IMT Intima-media thickness

There are no detailed clinical studies, and most USG devices do not have probes that sufficiently penetrate tissue in adult DM patients. Hence, A-IMT measurement is not a routine evaluation in adults. With the new USG devices and high-resolution probes, abdominal aorta visualization is much better and A-IMT can be measured by easily. It may be a useful approach to use A-IMT instead of C-IMT to determine subclinical organ damage in type II DM patients.

In our study, we found that both IMT values were significantly higher in type II DM patients, with A-IMT being more prominent. In a previous study, increased C-IMT in type II DM patients was associated with older age, male sex, smoking, and pulse pressure [22]. It has also been reported that advanced glycation end products, which are the result of DM disease, are associated with C-IMT [2]. In our study, we found that the age, systolic blood pressure, increased HbA1c and DM diagnosis time and A-IMT increase were closely related and correlated with the literature. In addition, low hemoglobin levels and increased A-IMT were closely related in our study.

Limitation

This study investigated the relationship between DM and A-IMT cross-sectionally. We have included a relatively small number of patients, but we have shown that A-IMT is significantly increased in DM patients. DM patients in our study had an average 5 years of diagnosis. This can be very early for the development of macrovascular complications in patients with DM. Because DM is a long-term disease and macrovascular complications occur after many years. For this reason, the follow-up of these patients should continue. The increase in IMT is also related to the cardiovascular events [23]. However, we did not evaluate prognosis in our study. Previous studies have shown that C-IMT is regressed by medical therapy in DM patients. Our study is not a follow-up study and therefore no disease control C-IMT and A-IMT assessments have been performed [24]. There is no study with A-IMT but the C-IMT measurement can be measured automatically and semi-automatically with new software programs, resulting in a lower average value than the manual measurement [25, 26]. This automatic measurement especially removes operator dependence and is more useful for repetitive measurements. However, our high-resolution device did not have this software program so we could not make this evaluation. In our study, if IMT could be measured automatically and semi-automatically, more objective and meaningful results could be obtained. The latest technological devices and high frequency probes are used in our study. For this reason, it may not be possible to obtain similar results with low-frequency and low-resolution devices.

Conclusions

As in pediatric DM patients, A-IMT is also increased by 22.8% in adult DM patients, and A-IMT can be easily measured with new model USG devices. According to the results of our study, A-IMT, which shows macrovascular organ involvement relatively early in DM, is more useful than C-IMT. A part of the abdominal USG, which is a routine examination in adult DM patients, should include the A-IMT measurement and the A-IMT value should be reported at the end of the abdominal USG. A-IMT is a cheap, easy, reproducible and non-invasive parameter that may be used to detect subclinical atherosclerosis, an early macrovascular complication of adult type II DM.

Abbreviations

A-IMT: Aortic intima media thickness; BMI: Body mass index; BUN: Blood urea nitrogen; CAD: Coronary artery disease; C-IMT: Carotid intima media thickness; DM: Diabetes mellitus; HDL: High density lipoprotein; hs-CRP: high sensitive C reactive protein; HT: Hypertension; LDL: Low density lipoprotein; USG: Ultrasonography

Acknowledgements
There is nothing to declare with this study.

Funding
This research received no specific grant from any funding agency.

Authors' contributions
ASK and HES made substantial contributions to patient inclusion, to data analysis and data interpretation. All authors have contributed in writing and correcting the manuscript and approved the submission of the manuscript.

Consent for publication
Not applicable.

Competing interests
The authors declare that they have no competing interests.

Author details
[1]Department of Radiology, University of Health Sciences - Adana Health Practices and Research Center, Adana, Turkey. [2]Department of Internal Medicine, University of Health Sciences - Adana Health Practices and Research Center, Adana, Turkey.

References

1. McCloskey K, Vuillermin P, Ponsonby AL, Cheung M, Skilton MR, Burgner D. Aortic intima-media thickness measured by trans-abdominal ultrasound as an early life marker of subclinical atherosclerosis. Acta Paediatr. 2014;103:124–30.
2. Lilje C, Cronan JC, Schwartzenburg EJ, Owers EM, Clesi P, Gomez R, et al. Intima-media thickness at different arterial segments in pediatric type 1 diabetes patients and its relationship with advanced glycation end products. Pediatr Diabetes. 2017; https://doi.org/10.1111/pedi.12557.
3. Astrand H, Rydén-Ahlgren A, Sundkvist G, Sandgren T, Länne T. Reduced aortic wall stress in diabetes mellitus. Eur J Vasc Endovasc Surg. 2007;33:592–8.
4. Su Y, Liu W, Wang D, Tian J. Evaluation of abdominal aortic elasticity by strain rate imaging in patients with type 2 diabetes mellitus. J Clin Ultrasound. 2014;42:475–80.
5. Shin PS, Kim DS. Histochemical studies of fetal arteries of Koreans with special reference to atherogenesis in adults. Yonsei Med J. 1963;4:37–42.
6. Nakashima Y, Chen YX, Kinukawa N, Sueishi K. Distributions of diffuse intimal thickening in human arteries: preferential expression in atherosclerosis-prone arteries from an early age. Virchows Arch. 2002;441:279–88.
7. Jarvisalo MJ, Jartti L, Nanto-Salonen K, Irjala K, Ronnemaa T, Hartiala JJ, et al. Increased aortic intima-media thickness: a marker of preclinical atherosclerosis in high-risk children. Circulation. 2001;104:2943–7.
8. Belhassen L, Carville C, Pelle G, Monin JL, Teiger E, Duval-Moulin AM, et al. Evaluation of carotid artery and aortic intima-media thickness measurements for exclusion of significant coronary atherosclerosis in patients scheduled for heart valve surgery. J Am Coll Cardiol. 2002;39:1139–44.
9. Koc AS, Gorgulu FF, Donmez Y, Icen YK. There is a significant relationship between morning blood pressure surge and increased abdominal aortic intima-media thickness in hypertensive patients. J Med Ultrason. 2001;2018 https://doi.org/10.1007/s10396-018-0877-y.
10. 2013 ESH/ESC. Guidelines for the management of arterial hypertension. Eur Heart J. 2013;34:2159–219.
11. Handa N, Matsumoto M, Maeda H, Hougaku H, Ogawa S, Fukunaga R, et al. Ultrasonic evaluation of early carotid atherosclerosis. Stroke. 1990;21:1567–72.
12. Heiss G, Sharrett AR, Barnes R, Chambless LE, Szklo M, Alzola C. Carotid atherosclerosis measured by B-mode ultrasound in populations: associations with cardiovascular risk factors in the ARIC study. Am J Epidemiol. 1991;134:250–6.
13. Wofford JL, Kahl FR, Howard GR, McKinney WM, Toole JF, Crouse JR 3rd. Relation of extent of extracranial carotid artery atherosclerosis as measured by B-mode ultrasound to the extent of coronary atherosclerosis. Arterioscler Thromb. 1991;11:1786–94.
14. O'Leary DH, Polak JF, Kronmal RA, Manolio TA, Burke GL, Wolfson SK Jr. The cardiovascular health study collaborative research group. Carotid-artery intima and media thickness as a risk factor for myocardial infarction and stroke in older adults. N Engl J Med. 1999;340:14–22.
15. Berenson G, Srinivasan S, Bao W, Newman WP 3rd, Tracy RE, Wattigney WA. Association between multiple cardiovascular risk factors and atherosclerosis in children and young adults. New Eng J Med. 1998;338:1650–5.
16. Enos WJ, Beyer J, Holmes R. Pathogenesis of coronary disease in American soldiers killed in Korea. JAMA. 1955;158:912–4.
17. Aloi M, Tromba L, Rizzo V, D'Arcangelo G, Dilillo A, Blasi S, et al. Aortic intima-media thickness as an early marker of atherosclerosis in children with inflammatory bowel disease. J Pediatr Gastroenterol Nutr. 2015;61:41–6.
18. Davis PH, Dawson JD, Blecha MB, Mastbergen RK, Sonka M. Measurement of aortic intimal-medial thickness in adolescents and young adults. Ultrasound Med Biol. 2010;36:560–5.
19. Kallio K, Jokinen E, Saarinen M, Hamalainen M, Volanen I, Kaitosaari T, et al. Arterial intima-media thickness, endothelial function, and apolipoproteins in adolescents frequently exposed to tobacco smoke. Circ Cardiovasc Qual Outcomes. 2010;3:196–203.
20. Meena D, Prakash M, Gupta Y, Bhadada SK, Khandelwal N. Carotid, aorta and renal arteries intima-media thickness in patients with sporadic idiopathic hypoparathyroidism. Indian J Endocrinol Metab. 2015;19:262–6.
21. Sartorato P, Zulian E, Benedini S, Mariniello B, Schiavi F, Bilora F, et al. Cardiovascular risk factors and ultrasound evaluation of intima-media thickness at common carotids, carotid bulbs, and femoral and abdominal aorta arteries in patients with classic congenital adrenal hyperplasia due to 21-hydroxylase deficiency. J Clin Endocrinol Metab. 2007;92:1015–8.

22. Cardoso CR, Marques CE, Leite NC, Salles GF. Factors associated with carotid intima-media thickness and carotid plaques in type 2 diabetic patients. J Hypertens. 2012;30:940–7.

23. Lorenz MW, Markus HS, Bots ML, Rosvall M, Sitzer M. Prediction of clinical cardiovascular events with carotid intima-media thickness: a systematic review and meta-analysis. Circulation. 2007;115:459–67.

24. Mita T, Katakami N, Shiraiwa T, Yoshii H, Gosho M, Shimomura I, et al. Dose-dependent effect of Sitagliptin on carotid atherosclerosis in patients with type 2 diabetes mellitus receiving insulin treatment: a post hoc analysis. Diabetes Ther. 2017;8:1135–46.

25. Novo G, Di Miceli R, Orlando D, Lunetta M, Pugliesi M, Fiore M, et al. Carotid intima-media thickness measurement through semi-automated detection software and analysis of vascular walls. Int Angiol. 2013;32:349–53.

26. Shenouda N, Proudfoot NA, Currie KD, Timmons BW, MacDonald MJ. Automated ultrasound edge-tracking software comparable to established semi-automated reference software for carotid intima-media thickness analysis. Clin Physiol Funct Imaging. 2018;38:396–401.

13

Diagnostic performance of multi-organ ultrasound with pocket-sized device in the management of acute dyspnea

Alfonso Sforza[1,4†], Costantino Mancusi[1,2†], Maria Viviana Carlino[1,3], Agostino Buonauro[1], Marco Barozzi[4], Giuseppe Romano[4], Sossio Serra[4] and Giovanni de Simone[1,3*]

Abstract

Background: The availability of ultra-miniaturized pocket ultrasound devices (PUD) adds diagnostic power to the clinical examination. Information on accuracy of ultrasound with handheld units in immediate differential diagnosis in emergency department (ED) is poor. The aim of this study is to test the usefulness and accuracy of lung ultrasound (LUS) alone or combined with ultrasound of the heart and inferior vena cava (IVC) using a PUD for the differential diagnosis of acute dyspnea (AD).

Methods: We included 68 patients presenting to the ED of "Maurizio Bufalini" Hospital in Cesena (Italy) for AD. All patients underwent integrated ultrasound examination (IUE) of lung-heart-IVC, using PUD. The series was divided into patients with dyspnea of cardiac or non-cardiac origin. We used 2 × 2 contingency tables to analyze sensitivity, specificity, positive predictive value and negative predictive value of the three ultrasonic methods and their various combinations for the diagnosis of cardiogenic dyspnea (CD), comparing with the final diagnosis made by an independent emergency physician.

Results: LUS alone exhibited a good sensitivity (92.6%) and specificity (80.5%). The highest accuracy (90%) for the diagnosis of CD was obtained with the combination of LUS and one of the other two methods (heart or IVC).

Conclusions: The IUE with PUD is a useful extension of the clinical examination, can be readily available at the bedside or in ambulance, requires few minutes and has a reliable diagnostic discriminant ability in the setting of AD.

Keywords: Acute dyspnea, Multi-organ ultrasound, Pocket-sized device, Emergency department

Background

Acute dyspnea is one of the most frequent symptoms of patients presenting to the emergency department (ED), with about 4–5 million hits per year in the United States [1]. The differential diagnosis is often challenging especially to distinguish between dyspnea of cardiac origin (CD) and dyspnea of other causes. Medical history, physical examination, blood gas analysis, electrocardiogram,

laboratory tests and chest X-rays are essential in the diagnostic process, but sometimes not enough and often difficult to obtain instantaneously. For these reasons, about 20% of patients who logs in ED for dyspnea receive incorrect diagnosis and consequently inadequate therapy [2].

Focused cardiac ultrasound plays an important role in the diagnostic evaluation of the patient at bedside and it is important for triage decisions and emergency treatment [3]. Large amount of information can be also obtained using lung ultrasound (LUS) especially in the identification and evaluation of pleuro-pulmonary diseases and in the evaluation of extra-vascular lung water [4, 5]. Utility of LUS has been recently tested to help discriminating causes of acute dyspnea in ED, with or without simultaneous

* Correspondence: simogi@unina.it
†Equal contributors
[1]Hypertension Research Center, Federico II University Hospital of Naples, Via Pansini 5, bld #1, 80131 Naples, Italy
[3]Department of Traslational Medical Science. Federico II University Hospital, Naples, Italy
Full list of author information is available at the end of the article

evaluation of heart and inferior vena cava (IVC) [6, 7]. Using pocket-size imaging device also the assessment of extravascular lung water with evaluation of B-lines and pleural effusion is feasible and reliable [8].

In the setting of ED standard echocardiographic equipment may be heavy and difficult to handle while hand-carried ultrasound devices have been developed for bedside use. In particular, the ultrasound technology pool has been enriched with pocket ultrasound devices that offer advantages in terms of portability and speed, and are able to reproduce images with standard ultrasound and color Doppler. These devices can be used as first ultrasound approach in ED and ambulance and confer added diagnostic power to the clinical examination in populations of patients with no history of cardiovascular disease [9, 10].

Informations on accuracy of first diagnostic assessment with pocket ultrasound device in immediate differential diagnosis for acute dyspnea in ED are still deficient. The aim of this study is to test the utility and accuracy of LUS alone or combined with ultrasound of the heart and IVC in the identification of CD with pocket ultrasound device in ED.

Methods

From November 2014 to August 2015 we enrolled 68 patients presenting to the ED of "Maurizio Bufalini" hospital in Cesena (Italy) for acute dyspnea or sudden worsening of chronic dyspnea within the previous 48 h. All patients underwent clinical exam, blood gas analysis, chest X-Ray, ECG, routine blood tests and integrated ultrasound examination of lung-heart-IVC with pocket size device Vscan (General Electric Healthcare) with a single probe (1.7–3.8 MHz), using abdominal preset for lung and cardiac preset for heart and IVC. Ultrasound examination was performed in semi sitting or supine position by one emergency physician expert in transthoracic echocardiography (ASE level III) and with good experience of LUS who was not taking care of the patient (Fig. 1). The ultrasound examination was done within 30 min from the arrival of the patients in ED.

Thorax was examined following a simplified protocol that provides two scans at each side: anteriorly on the II intercostal space, midclavicular line and lateral on the V intercostal space, midaxillary line, to sample upper and lower lungs [5, 11]. The presence or the absence of interstitial syndrome (IS, defined as the presence of at least 3 B-lines for field) and the presence or the absence of pleural effusion (defined as a hypo-anechoic space between the parietal and visceral pleura) were evaluated. LUS was defined positive for bilateral IS and/or effusion if any IS and/or effusion was present in at least 1 scan per side and symmetrically [12]. By symmetrical we mean the presence of IS and/or effusion in the same scans in both sides of the lungs.

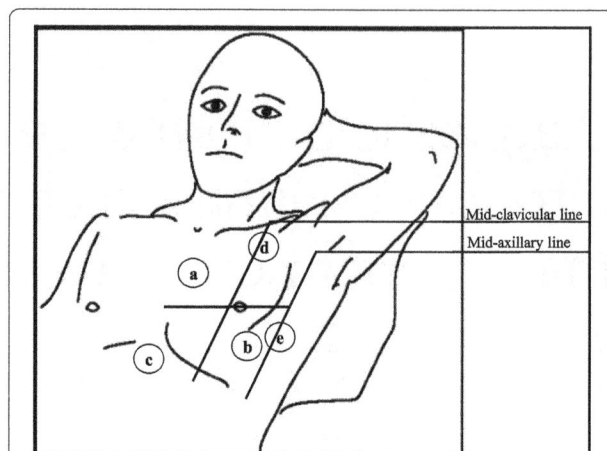

Fig. 1 Integrated ultrasound examination. **a**, **b**, **c**: heart and IVC examination. **d**, **e** lung ultrasound examination. **a**: parasternal long/short axis viex; **b**: apical view; **c**: subcostal view; **d**: anteriorly on the II intercostal space, midclavicular line; **e**: V intercostal space, midaxillary line

The heart was examined in at least one projection (parasternal long/short axis view and/or apical view and/or subcostal view) allowing qualitative evaluation of left ventricular systolic function, size of chambers and the presence or absence of pericardial effusion. Ejection fraction (EF) was estimated visually and categorized as preserved if >40% or reduced if ≤40% [13].

The IVC was explored in subcostal view and evaluated by the presence or absence of dilatation (> 2 cm) and hypo-reactivity with breathing (variation of size <50%) [3].

The final diagnosis of acute dyspnea was determined by an independent emergency physician (blind to the integrated ultrasound examination) who has followed each patient, taking into account all the clinical investigations performed (clinical exam, blood gas analysis, chest X-Ray, ECG, routine blood tests) and the evolution of the patients (response to diuretics, vasoactive agents, non-invasive ventilation, corticosteroids, etc.). Without knowledge of the ultrasound data collected in the ED, he had to classify patients into 2 groups: cardiogenic dyspnea (CD) and dyspnea of non-cardiac origin (non-CD). The primary end point was to compare the diagnostic performance of cardiopulmonary ultrasound with pocket size device and standard examinations (clinical, laboratory, chest x-ray, ECG) for the diagnosis of CD. Specifically, for the diagnosis of CD, the Boston-score diagnostic criteria (points 5–12) have been always satisfied [14].

In patients with coexistence of heart failure and another cause of dyspnea the main diagnosis was considered CD [15].

Another emergency physician expert in lung and cardiac ultrasound read all images, blind to the final diagnosis from the ED.

Statistics

Data were analyzed using SPSS version 21.0 (SPSS, Chicago, Illinois, USA). Continuous data are expressed as mean ± 1 standard deviation and categorical variables as percentages. Quantitative variables were compared by using Student's t-test while χ^2 distribution was used to compare categorical variables.

The population was divided into patients with CD and patients with non-CD. Contingency tables were produced to analyze sensitivity, specificity, positive predictive value and negative predictive value of the three ultrasonic findings obtained with pocket size device and their various combinations for the diagnosis of CD, based on the final diagnosis made by the emergency physician. Receiver operating characteristic (ROC) curves (AUC) are used to describe and compare the performance of each different ultrasound modality (Lung, Heart, IVC) and the combination between bilateral IS/effusion and only 1 of the cardiovascular abnormalities (EF ≤40% OR dilated and not collapsing IVC) versus the final ED diagnosis [16].

A p-value <0.05 was considered statistical significant.

Results

Our study population included 68 patients (43 males) with a mean age of 78 years. Table 1 shows the baseline

characteristics of the population at arrival in ED. An integrated ultrasound examination was feasible in all patients except 4 who were excluded from the IVC evaluation because under CPAP at arrival in ED. The ultrasound examination time was always less than 3 min.

Table 2 displays the definitive diagnosis of patients, 40% of whom had CD, while 60% had non-CD. Patients with CD show lower body temperature and percentage of neutrophils on white blood cell count (both $p < 0.05$) and have tendencies to have higher Lactate and creatinine levels and lower C-reactive protein compared to patients with non-CD (Table 1).

Table 3 shows the sensitivity, specificity, positive predictive value (PPV), negative predictive value (NPV) and accuracy for the diagnosis of CD of various ultrasound markers taken individually or in combination. LUS positivity for bilateral IS and/or effusion exhibited good sensitivity and good specificity. The maximum accuracy (90%) for the diagnosis of CD was obtained in the combination of LUS positivity for bilateral IS and/or effusion AND reduced EF OR dilated and hypo-reactive IVC, while the contemporary presence of all three ultrasound abnormalities did not give an optimal accuracy, especially because of the poor sensitivity.

Figure 2 shows receiving operating characteristics (ROC) curves (AUC) of the different ultrasound diagnostic approaches evaluated. The combined presence of bilateral IS/effusion AND only 1 other cardiovascular abnormalities (EF ≤40% OR dilated and not collapsing IVC) has the highest AUC for the identification of patients with dyspnea of cardiac origin. Although the difference is not statistically significant from the LUS alone, specificity is maximized.

Discussion

In a population of patients presenting to the ED for the recent onset of acute dyspnea the integrated ultrasound examination of Lung-Heart-IVC with a pocket size

Table 1 Baseline characteristics and in-hospital arrival vital signs of the study population

Characteristics	Total study population ($n = 68$)	Dyspnea of cardiac origin ($n = 27$)	Dyspnea of non-cardiac origin ($n = 41$)
Age (years)	78 ± 12	80 ± 9	77 ± 14
Men (%)	62	56	66
Heart Rate (bpm)	97 ± 25	91 ± 27	100 ± 24
Systolic BP (mmHg)	135 ± 24	138.7 ± 26.4	132.9 ± 22.6
Diastolic BP (mmHg)	78 ± 15	81.8 ± 14.9	75.3 ± 14.3
Respiratory rate (breaths/min)	24 ± 6	22 ± 6	25 ± 6
Oxygen saturation (%)	92 ± 6	93 ± 4	92 ± 7
PaO_2/Fio_2	269 ± 92	292 ± 75	254 ± 100
Body temperature (°C)	37 ± 1	36 ± 1*	37 ± 1
White Blood cell (×10^3/ml)	12.0 ± 5.8	10.4 ± 5.5	13.1 ± 5.7
Neutrophils (%)	77 ± 11	73 ± 10*	79 ± 11
Hemoglobin (g/dl)	12.7 ± 2.3	12.3 ± 2.1	12.9 ± 2.4
C reactive protein (mg/dl)	66 ± 79	51 ± 71	73 ± 82
Lactate (mmol/L)	2.4 ± 2.1	2.6 ± 2.9	2.3 ± 1.3
Creatinine (mg/dl)	1.2 ± 0.9	1.48 ± 1.21	1.09 ± 0.47
History of Chronic Obstructive Pulmonary disease (%)	49	32*	59
History of Heart Failure (%)	41	60*	29

BP Blood Pressure

*p > 0.05 vs dyspnea of non-cardiac origin

Table 2 Final diagnosis at ED discharge

	Cases
Final diagnosis	
Acute heart failure	25 (36.8%)
Pneumonia	18 (26.5%)
Acute or re-exacerbation of COPD	17 (25%)
Acute heart failure + Pneumonia	2 (2.9%)
Others: (3) lung cancer, (2) pulmonary embolism, (1) pneumothorax	6 (8.8%)
Identification of dyspnea of cardiac origin	
Dyspnea of cardiac origin	27 (39.7%)
Dyspnea of non-cardiac origin	41 (60.3%)

COPD Chronic Obstructive Pulmonary Disease

Table 3 Sensitivity, specificity, positive and negative predictive value and accuracy of the Chest X-ray, Boston score (points 8–12), lung, heart and IVC ultrasound and their combinations in the diagnosis of dyspnea of cardiac origin

Parameter	Sensitivity (%)	Specificity (%)	PPV (%)	NPV (%)	Accuracy (%)
Chest X-ray	75 (52.9–89.3)	85.4 (70.1–93.9)	75 (52.9–89.4)	85.4 (70.1–93.9)	82
Boston score (points 8–12)	79.2 (57.3–92)	70.7 (54.3–83.3)	61.3 (42.3–77.6)	85.3 (68.2–94.4)	74
IS/ effusion	92,6 (74.2–98.7)	80,5 (64.6–90.6)	75,8 (57.4–88.2)	94,3 (79.5–99)	85,3
IVC dilated and not collapsing	65,4 (44.3–82)	88,2 (71.6–96.2)	81 (57.4–93.7)	76,9 (60.2–88.2)	78,3
EF ≤ 40%	66,7 (46–82.7)	87,2 (71.7–95.2)	78,3 (55.8–91.7)	79,1 (63.5–89.4)	78,8
IS/effusion OR IVC dilated and not collapsing	100 (84.4–100)	71.4 (53.4–84.7)	72.9 (55.6–85.6)	100 (83.4–100)	85
IS/effusion OR EF ≤ 40%	92,3 (74.2–98.7)	70,7 (54.3–83.3)	67.5 (50.1–81.4)	93.5 (77.2–98.9)	80
IS/effusion AND IVC dilated and not collapsing	57,7 (37.2–76)	94,1 (78.9–98.9)	88,2 (62.2–97.9)	74,4 (58.6–86)	78,3
IS/effusion AND EF ≤ 40%	66.6 (46–82.7)	97,5 (85.5–99.8)	94,7 (71.8–99.7)	81.6 (71.8–99.7)	85
IS/effusion AND EF ≤ ≤40% AND IVC dilated and not collapsing	40.7 (23–60.9)	97,6 (85.6–99.8)	91,6 (59.7–99.5)	71.4 (57.6–82.3)	73,3
IS/effusion AND (EF ≤ 40% OR IVC dilated and not collapsing)	81.4 (61.2–92.3)	95.1 (82.2–99.2)	91.7 (71.6–98.6)	88.6 (74.6–95.7)	90

PPV Positive Predictive Value, *NPV* Negative Predictive Value, *IS* Bilateral and symmetrical Interstitial Syndrome, *IVC* Inferior Vena Cava, *EF* Ejection Fraction

device is feasible and has reliable diagnostic value for the diagnosis of dyspnea of cardiac origin.

Among clinical manifestations of cardiovascular disease, heart failure is increasing in prevalence and incidence, and is among the leading causes of hospitalization and death. Despite advances in recognize subclinical findings of impaired left ventricular function, in acute heart failure the

diagnosis is challenging [17–19]. Diastolic dysfunction of the left ventricle, present in all the types of heart failure, regardless of the values of EF, is characterized by increased left ventricular filling pressure with congestion or pulmonary edema and consequent respiratory symptoms. The dysfunction of the right heart, usually secondary to increase in pulmonary arterial pressure, is responsible for

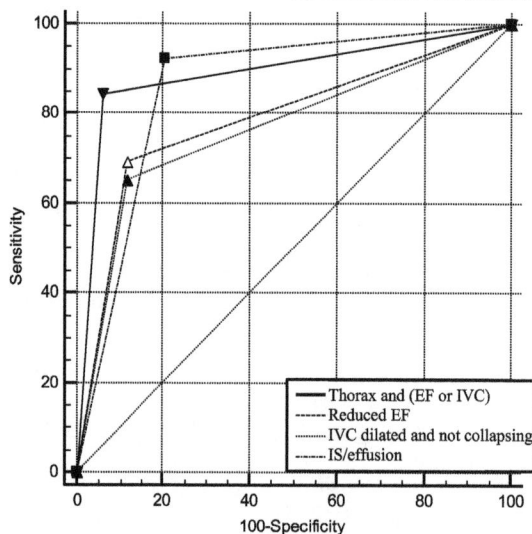

Parameter	Area under curve (AUC)	95% CI	p
IS/ effusion AND (EF ≤ 40% OR IVC dilated and not collapsing)	0.894	0.787–0.958	–
IS/ effusion	0.859	0.744–0.935	0.39
IVC dilated and not collapsing	0.768	0.641–0.867	0.03
EF ≤ 40%	0.787	0.662–0.882	0.02

Fig. 2 Receiver operating characteristic (ROC) curve comparing accuracy of different ultrasound modalities. p vs IS/effusion AND EF ≤ 40% OR IVC dilated and not collapsing

the appearance of the signs of peripheral congestion in heart failure (peripheral edema, liver stasis and distended jugular veins).

Even in the ED diagnosis of acute heart failure is mostly based on clinical examination. However, signs and symptoms of acute heart failure are not specific. Even chest x-ray may be falsely negative in 20% of cases [20]. The Boston score that we adopted has a validated prognostic value in Italy and has proved to be more accurate in predicting poor prognosis than other criteria [21].

In our study the diagnostic accuracy of chest X-ray and Boston clinical criteria risk score ≥ 8 was suboptimal for detection of patients with acute heart failure and was much lower compared to integrated ultrasound examination of Lung-Heart-IVC. As already demonstrated, LUS performs better than Chest X-ray in identification of patients with acute heart failure, probably because of poor quality of X-ray in the setting of ED [15, 20].

LUS can be of great help in differentiating CD from non-CD, especially in the case of borderline Boston score (between 5 and 7). The presence of numerous B-lines, sometimes confluent, configures the framework of an alveolar-interstitial syndrome [22]. It may reflect the presence of either cardiogenic or inflammatory edema, or fibrosis [12]. Pleural effusion may instead be the result of inflammation of the lung parenchyma or heart failure with increased central venous pressure [23].

In our analysis, the presence of bilateral IS and/or effusion exhibits a high sensitivity for the diagnosis of CD, with a high negative predictive value, confirming the pathophysiological assumption that in acute heart failure interstitial edema or effusion are present bilaterally and confirming the diagnostic importance of LUS in patients with decompensated heart failure [24, 25]. Among patients with heart failure in whom bilateral IS is absent, right heart dysfunction might be prevalent. In addition, specificity and, especially, positive predictive value are suboptimal, probably due to presence of lung IS also in the case of pulmonary fibrosis, acute respiratory distress syndrome, interstitial pneumonia, bilateral pneumonia. Although there are ultrasound signs to help differentiating cardiogenic pulmonary edema from ARDS, these are not easily recognizable, especially in an emergency setting with portable devices with cardiac probe [26]. One limitation of our approach in LUS should be highlighted: we decided to adopt a simplified protocol with only four zone scanning protocol to speed up the echo examination time. In the setting of ED this has already been done using a simplified six zone scanning protocol obtaining a sensitivity for LUS alone comparable to what we have found [23]. A more comprehensive scanning would have been optimal but also time consuming and so not feasible facing patients in critical condition.

The presence of EF less than or equal to 40% has a low sensitivity for the diagnosis of dyspnea related to acute cardiac decompensation. This reflects the fact that a significant proportion of patients with HF presents with preserved EF [27]. However, as expected, the specificity is good.

The presence of dilated and not collapsing IVC is typically an accurate index of increased right atrial pressure that can be a result of either an increased pulmonary arterial pressure or right ventricular dysfunction with or without significant tricuspid regurgitation [28]. In our study, this index exhibits low sensitivity for the diagnosis of cardiogenic dyspnea. This is probably because a sudden increase in pulmonary capillary wedge pressure has no immediate effect on the pulmonary arterial circulation. However, the combination of dilation and hypo-reactivity of the IVC carries good specificity for the diagnosis of cardiogenic dyspnea with an acceptable positive predictive value. Thus we partially confirm the finding that a dilated and not collapsing IVC has acceptable correlation with increased left ventricular pressure [29], though IVC can be dilated and not collapsing also in different acute (pulmonary embolism, pneumonia with severe hypoxemia) or chronic (pulmonary hypertension in chronic heart failure, chronic pulmonary heart disease) conditions as well as in myocardial infarction with right ventricular dysfunction [28].

The combination of bilateral IS/effusion and EF ≤40% has a better accuracy than the association between bilateral IS/effusion and dilated and not collapsing IVC for the diagnosis of CD. The contemporary presence of all three ultrasound abnormalities has not an optimal accuracy, especially because of the poor sensitivity.

In the diagnosis of acute heart failure the combination of reduced left ventricular EF and poor collapsibility of IVC has been demonstrated to have high specificity and sensitivity for the diagnosis of HF [30], with an adjunctive specificity value for the LUS. In our paper we expand this finding demonstrating that a combination of positive LUS examination and reduced EF or IVC dilated and not collapsing demonstrates the best accuracy in the diagnosis of dyspnea of cardiac origin, mainly due to the ability of this combination to maximize specificity compare to LUS alone.

Consistently, the association between bilateral IS/effusion and only 1 of the cardiovascular abnormalities (EF ≤40% or dilated and not collapsing IVC) improves the sensitivity and accuracy compared to the association between bilateral IS/effusion and EF ≤ 40%, because it captures also patients with HF with preserved ejection fraction among whom many have dilated and not collapsing IVC.

The diagnostic value of lung-cardiac-IVC integrated ultrasound was recently tested by *Kajimoto* et al. who showed accuracy (93.3%) slightly greater than our study. This difference possibly reflects the fact that in our protocol color Doppler was not available and only EF was the parameter of LV function detectable during cardiac ultrasound, whereas in their protocol cardiac ultrasound was considered diagnostic also with EF >40% when associated with moderate to severe mitral regurgitation [7] expanding the spectrum of types of recognizable heart failure.

Limitations

Our study has some limitations. First, the population sample could be larger. However our findings are consistent with previous reports [7, 12]. It was not possible to follow the clinical course of all enrolled patients because 7 of them were admitted to a different hospital after the ED evaluation. In the remaining 61 patients the EP diagnosis has been confirmed in 93.4% of the cases at the final hospital discharge. Since our aim was to evaluate the diagnostic accuracy of ultrasound in the ED we decided to adopt as diagnostic gold standard the EP diagnosis. Also it is not yet possible with the pocket ultrasound device to examine the diastolic function of the left ventricle.

Conclusions

Overall, the integrated lung-heart-IVC ultrasound examination improves the accuracy of LUS alone, by maximizing specificity, and allowing to capture different types of heart failure. This makes pocket ultrasound devices useful for the efficiency and speed in the differential diagnosis of acute dyspnea in the ED.

The IUE of lung-heart-inferior vena cava with pocket ultrasound devices is an extension of the clinical examination and can be realized with a protocol that provides 4 thoracic scans (2 front and 2 lateral), at least one view (parasternal and/or apical and/or subcostal) which enables the assessment of LV systolic function and the subcostal view for the inferior vena cava. This method is readily available at bedside or even in ambulance, requires few minutes and has reliable diagnostic accuracy in the management of acute dyspnea.

Abbreviations
AD: Acute dyspnea; CD: Cardiac dyspnea; ED: Emergency department; EF: Ejection fraction; HF: Heart failure; IS: Interstitial syndrome; IUE: Integrated ultrasound examination; IVC: Inferior vena cava; LUS: Lung ultrasound; NPV: Negative predictive value; PPV: Positive predictive value; PUD: Pocket size device

Acknowledgements
None.

Funding
All the Authors do not receive any founding related to this manuscript.

Authors' contributions
AS selected the patients, performed US and supervised data collections. AS and CM conceived the manuscript and coordinate to draft the manuscript, MVC, AB, MB, SS and GdS helped to draft the manuscript, gave conceptual help and prepared the tables, GdS provided statistical advice, managed quality control and manuscript revision. All authors read and approved the final manuscript.

Competing interests
The authors declare that they have no competing of interests.

Consent for publication
Not applicable.

Author details
[1]Hypertension Research Center, Federico II University Hospital of Naples, Via Pansini 5, bld #1, 80131 Naples, Italy. [2]Department of Advanced Biomedical Science, Federico II University Hospital, Naples, Italy. [3]Department of Traslational Medical Science. Federico II University Hospital, Naples, Italy. [4]Emergency Department, Bufalini Hospital, Cesena, Italy.

References
1. Wang CS, FitzGerald JM, Schulzer M, Mak E, Ayas NT. Does this dyspneic patient in the emergency department have congestive heart failure? JAMA. 2005;294:1944.
2. Ray P, Birolleau S, Lefort Y, Becquemin MH, Beigelman C, Isnard R, et al. Acute respiratory failure in the elderly: etiology, emergency diagnosis and prognosis. Crit Care. 2006;10:R82.
3. Labovitz AJ, Noble VE, Bierig M, Goldstein SA, Jones R, Kort S, et al. Focused cardiac ultrasound in the emergent setting: a consensus statement of the American Society of Echocardiography and American College of Emergency Physicians. J Am Soc Echocardiogr. 2010;23(12):1225–30.
4. Copetti R, Soldati G. (2012). Ecografia Toracica seconda edizione. C.G. Edizioni Medico Scientifiche.
5. Picano E, Pellikka PA. Ultrasound of extravascular lung water: a new standard for pulmonary congestion. Eur Heart J. 2016;37(27):2097–104.
6. Cibinel GA, Casoli G, Elia F, Padoan M, Pivetta E, Lupia E, et al. Diagnostic accuracy and reproducibility of pleural and lung ultrasound in discriminating cardiogenic causes of acute dyspnea in the Emergency Department. Intern Emerg Med. 2012;7:65.
7. Kajimoto K, Madeen K, Nakayama T, Tsudo H, Kuroda T, Abe T. Rapid evaluation by lung-cardiac-inferior vena cava (LCI) integrated ultrasound for differentiating heart failure from pulmonary disease as the cause of acute dyspnea in the emergency setting. Cardiovasc Ultrasound. 2012;10:49.
8. Sicari R, Galderisi M, Voigt JU, Habib G, Zamorano JL, Lancellotti P, et al. The use of pocket-size imaging devices: a position statement of the European Association of Echocardiography. Eur J Echocardiogr. 2011;12(2):85–7.
9. Galderisi M, Santoro A, Versiero M, Schiano Lomoriello V, Esposito R, Raia R, et al. Improved cardiovascular diagnostic accuracy by pocket size imaging device in non-cardiologic outpatients: the NaUSiCa (Naples Ultrasound Stethoscope in Cardiology) study. Cardiovasc Ultrasound. 2010;8:51.
10. Testuz A, Müller H, Keller PF, Meyer P, Stampfli T, Sekoranja L, et al. Diagnostic accuracy of pocket-size handheld echocardiographs used by cardiologists in the acute care setting. Eur Heart J Cardiovasc Imaging. 2013; 14(1):38–42.
11. Volpicelli G, Elbarbary M, Blaivas M, Lichtenstein DA, Mathis G, Kirkpatrick AW, et al. International evidence-based recommendations for point-of-care lung ultrasound. Intensive Care Med. 2012;38(4):577–91.
12. Gargani L. Lung ultrasound: a new tool for the cardiologist. Cardiovasc Ultrasound. 2011;9:6.

13. Kimura BJ, Yogo N, O'Connell CW, Phan JN, Showalter BK, Wolfson T. Cardiopulmonary limited ultrasound examination for "quick-look" bedside application. Am J Cardiol. 2011;108(4):586–90.

14. Remes J, Miettinen H, Reunanen A, Pyorala K. Validity of clinical diagnosis of heart failure in primary health care. Eur Heart J. 1991;12:315.

15. Pirozzi C, Numis FG, Pagano A, Melillo P, Copetti R, Schiraldi F. Immediate versus delayed integrated point-of-care-ultrasonography to manage acute dyspnea in the emergency department. Crit Ultrasound J. 2014;6(1):5.

16. Hanley JA, McNeil BJ. A method of comparing the areas under receiver operating characteristic curves derived from the same cases. Radiology. 1983;148(3):839–43.

17. Mancusi C, Gerdts E, de Simone G, Midtbø H, Lønnebakken MT, Boman K, et al. Higher pulse pressure/stroke volume index is associated with impaired outcome in hypertensive patients with left ventricular hypertrophy the LIFE study. Blood Press. 2017;26(3):150–5.

18. De Marco M, Gerdts E, Mancusi C, Roman MJ, Lønnebakken MT, Lee ET, et al. Influence of left ventricular stroke volume on incident heart failure in a population with preserved ejection fraction (from the strong heart study). Am J Cardiol. 2017;119(7):1047–52.

19. de Simone G, Izzo R, Losi MA, Stabile E, Rozza F, Canciello G, Mancusi C, Trimarco V, De Luca N, Trimarco B. Depressed myocardial energetic efficiency is associated with increased cardiovascular risk in hypertensive left ventricular hypertrophy. J Hypertens. 2016;34(9):1846–1853.

20. Collins SP, Lindsell CJ, Storrow AB, Abraham WT. Prevalence of negative chest radiography results in the emergency department patient with decompensated heart failure. Ann Emerg Med. 2006;47:13.

21. Di Bari M, Pozzi C, Cavallini MC, Innocenti F, Baldereschi G, De Alfieri W, et al. The diagnosis of heart failure in the community. J Am Coll Cardiol. 2004;44:1601.

22. Lichtenstein D, Mézière G, Biderman P, Gepner A, Barré O. The comet-tail artifact: an ultrasound sign of alveolar-interstitial syndrome. Am J Respir Crit Care Med. 1997;156:1640.

23. Natanzon A, Kronzon I. Pericardial and pleural effusions in congestive heart failure-anatomical, pathophysiologic, and clinical considerations. Am J Med Sci. 2009;338(3):211–6.

24. Pivetta E, Goffi A, Lupia E, Tizzani M, Porrino G, Ferreri E, et al. Lung ultrasound-implemented diagnosis of acute decompensated heart failure in the ED: a SIMEU multicenter study. Chest. 2015;148(1):202–10.

25. Miglioranza MH, Gargani L, Sant'Anna RT, Rover MM, Martins VM, Mantovani A, et al. Lung ultrasound for the evaluation of pulmonary congestion in outpatients: a comparison with clinical assessment, natriuretic peptides, and echocardiography. JACC Cardiovasc Imaging. 2013;6(11):1141–51.

26. Copetti R, Soldati G, Copetti P. Chest sonography: a useful tool to differentiate acute cardiogenic pulmonary edema from acute respiratory distress syndrome. Cardiovasc Ultrasound. 2008;6:16.

27. Nieminen MS, Brutsaert D, Dickstein K, Drexler H, Follath F, Harjola VP, et al. EuroHeart Failure Survey II (EHFS II): a survey on hospitalized acute heart failure patients: description of population. Eur Heart J. 2006;27(22):2725–36.

28. Brennan JM, Blair JE, Goonewardena S, Ronan A, Shah D, Vasaiwala S, et al. Reappraisal of the use of inferior vena cava for estimating right atrial pressure. J Am Soc Echocardiogr. 2007;20:857.

29. Blair JE, Brennan JM, Goonewardena SN, Shah D, Vasaiwala S, Spencer KT. Usefulness of hand-carried ultrasound to predict elevated left ventricular filling pressure. Am J Cardiol. 2009;103(2):246–7.

30. Anderson KL, Jenq KY, Fields JM, Panebianco NL, Dean AJ. Diagnosing heart failure among acutely dyspneic patients with cardiac, inferior vena cava, and lung ultrasonography. Am J Emerg Med. 2013;31(8):1208–14.

14

Clinical and echocardiographic predictors of mortality in acute pulmonary embolism

Talal Dahhan[1,6], Irfan Siddiqui[2], Victor F. Tapson[3], Eric J. Velazquez[4], Stephanie Sun[5], Clemontina A. Davenport[5], Zainab Samad[4] and Sudarshan Rajagopal[4,6*]

Abstract

Purpose: The aim of this study was to evaluate the utility of adding quantitative assessments of cardiac function from echocardiography to clinical factors in predicting the outcome of patients with acute pulmonary embolism (PE).

Methods: Patients with a diagnosis of acute PE, based on a positive ventilation perfusion scan or computed tomography (CT) chest angiogram, were identified using the Duke University Hospital Database. Of these, 69 had echocardiograms within 24–48 h of the diagnosis that were suitable for offline analysis. Clinical features that were analyzed included age, gender, body mass index, vital signs and comorbidities. Echocardiographic parameters that were analyzed included left ventricular (LV) ejection fraction (EF), regional, free wall and global RV speckle-tracking strain, RV fraction area change (RVFAC), Tricuspid Annular Plane Systolic Excursion (TAPSE), pulmonary artery acceleration time (PAAT) and RV myocardial performance (Tei) index. Univariable and multivariable regression statistical analysis models were used.

Results: Out of 69 patients with acute PE, the median age was 55 and 48 % were female. The median body mass index (BMI) was 27 kg/m^2. Twenty-nine percent of the cohort had a history of cancer, with a significant increase in cancer prevalence in non-survivors (57 % vs 29 %, $p = 0.02$). Clinical parameters including heart rate, respiratory rate, troponin T level, active malignancy, hypertension and COPD were higher among non-survivors when compared to survivors ($p \leq 0.05$). Using univariable analysis, NYHA class III symptoms, hypoxemia on presentation, tachycardia, tachypnea, elevation in Troponin T, absence of hypertension, active malignancy and chronic obstructive pulmonary disease (COPD) were increased in non-survivors compared to survivors ($p \leq 0.05$). In multivariable models, RV Tei Index, global and free (lateral) wall RVLS were found to be negatively associated with survival probability after adjusting for age, gender and systolic blood pressure ($p \leq 0.05$).

Conclusion: The addition of echocardiographic assessment of RV function to clinical parameters improved the prediction of outcomes for patients with acute PE. Larger studies are needed to validate these findings.

Keywords: Echocardiography, Pulmonary embolism, Right ventricular function, Speckle-tracking echocardiography

Background

Acute pulmonary Embolism (PE) is a major cause of morbidity and mortality in the United States and Europe, accounting for 100,000 and 300,000 deaths annually, respectively [1, 2]. PE can be classified as massive, submassive or nonmassive based on the hemodynamic status and right ventricular (RV) function of the patient. Massive PE is characterized by systemic hypotension or cardiogenic shock, submassive PE is characterized by RV dysfunction without hypotension, and nonmassive PE has neither systemic hypotension nor RV dysfunction [2]. Massive PE is associated with an in-hospital mortality of 25–50 %, submassive PE with a mortality rate of 3–15 %, while nonmassive PE is associated with mortality of 5 % or less [3]. Risk assessment in patients with submassive PE can be difficult, as the mortality rates for submassive PE can approach that of massive PE [4]. While there is a consensus that systemic thrombolysis,

* Correspondence: sudarshan.rajagopal@duke.edu;
sudarshan.rajagopal@dm.duke.edu
[4]Department of Medicine, Division of Cardiology, Duke University, Durham, NC, USA
[6]Center for Pulmonary Vascular Disease, Box 102351, DUMC, Durham, NC 27710, USA
Full list of author information is available at the end of the article

catheter-directed interventions, or surgery are indicated in patients with massive PE, the management of patients with submassive PE remains controversial. Therefore, there remains a challenge in the clinical management of patients who have stable hemodynamics but demonstrate evidence of RV dysfunction, either by electrocardiogram, echocardiogram, computed tomography (CT) scan or cardiac biomarkers [2]. The benefit of thrombolytic or invasive therapies relative to the risk of bleeding is unclear among such patients [5]. An improved approach to risk assessment could therefore allow the identification of those patients presenting with submassive PE who would benefit most from therapy.

To address this, risk assessments based on clinical and imaging parameters have been developed. The Pulmonary Embolism Severity Index (PESI) is an excellent clinical predictor of outcomes in patients with PE [6]. It is based on 11 clinical criteria including age, sex, history of cancer and hemodynamic parameters. Five risk categories are included, ranging from very low risk, with 30-day mortality of less than 2 %, to very high risk, with 10.0–24.5 % mortality [6]. The simplified PESI (sPESI) was subsequently developed, with only six, rather than 11, clinical criteria. In this index, only two risk categories were included, with low risk associated with 1.1 % mortality and high risk associated with an 8.9 % risk of death [7]. Quantitative echocardiographic assessment has been gaining importance in patients with RV dysfunction, including those with congenital heart disease, pulmonary hypertension and pulmonary embolism [8, 9]. A number of studies [10–21] have tested the utility of novel echocardiographic or serum biomarkers for risk assessment in acute PE, but only a few studies have tested whether such parameters provide additional benefit to clinical predictors [22, 23]. We hypothesized that the addition of quantitative echocardiographic markers of RV function would add to clinical parameters to predict outcomes in patients with acute PE.

Methods
Study population
We retrospectively identified patients who had a diagnosis of acute PE between January 2010 and April 2014, confirmed by contrasted computed tomography (CT) scan of the chest and/or ventilation-perfusion (VQ) nuclear medicine imaging at Duke University Medical Center (Durham, NC, USA) using the Duke Enterprise Data Unified Content Explorer (DEDUCE) [24]. Subjects were included in the study if they had an echocardiogram performed within 24–48 h of diagnosis of acute PE. Subjects were excluded if their echocardiographic images were suboptimal for RV strain measurement due to poor image quality or poor RV views. Clinical data including demographics, medical history, comorbidities,

systemic blood pressure, heart rate, respiratory rate, oxygen saturation on room air and with supplemental oxygen, were collected from the medical record. The Duke University Medical Center Institutional Review Board approved this study.

Echo-derived parameters of RV function
All echocardiographic studies were performed on GE Vivid E9 using a 3.5 MHz probe (GE, Vingmed Ultrasound, Hortom, Norway) or Philips IE33 (Philips, Netherlands). Off-line analyses of images were performed in Xcelera (Philips, Andover, MA) and Image-Arena (TomTec Imaging Systems, Unterschleißheim, Germany) by a single experienced reader and analysis was confirmed by a separate experienced reader; inter-reader variability for these studies have been shown to be low [25]. TAPSE was determined from an M-mode through the lateral tricuspid annulus by calculating the amount of longitudinal motion of the annulus at peak systole [26] (Fig. 1a). RV Tei index was calculated as the RV isovolumic time (IVT) divided by the ejection time (ET) using the pulsed Doppler method [8] (Fig. 1c). IVT was calculated as the duration of tricuspid regurgitation from continuous wave Doppler across the tricuspid valve minus the ET from a single representative beat. ET was calculated as the duration of RV outflow on pulsed Doppler across the RVOT from a single representative beat (Fig. 1c). Care was taken to use beats with similar RR intervals to minimize errors in calculation. RV Fraction Area Change (FAC) [27] was calculated as the [(RV end-diastolic area – end-systolic area)/end-diastolic area] × 100 (Fig. 1d). The RV endocardium was traced in systole and diastole from the annulus, along the free wall, to the apex and back along the interventricular septum using the apical four-chamber view. Attempts were made to trace the free wall beneath trabeculations (Fig. 1d).

RV longitudinal strain
2D strain analysis was performed from the apical 4-chamber view as previously described [28] (Fig. 1b). The reference point for a single cardiac cycle was placed at the beginning of the QRS. Pulmonic valve closure was determined from the pulsed wave Doppler profile of the RV outflow tract. The endocardial border was traced in end systole and the region of interest was adjusted to exclude the pericardium. The quality of the tracking was confirmed visually from 2D images and from the strain traces. Segments with persistently inadequate tracking despite attempts at improving border definition and region of interest were excluded from analysis. The longitudinal strain of the RV free wall (RV_{free}) was calculated as the average of the three free wall segments and the longitudinal strain of the RV septum (RV_{sept}) was

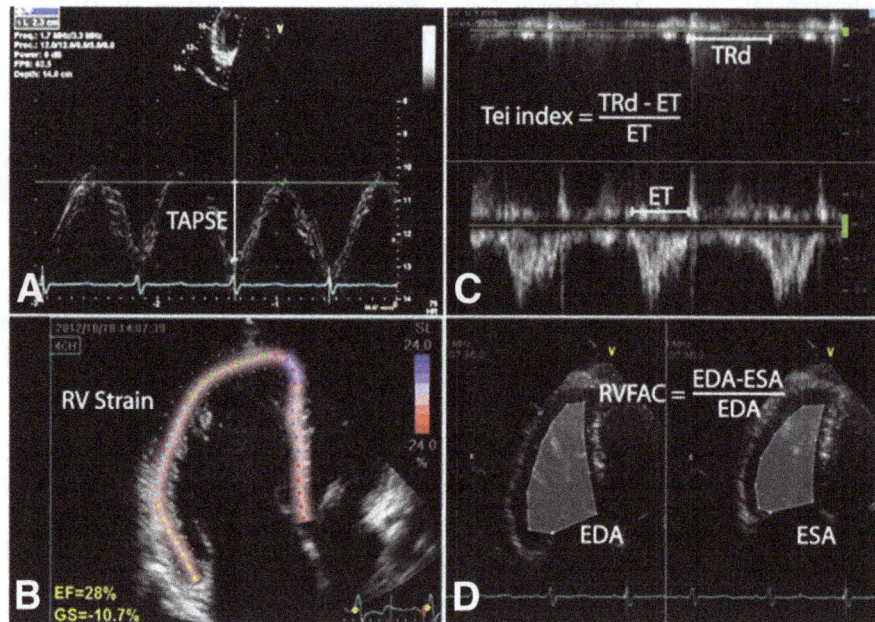

Fig. 1 Different 2D echocardiographic methods used in this study to assess RV function. **a** Tricuspid Annular Plane Systolic Excursion (TAPSE) is determined from an M-mode image through the lateral tricuspid annulus by calculating the amount of longitudinal motion of the tricuspid annulus at peak systole. **b** RV longitudinal strain is calculated from speckle-tracking of an RV focused apical 4-chamber view. **c** RV Tei index is calculated as the RV isovolumic time (equal to tricuspid regurgitation duration (TRd) – ejection time (ET)) divided by the ET using the pulsed Doppler method. **d** RV Fractional Area Change (RV FAC) was calculated as the [(RV end-diastolic area – end-systolic area)/end-diastolic area] × 100

calculated as the average of the three septal segments. Global RVLS was calculated as the average of strains from all segments. All strain and other 2D echo-derived parameter analyses were performed blinded to clinical data.

Statistical analysis

Demographic and clinical characteristics of participants were presented in the study by survival status and the two groups were compared using Fisher's exact test for categorical variables and a Kruskal-Wallis rank sum test for continuous variables. Continuous variables were summarized by the median and interquartile range and categorical variables were summarized by counts and percentages (Tables 1 and 2). Table 3 displays the odds ratios and 95 % confidence intervals resulting from uni-variable logistic regression modeling the probability of survival. These models investigated the association between clinical characteristics, cardiac biomarkers, specific echocardiographic features and PESI predictor score on the probability of survival and no adjustment for multiple testing was done. Multivariable models were fit to investigate the effects of some clinical features with echocardiographic parameters on survival, and the results are shown in Table 4. Statistical analyses were performed using SAS 9.4 (SAS, Cary, NC) and R (R Core Team (2015), Vienna, Austria).

Results

During the study period, 135 patients were admitted with a clinical diagnosis of acute PE. Among these, 95 patients diagnosed with an acute PE had a transthoracic echocardiogram within the initial 24–48 h of admission. 26 patients did not have suitable images for offline analysis, resulting in a cohort of 69 analyzed subjects. Six of the subjects underwent thrombolysis. At 30 days, of these 69 subjects, 14 had died and 55 survived. (Table 1).

Baseline characteristics and presentation

The baseline characteristics of all 69 patients are listed in Table 1. The median age was 55 years old (range 16–95) and 48 % ($n = 38$) of patients were females. The median body mass index (BMI) was 27 kg/m^2 (range 20–68). With respect to comorbidities, 29 % ($n = 20$) of the cohort had a history of cancer, with a significantly higher prevalence in non-survivors compared to survivors (57 % vs. 29 %, $p = 0.02$). The only other significant difference in comorbidities between non-survivors and survivors was in the prevalence of hypertension (non-survivors, 64 %, vs. survivors, 25 %, $p = 0.03$). 13 % of patients ($n = 9$) had a history of prior venous thromboembolism. On presentation, 90 % ($n = 62$) had NYHA class III symptoms (Table 1). Hypoxemia on presentation, tachycardia, tachypnea, elevation in Troponin T, absence of hypertension, active malignancy and chronic

Table 1 Baseline characteristics for the cohort of patients with acute PE

Parameter (n)	All patients 69	Non-Survivors 14	Survivors 55	p-Value
Age at Diagnosis (69)	55 [43–72]	60 [53.5–69.8]	50 [42.5–72]	0.11
Female Gender (69)	33 (48)	6 (42.86)	27 (49.09)	0.77
Body Mass Index (69)	27 [23–28]	26.5 [22.2–27]	27 [23–28]	0.42
Vital Signs:				
Systolic Blood Pressure (66)	118 [107–137]	111 [99.5–144.8]	118 [109–136.5]	0.38
Diastolic Blood Pressure (66)	73 [61.5–81.5]	65 [60.8–71]	75.5 [63.5–83.8]	0.08
Heart Rate (66)	94 [84–111.5]	115 [102.2–125.5]	90 [81.8–105.8]	0.02
Respiratory Rate (66)	20 [18–24]	24 [21.5–28]	20 [18–24]	0.01
Fraction of Inspired Oxygen (69)	0.2 [0.2–0.3]	0.3 [0.2–0.4]	0.2 [0.2–0.3]	0.01
Troponin T level (ng/mL) (23)	0.1 [0–0.3]	0.6 [0.5–0.7]	0.1 [0–0.2]	<0.01
Medical History				
Essential Hypertension (69)	25 (36.23)	9 (64.29)	16 (29.09)	0.03
Type II Diabetes (69)	4 (5.8)	1 (7.14)	3 (5.45)	>0.99
Hypothyroidism (69)	6 (8.7)	1 (7.14)	5 (9.09)	>0.99
Chronic Kidney Disease (69)	3 (4.35)	1 (7.14)	2 (3.64)	0.5
Previous Venous Thromboembolism (69)	9 (13.04)	0 (0)	9 (16.36)	0.19
Connective Tissue Disease (69)	2 (2.9)	1 (7.14)	1 (1.82)	0.37
Active Malignancy (69)	20 (28.99)	8 (57.14)	12 (21.82)	0.02
Orthopedic Fracture or Injury (69)	5 (7.25)	0 (0)	5 (9.09)	0.58
Chronic Obstructive Pulmonary Disease (69)	5 (7.25)	3 (21.43)	2 (3.64)	0.05
Shortness of Breath:				
NYHA class1	2 (2.9)	0 (0)	2 (3.64)	
NYHA class2	5 (7.25)	1 (7.14)	4 (7.27)	
NYHA class3	15 (21.74)	1 (7.14)	14 (25.45)	
NYHA class4	47 (68.12)	12 (85.71)	35 (63.64)	
Pulmonary Embolism Severity Index (PESI) class (69)				<0.01
Class 1	32 (46.38)	1 (7.14)	31 (56.36)	
Class 2	10 (14.49)	2 (14.29)	8 (14.55)	
Class 3	17 (24.64)	5 (35.71)	12 (21.82)	
Class 4	10 (14.49)	6 (42.86)	4 (7.27)	

Shown are median and inter-quartile range in brackets or number of patients with percent of patients in parentheses. P-value denotes comparison between non-survivors and survivors

Abbreviations: NYHA New York Heart Association

obstructive pulmonary disease (COPD) were statistically significantly different ($p \leq 0.05$) between non-survivors and survivors (Table 1).

Echocardiographic assessment of RV function in acute PE
A number of echocardiographic parameters were assessed in our cohort (Table 2). These included parameters that are thought to quantify RV systolic function (TAPSE, global, regional and free wall RV longitudinal strain (RVLS), RV myocardial performance (Tei) Index, RV fraction area change (RVFAC), and subjective echocardiographic evaluation of RV function) and RV size (RV/LV ratio in systole and diastole, diameters of RV and LV in systole and diastole). RVFAC, Tei Index, global and free wall RVLS were significantly different between survivors and nonsurvivors ($p \leq 0.05$). For example, a significant proportion of non-survivors had global and free wall RVLS of more than −12.5 (Fig. 2), a value which has been demonstrated to be associated with worse outcomes in pulmonary hypertension [29]. TAPSE, subjective RV dilation and subjective RV dysfunction were not statistically different between survivors and non-survivors ($p > 0.05$).

Table 2 Echocardiographic parameters in survivors and nonsurvivors with acute PE

	Overall	Non-Survivors	Survivors	p-Value
Parameter (n)	69	14	55	
TAPSE (52) (cm)	1.9 [1.5–2.3]	2.1 [1.2–2.4]	1.9 [1.6–2.2]	0.82
Global RVLS (69) (%)	−18.1 [−20.8–14.9]	−15.7 [−19.2–12.1]	−18.6 [−21.8–15.6]	0.05
Average Septal RV Wall strain (69) (%)	−17.8 [−22.7–13.9]	−16.8 [−18.6–9.3]	−17.8 [−22.9–14.7]	0.20
Average Free Wall RV Wall strain (69) (%)	−18.2 [−22.8–13.9]	−15 [−18.7–10.3]	−19.2 [−23.2–14.3]	0.04
RV Tei Index (59)	0.5 [0.4–0.5]	0.5 [0.5–0.6]	0.5 [0.4–0.5]	0.01
Pulmonary Artery Acceleration Time (64) (ms × 10)	9.5 [7–12]	9 [7–10]	10 [7–12]	0.58
RV/LV ratio in systole (52)	1 [0.8–1.4]	1.1 [1–1.4]	1 [0.8–1.5]	0.74
RV/LV ratio in diastole (52)	0.7 [0.6–0.9]	0.8 [0.7–1]	0.7 [0.6–0.9]	0.35
RV base (42) (cm)	3.8 [3.3–4.3]	4.2 [3.5–4.3]	3.7 [3.3–4.3]	0.61
RV middle (39) (cm)	3.3 [2.9–3.6]	3.5 [3–4.5]	3.3 [2.9–3.6]	0.31
RV length (39) (cm)	7.5 [7–7.9]	7.5 [7.2–7.8]	7.5 [6.9–7.9]	0.61
RV diastolic diameter (52) (cm)	2.7 [2.1–3.1]	2.7 [2.3–3.1]	2.7 [2.1–3.2]	0.41
LV diastolic diameter (52) (cm)	3.5 [2.9–4.1]	3.2 [2.9–3.8]	3.6 [3–4.2]	0.63
RV systolic diameter (52) (cm)	2.4 [2.1–2.9]	2.6 [2.2–2.9]	2.4 [2–2.9]	0.57
LV systolic diameter (34) (cm)	2.3 [1.9–2.7]	2.2 [1.9–3]	2.4 [2–2.6]	0.65
RV fractional area change (67) (%)	34.4 [27.6–43.1]	27.9 [19.6–35.8]	38.6 [28.9–43.8]	0.02
RV area in diastole (67) (cm²)	24.3 [19.9–31]	25 [22–44]	24.1 [19.3–29.8]	0.22
RV area in Systole (67) (cm²)	16.8 [11.4–19.6]	16.8 [14.6–26.3]	16.9 [11.1–19.4]	0.20
RV basal free wall strain (69) (%)	−21.4 [−27.4–13.5]	−14.8 [−23.9–10.9]	−22.4 [−28.2–16.1]	0.06
RV middle free wall strain (69) (%)	−16.3 [−22.6–9.5]	−12.4 [−14.5–9.2]	−17.9 [−23.5–9.8]	0.10
RV apical free wall strain (69) (%)	−13.9 [−21.4–8.3]	−11.4 [−15.2–7.7]	−14.9 [−21.4–9.2]	0.33
RV basal septal strain (69) (%)	−19 [−24.5–13.9]	−17.1 [−20.1–13]	−19.6 [−24.8–13.9]	0.23
RV middle septal strain (69) (%)	−18.4 [−23.3–13.7]	−15.6 [−22.8–8.5]	−19 [−22.8–14.2]	0.32
RV apical septal strain (69) (%)	−16 [−19.7–9.5]	−12.1 [−17.7–7]	−16.4 [−19.9–9.8]	0.15
RV subjective size				0.28
Normal RV size	39 (56.52)	7 (50)	32 (58.18)	
Mild RV dilation	11 (15.94)	3 (21.43)	8 (14.55)	
Moderate RV dilation	12 (17.39)	1 (7.14)	11 (20)	
Severe RV dilation	7 (10.14)	3 (21.43)	4 (7.27)	
RV subjective function				0.60
Normal RV function	38 (55.07)	6 (42.86)	32 (58.18)	
Mildly reduced RV function	10 (14.49)	2 (14.29)	8 (14.55)	
Moderately reduced RV function	15 (21.74)	4 (28.57)	11 (20)	
Severely reduced RV function	6 (8.7)	2 (14.29)	4 (7.27)	
LV ejection fraction (69)				0.07
LV ejection fraction < 40 %	6 (8.7)	3 (21.43)	3 (5.45)	
LV ejection fraction 40–50 %	6 (8.7)	2 (14.29)	4 (7.27)	
LV ejection fraction >50 %	57 (82.61)	9 (64.29)	48 (87.27)	

Shown are median and inter-quartile range in brackets or number of patients with percent of patients in parentheses. *P*-value denotes comparison between non-survivors and survivors

Abbreviations: *RV* right ventricle, *LV* left ventricle, *TAPSE* tricuspid annular plane systolic excursion, *RVLS* RV longitudinal strain

Table 3 Univariable analysis of clinical and echocardiographic parameters in predicting outcome in acute PE

	OR	2.5 %	97.5 %	Estimate	SE	Z	p-value
Age at Diagnosis (69) (years)	0.98	0.94	1.01	−0.02	0.02	−1.44	0.15
Female Gender (69)	1.29	0.39	4.20	0.25	0.60	0.42	0.68
Body Mass Index (69) (kg/m^2)	1.06	0.93	1.20	0.06	0.06	0.87	0.39
Systolic blood pressure (66) (mmHg)	1.01	0.99	1.04	0.01	0.01	0.91	0.36
Diastolic blood pressure (66) (mmHg)	1.04	1.00	1.10	0.04	0.02	1.80	0.07
Malignancy (69)	0.21	0.06	0.72	−1.56	0.63	−2.48	0.01
Troponin T (23) (ng/mL)	0.00	0.00	0.52	−13.18	6.39	−2.06	0.04
CK-MB (50) (ng/mL)	0.99	0.93	1.04	−0.01	0.03	−0.52	0.60
Mild subjective RV dilation (69)	0.58	0.12	2.77	−0.54	0.80	−0.68	0.50
Moderate subjective RV dilation (69)	2.41	0.27	21.81	0.88	1.12	0.78	0.43
Severe subjective RV dilation (69)	0.29	0.05	1.61	−1.23	0.87	−1.42	0.16
Mild subjective RV dysfunction (69)	0.75	0.13	4.44	−0.29	0.91	−0.32	0.75
Moderate subjective RV dysfunction (69)	0.52	0.12	2.17	−0.66	0.73	−0.90	0.37
Severe subjective RV dysfunction (69)	0.37	0.06	2.53	−0.98	0.97	−1.01	0.31
LV ejection fraction 40–50 % (69)	2.00	0.19	20.61	0.69	1.19	0.58	0.56
LV ejection fraction > 50 %(69)	5.33	0.93	30.74	1.67	0.89	1.87	0.06
Global RVLS (69) (%)	0.88	0.78	0.99	−0.13	0.06	−2.13	0.03
Free wall RV strain (69) (%)	0.90	0.82	1.00	−0.10	0.05	−2.00	0.05
TAPSE (52) (cm)	1.47	0.43	4.96	0.38	0.62	0.62	0.54
RV/LV ratio in systolic (52)	1.10	0.23	5.22	0.10	0.79	0.12	0.90
RV/LV ratio in diastolic (52)	0.39	0.02	6.50	−0.95	1.44	−0.66	0.51
RV Tei index (59)	0.00	0.00	0.34	−7.00	3.02	−2.32	0.02
RVFAC (67)	1.05	1.00	1.12	0.05	0.03	1.81	0.07
PAAT (64) (ms × 10)	1.07	0.89	1.30	0.07	0.10	0.72	0.47
PESI class 3 (69)	0.13	0.01	1.61	−2.05	1.29	−1.59	0.11
PESI class 4 (69)	0.08	0.01	0.73	−2.56	1.15	−2.23	0.03
PESI class 5 (69)	0.02	0.00	0.23	−3.84	1.20	−3.19	<0.01

Odds ratio (survival over non-survival), 95 % confidence interval, estimate, standard error, and p-value of the univariable logistic regression models are shown
Abbreviations: *CK-MB*, creatine kinase-myocardial band, *RV* right ventricle, *LV* left ventricle, *RVLS* RV longitudinal strain, *TAPSE* tricuspid annular plane systolic excursion, *RVFAC* RV fractional area change, *PAAT* pulmonary artery acceleration time, *PESI* pulmonary embolism severity index

Univariable and multivariable predictors of outcome in acute PE

On univariable analysis, a number of clinical and echo-cardiographic parameters were statistically significantly ($p \leq 0.05$) associated with 30 day mortality. These included active malignancy, serum troponin, global and free wall RVLS, RV Tei Index, and patients with PESI classes four and five. For multivariable regression analysis, we attempted to include PESI as a clinical predictor with selected echo parameters, but could not because PESI score (whether categorical or continuous) demonstrated non-trivial collinearity with global and free wall RVLS and RV Tei index, resulting in unstable standard errors of estimates. Similarly, both heart rate and systolic blood pressure displayed significant collinearity, so only systolic blood pressure was included as it was a predictor in the univariable model. As the

multivariable models could not include those clinical and echocardiographic predictors together, we instead used a multivariable model that included parameters used to calculate PESI [6], namely age, gender and systolic blood pressure. With this multivariable regression model, global and free wall RVLS and RV Tei index all predicted outcome with statistical significance ($p \leq 0.05$).

Discussion

This study demonstrates that the addition of selected echocardiographic estimates of RV function to clinical parameters in patients with acute PE improved prediction of 30-day mortality in a cohort of patients with acute PE. In our cohort, global, free wall RVLS and RV Tei index analyses were independently associated with mortality on univariable and multivariable analysis. However, other assessments of RV function, including

Table 4 Multivariable analysis of clinical and echocardiographic parameters in predicting outcome in acute PE

	OR	2.5 %	97.5 %	Estimate	SE	Z	p-value
Global RVLS model							
Age	0.99	0.95	1.02	−0.01	0.02	−0.74	0.46
Female Gender	1.20	0.32	4.58	0.18	0.68	0.27	0.79
Systolic Blood Pressure	1.01	0.99	1.04	0.01	0.01	0.97	0.33
Global RVLS	0.87	0.77	1.00	−0.14	0.07	−2.01	0.04
Free wall RVLS model							
Age	0.99	0.95	1.03	−0.01	0.02	−0.68	0.50
Female Gender	1.21	0.32	4.61	0.19	0.68	0.28	0.78
Systolic Blood Pressure	1.01	0.98	1.04	0.01	0.01	0.67	0.50
Free wall RVLS	0.89	0.80	1.00	−0.11	0.06	−1.95	0.05
RV Tei Index model							
Age at Diagnosis	0.99	0.95	1.03	−0.01	0.02	−0.53	0.60
Female Gender	0.78	0.17	3.47	−0.26	0.76	−0.33	0.74
Systolic Blood Pressure	1.02	0.99	1.05	0.02	0.02	1.19	0.23
RV Tei Index	0.00	0.00	0.36	−7.82	3.46	−2.26	0.02

Odds ratio (survival over non-survival), 95 % confidence interval, estimate, standard error, and p-value of the multivariable logistic regression models are shown

TAPSE, RVFAC, and subjective evaluations of RV size and function were not associated with mortality on univariable analysis. At this time, there are no clear guidelines as to which parameters should be used to assess RV function [8], and significant inter-rater variability exists in subjective evaluation of the RV [9]. The objective echocardiographic assessment of RV function with qualitative parameters, such as RVLS, may reduce inter-rater variability [25] and have utility in identifying submassive PE patients who may benefit most from consideration of aggressive therapies.

The European Society of Cardiology [2] and the American College of Chest Physicians guidelines [30] emphasize the importance of the assessment of RV function and cardiac biomarkers in risk assessment of acute PE, as they may allow the identification of high-risk patients before they clinically deteriorate. An alternative strategy has been the use of clinical risk prediction algorithms, such as PESI and sPESI [6, 7]. In our analysis, we found significant collinearity between PESI and RVLS and Tei index, suggesting that these echocardiographic and clinical parameters are all associated with high risk features. While global and free wall RVLS require special software and analysis to obtain, RV Tei index is relatively straightforward to acquire and could be used broadly. Vitarelli et al. found an association of a number of parameters of RV function with 6 month adverse outcomes in acute PE patients on univariate analysis [27]. Moreover, they found that mid-free wall RVLS, RVSP and 3D RV ejection fraction were associated with adverse outcome on multivariate analysis. While we observed large absolute numerical differences in basal free wall strain between survivors and nonsurvivors, they did not reach statistical significance due to large variance. It is likely that they would have been significant in a larger study. Overall, the results here extend the findings of Vitarelli et al., as we found that both global and free wall RVLS were associated with outcome on multivariable analysis after accounting for age, gender and systolic blood pressure.

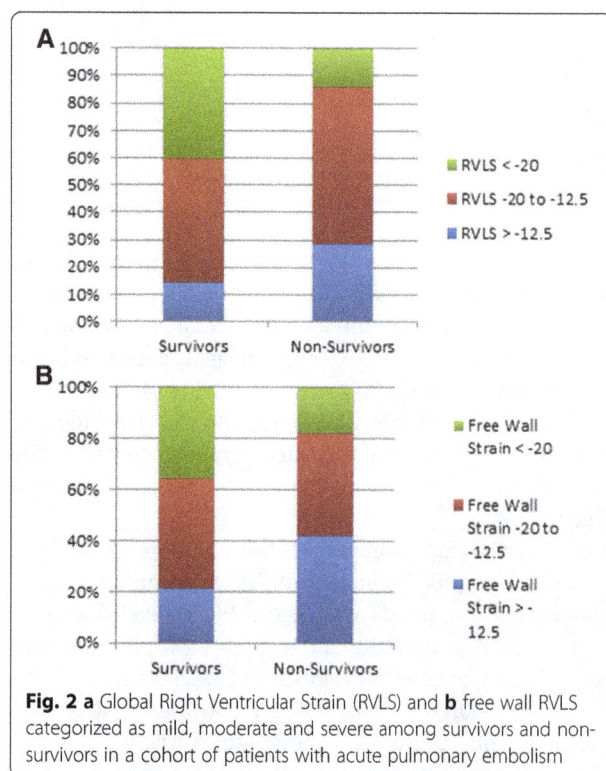

Fig. 2 a Global Right Ventricular Strain (RVLS) and **b** free wall RVLS categorized as mild, moderate and severe among survivors and non-survivors in a cohort of patients with acute pulmonary embolism

While subjective RV dysfunction has been associated with worse outcomes in PE [31], a number of studies suggest that quantifiers of RV function may better identify high-risk patients, although most of these studies did not test the utility of such parameters in combination with clinical characteristics [11, 13–21]. For example, RV dysfunction, as assessed by tricuspid annular plane systolic excursion (TAPSE) and RV myocardial performance (Tei) index, has been characterized in patients with PE [32, 33]. Another recent study identified the ratio of RV to LV end-diastolic diameter, RV systolic pressure, tricuspid annular plane systolic excursion, and inferior vena cava collapsibility to be independently associated with mortality in patients presenting with acute PE [11]. Abnormal RV global and free wall speckle-tracking strains have been associated with adverse events in patients with PE [27]. Ozsu and coworkers demonstrated a correlation of Tei index with treatment response in acute PE [33]. Park and coworkers demonstrated that TAPSE correlated with other parameters of RV function and BNP in acute PE [32]. RV ejection fraction and regional mid wall strain has been prospectively assessed in patients with PE, with a potential to assess a therapeutic response [27]. Thus, there are a number of parameters of RV function that have been shown to correlate with outcomes in acute PE.

Conclusions

Although our cohort of patients is small, we found an association of free-wall, global RV strain and RV Tei index with mortality. Notably, we did not find such a relationship between other measures, including TAPSE, RV size and RV/LV ratio. The associations we found were still significant after the inclusion of clinical risk factors [6, 7]. These findings suggest that the addition of echocardiographic parameters to clinical parameters may improve risk prediction in acute PE.

Limitations

Our study is a retrospective, single center study with a small cohort of patients, which may limit the generalizability of these findings. Patient care was variable, resulting in significant differences in studies that were performed, such as troponin T, which was only performed in 23 of the 69 subjects included in the final analysis. As there was no set protocol for RV imaging in this retrospective study, there was a relatively low suitability (72.6 %) of images for offline analysis and poor tracking observed in the basal and mid-free wall segments. In our analysis, we found significant collinearity between PESI and RVLS and Tei index, preventing us from combining our echo predictors with PESI score. Therefore, it is possible that echo predictors do not add significant information to the PESI score. Previous

studies from our group have demonstrated small inter- and intra-observer variability in assessment of RV strain [34], so such analyses were not included in this study. Future prospective, multi-center studies that address objective RV function assessment in relation to outcomes in patients with PE are needed to validate these findings.

Abbreviations
2D: Two dimensional; 3D: Three dimensional; BNP: Brain natriuretic peptide; COPD: Chronic obstructive pulmonary disease; CT: Computed tomography; DEDUCE: Duke Enterprise Data Unified Content Explorer; EF: Ejection fraction; ET: Ejection time; GE: General electric; IVT: Iso volumic time; LV: Left ventricle; PAAT: Pulmonary artery acceleration time; PE: Pulmonary embolism; PESI: Pulmonary embolism severity index; RV: Right ventricle; RVFAC: Right ventricular fraction area change; RVLS: Right ventricular longitudinal strain; RVOT: Right ventricular outflow tract; SAS: Statistical analysis system software; sPESI: simplified pulmonary embolism severity index; TAPSE: Tricuspid annular plane systolic excursion; VQ: Ventilation perfusion

Competing interests
The authors declare that they have no competing interests.

Funding
Funding was obtained from NIH grants K08HL114643, Gilead Research Scholars in Pulmonary Arterial Hypertension and a Burroughs Welcome Career Award for Medical Scientists supporting Sudarshan Rajagopal, the corresponding author. Clemontina Davenport is partially supported by Duke CTSA grant UL1TR001117.

Authors' contributions
TD, ZS and SR designed the study. TD collected data and wrote the manuscript. IS collected data, performed the echocardiographic analysis. SS and CD performed the statistical analysis. VT, EV, ZS and SR reviewed and edited the manuscript. All authors read and approved the final manuscript.

Author details
[1]Department of Medicine, Division of Pulmonary, Allergy and Critical Care Medicine, Duke University, Durham, NC, USA. [2]Department of Medicine, East Carolina University, Greenville, NC, USA. [3]Department of Medicine, Division of Pulmonary and Critical Care Medicine, Cedars Sinai Medical Center, Los Angeles, CA, USA. [4]Department of Medicine, Division of Cardiology, Duke University, Durham, NC, USA. [5]Department of Biostatistics and Bioinformatics, Duke University Medical Center, Durham, NC, USA. [6]Center for Pulmonary Vascular Disease, Box 102351, DUMC, Durham, NC 27710, USA.

References
1. Horlander KT, Mannino DM, Leeper KV. Pulmonary embolism mortality in the United States, 1979–1998: an analysis using multiple-cause mortality data. Arch Intern Med. 2003;163(14):1711–7.
2. Konstantinides SV, Torbicki A, Agnelli G, et al. 2014 ESC guidelines on the diagnosis and management of acute pulmonary embolism. Eur Heart J. 2014;35(43):3033–69. 3069a-3069k.
3. Torbicki A, Perrier A, Konstantinides S, et al. Guidelines on the diagnosis and management of acute pulmonary embolism: the Task Force for the Diagnosis and Management of Acute Pulmonary Embolism of the European Society of Cardiology (ESC). Eur Heart J. 2008;29(18):2276–315.
4. Goldhaber SZ, Visani L, De Rosa M. Acute pulmonary embolism: clinical outcomes in the International Cooperative Pulmonary Embolism Registry (ICOPER). Lancet. 1999;353(9162):1386–9.
5. Meyer G, Vicaut E, Danays T, et al. Fibrinolysis for patients with intermediate-risk pulmonary embolism. N Engl J Med. 2014;370(15):1402–11.

6. Aujesky D, Obrosky DS, Stone RA, et al. Derivation and validation of a prognostic model for pulmonary embolism. Am J Respir Crit Care Med. 2005;172(8):1041–6.

7. Jimenez D, Aujesky D, Moores L, et al. Simplification of the pulmonary embolism severity index for prognostication in patients with acute symptomatic pulmonary embolism. Arch Intern Med. 2010;170(15):1383–9.

8. Rudski LG, Lai WW, Afilalo J, et al. Guidelines for the echocardiographic assessment of the right heart in adults: a report from the American Society of Echocardiography endorsed by the European Association of Echocardiography, a registered branch of the European Society of Cardiology, and the Canadian Society of Echocardiography. J Am Soc Echocardiogr. 2010;23(7):685–713. quiz 786–688.

9. Lang RM, Bierig M, Devereux RB, et al. Recommendations for chamber quantification: a report from the American Society of Echocardiography's Guidelines and Standards Committee and the Chamber Quantification Writing Group, developed in conjunction with the European Association of Echocardiography, a branch of the European Society of Cardiology. J Am Soc Echocardiogr. 2005;18(12):1440–63.

10. Dursunoglu N, Dursunoglu D, Yildiz AI, Rota S. Evaluation of cardiac biomarkers and right ventricular dysfunction in patients with acute pulmonary embolism. Anadolu Kardiyol Derg. 2014.

11. Khemasuwan D, Yingchoncharoen T, Tunsupon P, et al. Right ventricular echocardiographic parameters are associated with mortality after acute pulmonary embolism. J Am Soc Echocardiogr. 2015;28(3):355–62.

12. Weekes AJ, Thacker G, Troha D, et al. Diagnostic accuracy of right ventricular dysfunction markers in normotensive emergency department patients with acute pulmonary embolism. Ann Emerg Med. 2016.

13. George E, Kumamaru KK, Ghosh N, et al. Computed tomography and echocardiography in patients with acute pulmonary embolism: part 2: prognostic value. J Thorac Imaging. 2014;29(1):W7–12.

14. Lee JH, Park JH, Park KI, et al. A comparison of different techniques of two-dimensional speckle-tracking strain measurements of right ventricular systolic function in patients with acute pulmonary embolism. J Cardiovasc Ultrasound. 2014;22(2):65–71.

15. Lobo JL, Holley A, Tapson V, et al. Prognostic significance of tricuspid annular displacement in normotensive patients with acute symptomatic pulmonary embolism. J Thromb Haemost. 2014;12(7):1020–7.

16. Platz E, Hassanein AH, Shah A, Goldhaber SZ, Solomon SD. Regional right ventricular strain pattern in patients with acute pulmonary embolism. Echocardiography. 2012;29(4):464–70.

17. Pruszczyk P, Goliszek S, Lichodziejewska B, et al. Prognostic value of echocardiography in normotensive patients with acute pulmonary embolism. JACC Cardiovasc Imaging. 2014;7(6):553–60.

18. Rodrigues AC, Cordovil A, Monaco C, et al. Right ventricular assessment by tissue-Doppler echocardiography in acute pulmonary embolism. Arq Bras Cardiol. 2013;100(6):524–30.

19. Rodrigues AC, Cordovil A, Monaco CG, et al. Assessing prognosis of pulmonary embolism using tissue-Doppler echocardiography and brain natriuretic peptide. Einstein (Sao Paulo). 2013;11(3):338–44.

20. Rydman R, Soderberg M, Larsen F, Caidahl K, Alam M. Echocardiographic evaluation of right ventricular function in patients with acute pulmonary embolism: a study using tricuspid annular motion. Echocardiography. 2010;27(3):286–93.

21. Stergiopoulos K, Bahrainy S, Strachan P, Kort S. Right ventricular strain rate predicts clinical outcomes in patients with acute pulmonary embolism. Acute Card Care. 2011;13(3):181–8.

22. Vitarelli A, Barilla F, Capotosto L, et al. Right Ventricular Function in Acute Pulmonary Embolism: A Combined Assessment by Three-Dimensional and Speckle-Tracking Echocardiography. J Am Soc Echocardiogr. 2014;27(3):329-38.

23. Pruszczyk P, Goliszek S, Lichodziejewska B, et al. Prognostic Value of Echocardiography in Normotensive Patients With Acute Pulmonary Embolism. JACC Cardiovasc Imaging. 2014.

24. Horvath MM, Winfield S, Evans S, Slopek S, Shang H, Ferranti J. The DEDUCE Guided Query tool: providing simplified access to clinical data for research and quality improvement. J Biomed Inform. 2011;44(2):266–76.

25. Forsha DE, Risum N, Smith PB, et al. A Novel Comprehensive RV Strain Analysis: Echocardiographic Approach to Define a Normal Adult Population. J Am Soc Echocardiogr. 2014:In press.

26. Kaul S, Tei C, Hopkins JM, Shah PM. Assessment of right ventricular function using two-dimensional echocardiography. Am Heart J. 1984;107(3):526–31.

27. Vitarelli A, Barilla F, Capotosto L, et al. Right ventricular function in acute pulmonary embolism: a combined assessment by three-dimensional and speckle-tracking echocardiography. J Am Soc Echocardiogr. 2014;27(3):329–38.

28. Risum N, Jons C, Olsen NT, et al. Simple regional strain pattern analysis to predict response to cardiac resynchronization therapy: rationale, initial results, and advantages. Am Heart J. 2012;163(4):697–704.

29. Sachdev A, Villarraga HR, Frantz RP, et al. Right ventricular strain for prediction of survival in patients with pulmonary arterial hypertension. Chest. 2011;139(6):1299–309.

30. Guyatt GH, Norris SL, Schulman S, et al. Methodology for the development of antithrombotic therapy and prevention of thrombosis guidelines: Antithrombotic Therapy and Prevention of Thrombosis, 9th ed: American College of Chest Physicians Evidence-Based Clinical Practice Guidelines. Chest. 2012;141(2 Suppl):53s–70.

31. McConnell MV, Solomon SD, Rayan ME, Come PC, Goldhaber SZ, Lee RT. Regional right ventricular dysfunction detected by echocardiography in acute pulmonary embolism. Am J Cardiol. 1996;78(4):469–73.

32. Park JH, Kim JH, Lee JH, Choi SW, Jeong JO, Seong IW. Evaluation of right ventricular systolic function by the analysis of tricuspid annular motion in patients with acute pulmonary embolism. J Cardiovasc Ultrasound. 2012; 20(4):181–8.

33. Ozsu S, Kiris A, Bulbul Y, et al. Relationship between cardiac troponin-T and right ventricular Tei index in patients with hemodynamically stable pulmonary embolism: an observational study. Anadolu Kardiyol Derg. 2012; 12(8):659–65.

34. Forsha D, Risum N, Kropf PA, et al. Right ventricular mechanics using a novel comprehensive three-view echocardiographic strain analysis in a normal population. J Am Soc Echocardiogr. 2014;27(4):413–22.

15

The impact of preload on 3-dimensional deformation parameters: principal strain, twist and torsion

Hyo-Suk Ahn[1], Yong-Kyun Kim[2], Ho Chul Song[2], Euy Jin Choi[2], Gee-Hee Kim[1], Jung Sun Cho[1], Sang-Hyun Ihm[1], Hee-Yeol Kim[1], Chan Seok Park[1]* and Ho-Joong Youn[1]

Abstract

Background: Strain analysis is feasible using three-dimensional (3D) echocardiography. This approach provides various parameters based on speckle tracking analysis from one full-volume image of the left ventricle; however, evidence for its volume independence is still lacking.

Methods: Fifty-eight subjects who were examined by transthoracic echocardiography immediately before and after hemodialysis (HD) were enrolled. Real-time full-volume 3D echocardiographic images were acquired and analyzed using dedicated software. Two-dimensional (2D) longitudinal strain (LS) was also measured for comparison with 3D strain values.

Results: Longitudinal (pre-HD: -24.57 ± 2.51, post-HD: -21.42 ± 2.15, $P < 0.001$); circumferential (pre-HD: -33.35 ± 3.50, post-HD: -30.90 ± 3.22, $P < 0.001$); and radial strain (pre-HD: 46.47 ± 4.27, post-HD: 42.90 ± 3.61, $P < 0.001$) values were significantly decreased after HD. The values of 3D principal strain (PS), a unique parameter of 3D images, were affected by acute preload changes (pre-HD: -38.10 ± 3.71, post-HD: -35.33 ± 3.22, $P < 0.001$). Twist and torsion values were decreased after HD (pre-HD: 17.69 ± 7.80, post-HD: 13.34 ± 6.92, $P < 0.001$; and pre-HD: 2.04 ± 0.86, post-HD: 1.59 ± 0.80, respectively, $P < 0.001$). The 2D LS values correlated with the 3D LS and PS values.

Conclusion: Various parameters representing left ventricular mechanics were easily acquired from 3D echocardiographic images; however, like conventional parameters, they were affected by acute preload changes. Therefore, strain values from 3D echocardiography should be interpreted with caution while considering the preload conditions of the patients.

Keywords: Three-dimensional echocardiography, Myocardial strain, Hemodialysis

Background

Two-dimensional (2D) echocardiography is the most widely used examination method for left ventricular (LV) dimension and function assessment, and the high frame rate of 2D speckle tracking echocardiography (STE) allows for the precise assessment of myocardial function through the analysis of myocardial deformation. Longitudinal, circumferential and radial movements, which represent dynamic LV changes during a cardiac cycle, can be measured from parasternal and apical echocardiographic windows.

However, assumptions about LV geometry were inevitably the limitation of this method [1].

Real-time three-dimensional (3D) echocardiography is better correlated with cardiac MRI than 2D echocardiography in the measurement of LV volumes [2]. It is particularly useful for evaluating cardiac volumes in patients with cardiomyopathies, whose hearts possess more complex structures than the normal heart, and allows for a more accurate measurement of LV volume even in cases of geometrically asymmetric LV aneurysms [3, 4]. Moreover, 3D echocardiography also proved to be superior to 2D echocardiography when evaluating cardiac valves [5]. Studies other than volume measurements can also be performed; for

* Correspondence: chanseok@catholic.ac.kr
[1]Divisions of Cardiology, College of Medicine, Catholic University of Korea, 222 Banpo-daero, Seocho-gu, Seoul 06591, Republic of Korea
Full list of author information is available at the end of the article

example, Yodwut et al. showed the clinical efficacy of 3D echocardiography for the assessment of LV diastolic function [6].

Recent studies have shown that 3D strain measurements of the left ventricle using speckle tracking can represent LV mechanical function and can be achieved using several types of vendor-dependent and independent software. Strain assessed by 3D STE can predict the prognosis of patients who have suffered acute myocardial infarction and heart failure [7, 8]. It can be measured even at frame rates as low as 18 frames/sec [9], and the rotational motion of the left ventricle can also be reliably measured from 3D echocardiography [10].

Principal strain (PS) is a newly introduced parameter in cardiology that can be obtained from 3D echocardiography. This is accomplished by recognizing the direction along which strain occurs (the so-called principal direction) and the entities of actual deformation along the principal direction. It characterizes 3D strain properties, including longitudinal and circumferential strain values as well as torsional shear deformation, and can therefore represent dynamic 3D movements of the left ventricle [11, 12].

Longitudinal and circumferential strain calculated by 2D STE was demonstrated to be affected by acute preload changes caused by normal saline infusion [13]. However, there are little data on the effects of preload on the various parameters that can be acquired from 3D STE, such as strain, twist and torsion. Moreover, it is not known whether the newly introduced echocardiographic parameter of PS is volume independent. Although twist can be measured from 2D STE, it is greatly affected by the position of the parasternal images [14]. Therefore, 3D STE is anticipated to be a useful tool for a more accurate analysis of twist and torsion.

We hypothesized that various kinds of strain values from 3D STE, including PS, twist and torsion, may be influenced by acute volume change. We attempted to test this in a group of patients with end-stage renal disease (ESRD) who underwent periodic hemodialysis (HD) and experienced a subsequent preload reduction.

Methods

Patients
Patients who were regularly undergoing HD at Bucheon St. Mary's Hospital in Bucheon, South Korea, were recruited. All subjects were enrolled on a prospective basis. Among the 98 patients who were regularly undergoing HD on a periodic basis for at least 1 month prior to enrollment in the institute, 63 patients volunteered. An experienced echocardiographer who was blinded to the study design performed screening echocardiography on all volunteer subjects. Before and after the screening echocardiography, the exclusion criteria were as follows:

(i) current acute coronary syndrome; (ii) previous cardiac surgery or device implantation; (iii) current presence or previous history of significant arrhythmia, such as atrial fibrillation; (iv) LV ejection fraction less than 50%; (v) evidence of major valvular heart disease (i.e., any degree of mitral or aortic stenosis; more than a mild degree of mitral, aortic, or tricuspid regurgitation; and the presence of a prosthetic valve); and (vi) a poor echocardiographic window that was not appropriate for interpretation.

Five patients were excluded after the screening echocardiography due to significant valve dysfunction ($n = 2$), arrhythmia detected during echocardiographic examination ($n = 1$), LV regional wall motion abnormalities ($n = 1$) and a poor echocardiographic window ($n= 1$); therefore, 58 subjects were finally enrolled in this analysis.

Echocardiographic examination
Transthoracic 2D and real-time 3D examinations were carried out by an experienced echocardiographer who was blinded to the study design while the patients were in the left lateral decubitus position.

A commercially available ultrasound machine (Vivid E9; General Electric Health Care, Milwaukee, WI) equipped with phased array transducers (M5S-D and 4 V–D) was applied for echocardiographic examination. Echocardiograms were performed immediately before and less than 30 min after a single dialysis session.

From the M-mode measurements, LV dimension and diastolic LV septal and posterior thickness were determined in the parasternal long-axis view. The 2D data were acquired from the parasternal long-axis and short-axis views and the three standard apical views. For each view, three consecutive cardiac cycles were recorded during quiet respiration. LV mass was determined using the area–length method and was corrected for body surface area. LV volume, ejection fraction and left atrial volume were determined using the modified Simpson's method from apical 4- and 2-chamber views. Pulsed Doppler echocardiography of transmitral velocities was used to determine the peak E velocity, peak A velocity and the ratio between peak E and A velocities (E/A ratio). LV early diastolic e' velocity and late diastolic a' velocity were determined at the septal and lateral portion of the mitral annulus by Doppler tissue imaging and then averaged for evaluation. These measurements were obtained by setting the sample volume at the septal and lateral annulus and then recording at a sweep of 100 mm/s. All examinations were performed according to the recommendations of the American Society of Echocardiography and the European Association of Cardiovascular Imaging [15].

Table 1 Baseline characteristics of patients

	Total (n = 58)
Age (years)	59 ± 12
Male (%)	29 (50)
Ultrafiltration rate (mL/kg/h)	11.5 ± 4.6
Hemoglobin (g/dL)	11.4 ± 1.1
Hematocrit (%)	33.4 ± 5.2
Albumin (g/dL)	4.1 ± 0.3
Calcium × phosphate product	48.7 ± 17.5
Cause of renal failure (%)	
Diabetes mellitus	36 (62)
Hypertension	17 (29)
Chronic glomerulonephritis	3 (5)
Others causes or cryptogenic	2 (4)
Stroke (%)	6 (10)
Current medication (%)	
ACEi[a]	0 (0)
ARB[b]	42 (72)
CCB[c]	34 (62)
Beta blocker	37 (64)
Statin	10 (17)

[a]ACEi angiotensin-converting enzyme inhibitor, [b]ARB angiotensin receptor blocker, [c]CCB calcium channel blocker

During 3D imaging, to achieve a high frame rate and the highest spatial resolution, the pyramidal scan volume was focused on the LV volume and the data sets were acquired during a single breath hold, taking care to include the whole left ventricle.

2D and 3D speckle tracking analysis
2D and 3D images were kept in a proprietary format (GE Healthcare, Milwaukee, WI) with Digital Imaging and Communications in Medicine Wrapper. Images were downloaded into a software package (EchoPAC version 12.0; GE Healthcare, Milwaukee, WI) and then exported into ImageArena Software (TomTec Imaging Systems; Unterschleissheim, Germany) for analysis, including 2D and 3D strain analyses. The 2D strain data were used to validate the 3D strain data. For this purpose, three apical B-mode sequences (2-, 3- and 4-

Table 2 Blood pressure and heart rate

	Pre-HD (n = 58)	Post-HD (n = 58)	P value
Blood pressure (mmHg)			
Systolic	155.4 ± 16.0	129.6 ± 19.4	<0.001
Diastolic	79.8 ± 13.1	74.4 ± 12.6	<0.001
Mean	105.0 ± 11.2	92.8 ± 13.1	<0.001
Heart rate (beats/min)	68.9 ± 10.1	70.6 ± 10.2	0.107

HD hemodialysis

chamber views) were recorded at an optimal frame rate (>30 frames/sec, also ensuring >30 frames/heartbeat) and optimal resolution for myocardium while focusing the image on the entire left ventricle; the images were kept in the DICOM format for post-processing. LS was assessed using the speckle tracking method at the endocardial level with Cardiac Performance Analysis software (Version 1.2, TomTec Imaging Systems; Unterschleissheim, Germany). Global values were then calculated as averages from the segments in each view.

Three-dimensional images were analyzed using commercially available vendor-independent software (4D LV analysis version 3.1; TomTec Imaging Systems; Unterschleissheim, Germany). First, the LV long axis was designated in the three apical views (four, three and two chamber) by the operator. The software distinguished the LV endocardial border and tracked it for an entire cardiac cycle. Last, the curves of PS strain were determined using the standard 16-segment model.

The reliability of the 3D measurements was estimated by comparing the 3D global longitudinal strain (LS) parameters with the corresponding parameter measured by 2D analysis from the relevant subjects. Correlations between 3D global PS and 2D global LS were also investigated. We also compared the differences in the 3D data analyzed by vendor-independent (4D LV analysis version 3.1; TomTec Imaging Systems, Unterschleissheim, Germany) and vendor-dependent (Echo PAC version 12.0; General Electric Health Care, Milwaukee, WI) software. Area strain (AS; i.e., area change ratio) could not be determined by vendor-independent software, and PS could not be calculated by vendor-dependent software. We directly compared only the values of 3D global longitudinal, circumferential, and radial strain that were acquired from the same 3D echocardiographic images using two different 3D image analysis systems. We also investigated the correlation between PS and AS.

Reproducibility
To evaluate intra-observer variability in the offline analysis, 20 patients were randomly selected and analyzed by the same operator with at least a 1-week interval between the two analyses. To assess the effect of inter-observer variability, the same 20 subjects were analyzed in a random order at different times using the same software by a second investigator who was blinded to the results from the first investigator.

Statistical analysis
All data analyses were performed using the statistical analysis software package R version 3.4.1 [16]. All continuous variables were shown as the mean ± standard deviation (SD). Differences in continuous variables between the pre- and post-HD states were estimated using

Table 3 Conventional echocardiographic parameters

	Pre-HD (n = 58)	Post-HD (n = 58)	P value
Septal thickness (mm)	10.9 ± 1.7	10.7 ± 2.0	0.292
Posterior wall thickness (mm)	10.3 ± 2.1	10.4 ± 1.8	0.692
LV end-diastolic dimension (mm)	51.4. ± 5.5	48.1 ± 5.7	<0.001
LV end-systolic dimension (mm)	31.2 ± 4.2	29.3 ± 4.5	<0.001
LV end-diastolic volume (mL/ m²)	67.4 ± 15.7	56.2 ± 17.9	<0.001
LV end-systolic volume (mL/ m²)	23.6 ± 6.5	20.6 ± 7.8	<0.001
Stroke volume (mL/m²)	42.2 ± 10.0	35.7 ± 10.8	0.033
LVEF (%)	65.1 ± 4.4	63.6 ± 4.3	0.023
LV mass index (g/m²)	119.9 ± 29.4	109.9 ± 30.0	<0.001
E wave (cm/s)	80.3 ± 24.7	58.4 ± 23.7	<0.001
A wave (cm/s)	87.5 ± 19.8	85.6 ± 29.1	0.685
E/A ratio	0.95 ± 0.34	0.74 ± 0.30	<0.001
DT (ms)	209.2 ± 43.1	224.0 ± 46.2	0.015
IVRT (ms)	84.4 ± 15.6	101.4 ± 23.8	<0.001
A wave duration (ms)	147.6 ± 17.7	148.9 ± 18.4	0.640
LA volume index (mL/m²)	49.7 ± 13.8	36.9 ± 14.4	<0.001
e' (cm/s)	6.61 ± 1.62	6.00 ± 1.50	0.001
a' (cm/s)	9.31 ± 2.52	8.91 ± 1.42	0.298
E/e'	12.83 ± 5.08	10.05 ± 4.22	<0.001

LV left ventricle, *LVEF* Left ventricular ejection fraction, E wave: Peak early diastolic mitral inflow velocity, A wave: Peak late diastolic mitral inflow velocity, *DT* Deceleration time of peak early diastolic mitral inflow velocity, *IVRT* Isovolumic relaxation time, *LA* left atrium, e': Average of peak early diastolic tissue velocity measured at septal and lateral mitral annulus, a': Average of peak late diastolic tissue velocity measured at septal and lateral mitral annulus, E/e': Ratio between peak early diastolic mitral inflow velocity and peak early diastolic tissue velocity

the paired t-test. The x^2 and Fisher's exact tests were applied to assess differences between categorical variables. The correlations between 3D PS, 3D LS and 2D LS were evaluated by Pearson's correlation coefficient. Linear regression analysis between the values of 2D and 3D strain was performed. The correlation between 3D PA and AS was also evaluated by Pearson's correlation coefficient and linear regression analysis [17].

Reliability was evaluated using the intra-class correlation coefficient (ICC) to determine both intra- and inter-observer variability using an R package for the ICC [18]. The inter-software variability was determined by the ICC. The clinical significance of the ICC was interpreted as follows: excellent, ICC ≥ 0.80; good, 0.60 ≤ ICC < 0.80; moderate, 0.40 ≤ ICC < 0.60; and poor, ICC < 0.40. Bland-Altman analyses were also

Table 4 Left ventricular volumes, strains, twist, and torsion in patients with end-stage renal disease (ESRD) before and after hemodialysis (HD) measured by 3-dimensional speckle tracking echocardiography

	Pre-HD (n = 58)	Post-HD (n = 58)	P value
Frame rates (/min)	26.3 ± 4.6	25.2 ± 4.7	0.120
LV end-diastolic volume (mL/m²)	73.0 ± 17.0	61.2 ± 15.2	<0.001
LV end-systolic volume (mL/m²)	25.9 ± 7.6	24.0 ± 6.9	<0.001
LV stroke volume (mL/ m²)	47.1 ± 10.4	37.2 ± 8.9	<0.001
LV ejection fraction	64.9 ± 3.9	61.0 ± 3.3	<0.001
Global principal strain (%)	−38.10 ± 3.71	−35.33 ± 3.22	<0.001
Global longitudinal strain (%)	−24.57 ± 2.51	−21.42 ± 2.15	<0.001
Global circumferential strain (%)	−33.35 ± 3.50	−30.90 ± 3.22	<0.001
Global radial strain (%)	47.67 ± 4.27	42.90 ± 3.61	<0.001
Twist (degree)	17.69 ± 7.80	13.34 ± 6.92	<0.001
Torsion (degree/s)	2.04 ± 0.86	1.59 ± 0.80	<0.001

LV Left ventricle

performed. The R package BlandAltmanLeh was used for this purpose [19]. *P*-values <0.05 were considered statistically significant.

Results

3D STE analysis successfully performed in all 58 patients, but the measurement of LS from 2D STE could not be performed due to poor image quality in one patient pre-HD and two patients post-HD.

The clinical characteristics of the subjects are summarized in Table 1. The mean ultrafiltration rate was 11.5 ± 4.6 mL/kg/h. The mean age of the subjects was 59 ± 12 years, and 50% of the participants were male (*n* = 29). The most common cause of ESRD was diabetes mellitus (*n* = 36, 62%), the second was hypertension

(*n* = 17, 29%), and the third was chronic glomerulonephritis (n = 3, 5%) (Table 1).

Table 2 presents the changes in blood pressure and heart rate after acute preload reduction caused by HD. Systolic, diastolic and mean blood pressure were significantly lowered after HD. The differences in heart rate based on HD status were statistically insignificant.

Conventional echocardiographic parameters are summarized in Table 3. Many echocardiographic parameters that depict LV systolic and diastolic function were changed after HD. The end-diastolic, end-systolic and stroke volumes of the left ventricle were decreased after HD. LV ejection fraction was also altered by preload reduction. Diastolic parameters were evaluated by pulsed-wave Doppler, including the peak E wave velocity, E/A

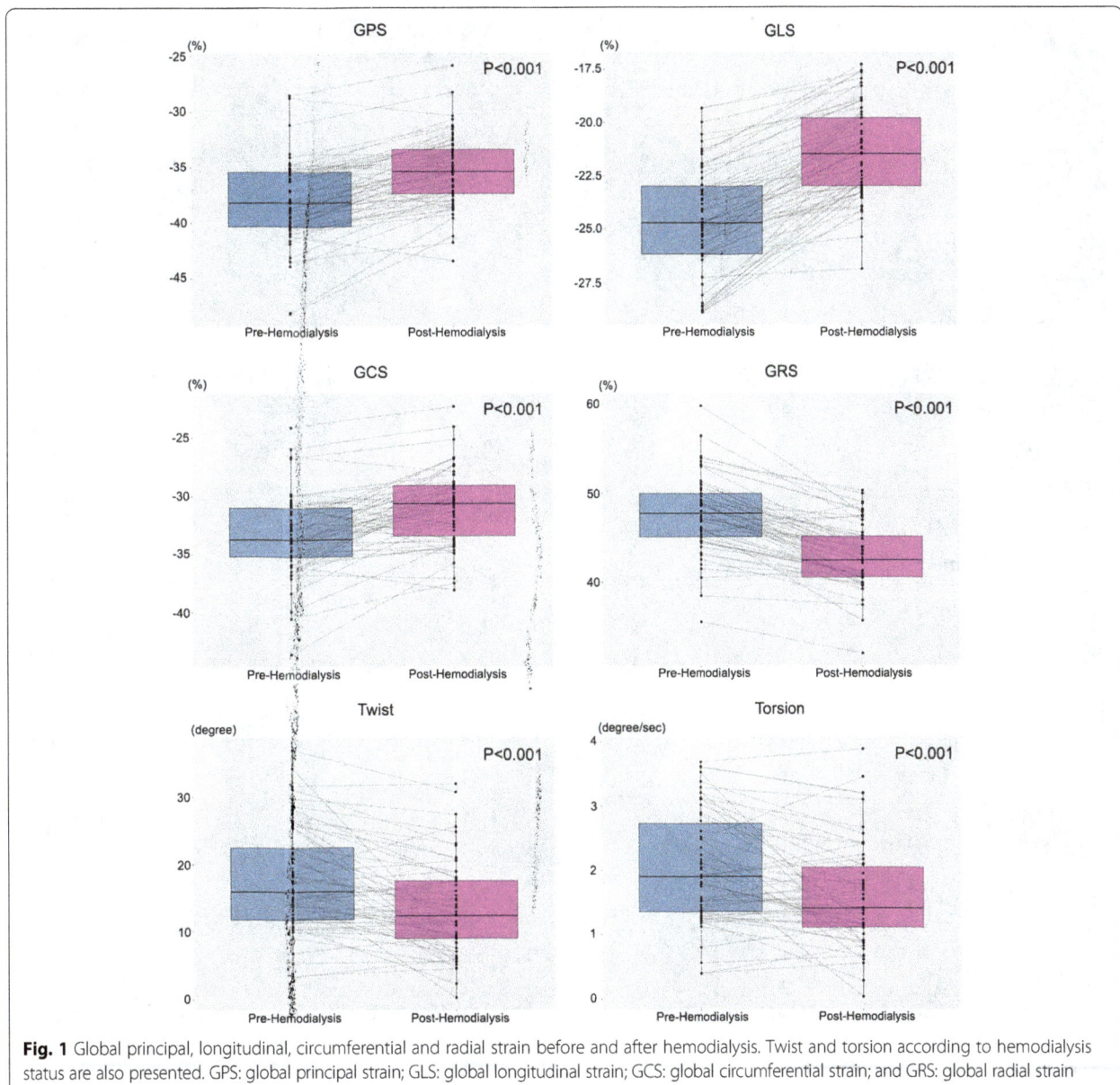

Fig. 1 Global principal, longitudinal, circumferential and radial strain before and after hemodialysis. Twist and torsion according to hemodialysis status are also presented. GPS: global principal strain; GLS: global longitudinal strain; GCS: global circumferential strain; and GRS: global radial strain

ratio, E wave deceleration time and isovolumetric relaxation time, which showed significantly different values based on HD status. Left atrial volume index, peak early diastolic tissue velocity (e') and the ratio between peak early diastolic mitral inflow velocity and peak early diastolic tissue velocity (E/ e') were also affected (Table 3).

Table 4 summarizes the LV volumes, strain, twist and torsion measured by 3D STE. The frame rates were not significantly different between pre- and post-HD patients. All parameters were easily obtained from one 3D LV full-volume image, and they were all affected by acute preload reduction. The novel parameter 3D PS was also changed after HD (pre-HD: −38.10 ± 3.71, post-HD: −35.33 ± 3.22, $P < 0.001$). The values of twist

and torsion were decreased according to the preload change caused by HD (pre-HD: 17.69 ± 7.80 post-HD:13.34 ± 6.92, $p < 0.001$; pre-HD: 2.04 ± 0.86 post-HD: 1.59 ± 0.80, respectively, $P < 0.001$) (Table 4, Figs. 1 and 2).

Table 5 compares the volumetric parameters measured by 2D and 3D echocardiography. End-diastolic and end-systolic volumes calculated by 3D echocardiography were significantly larger than those measured by 2D echocardiography. Linear analyses showed that values of 2D global LS were correlated with those of 3D global PS and LS (Fig. 3).

Table 6 shows that global LV strains in all directions are significantly different when analyzed by different

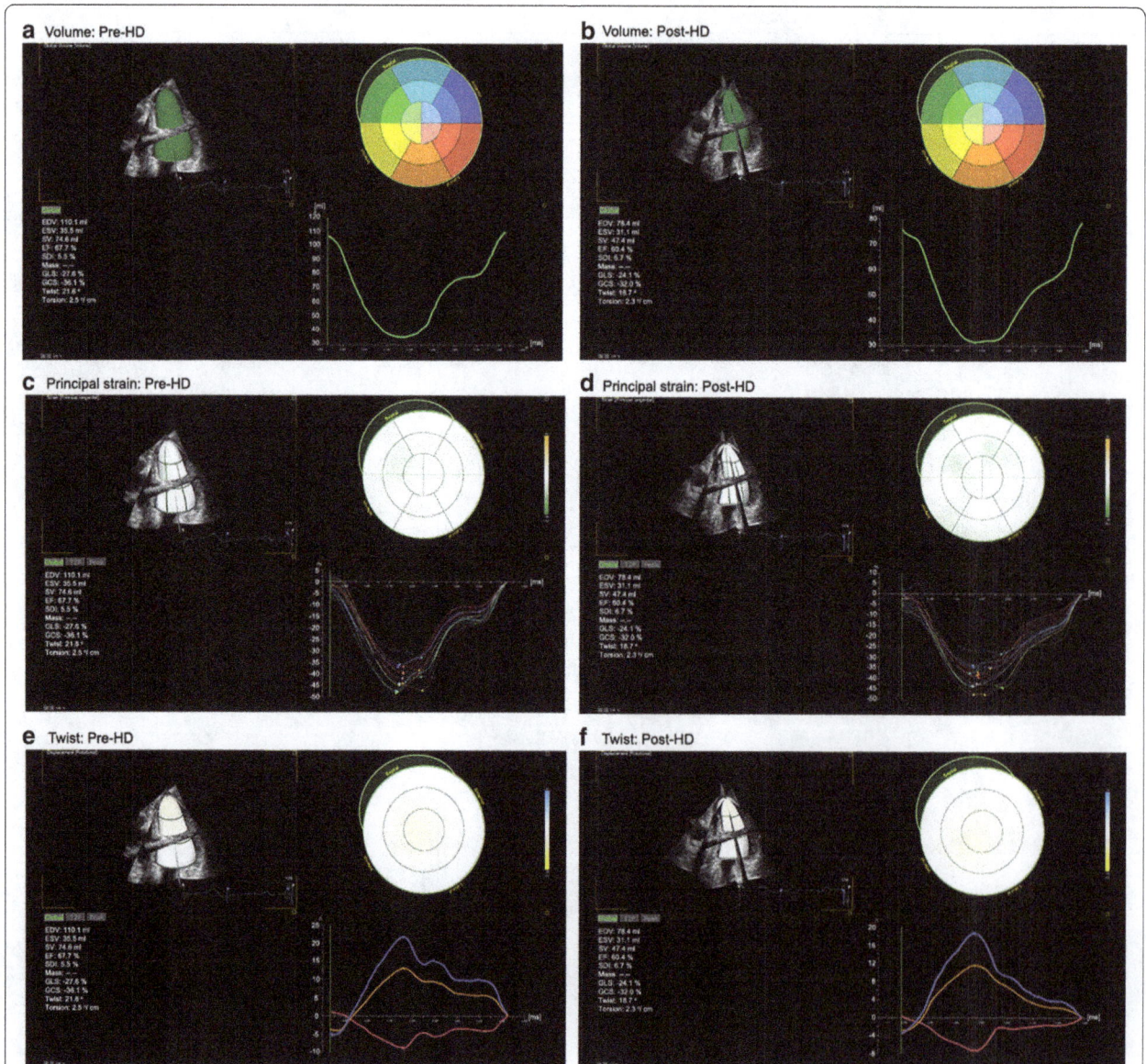

Fig. 2 Comparison of the volume, principal strain and torsion of the left ventricle based on the acute preload reduction. Pre-hemodialysis (**a**, **c** and **e**); and post-hemodialysis (**b**, **d** and **f**).

Table 5 Differences in left ventricular volumetric parameters measured by 2- and 3-dimensional echocardiography

	3D	2D	P value
Pre-HD (n = 58)			
End-diastolic volume (mL/m²)	73.0 ± 17.0	67.4 ± 15.7	<0.001
End-systolic volume (mL/m²)	25.9 ± 7.6	23.1 ± 6.7	<0.001
Stroke volume (mL/m²)	47.1 ± 10.4	43.7 ± 10.5	<0.001
Ejection fraction	64.9 ± 3.9	65.1 ± 4.4	0.770
Post-HD (n = 58)			
End-diastolic volume (mL/m²)	61.2 ± 15.2	56.5 ± 17.1	<0.001
End-systolic volume (mL/m²)	24.0 ± 6.9	20.8 ± 7.6	<0.001
Stroke volume (mL/m²)	37.2 ± 8.9	35.7 ± 10.4	0.029
Ejection fraction	61.0 ± 3.3	63.6 ± 4.3	<0.001

HD hemodialysis

analysis software although the same analyzer performed the analysis using the same images, and the correlations were weak or moderate. The correlation between PS and AS was weak in the pre-HD group, but a better correlation was observed in the post-HD group (Fig. 4).

Table 7 summarizes the ICCs of 3D STE strain for intra- and inter-observer measurements. All measurements were in excellent or good agreement, although some inter-observer variations were present, with relatively weak power. Bland-Altman plots for pre- and post-HD PS are presented in Fig. 5.

Discussion

2D speckle tracking is a useful method for cardiac evaluation. It has been applied in cases of subclinical cardiac dysfunction and for predicting prognosis. 2D echocardiographic images at higher frame rates enable the calculation of strain rate, and thus, it is possible to determine subtle changes in cardiac performance using this technique. However, at least six images should be obtained to

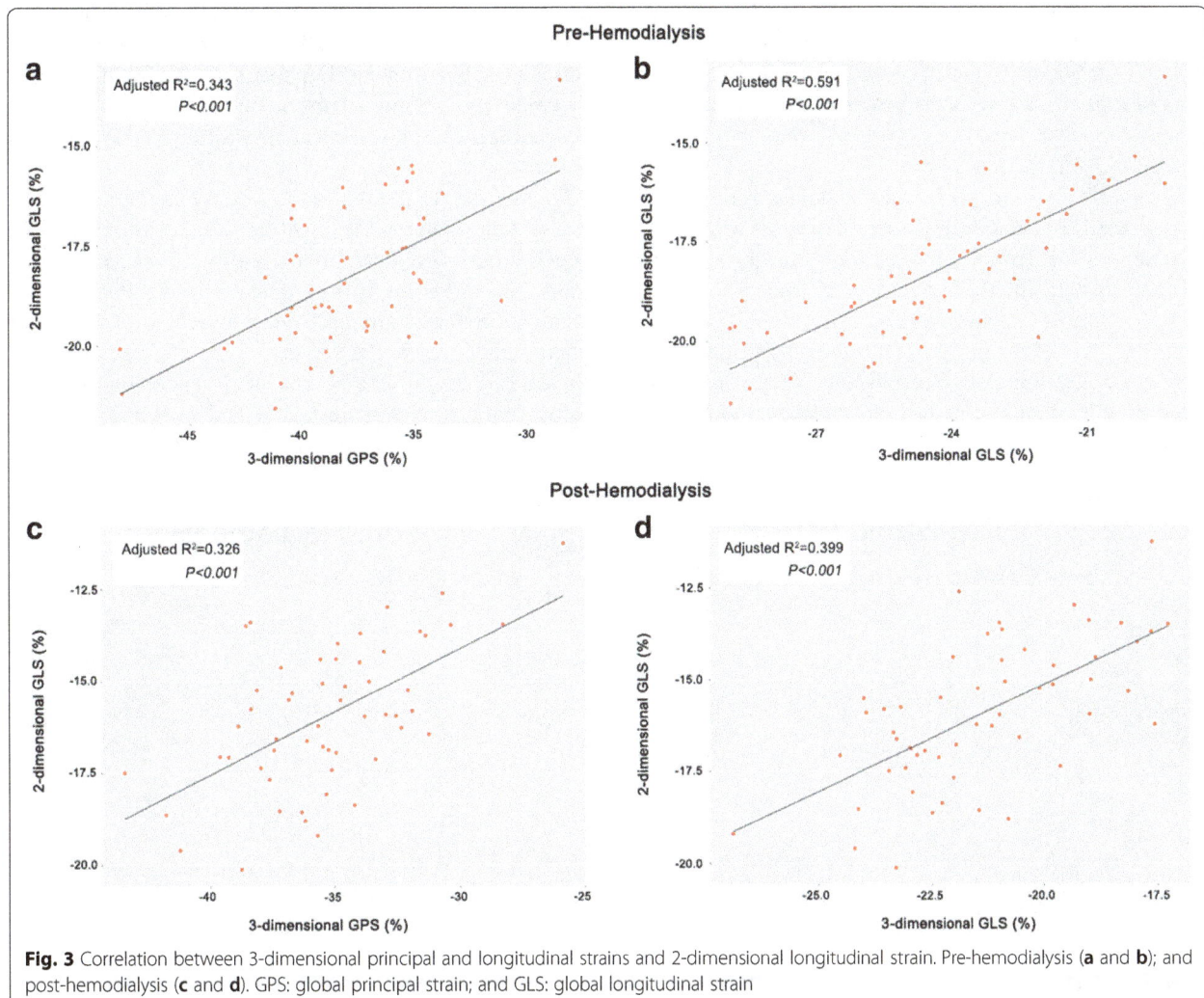

Fig. 3 Correlation between 3-dimensional principal and longitudinal strains and 2-dimensional longitudinal strain. Pre-hemodialysis (**a** and **b**); and post-hemodialysis (**c** and **d**). GPS: global principal strain; and GLS: global longitudinal strain

Table 6 Comparison of 3-dimensional left ventricular strains using two different software (4D LV analysis: version 3.1, EchoPAC: version 12.0)

	4D LV analysis	EchoPAC	P value	ICC	95% CI
Pre-HD (n = 58)					
Global longitudinal strain (%)	−24.57 ± 2.51	−17.10 ± 2.34	<0.001	−0.089	−0.840-0.355
Global circumferential strain (%)	−33.35 ± 3.50	−19.95 ± 2.51	<0.001	0.408	0.000–0.649
Global radial strain (%)	47.67 ± 4.27	53.45 ± 9.64	<0.001	−0.055	−0.783-0.376
Post-HD (n = 58)					
Global longitudinal strain (%)	−21.42 ± 2.15	−15.58 ± 3.21	<0.001	0.116	−0.494-0.477
Global circumferential strain (%)	−30.90 ± 3.22	−17.42 ± 3.71	<0.001	0.570	0.273–0.745
Global radial strain (%)	42.90 ± 3.61	45.79 ± 11.31	0.045	0.304	−0.176-0.588

ICC intra-class correlation coefficient, *CI* confidence interval, *HD* hemodialysis

measure the global strain and twist values from 2D echocardiography, and one type of strain cannot represent the dynamic cardiac motion. 2D speckle tracking also has limitations in measuring twist because its values are greatly affected by the position of image planes [14].

Real-time 3D echocardiography was first introduced in 1991 [20]. It has advantages for the measurement of LV volume, with a better correlation with cardiac MRI and fewer geometric assumption requirements. Consequently, 3D echocardiography has been suggested as a better option to measure LV volumes in cases of cardiomyopathy or aneurysmal changes that distort the geometry of the left ventricle [3, 4].

Recent advances in cardiovascular imaging techniques have made it possible to measure values of various types of strains from 3D echocardiographic images using the speckle tracking method, which is already widely used and has proven to have clinical importance in 2D imaging [21]. LV 3D strain was reported as a valuable predictor for LV function improvement after myocardial infarction [7] and can be an effective noninvasive method for assessing the twist motion of the left

ventricle, as it is less dependent on the position of the image plane [10]. A trial to determine normal reference values for real-time 3-dimensional STE has already been performed [22].

ESRD patients who are regularly undergoing HD have been used as a model for acute preload change in several previous studies. These studies showed that LV and atrial strain values were significantly decreased following preload reduction by HD [23, 24]. 3D echocardiography was also applied on ESRD patients for the evaluation of dynamic LV volume changes during HD [25], and it showed feasibility for clinical application in this group of patients.

PS analysis is a method for describing multidimensional deformations. It identifies the directions along which strain develops and the entity of actual contractions, and therefore, it is particularly well suited for biologic tissues with an underlying structure of muscular fibers along which the stress is generated, such as the heart [12]. In this study, we used vendor-independent software that was previously applied by several investigators [9, 26, 27]. This software was designed to track the

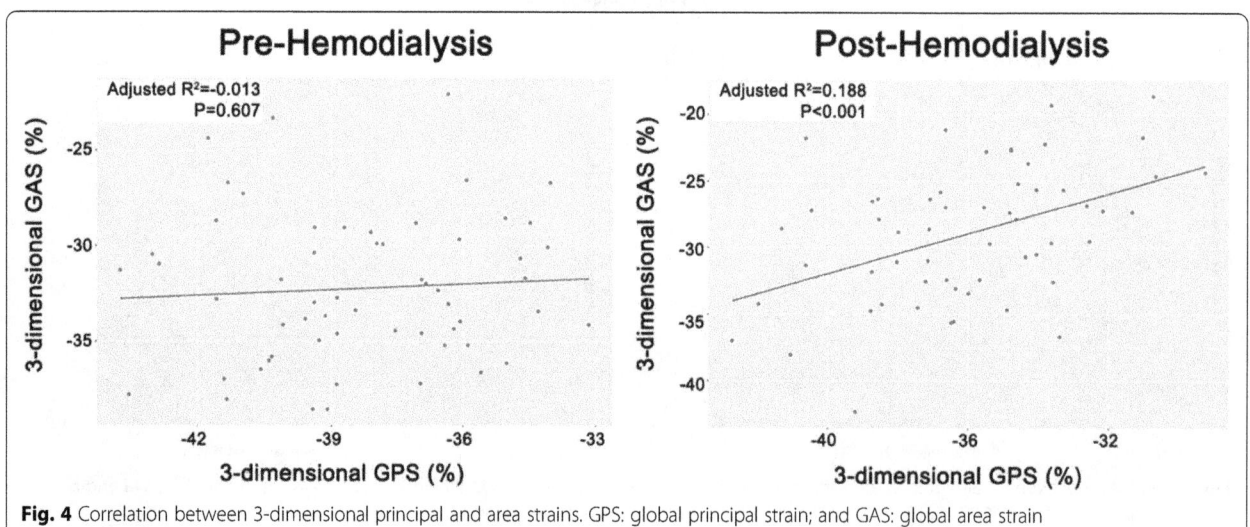

Fig. 4 Correlation between 3-dimensional principal and area strains. GPS: global principal strain; and GAS: global area strain

Table 7 Intra-class correlation coefficient (ICC) analysis of intra- and inter-observer variations for strains, twist and torsion of the left ventricle from 3D STE

	Intra-observer variation		Inter-observer variation	
	ICC	95% CI	ICC	95% CI
Pre-HD				
GPS	0.884	0.707–0.954	0.754	0.415–0.899
GLS	0.957	0.891–0.983	0.821	0.547–0.929
GCS	0.815	0.533–0.927	0.628	0.060–0.853
GRS	0.910	0.773–0.964	0.771	0.422–0.910
Twist	0.825	0.557–0.931	0.936	0.838–0.975
Torsion	0.868	0.666–0.948	0.949	0.870–0.980
Post-HD				
GPS	0.898	0.743–0.960	0.619	0.037–0.849
GLS	0.880	0.697–0.952	0.709	0.265–0.885
GCS	0.855	0.633–0.943	0.717	0.285–0.888
GRS	0.923	0.807–0.970	0.814	0.529–0.926
Twist	0.772	0.424–0.910	0.775	0.431–0.911
Torsion	0.713	0.276–0.887	0.746	0.358–0.899

CI confidence interval, *3D* three-dimensional, *STE* speckle tracking echocardiography, *HD* hemodialysis, *GPS* global principal strain, *GLS* global longitudinal strain, *GCS* global circumferential strain, *GRS* global radial strain

real-time 3D and 4D endocardial motion of the left ventricle. It provides the 3D PS value, which is unavailable from 2D images, as well as the traditional longitudinal, circumferential and radial strains.

Three-dimensional PS has proven to be effective in detecting subclinical cardiac abnormalities [26, 27]. AS is also a novel parameter for 3D echocardiographic images, but it only considers the longitudinal and circumferential movement of the left ventricle and does not represent the dynamic 3D motion of the left ventricle or have a correlation with myocardial muscle direction [21]. PS can represent more complex movements of the left ventricle because it considers not only longitudinal and circumferential movement but also twist movement during systole and diastole. It was also shown to correlate with cardiac muscle fiber arrangements. Therefore, it is a useful and novel parameter that can represent complex LV movements during the cardiac cycle.

In this study, twist and torsion calculated using 3D STE were also affected by acute preload changes. LV rotation plays an important role in LV contraction and relaxation. From 2D STE, the difference in the systolic rotation of the myocardium in the apical and basal short-axis planes is referred to as twist and reported in

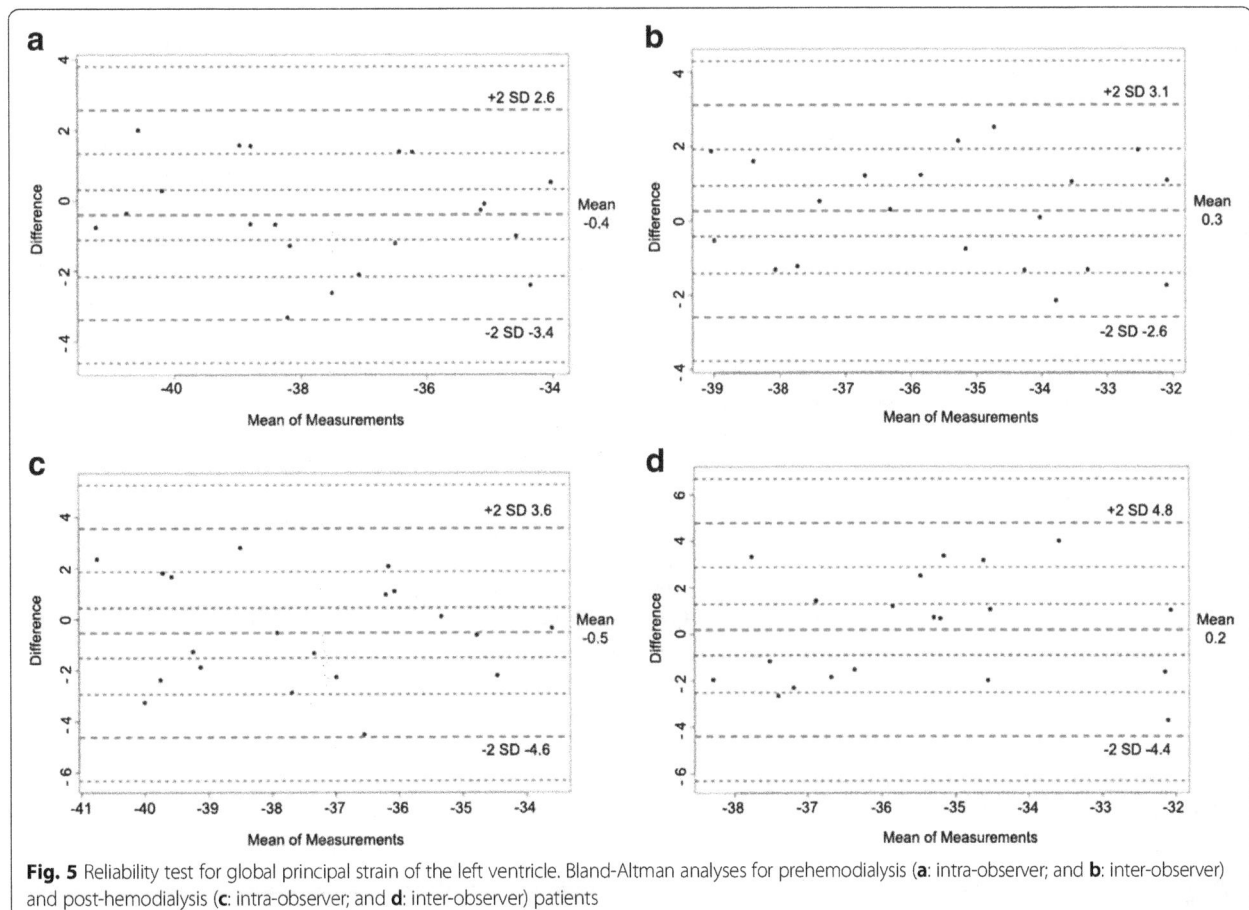

Fig. 5 Reliability test for global principal strain of the left ventricle. Bland-Altman analyses for prehemodialysis (**a**: intra-observer; and **b**: inter-observer) and post-hemodialysis (**c**: intra-observer; and **d**: inter-observer) patients

degrees. Data normalized to the distance between the respective image planes are referred to as torsion and reported in degrees/cm [14]. Weiner et al. reported that the rotational movement of the left ventricle measured by 2D STE was affected by preload changes caused by normal saline infusion [28]. However, the measurement of twist using 2D STE requires two apical and basal slices in two different cardiac cycles, and the dependence on the position of two image planes results in a less accurate analysis. The 3D STE used in this study will be a promising tool for further investigations of the rotational movement of the left ventricle.

This study has several strong points compared to other studies investigating changes in the echocardiographic parameters based on preload changes [13, 23, 24, 28].

First, we used newly developed novel strain values for the evaluation of preload reduction. Other strain values, which can be obtained from 2D STE, were also easily and simultaneously calculated during the same cardiac cycle. This benefit made it possible to measure various parameters representing cardiac mechanics more accurately.

Second, the software used was newly introduced vendor-independent software for 3D echocardiographic image analysis. There are several types of software for 3D strain evaluation on the market, but they yield different values in the measurement of 3D strain, even within the same patients [29]. Our results also showed significant vendor dependency even when the same 3D images were analyzed. In the clinic, various types of echocardiographic machines are used for patient care, and 3D echocardiography is already recommended in several guidelines for the evaluation of cardiac function, such as during cancer therapy [30]. This limitation can hamper the application of this technique in the clinical setting. The software that we used in this study was previously used by several investigators and has proven efficacy in 3D echocardiographic image analyses among various types of patients.

Third, 3D strain values could have been acquired from all subjects even though we could not calculate the LS value in 3 subjects due to poor echocardiographic windows. For measurements of acceptable strain values, good-quality real-time 3D echocardiographic images are essential. In addition, a significant learning curve is required even for experienced physicians or echocardiographers.

However, there are also several weak points in this study. The major limitation of this study is that it was performed in a single center with a relatively small number of patients, although the number of individuals enrolled in this study was larger than that in other studies [13, 23, 24, 28].

Second, this study only tracked the endocardium and not the entire myocardium. Compared with the epicardium, endocardial shape change is known to be more associated with global shape change; epicardial, endocardial or global volume; and global rotation and global twist parameters [31].

Third, although the heart rate and frame rate were not significantly different between the pre- and post-HD phases, the relatively higher heart rate post-HD due to acute volume reduction might have affected the frame rate of the 3D echocardiographic images and ultimately led to a greater decrease in all LV mechanical parameters. The frame rates of both groups were greater than 25 frames/s in this study. Yodwut et al. previously demonstrated that frame rates greater than 18 frames/s did not affect the strain values [9]. The lower resolution of the 3D echocardiogram may also influence the quality of the strain analysis and principal strain analysis (PSA) results. We attempted to mitigate this limitation by performing multiple 3D tracking assessments and by validating our data to 2D LS results. Although a previous study reported significant differences in 2D and 3D strain values [32], in this study the values of LS measured by 3D STE were relatively well correlated with both PS and 2D LS. Additionally, 2D STE measurements were not possible in three patients whose 3D STE measurements were available for 3D strain evaluation.

Fourth, HD is not a simple process that leads to only acute volume reduction. During HD, activation of the sympathetic nervous system occurs for the invitation and maintenance of compensatory mechanisms to maintain blood pressure, especially mechanisms involving heart rate and peripheral vasoconstriction [33]. The heart rate was not significantly different after HD, but HD affected blood pressure in this study. The effects of a decrease in blood pressure on the echocardiographic parameters could not be excluded.

Fifth, a study that aimed to determine normal reference values of 3D echocardiographic strain showed that there were differences in normal values between different segments, walls and levels of the left ventricle. There is still no accepted reference value of 3D strain, and there are significant inter-vendor differences in the measured values [29]. We used vendor-independent software in this study and compared only global strain values before and after acute preload reduction in the same subjects; therefore, this limitation could be overcome in this study.

Conclusion

This study showed that deformation parameters measured from 3D echocardiographic images using the speckle tracking method are affected by acute preload changes. 3D echocardiography can be used to calculate strain, twist and torsion, which can represent complex

LV mechanics, from a single image. However, all parameters representing LV systolic function, including the novel parameter of PS, were affected by acute preload changes. Therefore, the values of strain, twist and torsion acquired from 3D STE should be interpreted with caution and with consideration of the preload status of the patient. The findings of this study are important for patients in critical settings, such as acute heart failure and shock patients, who are experiencing significant volume shifts due to the disease and the treatment. More studies are needed to explore the prognostic value of PS, a novel parameter that reflects actual deformation along the principal direction, especially in ESRD patients who are very susceptible to cardiovascular complications.

Acknowledgments
Not applicable.

Funding
None.

Authors' contributions
HSA, MD: Data analysis, data interpretation and concept/design. YKK, MD, PhD, HCS, MD, PhD, EJC, MD. PhD: Data collection. GHK, MD. PhD, JSC, MD. PhD: Drafting of the article. SHI, MD, PhD, HYK, MD, PhD: Approval of the article. CSP, MD. PhD: Concept/design, data collection, approval of the article and statistical analysis. HJY, MD. PhD: Drafting of the article and approval of the article. All authors read and approved the final manuscript.

Consent for publication
Not applicable.

Competing interests
The authors declare that they have no competing interests.

Author details
[1]Divisions of Cardiology, College of Medicine, Catholic University of Korea, 222 Banpo-daero, Seocho-gu, Seoul 06591, Republic of Korea. [2]Nephrology, College of Medicine, Catholic University of Korea, Seoul, South Korea.

References
1. Krenning BJ, Voormolen MM, Roelandt JR. Assessment of left ventricular function by three-dimensional echocardiography. Cardiovasc Ultrasound. 2003;1:12.
2. Lee D, Fuisz AR, Fan PH, Hsu TL, Liu CP, Chiang HT. Real-time 3-dimensional echocardiographic evaluation of left ventricular volume: correlation with magnetic resonance imaging–a validation study. J Am Soc Echocardiogr. 2001;14(10):1001–9.
3. Shiota T, McCarthy PM, White RD, Qin JX, Greenberg NL, Flamm SD, Wong J, Thomas JD. Initial clinical experience of real-time three-dimensional echocardiography in patients with ischemic and idiopathic dilated cardiomyopathy. Am J Cardiol. 1999;84(9):1068–73.
4. Qin JX, Jones M, Shiota T, Greenberg NL, Tsujino H, Firstenberg MS, Gupta PC, Zetts AD, Xu Y, Ping Sun J, et al. Validation of real-time three-dimensional echocardiography for quantifying left ventricular volumes in the presence of a left ventricular aneurysm: in vitro and in vivo studies. J Am Coll Cardiol. 2000;36(3):900–7.
5. Gurzun MM, Popescu AC, Ginghina C, Popescu BA. Management of organic mitral regurgitation: guideline recommendations and controversies. Korean Circ J. 2015;45(2):96–105.
6. Yodwut C, Lang RM, Weinert L, Ahmad H, Mor-Avi V. Three-dimensional echocardiographic quantitative evaluation of left ventricular diastolic function using analysis of chamber volume and myocardial deformation. Int J Cardiovasc Imaging. 2013;29(2):285–93.
7. Abate E, Hoogslag GE, Antoni ML, Nucifora G, Delgado V, Holman ER, Schalij MJ, Bax JJ, Marsan NA. Value of three-dimensional speckle-tracking longitudinal strain for predicting improvement of left ventricular function after acute myocardial infarction. Am J Cardiol. 2012;110(7):961–7.
8. Ma C, Chen J, Yang J, Tang L, Chen X, Li N, Liu S, Zhang Y. Quantitative assessment of left ventricular function by 3-dimensional speckle-tracking echocardiography in patients with chronic heart failure: a meta-analysis. J Ultrasound Med. 2014;33(2):287–95.
9. Yodwut C, Weinert L, Klas B, Lang RM, Mor-Avi V. Effects of frame rate on three-dimensional speckle-tracking-based measurements of myocardial deformation. J Am Soc Echocardiogr. 2012;25(9):978–85.
10. Tavakoli V, Sahba N. Assessment of age-related changes in left ventricular twist by 3-dimensional speckle-tracking echocardiozgraphy. J Ultrasound Med. 2013;32(8):1435–41.
11. Mangual JO, De Luca A, Toncelli L, Domenichini F, Galanti G, Pedrizzetti G. Three-dimensional reconstruction of the functional strain-line pattern in the left ventricle from 3-dimensional echocardiography. Circ Cardiovasc Imaging. 2012;5(6):808–9.
12. Pedrizzetti G, Kraigher-Krainer E, De Luca A, Caracciolo G, Mangual JO, Shah A, Toncelli L, Domenichini F, Tonti G, Galanti G, et al. Functional strain-line pattern in the human left ventricle. Phys Rev Lett. 2012;109(4):048103.
13. Burns AT, La Gerche A, D'Hooge J, MacIsaac AI, Prior DL. Left ventricular strain and strain rate: characterization of the effect of load in human subjects. Eur J Echocardiogr. 2010;11(3):283–9.
14. Voigt JU, Pedrizzetti G, Lysyansky P, Marwick TH, Houle H, Baumann R, Pedri S, Ito Y, Abe Y, Metz S, et al. Definitions for a common standard for 2D speckle tracking echocardiography: consensus document of the EACVI/ASE/ Industry Task Force to standardize deformation imaging. Eur Heart J Cardiovasc Imaging. 2015;16(1):1–11.
15. Lang RM, Badano LP, Mor-Avi V, Afilalo J, Armstrong A, Ernande L, Flachskampf FA, Foster E, Goldstein SA, Kuznetsova T, et al. Recommendations for cardiac chamber quantification by echocardiography in adults: an update from the American Society of Echocardiography and the European Association of Cardiovascular Imaging. Eur Heart J Cardiovasc Imaging. 2015;16(3):233–70.
16. Team RDC. A Language and Environment for Statistical Computing. Vienna, Austria: R Foundation for Statistical Computing; 2016.
17. Wickham H. ggplot2: Elegant Graphics for Data Analysis. New York: Springer-Verlag; 2009.
18. Wolak ME, Fairbairn DJ, Paulsen YR. Guidelines for Estimating Repeatability. In: Methods in Ecology and Evolution vol. 2012;3:129–37.
19. Lehnert B: BlandAltmanLeh: Plots (Slightly Extended) Bland-Altman Plots. R package version 0.3.1. https://cran.r-project.org/package=BlandAltmanLeh. In.; 2015.
20. Sheikh K, Smith SW, von Ramm O, Kisslo J. Real-time, three-dimensional echocardiography: feasibility and initial use. Echocardiography. 1991;8(1):119–25.
21. Seo Y, Ishizu T, Aonuma K. Current status of 3-dimensional speckle tracking echocardiography: a review from our experiences. J Cardiovasc Ultrasound. 2014;22(2):49–57.
22. Kleijn SA, Pandian NG, Thomas JD, Perez de Isla L, Kamp O, Zuber M, Nihoyannopoulos P, Forster T, Nesser HJ, Geibel A, et al. Normal reference values of left ventricular strain using three-dimensional speckle tracking echocardiography: results from a multicentre study. Eur Heart J Cardiovasc Imaging. 2015;16(4):410–6.
23. Choi JO, Shin DH, Cho SW, Song YB, Kim JH, Kim YG, Lee SC, Park SW. Effect of preload on left ventricular longitudinal strain by 2D speckle tracking. Echocardiography. 2008;25(8):873–9.
24. Park CS, Kim YK, Song HC, Choi EJ, Ihm SH, Kim HY, Youn HJ, Seung KB. Effect of preload on left atrial function: evaluated by tissue Doppler and strain imaging. Eur Heart J Cardiovasc Imaging. 2012;13(11):938–47.
25. Krenning BJ, Voormolen MM, Geleijnse ML, van der Steen AF, ten Cate FJ, le EH, Roelandt JR. Three-dimensional echocardiographic analysis of left ventricular function during hemodialysis. Nephron Clin Pract. 2007;107(2):c43–9.
26. Pedrizzetti G, Sengupta S, Caracciolo G, Park CS, Amaki M, Goliasch G, Narula J, Sengupta PP. Three-dimensional principal strain analysis for characterizing subclinical changes in left ventricular function. J Am Soc Echocardiogr. 2014;27(10):1041–50. e1041.
27. Stefani L, De Luca A, Toncelli L, Pedrizzetti G, Galanti G. 3D Strain helps relating LV function to LV and structure in athletes. Cardiovasc Ultrasound. 2014;12:33.

28. Weiner RB, Weyman AE, Khan AM, Reingold JS, Chen-Tournoux AA, Scherrer-Crosbie M, Picard MH, Wang TJ, Baggish AL. Preload dependency of left ventricular torsion: the impact of normal saline infusion. Circ Cardiovasc Imaging. 2010;3(6):672–8.

29. Yuda S, Sato Y, Abe K, Kawamukai M, Kouzu H, Muranaka A, Kokubu N, Hashimoto A, Tsuchihashi K, Watanabe N, et al. Inter-vendor variability of left ventricular volumes and strains determined by three-dimensional speckle tracking echocardiography. Echocardiography. 2014;31(5):597–604.

30. Plana JC, Galderisi M, Barac A, Ewer MS, Ky B, Scherrer-Crosbie M, Ganame J, Sebag IA, Agler DA, Badano LP, et al. Expert consensus for multimodality imaging evaluation of adult patients during and after cancer therapy: a report from the American Society of Echocardiography and the European Association of Cardiovascular Imaging. Eur Heart J Cardiovasc Imaging. 2014;15(10):1063–93.

31. Piras P, Evangelista A, Gabriele S, Nardinocchi P, Teresi L, Torromeo C, Schiariti M, Varano V, Puddu PE. 4D-analysis of left ventricular heart cycle using procrustes motion analysis. PLoS One. 2014;9(1):e86896.

32. Saito K, Okura H, Watanabe N, Hayashida A, Obase K, Imai K, Maehama T, Kawamoto T, Neishi Y, Yoshida K. Comprehensive evaluation of left ventricular strain using speckle tracking echocardiography in normal adults: comparison of three-dimensional and two-dimensional approaches. J Am Soc Echocardiogr. 2009;22(9):1025–30.

33. Rubinger D, Backenroth R, Sapoznikov D. Sympathetic nervous system function and dysfunction in chronic hemodialysis patients. Semin Dial. 2013;26(3):333–43.

16

Quantitative evaluation of longitudinal strain in layer-specific myocardium during normal pregnancy in China

Juan Cong[1][*], Zhibin Wang[1], Hong Jin[2], Wugang Wang[1], Kun Gong[1], Yuanyuan Meng[1] and Yong Lee[1]

Abstract

Background: The myocardial wall of the left ventricle is a complex, multilayered structure and is not homogenous. The aim of this study was to determine longitudinal strain (LS) in the three myocardial layers in normal pregnant women according to gestation proceedings.

Methods: The advanced two-dimensional speckle tracking echocardiography (2D STE) was performed on 62 women during each pregnancy trimester and 6 to 9 weeks after delivery, while 30 age-matched, healthy, nonpregnant women served as controls. LS on endocardial, mid-myocardial and epicardial layers at 18 cardiac segments were measured.

Results: As gestation proceeded, all of layer-specific LS and global LS progressively decreased, which subsequently recovered postpartum ($P < 0.05$), and the LS gradient between inner and outer myocardium became greater, which reached its maximum in the late pregnancy. Peak systolic LS was the highest at endocardium and the lowest at epicardium, while the highest at the apical level and the lowest at the base ($P < 0.05$). In the early pregnancy and postpartum, LS at basal level was homogenous, meanwhile layer-specific LS showed significant differences at mid-ventricular and apical level throughout the progress of normal pregnancy ($P < 0.05$).

Conclusions: Using 2D STE, three-layer assessment of LS can be performed in pregnant women and shall give us new insights into the quantitative analysis of global and regional LV function during pregnancy. Future studies on the detection of pregnancy related heart disease would require these parameters as reference values for each time point of a normal pregnancy.

Keywords: Pregnancy, Myocardium, Layer, Strain, Speckle-tracking

Background

The cardiovascular system undergoes a number of changes during normal pregnancy, including increase in cardiac output and extracellular fluid volume as well as decrease in blood pressure, which are necessary for proceeding of a successful pregnancy. However, dramatical expansion in blood volume during gestation not only can meet the increased metabolic demands of tissue but also can exacerbate cardiac conditions of pregnant women. Although maternal heart disease just complicates a small number of pregnancies overall, it is the leading cause of nonobstetric

mortality during pregnancy [1]. So the comprehensive understanding of maternal cardiac function during non-complicated pregnancy is essential to the recognition of cardiac pathology and appropriate monitoring obstetrical patients.

Reduction of myocardial deformation accompanied with progressive cardiac hypertrophy according to gestation period has been described in previous studies [2–4]. These reports focus on the global myocardial wall thickness rather than different layers of the myocardium ranging from endocardium to epicardium. However, the myocardial wall of the left ventricle (LV) is a complex, multilayered structure and is not homogenous [5]. Until recently, speckle tracking echocardiography (STE) has been upgraded, which allows to quantify myocardial function in three

* Correspondence: congjuanmd@126.com
[1]Department of Echocardiography, The Affiliated Hospital of Qingdao University, Qingdao, Shandong Province, China
Full list of author information is available at the end of the article

layers [6]. Layer-specific differences of myocardial performance and deformation have been analyzed in normal subjects and different heart diseases [6–9]. However, still little is known about how differently multilayer myocardium contributes to myocardial deformation throughout the progress of normal pregnancy. In this study, we used the advanced two-dimensional (2D) STE to evaluate myocardial deformation within each of three myocardial layers, an endocardial, mid-myocardial, and epicardial layer. The aim of this study was to determine longitudinal strain (LS) in each of the three myocardial layers in normal pregnant women according to gestation proceeding.

Methods

Sixty-two of 71 subjects with singleton pregnancy (mean age, 28.2 ± 6.6 years; range, 24–36 years) and 30 age-matched, healthy, nonpregnant women were involved after informed consent and with approval from the Affiliated Hospital of Qingdao University Ethics Committee. Four visits were planned during the study: trimester 1, 12–14 weeks; trimester 2, 22–28 weeks; trimester 3, 36–40 weeks and 6–9 weeks after delivery. Enrolled criteria of healthy pregnant women was that they were without medical diseases, such as cardiovascular disorders, renal disease etc., and without obstetrical complications, such as gestational diabetes mellitus or pregnancy-induced hypertension. Subjects who had poor echo quality or any fetal abnormalities were excluded from the study.

Subjects underwent standard 2D echocardiographic examinations using commercially available ultrasound machine (Vivid E9; GE Healthcare, Horten, Norway) equipped with a M5S transducer. The following parameters were performed by M-Mode in the parasternal long-axis view as recommended [10]: interventricular septum (IVSd), posterior wall (PWd), left ventricular end-diastolic (LVEDd) and endsystolic (LVEDs) diameters. LV ejection fraction and stroke volume were calculated as previously described. Relative wall thickness (RWT) was calculated as (IVSd + PWd)/LVEDd. Cardiac indices were normalized for body surface area. Three apical long-axis scans were obtained at the apical four-chamber, two-chamber, and long-axis planes. Moreover, standard short-axis views were acquired at the basal, mid-ventricular and apical level. Tissue pulsed Doppler was recorded in the apical four- and two- chamber view. The average of peak systolic velocities (Sm), early diastolic velocities (Em), and late diastolic velocities (Am) at the septal, lateral, anterior, and inferior at mitral annulus were computed. The LV was divided into 18 cardiac segments: 6 segments (anterior, anteroseptal, inferior, lateral, posterior, and septal) at 3 levels (basal, mid, and apical). The frame rate was 52–94 frames/s. Peak systolic LS was obtained in three myocardial layers from the apical views.

All image acquisitions were performed throughout three consecutive cardiac cycles during breath-holds.

All grayscale images of the apical long-axis 2D echocardiography were analyzed frame by frame using an off-line software package (EchoPAC, PC version 113.1). The endocardial borders were delineated in the end-systolic frame of the images at the 3 apical views. Subsequently, the myocardial wall was automatically defined with multiple chains of nodes for allowing assessment of longitudinal endocardial, mid-myocardial and epicardial strains (Fig. 1). Then, quantitative myocardial parameters for each segment were evaluated in an 18 segment LV model (six segments at each level) at all three acquired apical long-axis views (Fig. 2). Deformation parameters were determined as average of the three consecutive beats. The myocardial deformation at the basal, mid-ventricular and apical levels were averaged to global longitudinal strain (GLS) in the endocardial layer (GLS-endo), in the mid-myocardial layer (GLS-mid) and in the epicardial layer (GLS-epi), respectively. All segmental values were averaged to ventricular GLS.

Statistical analysis was performed with SPSS (version 17.0). Data were shown as mean ± SD. LS was presented in its absolute value. Comparison of continuous variables was performed with independent sample t tests or ANOVA as appropriate. Reproducibility was assessed by the mean percentage error (absolute difference divided by the mean of the 2 observations). $P < 0.05$ was considered to indicate statistical significance.

Results

Table 1 shows the clinical and hemodynamic characteristics of the pregnant women and controls. As the pregnancy progressed, diastolic blood pressure and mean blood pressure were slightly reduced but followed by a mild increase toward the third trimester. Due to late increase in heart rate and in stroke volume, the cardiac index increased progressively by a mean of 33 % between the first and third trimesters.

Table 2 summarizes the parameters of LV geometry and function in the study population. There was a progressive increase in LV volume and LV wall thickness, which resulted in slightly eccentric hypertrophy during pregnancy. From the first trimester to the third trimester, ejective fraction and peak myocardial velocity of mitral annulus Sm decreased by 4.44 and 8.37 %, respectively. Those changes had almost returned to control levels in the postpartum study.

Data of layer-specific GLS in pregnant women is depicted in Table 3. Among 4464 segments with pregnant women, 4132 (92.56 %) segments were successfully analyzed while 512 (94.81 %) out of 540 segments with control subjects were assessed by modified speckle-tracking imaging. All of GLS showed significant decrease

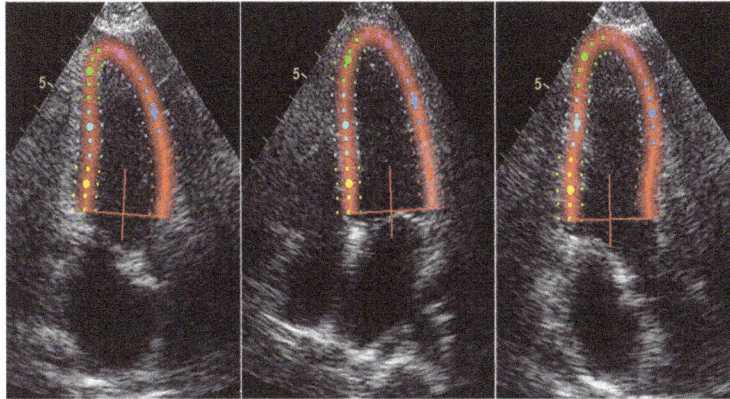

Fig 1 Multiple-dotted lines in three myocardial layers at the three parasternal long-axis scans. The endocardial borders are delineated in the end-systolic frame of the images at the apical four-chamber, two-chamber, and long-axis planes. Subsequently, the myocardial wall is automatically defined with multiple chains of nodes for allowing assessment of longitudinal endocardial, mid-myocardial and epicardial strains

in late pregnancy, consistent with the slightly decline of ejective fraction, and followed by a recovery postpartum. During normal pregnancy, GLS was the highest at endocardium, lower at mid-myocardium, and the lowest at epicardium and the deformation of all three-layer myocardial wall showed a decreasing tendency in the third trimester, which subsequently recovered after delivery (Fig. 3). As the gestation proceeded, the absolute difference in GLS-endo and GLS-epi became greater, which reached its maximum in the late pregnancy. The global epicardial-to-endocardial gradient was 21.21 % in trimester 1, 22.37 % in trimester 2, 24.81 % in trimester 3, and 20.40 % postpartum, respectively.

The peak LS of three myocardial layers at the basal, mid-ventricular, and apical levels of the LV in pregnancy are reported in Table 4. Considering a layer-specific

analysis of myocardial deformation in normal pregnancy, all of the peak systolic LS in the endocardium, mid-myocardium and epicardium were gradually increased from the base to the apex, the greatest in the apical level and the lowest in the base (Fig. 4). Moreover, the difference between inner and outer myocardium at each level increased during pregnancy. The epicardial-to-endocardial gradient was 5.26, 21.53 and 33.65 % at the basal, mid-ventricular and apical level in the first trimester, 6.66, 22.04 and 36.26 % in the second trimester, 7.51, 22.37 and 38.08 % in the third trimester, respectively, meanwhile it was 5.98, 22.76 and 33.51 % postpartum compared with 3.97, 23.29 and 38.15 % in the control subjects, respectively. In the trimester 1 and the post delivery period, peak systolic LS in the three layers were similar at the basal level. However, at both mid-ventricular and apical level,

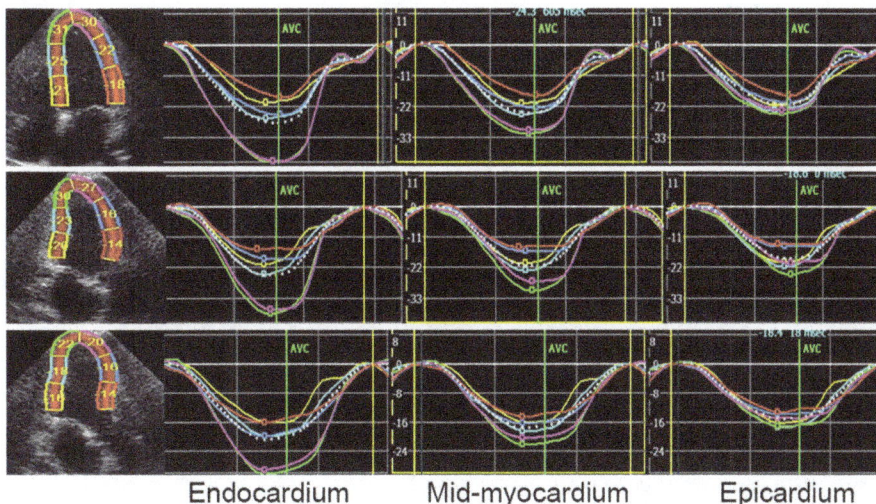

Endocardium   Mid-myocardium   Epicardium

Fig 2 Layer-specific strain curves in each segment. Quantitative myocardial parameters for each segment are evaluated in an 18 segment LV model (six segments at each level) at all three acquired parasternal long-axis views

Table 1 Clinical and hemodynamic characteristics in pregnant women

Variable	Controls	Trimester 1	Trimester 2	Trimester 3	Postpartum
	-	(13.6 ± 2.2)wk	(24.8 ± 3.4)wk	(38.1 ± 2.6)wk	(7.4 ± 2.4)wk
No. participants	30	62	62	62	62
Weight(kg)	59.3 ± 11.4	61.1 ± 9.6	68.2 ± 8.5*[†‡§]	72.8 ± 7.0*[†]	62.8 ± 13.5[‡]
BSA(m^2)	1.63 ± 0.12	1.64 ± 0.20	1.66 ± 0.11[‡]	1.74 ± 0.10*[†]	1.66 ± 0.18[‡]
Heart rate(bpm)	81.1 ± 14.3	82.6 ± 12.4	85.1 ± 17.2	90.1 ± 9.8*[†]	81.3 ± 14.2[‡]
SBP(mmHg)	104.2 ± 10.7	105.1 ± 8.7	102.9 ± 11.5	107.6 ± 9.6	110.2 ± 10.3
DBP(mmHg)	64.4 ± 8.0	64.3 ± 6.9	61.3 ± 6.8[‡§]	67.2 ± 7.9	68.6 ± 6.2
MBP(mmHg)	79.3 ± 8.5	80.5 ± 7.0	76.5 ± 6.2[‡§]	81.7 ± 7.7	83.3 ± 8.1
CI (l·min^{-1}·m^{-2})	2.98 ± 0.76	3.01 ± 0.66	3.59 ± 0.79*	4.06 ± 0.72*[†]	3.36 ± 0.72[‡]
SVI(ml/m^2)	34.58 ± 6.23	35.11 ± 9.60	37.56 ± 8.52	39.03 ± 5.34*[†]	36.56 ± 7.54

Data are given as mean ± SD, BSA indicates Body surface area
SBP systolic blood pressure, *DBP* diastolic blood pressure, *MBP* mean blood pressure, *CI* cardiac index, *SVI* stroke volume index
*P < 0.05 vs. Controls; [†]P < 0.05 vs. Trimester 1; [‡]P < 0.05 vs. Trimester 3; [§]P < 0.05 vs. Postpartum

there was significantly difference among layer-specific myocardial deformation during the gestation period and postpartum.

Table 5 summarizes the univariate relations of layer-specific strain in the third trimester during pregnancy. The GLS in the endocardial, mid-myocardial and epicardial layers showed significant associations with gestation period, maternal age, BSA and with other ventricular parameters as LVEDd, RWT, sphericity index as well as LVEF.

For deformational assessments of the endocardial, mid-myocardial, and epicardial layers, intraobserver and interobserver variability were 11.7 %, 12.3 %, 12.4 %, respectively, and 12.3 %, 12.8 %, 12.6 %, respectively.

Discussion

A comprehensive evaluation of systolic LV function requires the consideration of all of the parameters on the global and local level. The indices of LV myocardial strain describe ventricular deformation at regional level, which have been demonstrated to be more sensitive and accurate in the identification of LV functional impairment compared with global performance of the heart [11, 12]. A number of studies on maternal myocardial deformation during pregnancy have been published, but there is still controversy regarding the changes in LV performance [2–4, 13, 14]. Moreover, these findings analyzed the myocardial function considering the complete wall thickness without further distinction between

Table 2 The morphological and functional changes in the left ventricle in pregnant women

Variable	Controls	Trimester 1	Trimester 2	Trimester 3	Postpartum
	-	(13.6 ± 2.2)wk	(24.8 ± 3.4)wk	(38.1 ± 2.6)wk	(7.4 ± 2.4)wk
LVEDd (mm)	44.18 ± 2.50	45.28 ± 2.83	46.88 ± 3.40	48.84 ± 3.26*[†]	46.31 ± 3.14
LVEDs (mm)	28.08 ± 2.84	28.24 ± 3.21	29.62 ± 2.91	30.46 ± 2.81*	28.72 ± 2.51
RWT	0.25 ± 0.09	0.27 ± 0.07	0.28 ± 0.05	0.29 ± 0.06*	0.26 ± 0.06
LVMi (g/m^2)	59.25 ± 18.00	62.57 ± 24.81	66.37 ± 16.74	71.23 ± 14.46*[†]	63.14 ± 16.08[‡]
Sphericity index	0.27 ± 0.04	0.31 ± 0.07*	0.32 ± 0.05*[§]	0.32 ± 0.06*	0.28 ± 0.06[‡]
LVEDV(ml)	76.14 ± 21.20	81.39 ± 19.54	83.78 ± 14.58	87.72 ± 17.18*[†]	82.77 ± 16.85[‡]
LVESV(ml)	32.00 ± 7.29	33.91 ± 6.16	36.30 ± 7.96*	39.67 ± 7.98*	34.08 ± 8.32
LVEDV index (ml/m^2)	44.06 ± 17.44	41.93 ± 18.61	49.33 ± 14.49[†]	51.67 ± 12.65*[†]	46.63 ± 16.49
EF (%)	67.57 ± 5.12	68.00 ± 5.21	65.46 ± 4.49[†]	64.98 ± 3.93*[†]	66.89 ± 4.91
Sm (cm/min)	7.01 ± 1.63	7.06 ± 1.24	6.82 ± 1.03	6.47 ± 1.21*[†]	6.93 ± 1.72
E/Em	8.33 ± 1.07	11.56 ± 2.08*	12.46 ± 3.18*	13.34 ± 4.33*	9.04 ± 4.05

Data are given as mean ± SD, LVEDd indicates left ventricular end-diastolic dimension
LVEDs left ventricular end-systolic dimension, *RWT* relative wall thickness, *LVMi* left ventricular mass index, *LVEDV* indicates left ventricular end-diastolic volume, *LVESV* left ventricular end-systolic volume, *EF* ejection fraction, *Sm* average of peak systolic velocities, *E* peak early diastole transmitral wave velocity, *Em* average of peak early diastolic velocities
*P < 0.05 vs. Controls; [†]P < 0.05 vs. Trimester 1; [‡]P < 0.05 vs. Trimester 3;[§]P < 0.05 vs. Postpartum

Table 3 Three-layer longitudinal strain evolution during pregnancy

	Controls	Trimester 1 (13.6 ± 2.2)wk	Trimester 2 (24.8 ± 4.4)wk	Trimester 3 (38.1 ± 2.6)wk	Postpartum (7.4 ± 2.4)mo
GLS-endo (%)	24.32 ± 4.11	24.10 ± 2.78	$23.97 ± 2.98^{\ddagger}$	$21.40 ± 3.07^{*\dagger}$	$24.02 ± 3.17^{\ddagger}$
GLS-mid (%)	21.15 ± 2.90	20.98 ± 3.20	$21.03 ± 3.21^{\ddagger}$	$18.34 ± 2.76^{*\dagger}$	$21.18 ± 2.26^{\ddagger}$
GLS-epi (%)	18.96 ± 2.84	19.01 ± 3.33	$18.61 ± 2.83^{\ddagger}$	$16.09 ± 2.57^{*\dagger}$	$19.12 ± 3.33^{\ddagger}$
Avg.GLS (%)	20.34 ± 2.97	21.09 ± 3.15	$21.21 ± 2.60^{\ddagger}$	$18.62 ± 2.81^{*\dagger}$	$20.95 ± 3.06^{\ddagger}$

Data are given as mean ± SD in absolute values. GLS indicates the global longitudinal strain; GLS-endo, the average value of global longitudinal strain in the endocardial layer at the basal, mid-ventricular and apical levels; GLS-mid, the average value of global longitudinal strain in the mid-myocardial layer at the basal, mid-ventricular and apical levels; GLS-epi, the average value of global longitudinal strain in the epicardial layer at the basal, mid-ventricular and apical levels
$^{*}P < 0.05$ vs. Controls; $^{\dagger}P < 0.05$ vs. Trimester 1; $^{\ddagger}P < 0.05$ vs. Trimester 3; $^{\S}P < 0.05$ vs. Postpartum

different layers of the myocardium. To the best of our knowledge, this study is the first to demonstrate the deformation of layer-specific myocardium, endocardial, mid-ventricular and epicardial layers during normal pregnancy using the modified 2D STE.

During pregnancy, a series of dramatic changes in cardiovascular system, including increases in blood volume and cardiac output as well as decreases in LV afterload, occur to meet the drastic increases in the metabolic demands and thus supply adequate blood to the growth of the fetus. In the present study, LV size gradually enlarged according to gestational weeks. From early to late pregnancy, cardiac index progressively elevated by about one third resulting from accelerated heart rate and increased stroke volume. Blood pressure, afterload of LV, slightly decreased during mid-pregnancy and tended to increase toward the third trimester. As a response to the changes in the volume and pressure, a slight cardiac hypertrophy occurred to enable the heart to fulfill its function during pregnancy. These changes slowly returned to normal value postpartum. Our data about hemodynamic and morphological changes during pregnancy is in concordance with the previous studies [2–4, 15].

The quantitative assessment of LS is an important part of echocardiophic analysis. The longitudinal behavior of ventricular wall is principal deformation of the heart [11], which represents as shortening and lengthening of

myocardial fibers from the base to the apex [16]. In the current study, we found the ventricular GLS decreased significantly in late pregnancy. This is similar to the previous studies, which had demonstrated that the global myocardial deformation in three dimensions, longitudinal, circumferential as well as radial strain, reduced markedly in the third trimester [2, 3]. Those reports considered multilayered structure of the ventricular wall as a total thickness. However, the LV wall is not homogenous, which is composed of three layers of myocardium ranging from endocardium to epicardium. Spatial configuration of ventricular myocardial fibers in the subendocardial and subepicardial layers provide sequential contractile activity of ventricle and contribute to the equal redistribution of stress and strain of heart [5, 17]. Furthermore, histologic analyses have proved that different diseases could injury the myocardial layers to a different extent and could result in alternated predominant dysfunction in specific layers [18, 19]. Thus, evaluation myocardial deformation just across the ventricular wall thickness is not able to provide comprehensive information of the cardiac function.

Our data showed that, with the pregnancy proceeding, all GLS in each of three myocardial layers, endocardium, mid-myocardium, and epicardium reduced and reached its lowest in the trimester 3, which recovered after delivery. An increased epicardial-to-endocardial gradient of LS were described from the basal to the apical level of

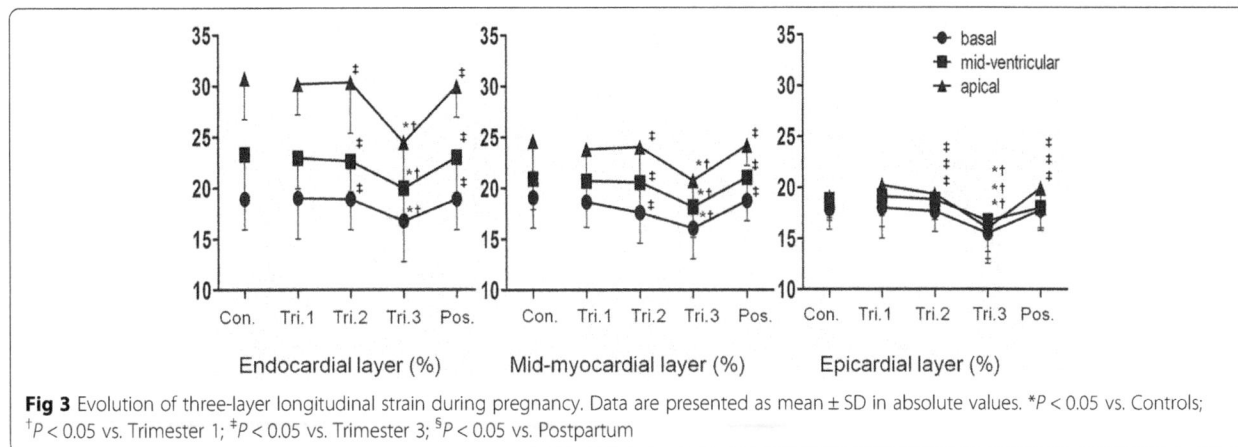

Fig 3 Evolution of three-layer longitudinal strain during pregnancy. Data are presented as mean ± SD in absolute values. $^{*}P < 0.05$ vs. Controls; $^{\dagger}P < 0.05$ vs. Trimester 1; $^{\ddagger}P < 0.05$ vs. Trimester 3; $^{\S}P < 0.05$ vs. Postpartum

Table 4 Three-layer longitudinal strain at the basal, mid-ventricular, and apical levels of the left ventricle in pregnancy

	Controls	Trimester 1 (13.6 ± 2.2)wk	Trimester 2 (24.8 ± 4.4)wk	Trimester 3 (38.1 ± 2.6)wk	Postpartum (7.4 ± 2.4) wk
Basal level (%)					
Endocardial layer (%)	18.62 ± 4.01	19.01 ± 5.67	18.91 ± 4.67‡	16.77 ± 4.91*†	18.91 ± 4.33‡
Mid-myocardial layer (%)	19.09 ± 4.61	18.65 ± 4.27	18.59 ± 4.67‡	16.08 ± 4.57*†	18.79 ± 5.07‡
Epicardial layer (%)	17.88 ± 3.72	18.01 ± 4.70	17.65 ± 4.70‡	15.51 ± 4.36*†	17.78 ± 4.22‡
P -value (between layers)	. > 0.05	>0.05	<0.05	< 0.05	> 0.05
Mid-ventricular level (%)					
Endocardial layer (%)	23.31 ± 5.16	22.95 ± 4.53	22.64 ± 4.11‡	19.98 ± 3.31*†	23.02 ± 5.26‡
Mid-myocardial layer (%)	20.92 ± 5.22	20.72 ± 4.31	20.57 ± 4.29‡	18.18 ± 3.80*†	21.07 ± 4.92‡
Epicardial layer (%)	17.88 ± 3.72	18.01 ± 4.70	17.65 ± 4.70‡	15.51 ± 4.36*†	17.78 ± 4.22‡
P-value (between layers)	< 0.01	< 0.01	< 0.001	< 0.001	< 0.01
Apical level (%)					
Endocardial layer (%)	30.77 ± 6.23	30.19 ± 5.65	30.36 ± 7.44‡	27.47 ± 6.97*†	29.96 ± 5.44‡
Mid-myocardial layer (%)	24.63 ± 6.05	23.83 ± 5.19	24.03 ± 6.06‡	20.77 ± 5.47*†	24.21 ± 6.46‡
Epicardial layer (%)	19.03 ± 4.77	20.03 ± 5.65	19.35 ± 5.30‡	17.01 ± 4.79*†	19.92 ± 4.82‡
P-value (between layers)	< 0.001	< 0.001	< 0.001	< 0.001	< 0.001

Data are given as mean ± SD in absolute values; *$P < 0.05$ vs. Controls; $^{\dagger}P < 0.05$ vs. Trimester 1; $^{\ddagger}P < 0.05$ vs. Trimester 3

the ventricle in pregnant women, which is in agreement with the findings of layer-specific LS in normal non-pregnant subjects [7, 9]. We noticed that the deformation of three-layer myocardium at the basal level was significantly different in the second and the third trimester, while it was almost homogenous in the early

pregnancy and postpartum as well as non-pregnant controls. This finding may be resulted from hemodynamic and cardiac morphological changes in the middle and late pregnancy.

Both ventricular GLS and layer-specific LS reflect myocardial function regulated by regional condition of

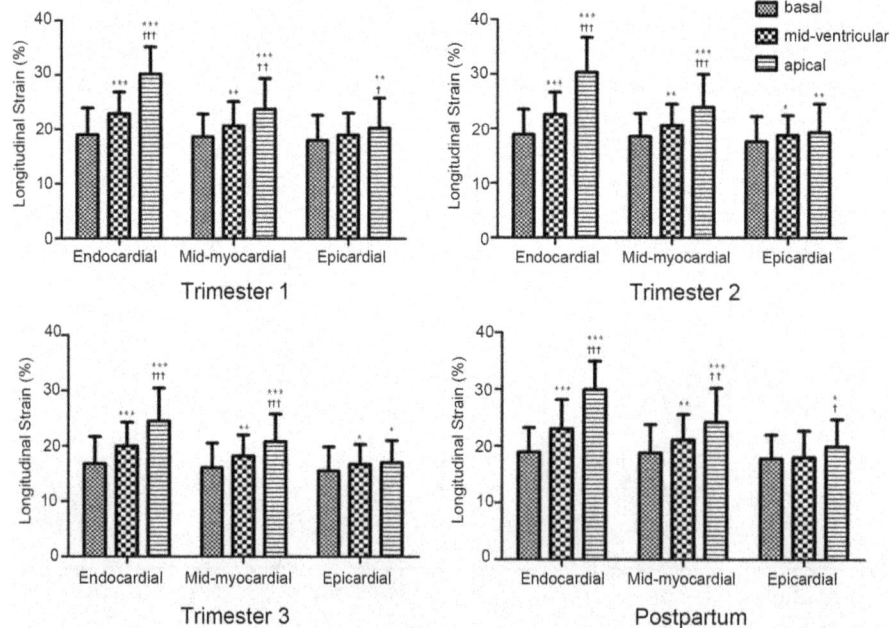

Fig 4 LV longitudinal strain of endocardial, mid-myocardial, and epicardial layers in normal pregnancy. Data are presented as mean ± SD in absolute values. *$P < 0.05$ vs. basal; **$P < 0.01$ vs. basal; ***$P < 0.001$ vs. basal; $^{\dagger}P < 0.05$ vs. mid-ventircular; $^{\dagger\dagger}P < 0.01$ vs. mid-ventricular; $^{\dagger\dagger\dagger}P < 0.001$ vs. mid-ventircular

Table 5 Univariate relations (r coefficient and significance) of layer-specific strain components in the third trimester during pregnancy

Variable	Avg.GLS (P-value)	GLS-endo (P-value)	GLS-mid (P-value)	GLS-epi (P-value)
Gestation period(w)	$0.385(P < 0.01)$	$0.290(P < 0.05)$	$0.472(P < 0.01)$	$0.487(P < 0.01)$
Age(year)	$0.368(P < 0.01)$	$0.291(P < 0.01)$	$0.372(P < 0.01)$	$0.473(P < 0.01)$
BSA(m^2)	$0.510(P < 0.01)$	$0.610(P < 0.01)$	$0.479(P < 0.01)$	$0.388(P < 0.01)$
LVEDd(mm)	$0.275(P < 0.05)$	$0.223(P < 0.05)$	$0.263(P < 0.05)$	$0.337(P < 0.01)$
RWT	$0.308(P < 0.01)$	$0.284(P < 0.05)$	$0.342(P < 0.01)$	$0.281(P < 0.05)$
Sphericity index	$0.265(P < 0.05)$	$0.297(P < 0.01)$	$0.232(P < 0.05)$	$0.244(P < 0.05)$
EF(%)	$0.686(P < 0.01)$	$0.640(P < 0.01)$	$0.682(P < 0.01)$	$0.707(P < 0.01)$

Abbreviations as in Tables 1, 2, and 3. Values of GLS, GCS, GRS and GAS considered as 'positive' (sign +) to build the univariate relations in order to homogenize the results of analyses and strengthen their clinical meaning: the higher the values, the better is the strain deformation independent of the plus/minus sign

ventricular loading and chamber morphology. To produce the same stroke volume, there is an inverse relationship between heart size and strain [20]. During early and middle pregnancy, a decreased cardiac afterload was balanced by an enlarged ventricular chamber and thus stroke volume index does not significantly increase. As a result, global and layer-specific strain keeps stable. Hypertrophy is commonly seen as a primary mechanism of the heart to reduce stress on the ventricular walls [21]. At the end of pregnancy, a mild cardiac hypertrophy happened, but it could not completely balance further increase in LV size and higher cardiac afterload. Therefore, longitudinal deformation both across total wall thickness and in multiple-layer myocardium significantly decreased despite an increasing stroke work.

In addition, LV hypertrophy during pregnancy is a complex process including a number of changes in extracellular matrix [2], the hormonal levels as well as the molecular mechanism. Recent studies have shown there is a unique system of molecular signaling pathway involved in pregnancy-induced hypertrophy [22–24]. The ubiquitin-proteasome system is known to play an important role in the degradation of damaged and misfolded proteins in the heart [25]. Both trypsin-like activity (β2) and chymotrypsin-like activity (β5), the subunit of the ubiquitin-proteasome system, were reported significantly elevated to the highest level in the subendocardium in a canine model of LV hypertrophy [26]. This possibly is one of the reasons for different strains in multiple myocardium during pregnancy. However, the precise role of molecular mechanism in physiological heart hypertrophy during pregnancy is still little known yet.

The present study on three-layer myocardial deformation in normal pregnancy can be essential for better understanding of different pathological or disease stage during pregnancy, and this is likely to give new insight into the clinically relevant therapies for pregnancy-induced cardiovascular complications, such as peripartum cardiomyopathy and pre-eclampsia.

The limitations of the present study are as follows. Firstly, the vendor-specific software to analyze layer-specific strain has not been validated by sonomicrometry. However, the current speckle tracking software has already been proved to be in coincidence with MRI both experimentally and clinically for detailed evaluation of layer-specific myocardial function. Secondly, due to continuity of myocardial fibers, the deformation parameters within the three layers are not completely isolated and absolute, and they influence each other. Thirdly, STE analysis depends on spatial resolution that tends to decrease with depth settings and higher frame rates. Fourthly, there are several dimensional movements of LV myocardium, longitudinal, circumferential and radial axis. The present study just focuses on the longitudinal deformation, the primary strain of the heart during pregnancy. Lastly, it doesn't have clear clinical implications of layer-specific LS, since at the moment it's hard to see a real utility in measuring a well-known physiological effect in normal pregnancies.

Conclusions

Using 2D STE, three-layer assessment of LS can be performed in pregnant women and shall give us new insights into the quantitative analysis of global and regional LV function during the pregnancy. Future studies on the detection of pregnancy related heart disease would require these parameters as reference values for each time point of a normal pregnancy.

Abbreviations
2D: Two-dimensional; Am: The average of late diastolic velocities at mitral annulus; Em: The average of early diastolic velocities at mitral annulus; GLS: Global longitudinal strain; GLS-endo: Global longitudinal strain in the endocardial layer; GLS-epi: Global longitudinal strain in the epicardial layer; GLS-mid: Global longitudinal strain in the mid-myocardial layer; IVSd: Interventricular septum; LS: Longitudinal strain; LV: Left ventricle; LVEDd: Left ventricular end-diastolic diameter; PWd: Posterior wall; RWT: Relative wall thickness; Sm: The average of peak systolic velocities at mitral annulus; STE: Speckle tracking echocardiography.

Acknowledgments
We thank Songyan Liu for contributing analysis tools.

Authors' contributions

JC conceived of the study, performed the experiments and draft the manuscript. ZBW participated in the design and performed the experiments. HJ participated in the experiments. WGW carried out the statistical analysis. KG participated in the statistical analysis and the experiments. YYM participated in the experiments. YL helped to draft the manuscript. All authors read and approved the final manuscript.

Competing interests

The authors declare that they have no competing interests.

Author details

[1]Department of Echocardiography, The Affiliated Hospital of Qingdao University, Qingdao, Shandong Province, China. [2]Department of Cardiology, The Affiliated Hospital of Shandong Medical College, Linyi, Shandong Province, China.

References

1. Presbitero P, Boccuzzi Giacomo G, Groot Christianne JM, Roos-Hesselink Jolien W. ESC textbook of cardiovascular medicine. Oxford: Oxford University Press; 2009.
2. Savu O, Jurcut R, Giusca S, van Mieghem T, Gussi I, Popescu BA, Ginghina C, Rademakers F, Deprest J, Voigt JU. Morphological and functional adaptation of the maternal heart during pregnancy. Circ Cardiovasc Imaging. 2012;5: 289–97.
3. Cong J, Fan T, Yang X, Squires JW, Cheng G, Zhang L, Zhang Z. Structural and functional changes in maternal left ventricle during pregnancy: a three-dimensional speckle-tracking echocardiography study. Cardiovasc Ultrasound. 2015;13:6.
4. Simmons LA, Gillin AG, Jeremy RW. Structural and functional changes in left ventricle during normotensive and preeclamptic pregnancy. Am J Physiol Heart Circ Physiol. 2002;283:H1627–33.
5. Torrent-Guasp F, Ballester M, Buckberg GD, Carreras F, Flotats A, Carrio I, Ferreira A, Samuels LE, Narula J. Spatial orientation of the ventricular muscle band: physiologic contribution and surgical implications. J Thorac Cardiovasc Surg. 2001;122:389–92.
6. Adamu U, Schmitz F, Becker M, Kelm M, Hoffmann R. Advanced speckle tracking echocardiography allowing a three-myocardial layer-specific analysis of deformation parameters. Eur J Echocardiogr. 2009;10:303–8.
7. Leitman M, Lysiansky M, Lysyansky P, Friedman Z, Tyomkin V, Fuchs T, Adam D, Krakover R, Vered Z. Circumferential and longitudinal strain in 3 myocardial layers in normal subjects and in patients with regional left ventricular dysfunction. J Am Soc Echocardiogr. 2010;23:64–70.
8. Sarvari SI, Haugaa KH, Zahid W, Bendz B, Aakhus S, Aaberge L, Edvardsen T. Layer-specific quantification of myocardial deformation by strain echocardiography may reveal significant CAD in patients with non-ST-segment elevation acute coronary syndrome. J Am Coll Cardiol Img. 2013;6:535–44.
9. Shi J, Pan C, Kong D, Cheng L, Shu X. Left Ventricular Longitudinal and Circumferential Layer-Specific Myocardial Strains and Their Determinants in Healthy Subjects. Echocardiography (Mount Kisco, NY). 2016;33:510–8.
10. Lang RM, Badano LP, Mor-Avi V, Afilalo J, Armstrong A, Ernande L, Flachskampf FA, Foster E, Goldstein SA, Kuznetsova T, Lancellotti P, Muraru D, Picard MH, Rietzschel ER, Rudski L, Spencer KT, Tsang W, Voigt JU. Recommendations for cardiac chamber quantification by echocardiography in adults: an update from the American Society of Echocardiography and the European Association of Cardiovascular Imaging. J Am Soc Echocardiogr. 2015;28:1–39. e14.
11. Reisner SA, Lysyansky P, Agmon Y, Mutlak D, Lessick J, Friedman Z. Global longitudinal strain: a novel index of left ventricular systolic function. J Am Soc Echocardiogr. 2004;17:630–3.
12. Leitman M, Lysyansky P, Sidenko S, Shir V, Peleg E, Binenbaum M, Kaluski E, Krakover R, Vered Z. Two-dimensional strain-a novel software for real-time quantitative echocardiographic assessment of myocardial function. J Am Soc Echocardiogr. 2004;17:1021–9.
13. Sengupta S. P., Bansal M., Hofstra L., Sengupta P. P. and Narula J. Gestational changes in left ventricular myocardial contractile function: new insights from two-dimensional speckle tracking echocardiography. Int J Cardiovasc Imaging. 2016. doi:10.1007/s10554-016-0977-y.
14. Ando T, Kaur R, Holmes AA, Brusati A, Fujikura K, Taub CC. Physiological adaptation of the left ventricle during the second and third trimesters of a healthy pregnancy: a speckle tracking echocardiography study. Am J Cardiovasc Dis. 2015;5:119–26.
15. Mesa A, Jessurun C, Hernandez A, Adam K, Brown D, Vaughn WK, Wilansky S. Left Ventricular Diastolic Function in Normal Human Pregnancy. Circulation. 1999;99:511–7.
16. D'Hooge J, Heimdal A, Jamal F, Kukulski T, Bijnens B, Rademakers F, Hatle L, Suetens P, Sutherland GR. Regional strain and strain rate measurements by cardiac ultrasound: principles, implementation and limitations. Eur J Echocardiogr. 2000;1:154–70.
17. Vendelin M, Bovendeerd PH, Engelbrecht J, Arts T. Optimizing ventricular fibers: uniform strain or stress, but not ATP consumption, leads to high efficiency. Am J Physiol Heart Circ Physiol. 2002;283:H1072–81.
18. Picano E, Pelosi G, Marzilli M, Lattanzi F, Benassi A, Landini L, L'Abbate A. In vivo quantitative ultrasonic evaluation of myocardial fibrosis in humans. Circulation. 1990;81:58–64.
19. Flameng W, Wouters L, Sergeant P, Lewi P, Borgers M, Thone F, Suy R. Multivariate analysis of angiographic, histologic, and electrocardiographic data in patients with coronary heart disease. Circulation. 1984;70:7–17.
20. Marciniak A, Claus P, Sutherland GR, Marciniak M, Karu T, Baltabaeva A, Merli E, Bijnens B, Jahangiri M. Changes in systolic left ventricular function in isolated mitral regurgitation. A strain rate imaging study. Eur Heart J. 2007;28:2627–36.
21. Hill JA, Olson EN. Cardiac plasticity. N Engl J Med. 2008;358:1370–80.
22. Eghbali M, Deva R, Alioua A, Minosyan TY, Ruan H, Wang Y, Toro L, Stefani E. Molecular and functional signature of heart hypertrophy during pregnancy. Circ Res. 2005;96:1208–16.
23. Eghbali M, Wang Y, Toro L, Stefani E. Heart hypertrophy during pregnancy: a better functioning heart? Trends Cardiovasc Med. 2006;16:285–91.
24. Gonzalez AM, Osorio JC, Manlhiot C, Gruber D, Homma S, Mital S. Hypertrophy signaling during peripartum cardiac remodeling. Am J Physiol Heart Circ Physiol. 2007;293:H3008–13.
25. Predmore JM, Wang P, Davis F, Bartolone S, Westfall MV, Dyke DB, Pagani F, Powell SR, Day SM. Ubiquitin proteasome dysfunction in human hypertrophic and dilated cardiomyopathies. Circulation. 2010;121:997–1004.
26. Depre C, Wang Q, Yan L, Hedhli N, Peter P, Chen L, Hong C, Hittinger L, Ghaleh B, Sadoshima J, Vatner DE, Vatner SF, Madura K. Activation of the cardiac proteasome during pressure overload promotes ventricular hypertrophy. Circulation. 2006;114:1821–8.

17

Feasibility of basic transesophageal echocardiography in hemorrhagic shock: potential applications during resuscitative endovascular balloon occlusion of the aorta (REBOA)

William A. Teeter[1], Bianca M. Conti[2], Phil J. Wasicek[3], Jonathan J. Morrison[4], Dawn Parsell[3], Bryan Gamble[5], Melanie R. Hoehn[6], Thomas M. Scalea[7] and Samuel M. Galvagno Jr[8*]

Abstract

Background: There are numerous studies in the cardiovascular literature that have employed transesophageal echocardiography (TEE) in swine models, but data regarding the use of basic TEE in swine models is limited. The primary aim of this study is to describe an echocardiographic method that can be used with relative ease to qualitatively assess cardiovascular function in a porcine hemorrhagic shock model using resuscitative endovascular balloon occlusion of the aorta (REBOA).

Methods: Multiplane basic TEE exams were performed in 15 during an experimental hemorrhage model using REBOA. Cardiac anatomical structure and functional measurements were obtained. In a convenience sample (two animals from each group), advanced functional cardiovascular measurements were obtained before and after REBOA inflation for comparison with qualitative assessments.

Results: Basic TEE exams were performed in 15 swine. Appropriate REBOA placement was confirmed using TEE in all animals and verified with fluoroscopy. Left ventricular volume was decreased in all animals, and left ventricular systolic function increased following REBOA inflation. Right ventricular systolic function and volume remained normal prior to and after hemorrhage and REBOA use. Mean ejection fraction (EF) decreased from 64% (S.D. 9.6) to 62.1 (S.D. 16.8) after hemorrhage and REBOA inflation ($p = 0.76$); fractional area of change (FAC) decreased from 49.8 (S.D. 9.0) to 48.5 (S.D. 13.6) after hemorrhage and REBOA inflation ($p = 0.82$).

Conclusion: Basic TEE, which requires less training than advanced TEE, may be employed by laboratory investigators and practitioners across a wide spectrum of experimental and clinical settings.

Background

The porcine model is commonly used in cardiovascular research related to experimental models of hemorrhagic shock [1, 2]. Swine are mammalian vertebrates with a cardiovascular system that is very similar to humans, and for this reason, have served as the dominant animal model for previous study designs published in the literature [3, 4].

For instance, with regard to vascular size, an 80–100 kg swine has an aortic diameter of 1.6–1.8 cm versus an aortic diameter of 1.6–2.4 cm in a similarly-sized human [1, 5]. However, several potentially significant differences exist. For example, porcine hearts are shaped more like a "valentine," have different orientations for insertion of the superior and inferior vena cava, and have dissimilar atrial components [5]. Table 1 summarizes some anatomical differences between swine and humans.

Transesophageal echocardiography (TEE) is an invasive diagnostic modality that carries minimal risk but requires

* Correspondence: sgalvagno@som.umaryland.edu
[8]Department of Anesthesiology, Divisions of Critical Care Medicine and Trauma Anesthesiology, University of Maryland School of Medicine, Baltimore, MD, USA
Full list of author information is available at the end of the article

Table 1 Major anatomical differences between porcine and human hearts

Features	Porcine Heart	Human Heart
Shape and Orientation	"Valentine shaped heart" which is oriented in line with the unguligrade stance of the pig	"Trapezoidal" shaped heart oriented in line with the orthograde posture of the human being
Presence of tubular appendage	Observed in the right atrium	Observed in the left atrium
Vena cava orientation	The superior and inferior vena cava opens into the right atrium at right angles to each other	The superior and inferior vena cava open into the right atrium in a straight line at 180 degrees
Pulmonary veins	Left atrium receives 2 pulmonary veins	Left atrium receives 4 pulmonary veins
Muscular moderator in right ventricle	Prominent and situated more superior in the right ventricle	Less prominent and situated more inferior in the right ventricle
Characteristic of Apical components	Contains coarse and broad trabeculations	Trabeculations are absent and apex is narrower
Aortic-Mitral fibrous continuity	Reduced as 2/3RD of aortic valve is supported by left ventricular musculature	Not reduced
Coronary Dominance	Left anterior descending coronary artery dominant	Right coronary dominant
Difference in right and left atrio-ventricular branches	Right atrio-ventricular branches are less developed than left-sided equivalents	No major differences exist between the right and left atrio-ventricular branches

extensive knowledge about anatomy, physiology, and physics for appropriate application [6]. There are numerous studies in the cardiovascular literature that have employed TEE in swine models, but nearly all of these studies have dealt with cardiovascular physiology related to cardiac surgery [7], valvular abnormalities [8], myocardial infarction [9, 10], or cardiopulmonary resuscitation [11]. Data regarding the use of TEE in swine models is limited; one of the few papers describing the technique was published over 20 years ago [2], and baseline anatomical and hemodynamic parameters for TEE use in swine models have only recently been defined [1]. Both three-dimensional [8] and transthoracic ultrasound [12] in swine models have been described, but use of basic TEE in a swine model of hemorrhagic shock has not. Herein, we describe our experience using basic multiplane TEE to characterize hemodynamic changes in a large closed chest experimental swine model of non-compressible hemorrhage using resuscitative endovascular occlusion of the aorta (REBOA). The primary aim of this study is to describe an echocardiographic method that can be used with relative ease to qualitatively assess cardiovascular function in a porcine hemorrhagic shock model.

Methods
Animal model
The overall objective of this in vivo study was to characterize changes in arterial waveforms that occur during hemorrhage and uses Yorkshire swine (*Sus scrofa*) weighing between 70 and 90 kg. Once animals were induced into hemorrhagic shock, animals were subsequently enrolled into various substudies which are reported separately. This study was study was undertaken at a certified laboratory, following Institutional Animal Care and Use Committee (IACUC)

approval. The study consisted of two phases: animal preparation and volume controlled hemorrhage.

General anesthesia was induced using intramuscular ketamine (10-15 mg/kg) and xylazine (1–2.2 mg/kg) followed by intravenous propofol and ketamine and maintained with isoflurane (minimum alveolar concentration [MAC] range 1–4%) by mask followed by tracheostomy intubation. Animals were ventilated using a volume-controlled mode of 6 cc/kg with an FiO2 of 40–100% to maintain SpO2 > 92%. The jugular veins were cannulated bilaterally to permit intravenous access and placement of a Swan-Ganz catheter. An open cystostomy was performed for urine drainage.

Hemorrhagic shock was induced by removing 40% of the animal's blood volume over the course of 20 min from a femoral venous catheter. The first 20% of blood volume was removed over 7 min, and the remaining 20% of blood volume was removed over 13 min.

In order to prevent hemorrhage induced cardiac arrest, animals were given fluid boluses with 500 mL of lactated ringers, if in the judgement of the anesthetist, the animal was deteriorating to the verge of cardiac arrest. The animals were euthanized at the end of the protocol. The study design is summarized in Fig. 1.

Resuscitative endovascular balloon occlusion of the aorta (REBOA)
Resuscitative Endovascular Balloon Occlusion of the Aorta (REBOA) is a hemorrhage control technique which allows for the attenuation of hemorrhage by temporarily occluding the aorta in order to support blood pressure until definitive hemostasis can be achieved [13, 14]. There has been considerable interest in performing REBOA closer to the point of injury and for prolonged durations

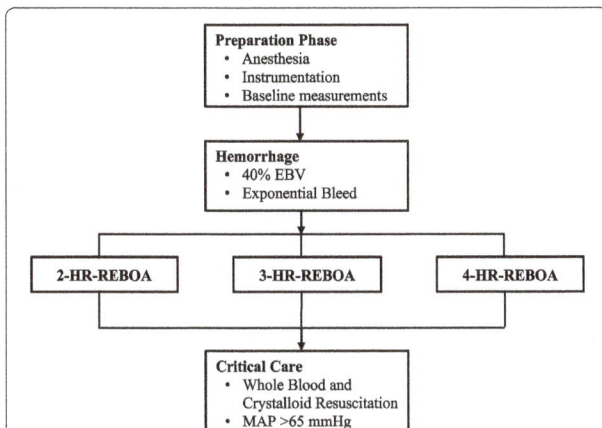

Fig. 1 Summary of the three experimental hemorrhage REBOA models. EBV-estimated blood volume. MAP-mean arterial pressure. REBOA-resuscitative endovascular balloon occlusion of the aorta. The time interval indicates the amount of time the REBOA balloon was inflated in zone I of the animal

in order to lessen the effects of extended transport time prolonged field care [15, 16]. The physiologic effects of REBOA inflation for extended periods of time on the myocardium remains unknown. In this study, Zone 1 aortic occlusion was performed at the end of the hemorrhage protocol, with inflation of the balloon in the thoracic aorta (Fig. 2).

Aortic occlusion was confirmed using fluoroscopy.

Multiplane TEE

Both baseline and post-hemorrhage multiplane TEE was performed under general anesthesia using a General Electrics LOGIQ e® ultrasound machine with a 6Tc-RS TEE probe (General Electrics Healthcare, Chicago, IL). TEE exams were performed by anesthesiologists certified by the National Board of Echocardiography; one investigator was certified at the basic TEE level (SG) and another at the advanced level (BC). For multiplane TEE, four maneuvers were used: [1] mechanical rotation of the variable plane phased array between 0° and 180°; [2] rotation of the shaft of the scope leftward and rightward; [3] advancement and withdrawal of the scope; and [4] tip anteflexion, retroflexion, and leftward and rightward flexion [2]. A basic TEE exam was performed using the 11 most relevant views recommended by the Consensus guidelines for basic perioperative TEE of the American Society of Echocardiography (ASE) and the Society of Cardiovascular Anesthesiologists (SCA) [6]. Specifically, the scope of practice for a basic TEE exam involves a limited application focused on intraoperative monitoring rather than specific diagnosis; a comprehensive exam, involving quantitative measurements is not within the scope of the basic perioperative TEE exam [6].

Insertion of TEE probe

The TEE probe was inserted as previously described by Ren et al. [2] A disposable transducer sheath (100 cm long) was placed over the TEE probe with gel filling the inside and covering the tip of the probe. The distal portion of the probe was lubricated with gel and the probe was introduced while an assistant provided manual tongue elevation and retraction. With the swine in a supine position, the TEE scope was inserted blindly with the transducer array at 0° rotation by directing the tip into the posterior part of the pharynx, gently allowing the

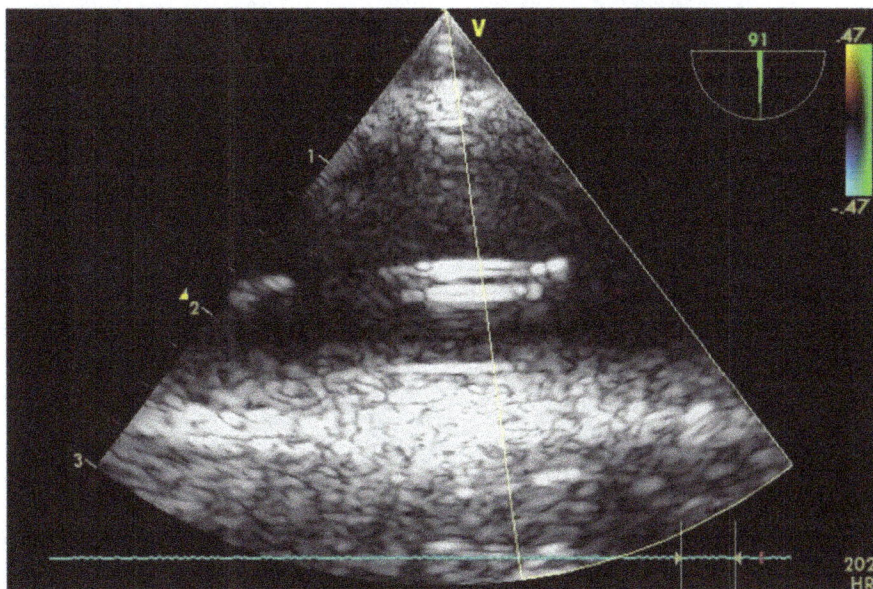

Fig. 2 Midesophageal descending aortic long axis view. The hyperechoic structure located in the middle of the plane is the REBOA catheter

probe to flex passively, and advanced until images were obtained (approximately 45–60 cm from the incisors).

Cardiac anatomical structure and function measurements
TEE images were recorded prior to experimental induction of bleeding and during occlusion with REBOA. The "iHeartScan™" Form was used to record qualitative and quantitative data (University of Melbourne, AUS). The iHeartScan™ is a limited echocardiography study that is qualitative and quantitative [17]. It is intended to be completed in approximately 10 min or 15 min for extended measurement. Components of the exam include qualitative assessments of ventricular volume in M-mode or 2D, systolic function (including both the right and left ventricle), left atrial filling pressure (assessed by observing interatrial sepal motion), valve assessment, presence of pericardial effusion, and estimation of overall hemodynamic state (i.e., vasodilated, primary systolic or diastolic failure, right ventricular failure) [17]. Extended aspects of the iHeartScan™ include calculation of ejection fraction, cardiac output, diastolic function (E/E', E/A ratios, etc.), and valve measurements. Advanced hemodynamic calculations were made for selected animals. Measurements of chambers and great vessel diameters were obtained as recommended by the ASE/SCA Consensus guidelines [6]. Ejection fraction (EF) was calculated when using the Teichholz method [18, 19]. Stroke volume was calculated by multiplying the left ventricular outflow tract (LVOT) diameter x LVOT velocity time integral (VTI) [π (LVOT diameter/2)^2 x LVOT VTI]; cardiac output was calculated by multiplying stroke volume x heart rate.

Statistical analysis
Descriptive statistics were employed as appropriate according to the parametric or nonparametric nature of the data. Continuous data are described with a mean ± standard deviation. A P value of < 0.05 was considered statistically significant. Data were analyzed using the R package (version 3.1.1) for statistical computing (R Foundation for Statistical Computing, Vienna, Austria).

Results
Basic TEE exams were performed in all 15 swine. The mean animal weight was 79.6 ± 5.5 kg. Heart rate significantly increased after REBOA inflation (76.8 [S.D. 21.3] vs. 151 [S.D. 47.1]; $p < 0.001$) with a corresponding significant increase in shock index, but mean arterial blood pressure did not change significantly. Qualitative basic TEE findings are summarized in Table 2.

With the exception of mean pulmonary artery systolic pressure in the 2-h experimental groups, no significant changes were observed in pulmonary artery pressures despite echocardiographic findings indicating hypovolemic shock. Similarly, there were no statistically significant differences in mean arterial blood pressure in any of the three study arms prior to and after REBOA inflation, despite experimental blood loss of 40%. In all animals, basic TEE qualitatively revealed increased LV function and hypovolemia as evidenced hyperdynamic physiology.

In a convenience sample (two animals from each group), advanced functional cardiovascular measurements were obtained before and after REBOA inflation for comparison with qualitative assessments. Mean ejection fraction (EF) decreased from 64% (S.D. 9.6) to 62.1 (S.D. 16.8) after hemorrhage and REBOA inflation ($p = 0.76$); fractional area of change (FAC) decreased from 49.8 (S.D. 9.0) to 48.5 (S.D. 13.6) after hemorrhage and REBOA inflation ($p = 0.82$). VTI and LVOT measurements were obtained in animals; mean cardiac output was 3.7 L/min prior to hemorrhage and REBOA inflation, and 7.6 L/min thereafter.

Midesophageal aortic long and short axis views were obtained to confirm correct REBOA catheter position (Figs. 2, 3, and 4). Catheter position was verified in all animals with basic TEE and confirmed with the use of fluoroscopy.

Discussion
In a porcine closed chest experimental swine model of non-compressible hemorrhage using REBOA, use of basic multiplane TEE detected hemodynamic changes that could

Table 2 Summary of basic TEE findings and overall hemodynamic state during three experimental models (n = 5 animals in each phase)

Model	Timing	Shock Index	Pulmonary Artery Pressure	Mean Arterial Pressure	LV ventricular volume	RV ventricular volume	LV systolic function	RV systolic function	Hemodynamic state
2 h	Pre-bleed	0.63	37/27	93.5 (13.6)	Normal	Normal	Normal	Normal	Normal
	REBOA inflation	1.24*	47*/26	111.7 (29.1)	Hypovolemic	Normal	Increased	Normal	Empty
3 h	Pre-bleed	0.58	35/26	115.3 (13.2)	Normal	Normal	Normal	Normal	Normal
	REBOA inflation	0.96*	38/29	114.3 (14.8)	Hypovolemic	Normal	Increased	Normal	Empty; mild diastolic failure
4 h	Pre-bleed	0.56	33/24	116.6 (31.2)	Normal	Normal	Normal	Normal	Normal
	REBOA inflation	0.91*	38/27	100.3 (20.6)	Hypovolemic	Normal	Increased	Normal	Empty; mild diastolic failure

Basic TEE exams were performed pre-bleed and post-bleed during REBOA inflation. Findings are summarized qualitatively for all animals; hemodynamic findings are described with means and standard deviation. Shock index = heart rate / systolic blood pressure. *P < 0.01

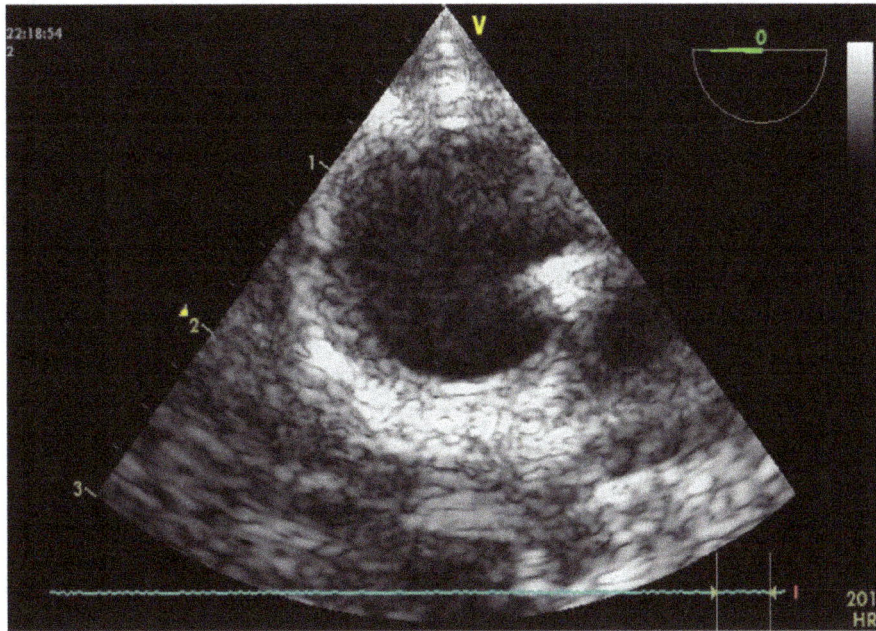

Fig. 3 Midesophageal descending aortic short axis view. The hyperechoic structure located in the right lower quadrant of the aorta is the REBOA catheter

not be verified with the use of mean arterial pressure and pulmonary artery catheter data. With the increasing use of REBOA in both experimental settings and clinical settings, methods to rapidly and accurately assess hemodynamics are required. The use of basic TEE is of interest to laboratory investigators and clinicians for several reasons. First, the goal of basic TEE is intraoperative monitoring; while TEE is invasive, at the basic level, TEE can be used by a wide variety of scientists and clinicians to observe hemodynamic changes associated with aortic occlusion and hemorrhage. Second, basic TEE may reveal earlier evidence of hypovolemia despite relatively normal

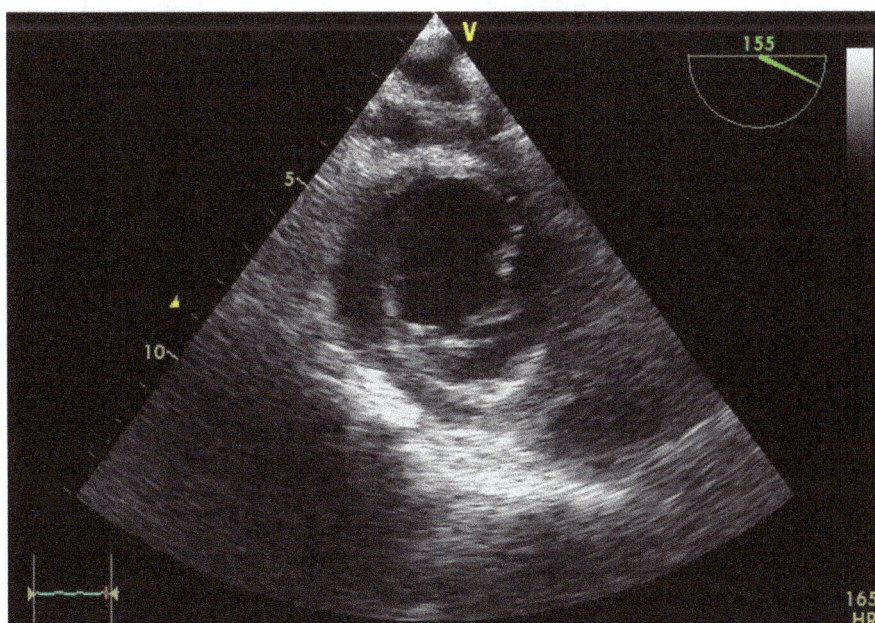

Fig. 4 A representative transgastric short axis transesophageal view. Such a view is useful for assessing early regional wall abnormalities indicative of myocardial dysfunction and overall volume status

vital signs. Third, basic TEE may be helpful for localizing and confirming REBOA position. The primary goal of the basic TEE exam is intraoperative monitoring. The exam is not designed for practitioners to use the full diagnostic potential of TEE; hence, training requirements are considerably less than required for the advanced TEE exam [6]. Performance of basic TEE may be feasible in a wide variety of settings, including the laboratory, intensive care unit, and austere medical environments. Currently, "certification" is only available for licensed physicians who have passed an exam and demonstrated supervised performance of exams, but such requirements do not preclude performance of basic TEE exams in the laboratory by properly supervised investigators.

Limited application of TEE is potentially useful in both experimental and clinical settings where REBOA is employed for hemorrhage control because cardiac dysfunction is common in critical illness, but the effects on porcine and human hearts during REBOA are uncertain [20]. Basic TEE was feasible for all animals in our study. Clear evidence of hypovolemia was observed in all animals despite normal systemic and pulmonary blood pressure measurements. In animals with prolonged balloon inflation, evidence of early diastolic dysfunction was also observed, although in the subset of animals where EF and FAC were measured, no statistically significant differences were observed. These findings indicated a hyperdynamic cardiovascular state consistent with compensated shock. Such findings would be of great importance for both laboratory investigators and clinicians because further decreases in heart function would likely signify the upper limit of REBOA insertion before instituting definitive blood component resuscitation and surgical correction of hemorrhage.

An additional advantage of using basic TEE is for confirmation of proper REBOA location when fluoroscopic methods are not available. In previous studies, the subxiphoid view from a Focused Abdominal Sonogram for Trauma (FAST) was shown to reliably identify a central aortic guidewire, but in situations where the abdomen or chest is opened, such an exam may not be practicable [21]. In austere or limited resource settings when REBOA may be required as a temporizing measure for severe hemorrhage, fluoroscopy will likely be unavailable whereas a modern, compact TEE machine might be. In our study, a portable ultrasound machine weighing 11.5 lbs. (5.2 kg) was used. Moreover, use of TEE for both hemodynamic assessment and proper REBOA positioning obviates any exposure to radiation. In situations where REBOA has been employed for life-threatening hemorrhage, TEE has been used to confirm guidewire placement in the descending aorta [22]. Malpositioned REBOA, including inappropriate advancement into the ascending aorta, has potentially catastrophic consequences, including arrhythmia,

carotid dissection, and coronary vasospasm [21]. Use of basic TEE is feasible with the advent of smaller, portable machines and probes, thus limiting radiation exposure and reducing the "footprint" associated with fluoroscopy.

There are several limitations to this work. Although the basic TEE exam requires less training and is easier to perform, advanced measurements, including functional measurement of stroke volume, cardiac output, stroke volume variation, and regional myocardial wall motion would likely be helpful to measure in future studies. Advanced calculations were obtained randomly in each experimental group for this study, but regular measurement of these parameters requires a more thorough exam performed by a practitioner with advanced TEE training. Basic TEE measurements were obtained prior to experimental hemorrhage and after REBOA inflation post-hemorrhage. Additional TEE exams conducted at regular intervals might have been more likely to reveal hemodynamic changes.

Conclusions
Basic TEE is feasible in porcine hemorrhagic shock models involving REBOA. This method can be performed with relative ease and may assist with early detection of hypovolemia and confirmation of precise proximal REBOA deployment. Basic TEE requires less training than advanced TEE and may be employed by laboratory investigators and practitioners across a wide spectrum of experimental and clinical settings.

Abbreviations
ASE: American Society of Echocardiography; AUS: Australia; EF: Ejection fraction; FAC: Fractional area of change; FAST: Focused abdominal sonogram for trauma; IACUC: Institutional animal care and use committee; LVOT: Left ventricular outflow tract; MAC: minimal alveolar concentration; REBOA: Resuscitative endovascular balloon occlusion of the aorta; S.D.: Standard deviation; SCA: Society of Cardiovascular Anesthesiologists; TEE: Transesophageal echocardiography; VTI: Velocity time integral

Funding
This study was supported by a grant (W81XWH-16-1-0116) from the Defense Medical Research and Development Program- Broad Agency, US Army Medical Research (Primary Investigator: Thomas Scalea, MD).

Authors' contributions
WAT, TMS, SMG, DP, MRH, and BG conceived and designed the study. WAT, PJW, JJM, BC, and SMG collected the data and performed the analysis. WAT, BC, and SMG drafted the manuscript. All authors critically reviewed the manuscript and data analysis. All authors read and approved the final manuscript.

Consent for publication
Data for this study was approved by release by the US Army Medical Research Directorate.

Competing interests

The authors declare that they have no competing interests.

Author details

[1]University of North Carolina, Raleigh, North Carolina, USA. [2]Department of Anesthesiology, Division of Trauma Anesthesiology, University of Maryland School of Medicine, Baltimore, MD, USA. [3]Department of Surgery, University of Maryland School of Medicine, Baltimore, MD, USA. [4]Department of Surgery, Program in Trauma, University of Maryland School of Medicine, Baltimore, MD, USA. [5]Department of Surgery, Walter Reed National Medical Center, United States Army, Bethesda, MD, USA. [6]Department of Surgery, Emory University, Atlanta, GA, USA. [7]University of Maryland, Program in Trauma, Baltimore, MD, USA. [8]Department of Anesthesiology, Divisions of Critical Care Medicine and Trauma Anesthesiology, University of Maryland School of Medicine, Baltimore, MD, USA.

References

1. Huenges K, Pokorny S, Berndt RCJ, Lutter G. Transesophageal echocardiography in swine: establishment of a baseline. Ultrasound Med Biol. 2017;43:974–80.
2. Ren JFSD, Lighty GW Jr, Menz VV, Michele JJ, Li KS, Dillon SM, Marchlinski FESB. Multiplane transesophageal and intracardiac echocardiography in large swine: imaging technique, normal values, and research applications. Echocardiography. 1997;14:135–48.
3. Morrison JJRJ, Rt H, Watson JD, Sokol KK, Rasmussen TE. Use of resuscitative endovascular balloon occlusion of the aorta in a highly lethal model of noncompressible torso hemorrhage. Shock. 2014;41:130–7.
4. Scott DJEJ, Villamaria C, Morrison JJ, Houston R 4th, Spencer JR, TE R. A novel fluoroscopy-free, resuscitative endovascular aortic balloon occlusion system in a model of hemorrhagic shock. J Trauma Acute Care Surg. 2013; 75:122–8.
5. Crick SJ, Sheppard MN, Ho SY, Gebstein L, Anderson RH. Anatomy of the pig heart: comparisons with normal human cardiac structure. J Anat. 1998; 193:105–19.
6. Reeves ST, Finley AC, Skubas NJ, et al. Basic perioperative transesophageal echocardiography examination: a consensus statement of the American Society of Echocardiography and the Society of Cardiovascular Anesthesiologists. J Am Soc Echocardiogr. 2013;26(5):443–56.
7. Bartel TMS, Caspari G, Erbel R. Intracardiac and intraluminal echocardiography: indications and standard approaches. Ultrasound Med Biol. 2002;28:997–1003.
8. Sündermann SHCN, Falk V, Bettex D. Two- and three-dimensional transoesophageal echocardiography in large swine used as model for transcatheter heart valve therapies: standard planes and values. Interact Cardiovasc Thorac Surg. 2016;22:580–6.
9. Ellenbroek GH vHG, Timmers L, Doevendans PA, Pasterkamp G, Hoefer IE. Primary outcome assessment in a pig model of acute myocardial infarction. J Vis Exp. 2016;(116):1–9.
10. Meybohm PGM, Renner J, Maracke M, Rossee S, Höcker J, Hagelstein SZK, Bein B. Assessment of left ventricular systolic function during acute myocardial ischemia: a comparison of transpulmonary thermodilution and transesophageal echocardiography. Minerva Anestesiol. 2011;77:132–41.
11. Anderson KLCM, Boudreau SM, Sharon DJ, Bebarta VS. Left ventricular compressions improve hemodynamics in a swine model of out-of-hospital cardiac arrest. Prehosp Emerg Care. 2017;21:272–80.
12. Kerut EKVC, Luka T, Pinkernell K, Delafontaine P, Alt EU. Technique and imaging for transthoracic echocardiography of the laboratory pig. Echocardiography. 2004;21:439–42.
13. Sridhar S, Gumbert SD, Stephens C, Moore LJ, Pivalizza EG. Resuscitative endovascular balloon occlusion of the aorta: principles, initial clinical experience, and considerations for the anesthesiologist. Anesth Analg. 2017; 125:884–90.
14. Russo RM, Williams TK, Grayson JK, et al. Extending the golden hour: partial resuscitative endovascular balloon occlusion of the aorta in a highly lethal swine liver injury model. J Trauma Acute Care Surg. 2016;80:372–8. discussion 8–80
15. Sadek S, Lockey DJ, Lendrum RA, Perkins Z, Price J, Davies GE. Resuscitative endovascular balloon occlusion of the aorta (REBOA) in the pre-hospital setting: an additional resuscitation option for uncontrolled catastrophic haemorrhage. Resuscitation. 2016;107:135–8.
16. Manley JD, Mitchell BJ, DuBose JJ, Rasmussen TEA. Modern Case Series of Resuscitative Endovascular Balloon Occlusion of the Aorta (REBOA) in an Out-of-Hospital, Combat casualty care setting. J Spec Oper Med. 2017;17:1–8.
17. iHeartScan. 2017. Retrieved on 26 June 2018 at www.iHeartScan.com.
18. Teichholz LE, Kruelen T, Herman MV, Gorlin R. Problems in echocardiographic volume determinations: echocardiographic-angiographic correlations in teh presence of absence of asynergy. Am J Cardiol. 1976;37:7–11.
19. Arora G, Morss AM, Piazza G, et al. Differences in left ventricular ejection fraction using teichholz formula and volumetric methods by cmr: implications for patient stratification and selection of therapy. J Carrdiovasc Magn Reson. 2010;12:P202.
20. Orde S, Slama M, Hilton A, Yastrebov K, McLean A. Pearls and pitfalls in comprehensive critical care echocardiography. Crit Care. 2017;21:1–10.
21. Guliani S, Amendola M, Strife B, et al. Central aortic wire confirmation for emergent endovascular procedurs: as fast as surgeon-performed ultrasound. J Trauma Acute Care Surg. 2015;79:549–54.
22. Lai CH, Wu HY. Resuscitation for an octogenarian with ruptured abdominal aortic aneurysm using endovascular balloon. Am J Emerg Med. 2008;26: 967e1–3.

18

Usefulness of carotid ultrasonography in the diagnosis of coronary artery disease in patients undergoing exercise echocardiography

Raúl Franco-Gutiérrez[1]* ⓘ, Alberto José Pérez-Pérez[1], Virginia Franco-Gutiérrez[2], Ana María Testa-Fernández[1], Rafael Carlos Vidal-Pérez[1], Manuel Lorenzo López-Reboiro[3], Víctor Manuel Puebla-Rojo[1], Melisa Santás-Álvarez[1], María Generosa Crespo-Leiro[4,5,6] and Carlos González-Juanatey[1]

Abstract

Background: Relationship between carotid and coronary artery disease (CAD) in patients undergoing invasive and non-invasive test is unclear. The aim of the study is to evaluate whether carotid disease is associated with CAD in patients submitted to exercise echocardiography (EE) and if it improves the EE ability to predict CAD.

Methods: We retrospectively studied 156 subjects without previous vascular disease who underwent EE, carotid ultrasonography and coronary angiography between 2002 and 2013. Positive EE was defined as exercise induced wall motion abnormalities, carotid disease according to Manheim and American Society of Echocardiography Consensus and significant CAD as stenosis ≥50%.

Results: Eighty-nine (57.1%) subjects had significant CAD. Factors associated with CAD in multivariate analysis were fasting plasma glucose (odds ratio [OR] 1.02, $p = 0.031$), pre-test probability of CAD > 65% (OR 3.71, $p < 0.001$), positive EE (OR 10.51, $p < 0.001$) and carotid plaque (CP) presence (OR 2.95, $p = 0.013$). There was neither statistical significant difference in area under the curve after addition of CP to EE results (0.77 versus 0.81, $p = 0.525$) nor sensitivity, specificity, predictive values or efficiency. CP presence reclassified as very high-risk according to Systematic COronary Risk Evaluation 13 patients (34.2%) with negative EE and 22 (33.3%) without CAD.

Conclusion: CP is associated with CAD in patients undergoing EE, however its addition to EE does not improve CAD prediction, probably due to insufficient statistical power. CP reclassified one third of patients to very high-risk category despite negative EE or CAD absence, these subjects benefit from aggressive primary prevention interventions.

Keywords: Stress echocardiography, Exercise test, Carotid artery disease, Coronary artery disease, Area under curve

Background

Ischaemic heart disease is a major problem due to its prevalence, health cost and mortality [1–3]. Stress echocardiography is a well-validated tool for diagnosis and risk stratification in patients with new onset chest pain, but it has some limitations that can impair its diagnostic capacity such as the dependence of pre-test probabilities

(PTP) of coronary artery disease (CAD), the need to achieve submaximal heart rate, the presence of suboptimal echocardiographic windows, the inability to detect non limiting flow coronary stenosis or pathologies that can produce wall motion abnormalities during exercise [2–4].

Carotid disease, defined as increased carotid intima-media thickness (CIMT) or the presence of atherosclerotic plaques (CP), has been associated with myocardial infarction, stroke and death [5–7]. Post-mortem studies have also demonstrated a correlation between carotid and CAD [8]. These findings encouraged

* Correspondence: raul.franco.gutierrez@sergas.es;
raulfrancogutierrez@yahoo.es
[1]Department of Cardiology, Hospital Universitario Lucus Augusti (HULA), Avenida doctor Ulises Romero n° 1, 27003 Lugo, Spain
Full list of author information is available at the end of the article

investigators to evaluate the possibility of using carotid disease in the diagnosis of CAD of patients undergoing invasive and non-invasive tests, however the studies published so far have shown inconsistent results [9–19]. In that sense a meta-analysis of 34 studies focused on the relation of CIMT with coronary atherosclerosis, 30 showed a positive but modest relationship with correlation positive coefficients between 0.12 and 0.51 with only one study being above 0.5 and some studies showed no relationship at all [19].

Our group has broad experience in the ultrasonographic assessment of carotid arteries, having demonstrated its usefulness as a marker of subclinical atherosclerosis in subjects with autoimmune diseases [20]. The studies mentioned before [5–8], along with our findings, led to the systematic use of carotid ultrasound in subjects with suspected CAD undergoing exercise echocardiography (EE) at our cardiovascular imaging laboratory since 2002. This approach has been endorsed by the European Society of Cardiology (ESC) stable CAD guidelines as a IIa level C recommendation [2].

A clinical study was designed to evaluate if carotid disease is associated with significant CAD in patients with suspected ischaemic heart disease undergoing treadmill exercise stress echocardiography at our institution and if it improves the EE ability to predict significant CAD.

Methods
Study population
Between Jan. 1st 2002 and Dec. 31st 2013 4024 consecutive Caucasian subjects older than 18 years with suspected CAD underwent EE and carotid ultrasonography at our institution. Of them, 390 patients (9.7%) were also submitted to a coronary angiography. 234 patients (60%) were excluded: 29 (7.4%) due to prior stroke, transient ischaemic attack or peripheral artery disease and 205 due to prior CAD (52.6%) defined as previous myocardial infarction [21], coronary revascularization or angiographic documentation of any coronary stenosis ≥50%. All patients signed informed consent before testing. The study was approved by the Regional Ethics Committee.

Demographic, clinical, baseline echocardiography, carotid ultrasonography and stress testing data were collected. PTP of CAD and Systematic COronary Risk Evaluation (SCORE) were assessed according to current ESC guidelines [1, 2].

Treadmill exercise stress echocardiography
Treadmill exercise was the stress modality chosen using a Philips Sonos 5500 ultrasound machine between 2002 and 2005 and a Philips iE33 after 2005 (Philips Medical Systems).

Heart rate, blood pressure and 12-lead electrocardiogram were obtained at baseline and at each exercise stage. EE was finished in case of physical exhaustion, disabling chest pain, significant arrhythmia and severe hypertensive or hypotensive response. Apical long-axis, apical 4- and 2-chamber and parasternal long- and short-axis views were obtained at rest, peak and immediately after exercise. Echocardiographic analysis was performed using a 17-segment model of the left ventricle to evaluate regional wall motion. Each segment was graded on a 4-point scale depending on its motion. Wall motion score index was calculated as the sum of the scores divided by the number of segments at rest and at peak exercise.

Ischaemic electrocardiographic abnormalities were defined as development of ST-segment deviation 80 msec after J point ≥1 mm. Echocardiographic ischaemia was defined as exercise induced new or worsening wall motion abnormalities, except worsening from akinesia to dyskinesia and isolated hypokinesia of the inferobasal segment. Extensive ischemia was defined as ischaemia involving ≥3 myocardial segments and multivessel ischemia as ischemia involving ≥2 different coronary territories [4].

Carotid ultrasonography
Carotid scans were performed immediately after stress testing in the same EE ultrasound equipment using a high-resolution, B-mode ultrasound system with a linear array (3–11 MHz) transducer. Measurement of the CIMT and CP definition were done following the ARIC protocol study [5] and expert consensus [22–25]. Semi-automated edge detection software was used (QLAB; Philips 110 Medical Systems, Andover, MA, USA).

Age- and sex-specific CIMT percentile values were obtained from previously published data in our country [26].

Both EE and carotid ultrasonography stored images were analysed by two imaging expert cardiologists blinded to angiography results. In case of disagreement a third expert was consulted.

Coronary angiography
The physician in charge of the patient carried out a coronary angiography considering the results of the EE and other conditions such as persistence of symptoms despite optimal medical treatment, patients' preferences and/or other clinical criteria. Coronary angiography was performed using standard technique. Significant angiographic disease was defined as stenosis ≥50% by visual assessment in any major epicardial arteries or in their branches.

Coronary angiography analysis was similar to ultrasonography.

Statistical analysis

Categorical variables were reported as percentages and comparison between groups were based on chi-square or Fisher's exact tests. Continuous variables were reported as mean (standard deviation) or median [interquartile range] when their distribution departed from normal and differences were assessed via the unpaired t test or the Mann-Whitney U test where appropriate. Binary and continuous quantitative variables were compared using logistic binary regression. To create predictive models for the presence of significant CAD, backward stepwise binary logistic regression was used with an entry set at 0.2 significance level and a retention set of 0.1. A p value of < 0.05 was considered statistically significant. ! DT V2009.06.26® macro for SPSS Statistics (Autonomous University of Barcelona) and IBM SPSS Statistics for Windows, Version 20.0. (Armonk, NY) was used to calculate sensitivity, specificity, positive (PPV) and negative predictive values (NPV), positive (PLR) and negative likelihood ratios (NLR) and efficiency of EE alone and combined with carotid ultrasonography. Area under the curve (AUC) was calculated by means of a receiver operating characteristic curve analysis; comparison between AUC was done by the DeLong method.

Results

One hundred fifty six patients were enrolled in the study. Mean age was 66.1 ± 10.4 years and 102 (65.4%) were men. There were no major complications during or after the tests.

Baseline characteristics are summarized in Table 1.

Prediction of CAD

Mean time between non-invasive tests and coronary angiography was 4.2 (3.2) months. Of the 156 patients 89 (57.1%) had significant CAD. This subgroup was older ($p = 0.045$), with male predominance ($p = 0.011$), had more frequently diabetes mellitus (DM), smoking habit ($p = 0.023$) and higher levels of fasting plasma glucose (FPG) ($p = 0.003$). Higher SCORE, PTP of CAD as well as positive EE and CP presence (all of them $p < 0.001$) were also significantly more frequent in patients with CAD.

In multivariate analysis FPG ($p = 0.031$), PTP > 65% ($p < 0.001$), positive EE ($p < 0.001$) and CP ($p = 0.013$) were predictors of significant CAD.

Comparisons of subgroups with and without significant CAD and multivariate analysis are represented in Tables 2 and 3 respectively.

Regarding the subgroup of 21 (13.6%) subjects with resting wall motion abnormalities 4 (19%) had global left ventricular hypokinesia. Of the 21 patients 17 (81.0%) developed worsening wall motion abnormalities during EE and all of them showed significant CAD in the angiography, 2 (9.5%) were defined as negative EE and did

not have significant CAD and 2 (9.5%) could not achieve submaximal predicted heart rate, both without significant CAD in the angiography.

AUC, sensitivity, specificity, predictive values, PLR and NLR and efficiency

AUC of EE alone was 0.77 (95% confidence interval [CI] 0.68–0.86), whereas AUC combining CP findings was 0.81 (95%CI 0.70–0.92) ($p = 0.525$). Results are summarized in Fig. 1 and Table 4.

Sensitivity, specificity, predictive values, PLR and NLR and efficiency of EE alone and EE combined with CP are also summarized in Table 4. Table 5 shows predictive values according to established intermediate PTP.

SCORE reclassification according to carotid ultrasound

According to European guidelines on cardiovascular disease prevention [1] 10 subjects (6.4%) had low-risk at the time of EE, 52 (33.3%) had moderate-risk, 47 (30.1%) had high-risk, 45 (28.8%) had very high-risk and 2 patients (1.3%) could not be classified. When carotid ultrasonography findings were applied 59 patients (37.8%) were reclassified as very high-risk according to CP presence. Focusing in the 62 patients with low or moderate SCORE risk, 28 (45.2%) had CP.

Of the 38 patients with negative EE 5 subjects (13.2%), 16 (42.1%), 10 (26.3%) and 7 (18.4%) had low, moderate, high and very high-risk respectively. Considering CP presence 13 patients (34.2%) were reclassified as very high-risk. Regarding the 21 patients with low or moderate SCORE risk and negative EE, 7 (33.3%) had CP being thereby considered as very high-risk.

Finally, of the 67 patients without CAD, 9 subjects (13.4%) had low-risk, 28 (41.8%) had moderate-risk, 19 (28.4%) had high-risk, 10 (14.9%) had very high-risk and 1 (1.5%) could not be classified. Considering CP results, 22 patients (33.3%) were classified as very high-risk despite normal angiography. Of the 37 patients without significant CAD initially classified as low or moderate SCORE risk 12 (32.4%) presented CP.

Discussion

This study correlates carotid disease with CAD in a real life cohort of patients without prior vascular disease undergoing EE. However, its addition to stress test does not improve CAD prediction by angiography. It is necessary to highlight the fact that nearly one third of patients with negative EE and without CAD are reclassified to high-risk group according to carotid ultrasonography findings.

Akosah et al. [13] found an association between carotid (CP or maximal CIMT ≥1 mm) and CAD in 236 patients referred for elective coronary angiography with a high NPV in case of both negative tests. However, only

Table 1 Baseline characteristics of patients

	Non-prior vascular disease (n = 156)
Age (years)	66.1 (10.4)
Male sex (%)	102 (65.4%)
Body mass index (Kg/m^2)	28.7 (4.0)
Hypertension	93 (59.6%)
Hypercholesterolemia	91 (58.3%)
DM	41 (26.3%)
Smoking habit	68 (43.6%)
Family history of premature CAD	22 (14.1%)
SCORE	
Low	10 (6.4%)
Moderate	52 (33.3%)
High	47 (30.1%)
Very high	45 (28.8%)
Chest pain	149 (95.5%)
Typical	82 (55.0%)
Atypical	65 (43.6%)
Non-anginal	2 (1.3%)
FPG levels (mg/dL)	114.3 (33.5)
GFR (ml//min/1.73 m^2)	78.3 (24.0)
Total Cholesterol levels (mg/dL)	189.2 (44.7)
Low-density lipoprotein levels (mg/dL)	114.4 (38.5)
High-density lipoprotein levels (mg/dL)	44.1 (11.7)
Triglyceride levels (mg/dL)	159.1 (94.1)
Drugs prior EE	
Beta-blockers	36 (23.1%)
Calcium channel blockers	40 (25.6%)
Nitrates	23 (14.7%)
Statins	68 (43.6%)
Antiplatelet drugs	51 (32.7%)
EE data	
Systolic BP (mmHg)	
Rest	141.5 (20.3)
Peak	184.9 (29.3)
Heart rate (beats/min)	
Rest	69.9 (13.1)
Peak	131.6 (18.6)
Rate-pressure (× 10^3 mmHg beats/min)	
Rest	9.9 (2.5)
Peak	24.4 (5.6)
Exercise time (min)	6.9 (2.7)
Positive EE	93 (59.6%)
Negative EE	38 (24.4%)
Failure to achieve submaximal predicted heart rate	25 (16.0%)

Table 1 Baseline characteristics of patients *(Continued)*

	Non-prior vascular disease (n = 156)
Metabolic equivalents	7.5 (2.6)
Left ventricular ejection fraction (%)	
Rest	62.5 (7.1)
Peak	64.3 (12.4)
Resting wall motion abnormality	21 (13.6%)
Wall motion score index	
Rest	1.04 (0.17)
Peak	1.22 (0.28)
Carotid ultrasound data	
Mean CIMT (mm)	0.88 (0.19)
Mean CIMT percentile Spanish population	
≤ 25th	18 (11.5%)
25th - 75th	40 (25.6%)
≥ 75th	98 (62.8%)
CP	95 (60.9%)
Calcified CP	47 (30.5%)

BP Blood pressure, *CAD* coronary artery disease, *CIMT* carotid intima-media thickness, *CP* carotid plaque, *DM* diabetes mellitus, *EE* exercise echocardiography, *FPG* fasting plasma glucose, *GFR* glomerular filtration rate, *SCORE* European Systematic COronary Risk Evaluation

162 (68.6%) subjects had stress test performed (the type was not described in their study) with a low PPV (36%) and also 95%CI were not reported. Kanwar et al. [14] reported a study on 50 symptomatic patients without prior CAD who underwent coronary angiography after stress testing. CP, especially those with heterogeneous composition, irregular surface or calcification, was a predictor of significant CAD showing a NPV of 100% in patients with negative/equivocal stress test and CP absence. In contrast to our study, 28% were non-Caucasians and they used different modalities of stress imaging test with a high incidence (64%) of equivocal results. Coskun et al. [15] identified hypertension and CIMT ≥1 mm as predictors of significant CAD in patients without previous CAD or stroke, scheduled for coronary angiography after a positive stress test. Similarly to Akosah et al. [13], the PPV of the stress test was lower compared to our results (61%). Finally, Ahmadvazir et al. [16] identified PTP, positive stress test and presence of CP as predictors of significant CAD in 591 patients with suspected CAD undergoing stress echocardiography. As in previous studies, the NPV combining stress test and carotid ultrasonography was high (80%) and, in agreement with our findings, nearly one third of the patients were reclassified for risk score according to CP results. However, only 35% of their patients were Caucasian, exercise as stress method was only used in 62% and only 83 (14%) underwent coronary angiography and, similar to the other

Table 2 Clinical, demographic, exercise and carotid ultrasound data in the subgroup of patients with and without CAD

	CAD ≥ 50% (n = 89)	CAD < 50% (n = 67)	p value
Age	67.6 (9.2)	64.1 (11.6)	0.045
Male sex	66 (74.2%)	36 (53.7%)	0.011
Body mass index	29.1 (4.2)	28.1 (3.7)	0.134
Hypertension	55 (61.8%)	38 (56.7%)	0.621
Hypercholesterolemia	56 (62.9%)	35 (52.2%)	0.193
DM	31 (34.8%)	10 (14.9%)	0.006
Smoking habit	46 (51.7%)	18 (32.8%)	0.023
Family history of early CAD	14 (15.7%)	8 (11.9%)	0.643
FPG levels	120.7 (38.7)	105.7 (22.4)	0.03
Total Cholesterol levels	192.0 (47.5)	185.5 (40.8)	0.379
Low-density lipoprotein levels	117.2 (40.7)	110.7 (36.1)	0.308
High-density lipoprotein levels	43.0 (11.3)	45.6 (12.1)	0.168
Triglyceride levels	160.6 (91.1)	157.2 (98.7)	0.824
GFR	75.6 (23.2)	81.1 (24.7)	0.105
SCORE			< 0.001
Low	1 (1.1%)	9 (13.6%)	
Moderate	24 (27.3%)	28 (42.4%)	
High	28 (31.8%)	19 (28.8%)	
Very high	35 (39.8%)	10 (15.2%)	
PTP of CAD			< 0.001
< 15%	0 (0%)	3 (4.5%)	
15–65%	31 (34.8%)	42 (62.7%)	
65–85%	55 (61.8%)	22 (32.8%)	
> 85%	3 (3.4%)	0 (0%)	
Positive EE	73 (82.0%)	20 (29.9%)	< 0.001
Mean CIMT (mm)	0.88 (0.21)	0.89 (0.18)	0.926
CIMT > 0.9 mm	38 (42.7%)	31 (46.3%)	0.745
CIMT > 75th percentile	52 (58.4%)	46 (68.7%)	0.242
CP	66 (74.2%)	29 (43.3%)	< 0.001
Calcified CP	32 (36.0%)	15 (22.4%)	0.079

PTP Pre-test probability. Rest of abbreviations as in Table 1

Table 3 Multivariate significant CAD analysis

Variable	B	p value	OR	95% CI Lower	95% CI Higher
Constant	−4.83	< 0.001	0.01		
Smoking habit	0.84	0.057	2.31	0.98	5.46
FPG	0.02	0.031	1.02	1.00	1.04
PTP of CAD > 65%	1.31	0.003	3.71	1.57	8.79
Positive EE	2.35	< 0.001	10.51	4.38	25.20
CP	1.08	0.013	2.95	1.25	6.93

CI confidence interval, *OR* odds ratio. Rest of abbreviations as in Tables 1 and 2

studies [13–15], CI or comparison between AUC were not reported. In contrast with previous results, Sachpekidis [17] did not find any statistical association between carotid and CAD (defined as positive dobutamine stress test) in 130 patients, 43% of them with previous CAD. However, the study population was small with only 38.5% yielding positive results, prior CAD could have hampered its findings and there was no comparison with angiography.

Atherosclerosis is a systemic disease and it is likely that patients with carotid disease also have CAD. This fact, as previously mentioned, was demonstrated in post-mortem studies [8] and in Bots' meta-analysis [19]. The highly variability of the association, with a correlation range between − 0.04 - 0.51 in the aforementioned meta-analysis, could be due to methodological differences in carotid ultrasound assessment and/or variability in atherosclerosis development between the vascular territories [19]. According to European and American guidelines on the management of stable CAD [2, 3] PTP of CAD must be established and then a non-invasive test must be performed for diagnostic or prognostic purposes depending on the degree of PTP. Both agree that a history of cerebrovascular or peripheral artery disease increases the likelihood of CAD [2, 3].

In our study most of the patients (96.2%) had intermediate PTP and, most importantly, none of them had previous vascular or CAD. Predictors positively associated with significant CAD were positive EE (OR = 10.51), PTP > 65% (OR = 3.71), CP (OR = 2.95) and FPG levels (OR = 1.02). It is interesting to mention that other important risk factors associated with CAD such as hypertension, hypercholesterolemia, cholesterol levels or smoking habit [1–3] were not significantly associated with CAD in our study, this fact can be explained due to insufficient statistical power and due to treatment effect, for example 42 patients (47.2%) with significant CAD were taking statins at the time of EE performance while only 26 (38.8%) of subjects without CAD were taking them, also 56 (62.9%) subjects with significant CAD where on antihypertensive drugs compared to only 35 (52.2%) of patients without CAD. FPG not DM was associated with CAD, the reason may be because the development of macrovascular disease occurs with insulin resistance, prior to DM diagnosis [27]; high or very high-risk SCORE was not also associated with CAD, probably because it is not designed to estimate it, just the risk of a fatal atherosclerotic event [1]. Although CP is the third in order in multivariable analysis after positive EE and PTP of CAD > 65%, it increases by nearly 3 the likelihood of having significant CAD so carotid ultrasound could be useful in case of intermediate PTP, where diagnosis must be

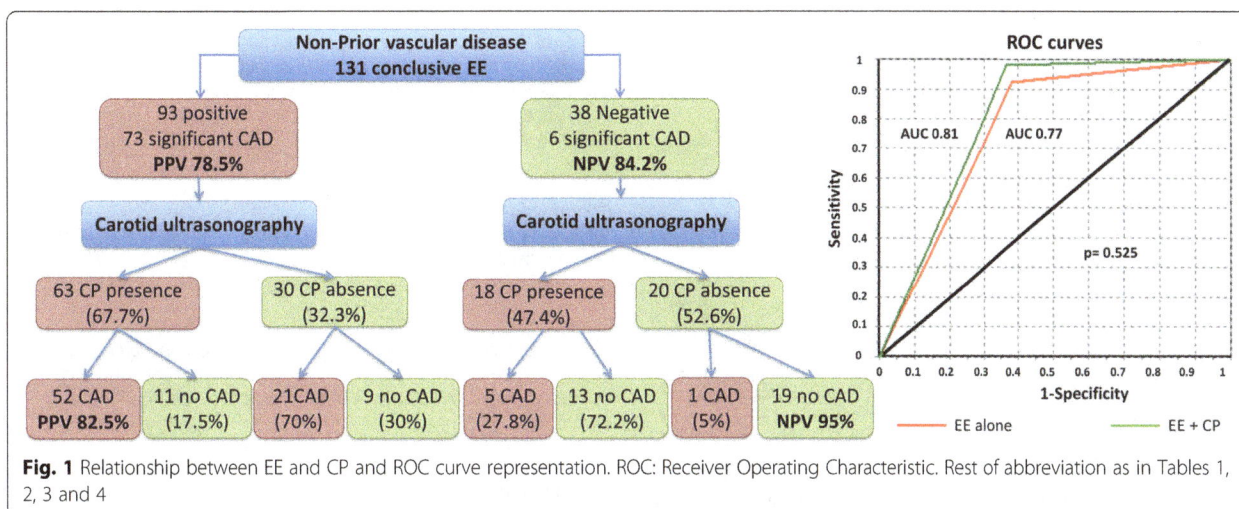

Fig. 1 Relationship between EE and CP and ROC curve representation. ROC: Receiver Operating Characteristic. Rest of abbreviation as in Tables 1, 2, 3 and 4

confirmed, or in equivocal EE. Moreover, and similar to Ahmadvazir et al. [16], CP presence reclassified around one third of patients to a high-risk category despite a negative EE or a normal coronary angiography. This is a very remarkable finding because these subjects benefit from aggressive primary preventive therapies [1] and, although ESC guidelines on cardiovascular disease prevention in clinical practice establish atherosclerotic plaque detection by carotid artery scanning in cardiovascular risk assessment as a IIb class level of evidence B recommendation [1], considering previously mentioned studies [7, 16] it might be changed to a IIa recommendation. Finally, although CP is associated with significant CAD its addition to EE did not improve AUC ($p = 0.525$), predictive values, efficiency and likelihood ratios due to CI overlap. These facts can be explained by insufficient statistical power, however it is important to mention the markedly but statistically non-significant increase in both NPV, especially in the moderate and high PTP of CAD groups, and in the NLR. These findings, although non-significant, are consistent to Kanwar et al. [14] and Ahmadvazir et al. [16] studies where CI were not reported. In this sense we considered our study only as hypothesis generating and increasing sample could corroborate it. Although there is a study addressing the utility of carotid ultrasonography for selecting patients who do not require coronary angiography before heart valve surgery [28], in our study 25.8% of patients with significant

CAD did not have CP and 43.3% of patients without significant CAD have CP in the carotid ultrasonography. For that reason we consider non-invasive stress test as the first line test in symptomatic patients with intermediate PTP and carotid ultrasonography as an additional tool for decision making. Unlike Kanwar et al. [14] we did not specifically analysed CP morphology, nevertheless we did not find significant association between calcified CP and significant CAD, this fact can be related to insufficient sample size.

Our study has some limitations. First of all, it is a retrospective single institution study with a low recruitment rate and therefore it is hampered by the use of different equipments and methods of image storage. One alternative could be a multicentre prospective study. Secondly, not all subjects with exercise and carotid tests were submitted to angiography. As a consequence, there are few patients with a negative EE (24.4%) in the sample and prevalence of CAD could be higher in our group than in the global population. Ideally, all subjects scheduled for EE and carotid ultrasonography should undergo angiography. However, it seems unethical to submit to an invasive, ionizing radiation exposing and expensive procedure asymptomatic people after optimal lifestyle and pharmacological management without bad-prognosis EE. Other important limitation is that the coronary artery stenosis percentage was assessed visually and not by using more accurate tools such as intravascular ultrasound or optical coherence tomography or by physiological

Table 4 Sensitivity, specificity, predictive values, AUC and likelihood ratios for CAD diagnosis

Conclusive EE ($N = 131$)								
	Sensitivity (95% CI)	Specificity (95%CI)	PPV (95% CI)	NPV (95% CI)	Efficiency (95% CI)	AUC (95% CI)	PLR	NLR
EE	92.4% (84.4–96.5)	61.5% (48.0–73.5)	78.5% (69.1–85.6)	84.2% (69.6–92.6)	80.2% (72.5–86.1)	0.77 (0.68–0.86)	2.40	0.12
EE + CP	98.1% (90.1–99.7)	63.3% (45.5–78.1)	82.5% (71.4–90.0)	95.0% (76.4–99.1)	85.5% (76.4–91.5)	0.81 (0.70–0.92)	2.68	0.03

AUC area under the curve, *NLR* negative likelihood ratio, *NPV* negative predictive value, *PLR* positive likelihood ratio, *PPV* positive predictive value. Rest of abbreviations as in Tables 1, 2 and 3

Table 5 Predictive values for significant CAD prediction depending on its prevalence

Prevalence of CAD	PPV (95%CI)	NPV (95%CI)
EE alone		
15%	29.8% (23.0–37.6)	97.9% (95.0–99.0)
65%	81.7% (75.9–86.4)	81.4% (66.3–90.7)
85%	93.2% (90.6–95.1)	58.8% (39.1–76.1)
EE + CP		
15%	32.1% (22.8–43.1)	99.5% (96.4–99.9)
65%	83.3% (75.6–88.9)	94.8% (71.8–99.2)
85%	93.8% (90.4–96.0)	85.6% (45.5–97.7)

Abbreviations as in Table 4

assessment of CAD stenosis in the cardiac catheterization laboratory (fractional flow reserve). This is a consequence of a retrospective study design, when some techniques were not available at the time of the angiography performance and it also reflects the usual clinical practice where intermediate stenosis are treated in case of a positive stress test and the methods mentioned before are used according to interventional cardiologist criteria, if negative or no stress test available. Comparison between carotid ultrasound and intracoronary imaging techniques in case of normal angiography could have helped to establish a better correlation between carotid and coronary artery disease, however the aim of the study was to find an association between carotid disease and significant and possibly flow limiting epicardial coronary stenosis causing chest pain. It is also important to keep in mind that this is a real life cohort study and using intravascular ultrasound or optical coherence tomography in people without intermediate CAD increases the cost and the duration of the procedure. Finally, there are 13.6% of patients with resting wall motion abnormalities, but we must consider that there are several conditions other than ischemic heart disease, such as cardiac sarcoidosis, myocarditis or cardiomyopathies that can also cause them.

Conclusions

In conclusion, our study shows that carotid disease, in particular the presence of CP, is associated with significant CAD in patients submitted to EE. Its addition to EE does not improve sensitivity, specificity, predictive values, likelihood ratios, efficiency and AUC for significant CAD diagnosis; probably due to insufficient statistical power. However, CP reclassified one third of patients to very high-risk SCORE category despite a negative EE or CAD absence and these subjects benefit from aggressive primary prevention interventions.

Abbreviations
AUC: Area under the curve; BP: Blood pressure; CAD: Coronary artery disease; CI: Confidence interval; CIMT: Carotid intima-media thickness; CP: Carotid

plaque; DM: Diabetes mellitus; EE: Exercise echocardiography; ESC: European Society of Cardiology; FPG: Fasting plasma glucose; GFR: Glomerular filtration rate; NLR: Negative likelihood ratio; NPV: Negative predictive value; OR: Odds ratio; PLR: Positive likelihood ratio; PPV: Positive predictive value; PTP: Pre-test probability; ROC: Receiver Operating Characteristic; SCORE: European Systematic COronary Risk Evaluation.

Acknowledgements
The authors want to thank Miss Leonor Ortega Fernández for her assistance in data collection.

Funding
This research was supported by the *Fundación Ramón Domínguez para la Investigación, el Desarrollo y la Innovación biosanitaria*, a non-profit foundation created by the merger of two Hospital Foundations: [Grant code ECOES].

Author's contributions
RFG (first author, corresponding author) and CGJ conceived and designed the research, RFG performed statistical analysis, CGJ handled funding and supervision, RFG, VFG, LOF and MLLR acquired the data, RFG, VFG and AJPP drafted the manuscript, all authors made critical revision of the manuscript for key intellectual content, and final approval of the manuscript submitted was done by CGJ and RFG. All authors read and approved the final manuscript.

Consent for publication
Not applicable.

Competing interests
The authors declare that they have no competing interests.

Author details
[1]Department of Cardiology, Hospital Universitario Lucus Augusti (HULA), Avenida doctor Ulises Romero n° 1, 27003 Lugo, Spain. [2]Department of Otolaryngology, Hospital Universitario Marqués de Valdecilla, Avenida Valdecilla n° 25, Santander 39008, Spain. [3]Department of Internal Medicine, Hospital Universitario Lucus Augusti (HULA), Avenida doctor Ulises Romero n° 1, Lugo 27003, Spain. [4]Department of Cardiology, Complejo Hospitalario Universitario A Coruña (CHUAC), As Xubias de Arriba n° 84, A Coruña 15006, Spain. [5]Intituto de Investigación Biomédica A Coruña (INIBIC), Xubias de Arriba n° 84, A Coruña 15006, Spain. [6]Universidad de La Coruña (UDC), Calle de la Maestranza n° 9, A Coruña 15001, Spain.

References
1. Piepoli MF, Hoes AW, Agewall S, Albus C, Brotons C, Catapano AL, et al. 2016 European Guidelines on cardiovascular disease prevention in clinical practice: The Sixth Joint Task Force of the European Society of Cardiology and Other Societies on Cardiovascular Disease Prevention in Clinical Practice (constituted by representatives of 10 societies and by invited experts): Developed with the special contribution of the European Association for Cardiovascular Prevention & Rehabilitation (EACPR). Eur Heart J. 2016;37:2315–81.
2. Montalescot G, Sechtem U, Achenbach S, Andreotti F, Arden C, Budaj A, et al. 2013 ESC guidelines on the management of stable coronary artery disease: the task force on the management of stable coronary artery disease of the European Society of Cardiology. Eur Heart J. 2013;34:2949–3003.
3. Fihn SD, Blankenship JC, Alexander KP, Bittl JA, Byrne JG, Fletcher BJ, et al. 2014 ACC/AHA/AATS/PCNA/SCAI/STS focused update of the guideline for the diagnosis and management of patients with stable ischemic heart disease: a report of the American College of Cardiology/American Heart Association Task Force on Practice Guidelines, and the American Association for Thoracic Surgery, Preventive Cardiovascular Nurses Association, Society for Cardiovascular Angiography and Interventions, and Society of Thoracic Surgeons. J Am Coll Cardiol. 2014;64:1929–49.

4. Pellikka PA, Nagueh SF, Elhendy AA, Kuehl CA, Sawada SG. American Society of Echocardiography recommendations for performance, interpretation, and application of stress echocardiography. J Am Soc Echocardiogr. 2007;20:1021–41.

5. Chambless LE, Heiss G, Folsom AR, Rosamond W, Szklo M, Sharrett AR, et al. Association of coronary heart disease incidence with carotid arterial wall thickness and major risk factors: the atherosclerosis risk in communities (ARIC) study, 1987-1993. Am J Epidemiol. 1997;146:483–94.

6. Lorenz MW, Markus HS, Bots ML, Rosvall M, Sitzer M. Prediction of clinical cardiovascular events with carotid intima-media thickness: a systematic review and meta-analysis. Circulation. 2007;115:459–67.

7. Inaba Y, Chen JA, Bergmann SR. Carotid plaque, compared with carotid intima-media thickness, more accurately predicts coronary artery disease events: a meta-analysis. Atherosclerosis. 2012;220:128–33.

8. Iwakiri T, Yano Y, Sato Y, Hatakeyama K, Marutsuka K, Fujimoto S, et al. Usefulness of carotid intima-media thickness measurement as an indicator of generalized atherosclerosis: findings from autopsy analysis. Atherosclerosis. 2012;225:359–62.

9. Heuten H, Claeys M, Goovaerts I, Ennekens G, Bosmans J, Vrints C. Can measurement of the intima-media thickness of the carotid artery improve the diagnostic value of exercise stress tests? Acta Cardiol. 2006;61:501–5.

10. Schroeder B, Francis G, Leipsic J, Heilbron B, John Mancini GB, Taylor CM. Early atherosclerosis detection in asymptomatic patients: a comparison of carotid ultrasound, coronary artery calcium score, and coronary computed tomography angiography. Can J Cardiol. 2013;29:1687–94.

11. Teragawa H, Kato M, Kurokawa J, Yamagata T, Matsuura H, Chayama K. Usefulness of flow-mediated dilation of the brachial artery and/or the intima-media thickness of the carotid artery in predicting coronary narrowing in patients suspected of having coronary artery disease. Am J Cardiol. 2001;88:1147–51.

12. Nowak J, Nilsson T, Sylven C, Jogestrand T. Potential of carotid ultrasonography in the diagnosis of coronary artery disease: a comparison with exercise test and variance ECG. Stroke. 1998;29:439–46.

13. Akosah KO, McHugh VL, Barnhart SI, Schaper AM, Mathiason MA, Perlock PA, et al. Carotid ultrasound for risk clarification in young to middle-aged adults undergoing elective coronary angiography. Am J Hypertens. 2006;19:1256–61.

14. Kanwar M, Rosman HS, Fozo PK, Fahmy S, Vikraman N, Gardin JM, et al. Usefulness of carotid ultrasound to improve the ability of stress testing to predict coronary artery disease. Am J Cardiol. 2007;99:1196–200.

15. Coskun U, Yildiz A, Esen OB, Baskurt M, Cakar MA, Kilickesmez KO, et al. Relationship between carotid intima-media thickness and coronary angiographic findings: a prospective study. Cardiovasc Ultrasound. 2009;7:59.

16. Ahmadvazir S, Zacharias K, Shah BN, Pabla JS, Senior R. Role of simultaneous carotid ultrasound in patients undergoing stress echocardiography for assessment of chest pain with no previous history of coronary artery disease. Am Heart J. 2014;168:229–36.

17. Sachpekidis V, Bhan A, Paul M, Gianstefani S, Smith L, Reiken J, et al. The additive value of three-dimensional derived left atrial volume and carotid imaging in dobutamine stress echocardiography. Eur J Echocardiogr. 2011;12:46–53.

18. Djaberi R, Schuijf JD, de Koning EJ, Rabelink TJ, Smit JW, Kroft LJ, et al. Usefulness of carotid intima-media thickness in patients with diabetes mellitus as a predictor of coronary artery disease. Am J Cardiol. 2009;104:1041–6.

19. Bots ML, Baldassarre D, Simon A, de Groot E, O'Leary DH, Riley W, et al. Carotid intima-media thickness and coronary atherosclerosis: weak or strong relations? Eur Heart J. 2007;28:398–406.

20. Gonzalez-Gay MA, Gonzalez-Juanatey C, Pineiro A, Garcia-Porrua C, Testa A, Llorca J. High-grade C-reactive protein elevation correlates with accelerated atherogenesis in patients with rheumatoid arthritis. J Rheumatol. 2005;32:1219–23.

21. Thygesen K, Alpert JS, Jaffe AS, Simoons ML, Chaitman BR, White HD, et al. Third universal definition of myocardial infarction. Circulation. 2012;126:2020–35.

22. Stein JH, Korcarz CE, Hurst RT, Lonn E, Kendall CB, Mohler ER, et al. Use of carotid ultrasound to identify subclinical vascular disease and evaluate cardiovascular disease risk: a consensus statement from the American Society of Echocardiography carotid intima-media thickness task force. Endorsed by the Society for Vascular Medicine. J Am Soc Echocardiogr. 2008;21:93–111 quiz 189-190.

23. Touboul PJ, Hennerici MG, Meairs S, Adams H, Amarenco P, Desvarieux M, et al. Mannheim intima-media thickness consensus. Cerebrovasc Dis. 2004;18:346–9.

24. Touboul PJ, Hennerici MG, Meairs S, Adams H, Amarenco P, Bornstein N, et al. Mannheim carotid intima-media thickness consensus (2004-2006). An update on behalf of the advisory board of the 3rd and 4th watching the risk symposium, 13th and 15th European stroke conferences, Mannheim, Germany, 2004, and Brussels, Belgium, 2006. Cerebrovasc Dis. 2007;23:75–80.

25. Touboul PJ, Hennerici MG, Meairs S, Adams H, Amarenco P, Bornstein N, et al. Mannheim carotid intima-media thickness and plaque consensus (2004-2006-2011). An update on behalf of the advisory board of the 3rd, 4th and 5th watching the risk symposia, at the 13th, 15th and 20th European stroke conferences, Mannheim, Germany, 2004, Brussels, Belgium, 2006, and Hamburg, Germany, 2011. Cerebrovasc Dis. 2012;34:290–6.

26. Grau M, Subirana I, Agis D, Ramos R, Basagana X, Marti R, et al. Carotid intima-media thickness in the Spanish population: reference ranges and association with cardiovascular risk factors. Rev Esp Cardiol (Engl Ed). 2012;65:1086–93.

27. Low Wang CC, Hess CN, Hiatt WR, Goldfine AB. Atherosclerotic cardiovascular disease and heart failure in type 2 diabetes – mechanisms, management, and clinical considerations. Circulation. 2016;133:2459–502.

28. Belhassen L, Carville C, Pelle G, Monin JL, Teiger E, Duval-Moulin AM, et al. Evaluation of carotid artery and aortic intima-media thickness measurements for exclusion of significant coronary atherosclerosis in patients scheduled for heart valve surgery. J Am Coll Cardiol. 2002;39:1139–44.

19

Comprehensive assessment of left ventricular myocardial function by two-dimensional speckle-tracking echocardiography

Vicente Mora[1]* (iD), Ildefonso Roldán[1], Elena Romero[1], Diana Romero[2], Javier Bertolín[1], Natalia Ugalde[2], Carmen Pérez-Olivares[1], Melisa Rodriguez-Israel[2], Jana Pérez-Gozalbo[1] and Jorge A. Lowenstein[2]

Abstract

Background: Left ventricular ejection fraction (LVEF) results from the combined action of longitudinal and circumferential contraction, radial thickening, and basal and apical rotation. The study of these parameters together may lead to an accurate assessment of the cardiac function.

Methods: Ninety healthy volunteers, categorized by gender and age (≤ 55 and > 55 years), were evaluated using two-dimensional speckle tracking echocardiography. Transversal views of the left ventricle (LV) were obtained to calculate circumferential strain and left ventricular twist, while three apical views were obtained to determine longitudinal strain (LS) and mitral annular plane systolic excursion (MAPSE). We established the integral myocardial function of the LV according to: 1. The Combined Deformation Parameter (CDP), which includes Deformation Product (DP) - Twist x LS (° x %) - and Deformation Index (DefI) -Twist / LS (° / %)-; and 2. the Torsion Index (TorI): Twist / MAPSE (° / cm).

Results: The mean age of our patients was 50.3 ± 11.1 years. CDP did not vary with gender or age. The average DP was -432 ± 172 ° x %, and the average DefI was -0.96 ± 0.36 ° / %. DP provides information about myocardial function (normal, pseudonormal, depressed), and the DefI quotient indicates which component (s) is/are affected in cases of abnormality. TorI was higher in volunteers over 55 years (16.5 ± 15.2 vs 13.1 ± 5.0 °/cm, $p = 0.003$), but did not vary with gender.

Conclusions: The proposed parameters integrate values of twisting and longitudinal shortening. They allow a complete physiological assessment of cardiac systolic function, and could be used for the early detection and characterization of its alteration.

Keywords: Deformation imaging, Speckle tracking, Ventricular torsion, Ventricular function, Myocardial strain

Background

Assessment of LV systolic function is the cornerstone of an echocardiographic examination. Many parameters can be used for clinical and research purposes, but LVEF is the most commonly employed. LVEF results from the combined action of longitudinal and circumferential contraction, radial thickening, and basal and apical rotation. However, LVEF has many limitations as a parameter, some of them related to imaging techniques and others to the definition itself [1, 2].

The particular double helical structure of myocardial fibers results in systolic rotation of the base and apex of the LV in opposite directions round its longitudinal axis, and the algebraic subtraction of this rotation causes twisting of the heart muscle. Due to this muscular movement, the base of the LV moves towards the apex, producing a longitudinal shortening of the LV [3]. Therefore, systolic ventricular contraction results from the combined and simultaneous action of twisting and shortening of the ventricle.

* Correspondence: vmoral@comv.es
[1]Cardiology Department, Hospital Dr Peset, Valencia, Spain
Full list of author information is available at the end of the article

Myocardial torsion - the consequence of these movements - is a fundamental component of cardiac function [4–6].

Speckle tracking echocardiography [7] (STE) is a useful echocardiographic tool for evaluating myocardial function, due its high temporal and spatial resolution, good inter and intraobserver reproducibility [8], the advantage of being independent of the insonation angle [9] and the fact that it is not affected by translational movements of the heart. Furthermore, due to its three-dimensional modality, it allows simultaneous assessment of the entire myocardium of the left ventricle [10].

Initially, rotational mechanics of the LV were measured using invasive approaches [11, 12]. However, during the last two decades, non-invasive imaging techniques have become available for this purpose, with cardiac magnetic resonance constituting the gold standard [13, 14]. The incorporation of STE into clinical practice has rekindled study of the LV's rotational mechanics [15–17], and a very good correlation with cardiac resonance has been reported ($r = 0.93$) [15, 16].

It has been suggested that, in the future, a combined approach in which both changes in LV rotational mechanics and longitudinal shortening are evaluated and interpreted in an integrated way will be necessary to establish normal reference values [18–20]. The calculation of ventricular torsion from rotation and longitudinal strain by means of STE can provide complementary information about systolic ventricular function in relation to the traditional parameters used in daily practice, such as LVEF [6].

We present values of strain and rotational mechanics obtained with STE in a healthy population. Based on these values, new parameters are proposed for the study of cardiac function, implying a more integral evaluation of the components involved in the mechanism of contraction.

Methods
Study population
This is an observational, prospective study in which 104 healthy volunteers were initially enrolled after being randomly selected among hospital staff. Inclusion criteria were: age > 18 years, absence of cardiovascular disease and/or risk factor, and normal physical and electrocardiographic examinations. Exclusion criteria were sports training and pregnancy.

The hospital's Clinical Research and Ethics Committee approved the study. The written informed consent of the participants was obtained.

Echocardiography
Two ultrasound systems (Vivid E9 and Vivid E95, GE Healthcare Medical Systems, Norway) equipped with 2.5 MHz transducer were used. Two-dimensional views of the apex (four, three and two chambers) were obtained to calculate longitudinal strain (LS). From the parasternal short axis perspective, transverse projections of the mitral valve, papillary muscles and apex facilitated calculation of radial strain, circumferential strain and rotational parameters. All images were obtained at a frequency of between 50 and 80 frames/second. The moment of aortic valvular closure was determined in the long axis apical projection. All images were transferred to a workstation for computer analysis (EchoPAC GE Healthcare software version 112.0.0).

The LV endocardial border was traced manually slightly within the myocardium to calculate myocardial strain. Then, with the help of the software, a second larger concentric circle was automatically generated near the epicardium to include the full thickness of the myocardial wall. The program automatically divided each projection into six equal segments and performed frame-by-frame speckle tracking, providing automated tracking confirmation (verified by the operator) and generating strain values, expressed as percentages.

Rotation is an angular displacement of a myocardial segment in a transverse projection around the longitudinal axis of the LV. Apical systolic rotation occurs in a counter-clockwise direction and is expressed in degrees with positive values when viewed from the vertex. Conversely, basal rotation is produced in a clockwise direction, with negative values. The twist that occurs as a consequence is the net difference, in degrees, between apical and basal rotation.

Care was taken to ensure that all ultrasound adjustments, including image depth and frame rate, were maintained for each individual's data collection. Images of four and two chambers were recorded for analysis of end-diastolic and end-systolic volumes, and LVEF was calculated using Simpson's biplane method.

In addition to LS, longitudinal shortening of the LV was estimated from the systolic excursion of the mitral annular plane (MAPSE) in the four-chamber projection by placing the M-mode cursor at the septal and lateral level of the ring and averaging both values. The base-apex distance (B-A) was determined in the four-chamber view, at the end-diastole and at the beginning of the QRS.

We evaluated the various parameters that contribute to LV myocardial function (Fig. 1):

a) Classic Torsion (CTor): Twist/B-A distance (degrees/cm)
b) Torsion Index (TorI): Twist/MAPSE (degrees/cm)
c) Combined Deformation Parameter (CDP):
   c.1 Deformation Product (DP): Twist x LS (degrees x %), and
   c.2 Deformation Index (DefI): Twist / LS (degrees / %).

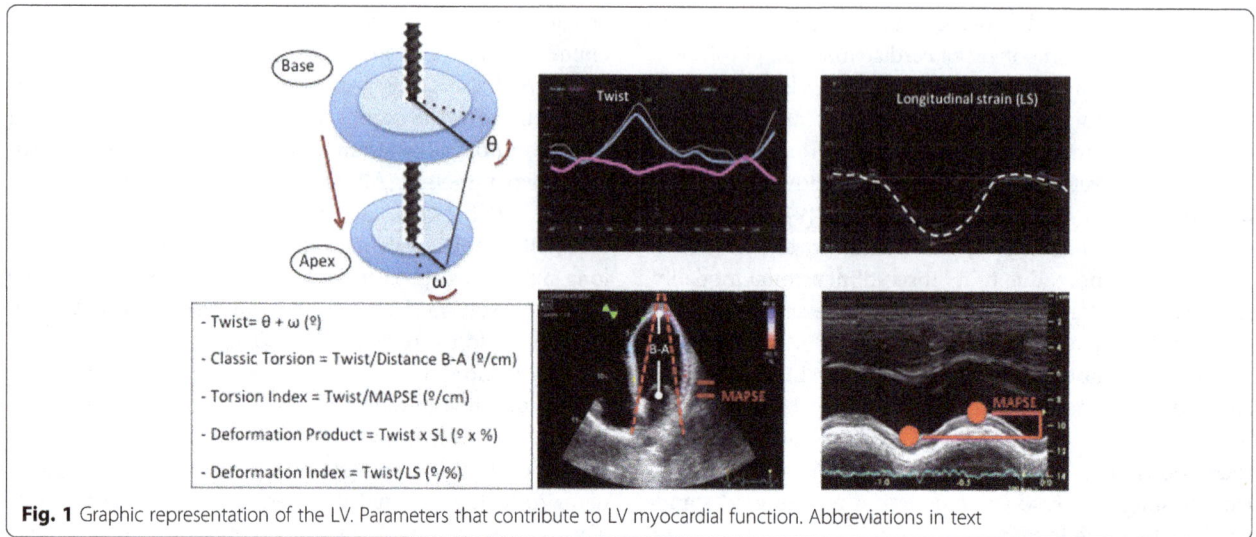

Fig. 1 Graphic representation of the LV. Parameters that contribute to LV myocardial function. Abbreviations in text

Statistical analysis

Continuous variables are expressed as mean and standard deviation, and proportions as percentages. We compared strain values according to gender and age (≤ 55 years and > 55 years) using a Student's t test. Normality of distribution of the studied parameters was confirmed. A p value of < 0.05 was considered statistically significant. The intraclass correlation coefficient was used to evaluate intraobserver and interobserver reproducibility of continuous variables, according to a random sample of 10 cases, with masking and measurements performed at different moments.

Statistical analyses were performed using the IBM SPSS Statistics v.19.0.0329 software package.

Results

Our study population was eventually composed of 90 healthy subjects after 14 of the original 104 were excluded due to a deficient ultrasonic window that made it impossible to obtain adequate measurements in all segments of the LV. Mean age was 50.3 ± 11.1 years, women 43.3%.

Table 1 details the population's characteristics. Women showed lower values for body surface, LV diameter and ventricular volume, while no gender differences were

observed in terms of ejection fraction. Patients over 55 years of age presented higher LVEF, despite having smaller ventricular diameters and volumes.

The mean values of LS, radial strain and circumferential strain are presented in Table 2. LS was the only of the 3 types of strain that was slightly higher in the female sex, while none showed differences according to age. MAPSE was higher among males and in the ≤55 year-old group. Neither the values of basal and apical rotation, nor the resulting twist, differed with gender or ages.

Behaviour of torsional parameters

CTor, TorI and DefI did not vary with sex, while age did have a bearing: CTor and TorI values were higher in older subjects (2.8 ± 0.9 vs 2.3 ± 1.0, $p = 0.05$, and 16.5 ± 15.2 vs 13.1 ± 5.0, $p = 0.003$, respectively), while no age differences were observed with respect to DefI (Table 2).

CDP showed no gender or age differences in either DP or DefI. The possible combinations between DP and DefI values appear in Table 3. Normal values of DP (– 432 ± 172 ° x %) and DefI (– 0.96 ± 0.36 °/%) relate to a cardiac function within normal limits. When there is myocardial

Table 1 Characteristics of the study population, differentiated by sex and age

	Total (n 90)	Men (n 52)	Women (n 38)	p	≤ 55 years (n 59)	> 55 years (n 31)	p
BS (m^2)	1.8 ± 0.2	1.9 ± 0.1	1.6 ± 0.1	0.01	1.8 ± 0.2	1.8 ± 0.1	0.42
HR (b/m)	65 ± 10	65 ± 11	66 ± 9	0.65	65 ± 11	67 ± 10	0.32
sBP (mmHg)	119 ± 16	121 ± 16	115 ± 15	0.07	117 ± 17	123 ± 15	0.11
LVd (mm)	45.5 ± 4.5	47.4 ± 4.2	43.0 ± 3.4	0.01	46.1 ± 4.5	44.3 ± 4.1	0.06
LVEDV (ml)	89.2 ± 28.4	101.1 ± 27.9	73.0 ± 20.1	0.01	96.1 ± 29.3	76.2 ± 21.7	0.01
LVESV (ml)	29.8 ± 11.1	34.1 ± 11.5	24.1 ± 7.5	0.01	32.9 ± 11.4	24.1 ± 8.1	0.01
LVEF (%)	66.6 ± 5.5	66.4 ± 5.4	66.9 ± 5.7	0.68	65.7 ± 5.3	68.4 ± 5.7	0.03

BS Body surface area, *HR* Heart rate, *sBP* systolic blood pressure, *LVd* Left ventricle end-diastolic diameter, *LVEDV* Left ventricular end-diastolic volume, *LVESV* Left ventricular end-systolic volume, *LVEF* Left ventricular ejection fraction

Table 2 Values of global longitudinal, radial and circumferential strain, and rotational parameters of the study population, differentiated by sex and age

	Total (n 90)	Men (n 52)	Women (n 38)	p	≤ 55 y (n 59)	> 55 y (n 31)	p
LS (%)	−21.1 ± 2.1	− 20.7 ± 2.0	−21.7 ± 2.1	0.02	−21.1 ± 1.8	−21.1 ± 2.5	0.98
RS (%)	33.5 ± 10.2	34.0 ± 9.9	32.8 ± 10.7	0.59	32.4 ± 9.6	35.6 ± 11.2	0.15
CS (%)	−21.6 ± 3.9	−21.9 ± 4.3	−21.3 ± 3.4	0.41	−21.2 ± 3.4	− 22.4 ± 4.7	0.16
MAPSE (cm)	1.4 ± 0.1	1.48 ± 0,1	1.36 ± 0.1	0.01	1.4 ± 0.2	1.3 ± 0.1	0.01
B-A (cm)	8.2 ± 0.8	8.6 ± 0.6	7.6 ± 0.6	0.01	8.3 ± 0.8	7.9 ± 0.8	0.04
Apical Rot (°)	14.4 ± 6.5	14.9 ± 7.0	13.7 ± 5.9	0.40	14.2 ± 1.0	14.7 ± 0.9	0.76
Basal Rot (°)	− 6.2 ± 3.6	−6.0 ± 3.5	−6.5 ± 3.8	0.50	−5.7 ± 3.4	− 7.3 ± 3.9	0.05
Twist (°)	20.3 ± 7.6	20.7 ± 7.9	19.6 ± 7.1	0.51	19.4 ± 7.9	21.9 ± 6.6	0.14
CTor (°/cm)	2.5 ± 1.0	2.4 ± 1.0	2.6 ± 1.0	0.39	2.3 ± 1.0	2.8 ± 0.9	0.05
TorI (°/cm)	14.2 ± 5.3	14.0 ± 5.4	14.5 ± 5.2	0.67	13.1 ± 5.0	16.5 ± 15.2	0.01
CDP							
DP (° x %)	−432 ± 172	− 431 ± 170	433 ± 177	0.96	− 415 ± 182	− 463 ± 149	0.21
DefI (° / %)	− 0.96 ± 0.36	−1.00 ± 0.39	−0.90 ± 0.31	0.18	−0.9 ± 0.3	−1.0 ± 0.3	0.09

LS Longitudinal Strain, *RS* Radial Strain, *CS* Circumferential Strain, *MAPSE* Mitral annular plane systolic excursion, *B-A* Base-Apex distance, *Rot.* Rotation, *CTor* Classic Torsion, *TorI* Torsion Index, *CDP* Combined Deformation Parameter, *DP* Deformation Product, *DefI* Deformation Index

dysfunction, the DP value can be pseudonormal or decreased, and so DefI is a better parameter of the origin in the involvement of LS, twisting or both. The DP is pseudormal when its value is maintained at the expense of a compensating increase of the twist, with LS diminished. When the DP is decreased, the DefI quotient will provide information on the origin of myocardial impairment in one (LS or twist) or both components.

Intraobserver and interobserver variability was suitable (Table 4), with intraclass correlation coefficients > 0.75.

Discussion

We describe values of new echocardiographic parameters that can be employed to perform a comprehensive evaluation of cardiac mechanics using a non-invasive technique - STE - in a sample of healthy subjects. In this way we intend to provide a full picture of the physiological components involved in ventricular contraction, and to determine which can serve as tools in the evaluation of different heart diseases.

STE is a useful technique to evaluate cardiac function [7], allowing each myocardial region to be visualized as a defined, relatively stable and unique speckle pattern, thus allowing it to be differentiated from other regions throughout the cardiac cycle. Nevertheless, calculating strain by means of this technique has its limitations, such as the dependence on frame speed for an adequate tracking of the marks [21], and on the quality of the two-dimensional image, as well as myocardium thickness heterogeneity, LV geometry, variations in the resolution of the lateral wall and suboptimal reproducibility [22].

The values obtained with STE are related specifically with LV myocardial function, and allow the mechanism of contraction and its components to be described, such as: longitudinal and circumferential shortening, radial thickening, and rotational movements [2].

The arrival of STE has revived interest in LV torsion, and research shows a very close correlation with cardiac resonance ($r = 0.93$) in humans [15, 16]. Cardiac torsion is a result of the peculiar architecture of the heart; several studies have highlighted the presence of obliquely oriented

Table 3 Combined Deformation Parameter. Possibilities of presentation

Combined deformation parameter			
Deformation Product (DP) (Twist x LS) (° x %)	Deformation Index (DefI) (Twist/LS) (° / %)	Status of Twist and LS	Myocardial function
Normal	Normal	Normal Twist + Normal LS	Normal
Pseudonormal	Increased	Increased Twist + LS diminished	Impaired
Diminished	Diminished	Diminished Twist + Normal LS	Impaired
	Increased	Normal Twist + LS diminished	Impaired
	Normal	Diminished Twist + LS diminished	Impaired

LS Longitudinal strain

Table 4 Intraobserver and interobserver variability

Intraclass correlation coefficient (95% CI)

		p
Intraobserver		
Global longitudinal strain	0.86 (0.53–0,96)	< 0.001
Twist	0.94 (0.65–0.98)	< 0.001
Classic Torsion	0.96 (0.84–0.99)	< 0.001
Torsion index	0.93 (0.63–0.98)	< 0.001
Strain product	0.97 (0.82–0.99)	< 0.001
Strain index	0.85 (0.52–0.96)	< 0.001
Interobserver		
Global longitudinal strain	0.87 (0.58–0.96)	< 0.001
Twist	0.85 (0.53–0.96)	< 0.001
Classic Torsion	0.87 (0.59–0.96)	< 0.001
Torsion index	0.80 (0.41–0.94)	< 0.001
Strain product	0.90 (0.65–0.97)	< 0.001
Strain index	0.77 (0.31–0.94)	0.003

muscle fibres in the subendocardium, which gradually change their angle so that they position themselves in the opposite direction to the subepicardium [3, 23, 24]. This spiral organization seems to be fundamental for both cardiac and diastolic systolic function [25, 26].

In the 1960s, Torrent-Guasp described myocardial architecture as a single band of muscle that forms a double helix [27], allowing simultaneous systolic rotation in opposite directions between the LV base and apex, around its longitudinal axis. At the same time, the ventricular base moves towards the apex, which induces a longitudinal shortening of the LV and, consequently, ventricular torsion [3, 28]. Therefore, systolic ventricular contraction results from the combined and simultaneous action of ventricular rotation and longitudinal shortening (Fig. 1). The two processes may not be affected in the same way by ventricular dysfunction [29], so their evaluation may represent a valuable tool for clinical practice, even in moderate pathological situations that are not detected by analysing classical hemodynamic parameters [17, 26, 30–32].

There is some semantic confusion in the literature surrounding the indistinct usage of the terms twist and torsion. Twist is the result of the algebraic difference between basal and apical rotation, and is expressed in degrees, while classic torsion (CTor) is usually defined by dividing the twist by the B-A distance during the final phase of the diastole, expressed in degrees/cm [33]. According to another definition, this formulation should be multiplied by the average radius of the base and the apex [34] to adjust for hearts of different longitudinal and transverse size. In both cases, the twist is normalized with respect to one or several "static" LV diameters, so

that one of the actions that take place simultaneously during the systole - namely, the shortening of the LV along its longitudinal axis - is not taken into account. However, it is possible to evaluate the "dynamic" longitudinal shortening of LV by calculating the MAPSE using conventional 2D echocardiography, and by estimating LS by means of EST.

The parameters proposed in this work for the evaluation of ventricular torsion, such as TorI and DefI, provide a more reliable representation of the components of cardiac systole. They involve quantification of longitudinal shortening and twist, as an expression of dynamic systolic events that occur simultaneously in an elastic organ such as the ventricular myocardium.

It is important to underline the difference between the meanings of the commonly used definition classic torsion (CTor) [34] and the proposed indexes of torsion (TorI and DefI). CTor refers to the twist per cm of the length of (B-A) of the LV, while TorI and DefI represent the rotation per unit of shortening and unit of longitudinal deformation of the LV, respectively. Basal and apical rotations, which produce the twist, are determined both by the segmental heterogeneity of the circumferential contraction and by its interaction with the simultaneous longitudinal contraction, which displaces the circumferential plane obliquely towards the apex during systole. The resulting LV torsion is the outcome of the longitudinal-circumferential shear.

The torsion generated as a result of this interaction, and which depends on the helical shape of the myocardial fibers, contributes to the thickening of the myocardium towards the ventricular centroid and the consequent ejection of the corresponding systolic volume. Therefore, with the proposed indices (TorI and DefI), we intend to provide a measure of intrinsic muscular torsion that is independent of cardiac size. CTor normalizes twist with respect to a static dimension such as the diastolic size of the LV. Thus, the extent of the torsion may be reduced according to its classical definition (with respect to the longitudinal size of the LV) (CTor) and increased when calculated by TorI and DefI, as can be appreciated in Table 5. This table shows the evolution of a patient with cardiac amyloidosis: a decrease in the twist, when accompanied, as it usually is, by a decrease in ventricular longitudinal shortening, can actually lead to an increase in intrinsic myocardial torsion known as "writhing", similar to the "squeezing" of a towel. In patients diagnosed with amyloidosis, an increase of TorI and DefI (greater "squeezing") justifies maintenance of the LVEF, despite the decreased twist and reduced contraction of the longitudinal axis. Hence, the indices we propose are more representative when defining the alterations of the ventricular torsion referred to as "squeezing", since they contemplate dynamic simultaneous actions like longitudinal shortening and twist.

Table 5 Evolution in a case of amyloidosis. Normal values of reference in Table 2

	Twist (°)	LS (%)	B-A (cm)	MAPSE (cm)	CTor (°/cm)	TorI (°/cm)	Combined deformation parameter		LVEF (%)
							DP (° x %)	DefI (° / %)	
Basal	20	−14	8	0.9	2.5 (N)	22.2 (↑)	− 280 (↓)	− 1.4 (↑)	55%
1 year	15	−10	8	0.7	1.8 (↓)	21.4 (↑)	− 150 (↓)	− 1.5 (↑)	55%
2 years	8	−8	8	0.6	1.0 (↓)	13.3 (N)	−64 (↓)	−1 (N)	48%
3 years	5	−7	8	0.5	0.6 (↓)	10.0 (↓)	−35 (↓)	−0.7 ↓	35%

From the beginning and throughout follow-up a low DP is an indicator of myocardial dysfunction, with normal LVEF. In the baseline diagnosis, a greater TorI and DefI are observed (with respect to the normal values in Table 2), reflecting an increase in myocardial torsion, which compensates to maintain the LVEF. This is not detected by the CTor measure, which appears normal. As the disease progresses, the normalization and subsequent diminishing of TorI and DefI are accompanied by lower LVEF, which reflects the exhaustion of the compensating mechanism. CTor shows less sensitivity in the detection of systolic dysfunction during follow-up
LS Longitudinal Strain, *B-A* Base-Apex distance, *MAPSE* Mitral annular plane systolic excursion, *T* Twist, *CTor* Classic Torsion, *TorI* Torsion Index, *DP* Deformation Product, *DefI* Deformation Index, *LVEF* Left Ventricular Ejection Fraction, *N* normal
↑: Increased, ↓: Diminished

However, MAPSE is not always feasible; namely, in patients with mitral prosthesis or calcification of the mitral annulus. As a result of this limitation, together with the fact that the LS and twist can be visualized with the same speckle tracking technology base, it is preferable to use DefI. In addition, MAPSE and LS do not always occur in parallel, and the latter has already demonstrated itself to be easily measured and to have prognostic capacity when considered in isolation [35–38].

We propose the "Combined Deformation Parameter" (CDP) for the estimation of myocardial function throughout the evaluation of the two fundamental components of contractile mechanics: twist and LS. The CDP consists of two aspects: first of all, the state of myocardial function, evaluated as the "Deformation Product" (Twist x LS), which quantifies the longitudinal deformation and the twist, both of which increase contractility. Secondly, the extent of the involvement of each component in ventricular function is assessed by the DefI quotient (Twist/LS). The different possible combinations are shown in Table 3. The "Deformation Product" may be normal, pseudormal (when its value is maintained at the expense of a compensating increase of the twist), or decreased. When the DP is pseudonormal or decreased, the DefI quotient will provide information on the origin of myocardial impairment in one or both components. These values may be altered before ventricular dysfunction occurs, and so may be of relevance for the early diagnosis and monitoring of some heart diseases.

The CDP may be useful for monitoring cardiopathies characterized by ventricular volume overload, in which LS may not represent the earliest alteration nor be the only alteration. Similarly, just as the study of cardiotoxicity in oncology is mainly based on the evaluation of EF and LS, the CDP may be an asset in the evaluation of transmural myocardial conditions that are not limited to LS.

In this sense, heart failure has also recently been classified according to alterations in the mechanical function of the LV [39]. After having observed anomalous specific patterns of ventricular myocardial mechanics in different subsets of patients with heart failure, an alternative approach has been proposed for its characterization [39, 40]. In this way, heart failure can be classified into three large subgroups: 1. Predominant longitudinal dysfunction; 2. Transmural dysfunction (longitudinal and circumferential); and 3. Predominant circumferential dysfunction. This classification is based on the orientation of the myocardial fibers of the LV, which are arranged obliquely in a double helix shape. Endocardial fibers, which are aligned in a more parallel fashion to the LV long axis, are mainly associated with longitudinal mechanics, while transmural fibers are mainly responsible for circumferential mechanics [41]. The action of the latter is predominant due to its greater radius of action.

Cardiac structural and functional changes during the early stages of heart failure can act as compensatory mechanisms. However, as the disease progresses, these mechanisms are often insufficient. When evaluated in isolation, LS has proven its prognostic capacity [42, 43] as the most important echocardiographic predictor of cardiovascular death and/or heart failure in the PARAMOUNT and TOPCAT trials of patients with heart failure and preserved EF [38, 44]. LVEF and global circumferential strain, the main determinant of ventricular twist, were preserved in the patient population, suggesting it acted as a compensatory mechanism. The echocardiographic characterization of these changes provides a framework for key management decisions [19, 45]. CDP could be useful in this respect due to their capacity to identify and quantify the normality or abnormality of myocardial function and to determine to what extent the different components of the heart are affected.

There is a consensus that future practice needs to adopt a combined approach in which changes in LV rotational mechanics and longitudinal shortening are considered and interpreted together, and normal values will need to be established if this to be possible [10, 19]. We show LV torsion to be a reliable integral measure of the early qualitative and quantitative detection of cardiac dysfunction. A standardized method of calculating LV torsion that is capable of providing reproducible and comparable measurements needs to be adopted before it can be used as a clinical tool for the diagnosis of myocardial dysfunction [17]. Likewise, the integration of complementary parameters of pumping and myocardial function should be considered for a more accurate evaluation of LV systolic function.

Conclusions

The proposed parameters integrate values of twisting and longitudinal shortening. In the present work, we provide reference values obtained in a population of healthy subjects. These parameters allow a complete physiological assessment of cardiac systolic function, and could be used for the early detection and characterization of its alteration.

Limitations

Despite the great advantages offered by 2D-STE, it does have several limitations. It depends on the quality of the image, produces inaccuracies due to planar movement, the quality of the tracking is usually lower at the distal level compared to nearby fields, and frames that are too high or too low are associated with poor tracking. Some limitations are overcome with 3D-STE [46], but a lower temporal resolution, greater susceptibility to image quality in the grey scale and lack of experience are among the remaining challenges.

The sample size is limited so that the new parameters deserve more extensive validation. Maybe a future, multicentre study could provide a definite answer regarding the usefulness of the proposed parameters. Likewise, the value of the new parameters should be validated against other methodologies, such as magnetic resonance imaging.

Abbreviations
B-A: Base-apex distance; CDP: Combined deformation parameter; CTor: Classic torsion; Defl: Deformation index; DP: Deformation product; LS: Longitudinal strain; LVEF: Left ventricular ejection fraction; MAPSE: Mitral annular plane systolic excursion; STE: Speckle tracking echocardiography; TorI: Torsion index

Funding
The authors declare that they have not received payments or assistance for any aspect of the work presented.

Authors' contributions
Manuscript design and plan: VM, IR, JAL. Data recording, data processing, quantification and analysis: VM, IR, ER, DR, JB, CP, NU, MR, JP, JAL. Discussion and synthesis of results: VM, IR, JAL. Manuscript writing: VM, IR, ER. All authors read and approved the final version of the manuscript.

Consent for publication
Not applicable.

Competing interests
Jorge A. Lowenstein has received medical fees for conferences on behalf of General Electric. All other authors declare no competing interest.

Author details
[1]Cardiology Department, Hospital Dr Peset, Valencia, Spain. [2]Cardiodiagnosis Department Medical Research of Buenos Aires, Buenos Aires, Argentina.

References
1. Zaca V, Ballo P, Galderisi M, Mondillo S. Echocardiography in the assessment of left ventricular longitudinal systolic function: current methodology and clinical applications. Heart Fail Rev. 2010;15:23–37.
2. Cameli M, Mondillo S, Solari M, Righini FM, Andrei V, Contaldi C, et al. Echocardiographic assessment of left ventricular systolic function: from ejection fraction to torsion. Heart Fail Rev. 2016;21:77–94.
3. Torrent-Guasp F, Ballester M, Buckberg GD, Carreras F, Flotats A, Carrió I, et al. Spatial orientation of the ventricular muscle band: physiologic contribution and surgical implications. J Thorac Cardiovasc Surg. 2001;122: 389–92.
4. Buckberg G, Hoffman JIE, Mahajan A, Saleh S, Coghlan C. Cardiac mechanics revisited. Circulation. 2008;118:2571–87.
5. Sengupta PP, Krishnamoorthy VK, Korinek J, Narula J, Vannan MA, Lester SJ, et al. Left ventricular form and function revisited: applied translational science to cardiovascular ultrasound imaging. J Am Soc Echocardiogr. 2007; 20:539–51.
6. Carreras F, García-Barnes J, Gil D, Pujadas S, Li Chi H, Suarez-Arias R, et al. Left ventricular torsion and longitudinal shortening: two fundamental components of myocardial mechanics assessed by tagged cine-MRI in normal subjects. Int J Cardiovasc Imaging. 2012;28:273–84.
7. Mondillo S, Galderisi M, Mele D, Cameli M, Lomoriello VS, Zaca V, et al. Echocardiography study group of the Italian society of C. Speckle tracking echocardiography: a new technique for assessing myocardial function. J Ultrasound Med. 2011;30:71–83.
8. Van Dalen BM, Soliman OI, Vletter WB, Kauer F, van der Zwaan HB, ten Cate FJ, Geleijnse ML. Feasibility and reproducibility of left ventricular rotation parameters measured by speckle tracking echocardiography. Eur J Echocardiogr. 2009;10:669–76.
9. Leitman M, Lysyansky P, Sidenko S, Shir V, Peleg E, Binenbaum M, Kaluski E, Krakover R, Vered Z. Two dimensional strain a novel software for real-time quantitative echocardiographic assessment of myocardial function. J Am Soc Echocardiogr. 2004;17:1021–9.
10. Teske AJ, De Boeck BW, Melman PG, Sieswerda GT, Doevendans PA, Cramer MJ. Echocardiographic quantification of myocardial function using tissue deformation imaging, a guide to image acquisition and analysis using tissue Doppler and speckle tracking. Cardiovasc Ultrasound. 2007;5:27.
11. Hansen DE, Daughters GT, Alderman EL, Ingels NB, Miller DC. Torsional deformation of the left ventricular midwall in human hearts with intramyocardial markers. Circ Res. 1988;62:941–52.
12. Ingels NB, Hansen DE, Daughters GT, Stinson EB, Alderman EL, Miller DC. Relation between longitudinal, circumferential, and oblique shortening and torsional deformation in the left ventricle of the transplanted human heart. Circ Res. 1989;64:915–27.
13. Axel L, Dougherty L. MR imaging of motion with spatial modulation of magnetization. Radiology. 1989;171:841–5.
14. Zerhouni EA, Parish DM, Rogers WJ, Yang A, Shapiro EP. Human heart: tagging with MR imaging. Radiology. 1988;169:59–63.
15. Helle-Valle T, Crosby J, Edvardsen T, et al. New noninvasive method for assessment of left ventricular rotation: speckle tracking echocardiography. Circulation. 2005;112:3149–56.
16. Notomi Y, Lysyansky P, Setser RM, et al. Measurement of ventricular torsion by two-dimensional ultrasound speckle tracking imaging. J Am Coll Cardiol. 2005;45:2034–41.
17. Russel IK, Götte MJW, Bronzwaer JG, Knaapen P, Paulus WJ, Van Rossum AC. Left ventricular torsion. An expanding role in the analysis of myocardial dysfunction. J Am Coll Cardiol Img. 2009;2:648–55.
18. Arts T, Meerbaum S, Reneman RS, Corday E. Torsion of the left ventricle during the ejection phase in the intact dog. Cardiovasc Res. 1984;18:183–93.
19. Van Mil AC, Drane A, Pearson J, McDonnell B, Cockcroft JR, Stöhr EJ. Interaction of LV twist with arterial haemodynamics during localised, non-

metabolic hyperaemia with and without blood flow restriction. Exp Physiol. 2016;101:509–20.

20. Sthör EJ, Shave RE, Baggish AL, Weiner RB. Left ventricular twist mechanics in the context of normal physiology and cardiovascular disease: a review of studies using speckle tracking echocardiography. Am J Physiol Heart Circ Physiol. 2016;311:H633–44.

21. Suffoletto MS, Dohi K, Cannesson M, Saba S, Gorcsan J. Novel speckle-tracking radial strain from routine black and white echocardiographic images to quantify dyssynchrony and predict response to cardiac resynchronization therapy. Circulation. 2006;113:960–8.

22. Geyer H, Caracciolo G, Abe H, Wilansky S, Carerj S, Gentile F, et al. Assessment of myocardial mechanics using speckle tracking echocardiography: fundamentals and clinical applications. J Am Soc Echocardiogr. 2010;23:351–69.

23. Torrent-Guasp F, Buckberg GD, Clemente C, Cox JL, Coghlan HC, Gharib M. The structure and function of the helical heart and its buttress wrapping. I. The normal macroscopic structure of the heart. Semin Thorac Cardiovasc Surg. 2001;13(4):301–19.

24. Torrent-Guasp F, Kocica MJ, Corno AF, Komeda M, Carreras-Costa F, Flotats A, et al. Towards new understanding of the heart structure and function. Eur J Cardiothorac Surg. 2005;27(2):191–201.

25. Arts T, Reneman RS, Veenstra PC. A model of the mechanics of the left ventricle. Ann Biomed Eng. 1979;7(3–4):299–318.

26. Cutrì E, Serrani M, Bagnoli P, Fumero R, Costantino ML. The cardiac torsion as a sensitive index of heart pathology: a model study. J Mech Behav Biomed Mater. 2010;55:104–19.

27. Torrent Guasp F. Sobre morfología y funcionalismo cardiacos (partes I, II y III). Rev Esp Cardiol. 1966;19:48–55. 56–71, 72–82

28. Moon MR, Ingels NB Jr, Daughters GT, Stinson EB, Hansen DE, Miller DC. Alterations in left ventricular twist mechanics with inotropic stimulation and volume loading in human subjects. Circulation. 1994;89:142–50.

29. Wang J, Khoury DS, Yue Y, Torre-Amione G, Nagueh SF. Preserved left ventricular twist and circumferential deformation, but depressed longitudinal and radial deformation in patients with diastolic heart failure. Eur Heart J. 2008;29:1283–9.

30. Marcelli E, Cercenelli L, Musaico M, Bagnoli P, Costantino ML, Fumero R, Plicchi G. Assessment of cardiac rotation by means of gyroscopic sensors. In: Comput Cardiol. 2008;35:389–92.

31. Esch BT, Warburton DER. Left ventricular torsion and recoil: implications for exercise performance and cardiovascular disease. J Appl Physiol. 2009;106(2):362–9.

32. Cutrì E, Bagnoli P, Marcelli E, Biondi F, Cercenelli L, Costantino ML, et al. A mechanical simulator of cardiac wall kinematics. ASAIO J. 2010;56(3):164–71.

33. Sorger JM, Wyman BT, Faris OP, Hunter WC, McVeigh ER. Torsion of the left ventricle during pacing with MRI tagging. J Cardiovasc Magn Reson. 2003;5:521–30.

34. Aelen FWL, Arts T, Sanders DGM, et al. Relation between torsion and cross-sectional area change in the human left ventricle. J Biomech. 1997;30:207–12.

35. Mondillo S, Galderisi M, Ballo P, Marino PN. Study Group of Echocardiography of the Italian Society of C. Left ventricular systolic longitudinal function: comparison among simple M-mode, pulsed, and M-mode color tissue Doppler of mitral annulus in healthy individuals. J Am Soc Echocardiogr 2006;19:1085–91.

36. Yuda S, Inaba Y, Fujii S, Kokubu N, Yoshioka T, Sakurai S et al. Assessment of left ventricular ejection fraction using long-axis systolic function is independent of image quality: a study of tissue Doppler imaging and M-mode echocardiography. Echocardiography 2006;23:846–52.

37. Shah AM, Claggett B, Sweitzer NK, Shah SJ, Anand IS, Liu L, et al. Prognostic importance of impaired systolic function in heart failure with preserved ejection fraction and the impact of spironolactone. Circulation. 2015;132:402–14.

38. Kraigher-Krainer E, Shah AM, Gupta DK, Santos A, Claggett B, Pieske B, et al. Impaired systolic function by strain imaging in heart failure with preserved ejection fraction. J Am Coll Cardiol. 2014;63:447–56.

39. Sengupta PP, Narula J. Reclassifying heart failure: predominantly subendocardial, subepicardial, and transmural. Heart Fail Clin. 2008;4:379–82.

40. Claus P, Omar AM, Pedrizzetti G, Sengupta PP, Nagel E. Tissue tracking technology for assessing cardiac mechanics: principles, normal values, and clinical applications. JACC Cardiovasc Imaging. 2015;8:1444–60.

41. Omar AMS, Bansal M, Sengupta PP. Advances in echocardiographic imaging in heart failure with reduced and preserved ejection fraction. Circ Res. 2016;119:357–74.

42. Hasselberg NE, Haugaa KH, Sarvari SI, Gullestad L, Andreassen AK, Smiseth OA, Edvardsen T. Left ventricular global longitudinal strain is associated with exercise capacity in failing hearts with preserved and reduced ejection fraction. Eur Heart J Cardiovasc Imaging. 2015;16:217–24.

43. Stampehl MR, Mann DL, Nguyen JS, Cota F, Colmenares C, Dokainish H. Speckle strain echocardiography predicts outcome in patients with heart failure with both depressed and preserved left ventricular ejection fraction. Echocardiography. 2015;32:71–8.

44. Komajda M, Lam CS. Heart failure with preserved ejection fraction: a clinical dilemma. Eur Heart J. 2014;35:1022–32.

45. Tribouilloy C, Rusinaru D, Mahjoub H, Goissen T, Lévy F, Peltier M. Impact of echocardiography in patients hospitalized for heart failure: a prospective observational study. Arch Cardiovasc Dis. 2008;101:465–73.

46. Pedrizzetti G, Sengupta S, Caracciolo G, Park CS, Amaki M, Goliasch G, et al. Three-dimensional principal strain analysis for characterizing subclinical changes in left ventricular function. J Am Soc Echocardiogr. 2014;27:1041–50.

20

Quality control of B-lines analysis in stress Echo 2020

Maria Chiara Scali[17,40], Quirino Ciampi[1,2*], Eugenio Picano[1], Eduardo Bossone[18], Francesco Ferrara[18], Rodolfo Citro[3], Paolo Colonna[4], Marco Fabio Costantino[5], Lauro Cortigiani[6], Antonello D'. Andrea[7], Sergio Severino[7], Claudio Dodi[8], Nicola Gaibazzi[9], Maurizio Galderisi[10], Andrea Barbieri[11], Ines Monte[12], Fabio Mori[13], Barbara Reisenhofer[14], Federica Re[15], Fausto Rigo[16], Paolo Trambaiolo[19], Miguel Amor[20], Jorge Lowenstein[21], Pablo Martin Merlo[21], Clarissa Borguezan Daros[22], José Luis de Castro e Silva Pretto[23], Marcelo Haertel Miglioranza[24], Marco A. R. Torres[25], Clarissa Carmona de Azevedo Bellagamba[25], Daniel Quesada Chaves[26], Iana Simova[27], Albert Varga[28], Jelena Čelutkienė[29], Jaroslaw D. Kasprzak[30], Karina Wierzbowska-Drabik[30], Piotr Lipiec[30], Paulina Weiner-Mik[30], Eva Szymczyk[30], Katarzyna Wdowiak-Okrojek[30], Ana Djordjevic-Dikic[31], Milica Dekleva[32], Ivan Stankovic[33], Aleksandar N. Neskovic[33], Angela Zagatina[34], Giovanni Di Salvo[35], Julio E. Perez[36], Ana Cristina Camarozano[37], Anca Irina Corciu[38], Alla Boshchenko[39], Fabio Lattanzi[40], Carlos Cotrim[41], Paula Fazendas[42], Maciej Haberka[43], Bozena Sobkowic[44], Wojciech Kosmala[45], Tomasz Witkowski[45], Piotr Gosciniak[46], Alessandro Salustri[47], Hugo Rodriguez-Zanella[48], Luis Ignacio Martin Leal[40], Alexandra Nikolic[49], Suzana Gligorova[50], Madalina-Loredana Urluescu[51], Maria Fiorino[52], Giuseppina Novo[53], Tamara Preradovic-Kovacevic[54], Miodrag Ostojic[49,54], Branko Beleslin[31], Bruno Villari[2], Michele De Nes[1], Marco Paterni[1], Clara Carpeggiani[1] and on behalf of Stress Echo 2020 study group of the Italian Society of Echocardiography and Cardiovascular Imaging (SIECVI)

Abstract

Background: The effectiveness trial "Stress echo (SE) 2020" evaluates novel applications of SE in and beyond coronary artery disease. The core protocol also includes 4-site simplified scan of B-lines by lung ultrasound, useful to assess pulmonary congestion.

Purpose: To provide web-based upstream quality control and harmonization of B-lines reading criteria.

Methods: 60 readers (all previously accredited for regional wall motion, 53 B-lines naive) from 52 centers of 16 countries of SE 2020 network read a set of 20 lung ultrasound video-clips selected by the Pisa lab serving as reference standard, after taking an obligatory web-based learning 2-h module (http://se2020.altervista.org). Each test clip was scored for B-lines from 0 (black lung, A-lines, no B-lines) to 10 (white lung, coalescing B-lines). The diagnostic gold standard was the concordant assessment of two experienced readers of the Pisa lab. The answer of the reader was considered correct if concordant with reference standard reading ±1 (for instance, reference standard reading of 5 B-lines; correct answer 4, 5, or 6). The a priori determined pass threshold was 18/20 (≥ 90%) with R value (intra-class correlation coefficient) between reference standard and recruiting center) > 0.90. Inter-observer agreement was assessed with intra-class correlation coefficient statistics.

(Continued on next page)

* Correspondence: qciampi@gmail.com
[1]CNR, Institute of Clinical Physiology, Biomedicine Department, Pisa, Italy
[2]Cardiology Division, Fatebenefratelli Hospital, Benevento, Italy
Full list of author information is available at the end of the article

(Continued from previous page)

Results: All 60 readers were successfully accredited: 26 (43%) on first, 24 (40%) on second, and 10 (17%) on third attempt. The average diagnostic accuracy of the 60 accredited readers was 95%, with R value of 0.95 compared to reference standard reading. The 53 B-lines naive scored similarly to the 7 B-lines expert on first attempt (90 versus 95%, $p = $ NS). Compared to the step-1 of quality control for regional wall motion abnormalities, the mean reading time per attempt was shorter (17 ± 3 vs 29 ± 12 min, $p < .01$), the first attempt success rate was higher (43 vs 28%, $p < 0.01$), and the drop-out of readers smaller (0 vs 28%, $p < .01$).

Conclusions: Web-based learning is highly effective for teaching and harmonizing B-lines reading. Echocardiographers without previous experience with B-lines learn quickly.

Keywords: Certification, Lung comets, Quality control, Stress echocardiography, Wall motion

Background

Stress echocardiography (SE) has some advantages over competing imaging techniques, including low cost, portability, radiation-free nature and versatility. Its major limitation is the dependence upon operator's expertise, which may impact on the quality and consistency of diagnostic results [1, 2]. This limitation is magnified when the technique is used for scientific purposes in a multi-center trial such as Stress Echo 2020 (SE2020) study, designed to provide effectiveness data in 10,000 patients from > 100 laboratories in a variety of conditions ranging from coronary artery disease to heart failure (with preserved or depressed ejection fraction), hypertrophic cardiomyopathy, repaired congenital heart disease, valvular heart disease and extreme physiology [3]. To achieve harmonization, one possible approach is the use of the core lab which analyses centrally images sent from all recruiting sites. This approach is typically the preferred choice in a clinical trial and minimizes the sources of measurement variability [4, 5]. The core lab option was discarded in SE 2020 for two reasons. First, it was too costly and logistically demanding. Second, it would provide efficacy data under ideal conditions, but our aim was to obtain effectiveness data realistically generated when the technique is deployed in the clinical arena, populated by real patients, real doctors and real problems [6]. A feasible approach to ensure consistency in data acquisition and interpretation in this challenging setting is to develop an upstream reading quality control for prospective centers willing to enter the study [7, 8]. In SE2020, this approach has already been implemented for regional wall motion abnormalities (RWMA), which remains the diagnostic cornerstone of SE [9]. However, a separate quality control needs to be performed for other aspects of contemporary SE practice, such as B-lines obtained with lung ultrasound (LUS) [10]. Also known as ultrasound lung comets, B-lines are a sign of accumulation of extra-vascular lung water [11] and can acutely increase during stress [12–14]. Their presence and/ or increase during stress places the patient in a higher risk subset for any level of RWMA [13] and indicates that

dyspnea is linked to acute backward heart failure [15]. B-lines assessment must be properly standardized and quality-controlled prior to dissemination and use for clinical and scientific purposes. The present report was part of the larger SE2020 study and focuses on the educational aspects of LUS-SE, describing the results of the upstream quality control and harmonization of B-lines reading criteria across 52 SE2020 centers.

Methods

The Pisa lab coordinated the quality control assessment for B-lines of all investigators who expressed their intention to participate in the study (Fig. 1). The coordinating center was in the National Research Council, Institute of Clinical Physiology in Pisa, Italy. The candidate centers included 52 centers (each with at least one certified reader) from 16 countries (Argentina, Brazil, Bulgaria, Costa Rica, Hungary, Italy, Lithuania, Mexico, Poland, Portugal, Romania, Qatar, Russia, Serbia, UK, USA). The selection criterion was that all readers had already passed the quality control for RWMA reading (step 1 in the "Road to SE 2020"). The B-lines reading was the step 2 in the "Road to SE 2020". The complete list of participants in the SE2020 consortium (as per January 20th, 2018) is reported in the Appendix. The study protocol was reviewed and approved by the institutional ethics committee as a part of the SE 2020 study (1487-CE Lazio-1, July 20, 2016). The study was funded with institutional funding of the Italian National Research Council and with travel grants of the Italian Society of Echocardiography and Cardiovascular Imaging with dedicated sessions during national meetings. No fort from industry was asked for or received.

An obligatory web-based educational platform was developed to facilitate the training process. Participating cardiologists were invited by email to join the platform, which was protected by user-specific passwords. The platform includes files and videos with detailed instructions on how to start the training and allows downloading and uploading of external files. The sequence of the certification process and web-based learning has already been

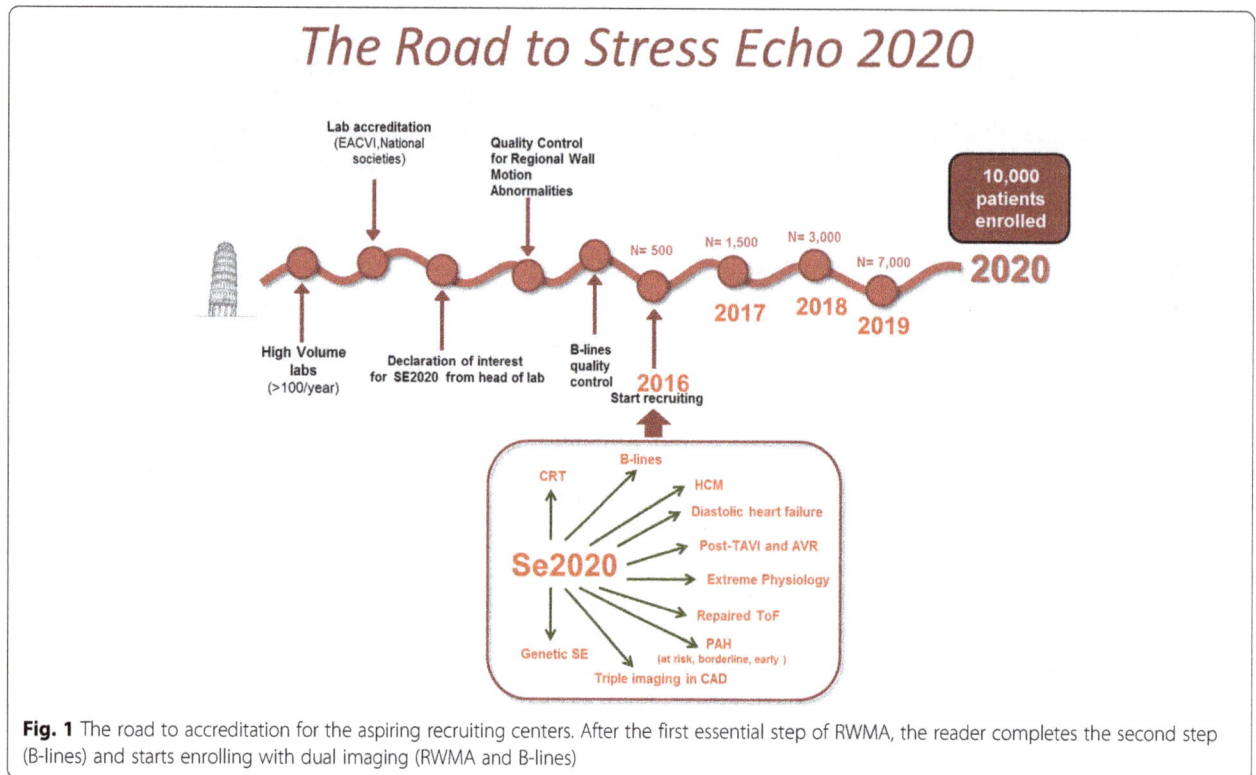

Fig. 1 The road to accreditation for the aspiring recruiting centers. After the first essential step of RWMA, the reader completes the second step (B-lines) and starts enrolling with dual imaging (RWMA and B-lines)

detailed and follows the same template used for RWMA [9]. We decided to have this platform mandatory and not optional as in the step-1 for RWMA, since in case of B-lines the technique is relatively young and recent advances in acquisition (with 4-site scan mode) and reporting were adopted in the SE2020 platform [16].

Study population of readers

Sixty readers from 52 different centers initially asked to enter the SE2020 study, had passed the RWMA test for quality control and therefore were allowed to enter the step-2 of SE2020.

All participants were clinical cardiologists and expert echocardiographers with ongoing high volume (> 100 tests per year) SE activity and the years of experience in SE ranged from 5 to 31 years (mean value 18 years). All were certified by national and/or international societies .

Lung ultrasound acquisition

To acquire lung ultrasound (LUS) images adopted for quality control test, we used commercially available ultrasound machines (IE 33, Philips, Medical Systems, Andover, Massachusetts, USA with a 2.5–3.5 MHz phased-array sector scan probe; Vivid E9, GE Healthcare, USA, manufactured in Horten, Norway, equipped or standard M5S transducer with second harmonic technology; Mylab Eight platform Esaote, Genova, Italy). The depth was adjusted according to the body habitus of the patient, with thin

patients requiring less depth and obese patients needing greater depth to visualize the pleural line. A B-line was defined with 4 constant criteria: vertical, laser-like, hyperechoic reverberation; arises from the pleural line extending to the bottom of the screen without fading; moves synchronously with lung sliding; and erases the A-lines, which are a part of the normal lung pattern as a horizontal, multiple reverberation artefact, equidistant from one another below the pleura, at exact multiples of the transducer-pleural line distance [17]. Detailed description of the scanning procedure and scanning sites is also available in a 2-min movie from our laboratory on YouTube (The incredible ULCs – ultrasound lung comets. Available at http://www.youtube.com/watch?v=7y_hUFBHStM. Accessed: July 10, 2018). LUS scanning was performed with the cardiac probe in the supine position at rest and soon after stress (with the patient again resuming the supine position). The 4-site simplified scan of the lung was used [16]. We analyzed the anterior and lateral hemithoraces, scanning along the anterior axillary (AA) and midaxillary (MA) lines on the third intercostal space (Fig. 2).

Web-based learning module

The 2-h web-based training module (http://se2020.alter vista.org) consisted of five sequential learning blocks: **a-** Selected readings of 3 recent review or original articles summarizing the evidences supporting the use of B-lines

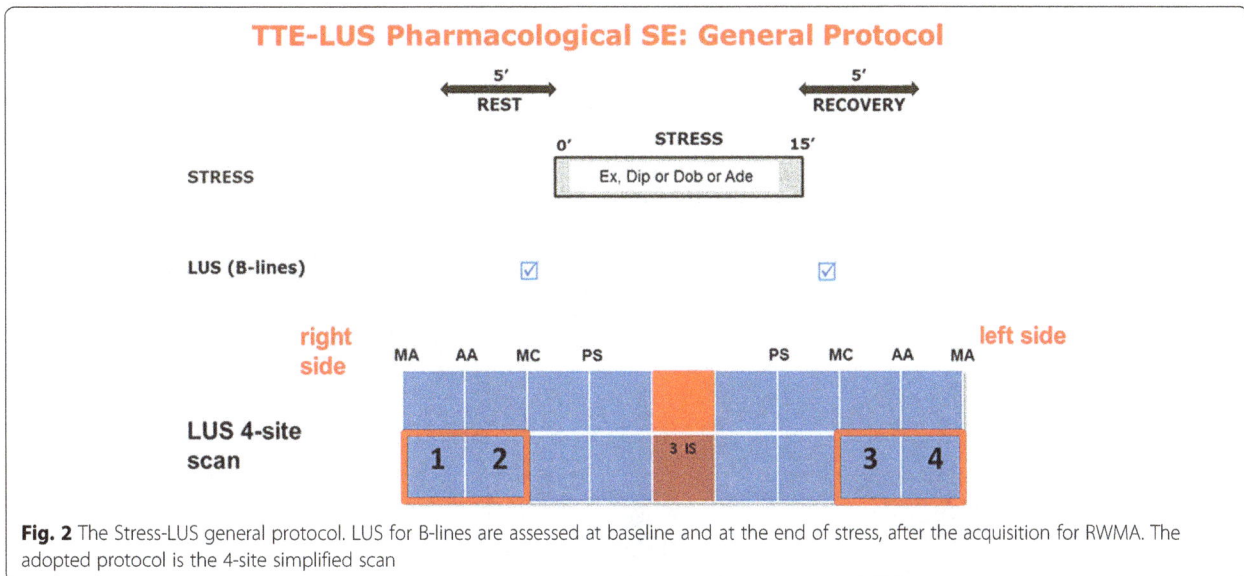

Fig. 2 The Stress-LUS general protocol. LUS for B-lines are assessed at baseline and at the end of stress, after the acquisition for RWMA. The adopted protocol is the 4-site simplified scan

during stress and the adopted scan technique and scoring criteria [8, 10, 13]; **b**- A power-point file of 25 slides summarizing key points and specific literature supporting the proposed reading policy illustrating tips and tricks highlighting the most frequent problems in B-lines interpretation with special focus on the technicalities of the 4-site simplified scanning technique; **c**- A theory self-assessment test with five questions with four answers each (only one correct) preliminary to video-clip reading; **d**- Short (< 15 s) video-clips of examinations with the same format of official test reading, with 5 min per reading with countdown clock, and one possible answer (from 0 to 10) for each video-clip (Fig. 3).

An expert trainer (QC or MCS) remained available to all readers for e-mail or phone contact to provide assistance with any issue concerning the training.

At all times there was the possibility of face-to-face discussion (via Skype) to address issues requiring special clarification with the principal investigator. After completing the web-based module the reader could take the test (maximum three attempts). After each attempt, the sequence of videos was mixed.

Reading sessions and pass threshold

We selected 20 cases of 10 patients (with rest and stress images) in which the presence and number of B-lines was documented by unanimous decision of 2 experienced observers (EP and QC). The privacy of patients during acquisition, storage, and transmission of the SE study was protected. All images were anonymized, and the identity of patients or the study condition (rest or stress) was not disclosed at any time to the readers. Each SE study was structured in a single video-clip of 10–15 s, with either resting or stress images. Each test clip was scored from 0 (black lung, A-lines, no B-lines) to 10

(white lung with coalescing B-lines). The diagnostic gold standard was the reading of Pisa lab. The answer of the reader was considered correct if concordant with reference standard reading ±1 (for instance, reference standard reading of 5 B-lines; correct answer 4, 5, or 6). The a priori determined pass threshold was 18/20 (≥ 90%) with R value of intra-class correlation coefficient > .90.

The LUS images were selected to represent the garden variety of stress testing modes, responses, results and image quality. They came from six different laboratories (Benevento, Lucca, Pisa, Porto Alegre, Rome, St Petersburg) in three countries (Brasil, Italy, Russian Federation), and showed the full spectrum of responses (from 0, $n = 7$; to 10, $n = 1$). All images were considered readable, with quality ranging from average-to-good ($n = 16$) to excellent ($n = 4$) in the assessment of the reference standard reading. The stress employed was exercise in 17 subjects, high dose accelerated dipyridamole (0.84 mg/kg over 6 min) in 2 and dobutamine (40 mcg/kg/min) in 1. The projection selected was the third intercostal space between left mid-axillary and anterior axillary lines in 4; third intercostal space between right mid-axillary and anterior axillary lines in 4; third intercostal space between right anterior-axillary and mid-clavicular lines in 4; third intercostal space between left anterior-axillary and mid-clavicular lines in 8.

After the pass or fail response

The response was pass (≥ 90% accuracy) or fail. With pass, the reader received a certificate of accreditation and could start recruiting with a written informed consent signed by each patient and after clearance by the local ethical committee. With fail, the unsuccessful reader could retake the test after 1 month. After the second fail, the reader could undergo training in a recommended center and try again after 1 year.

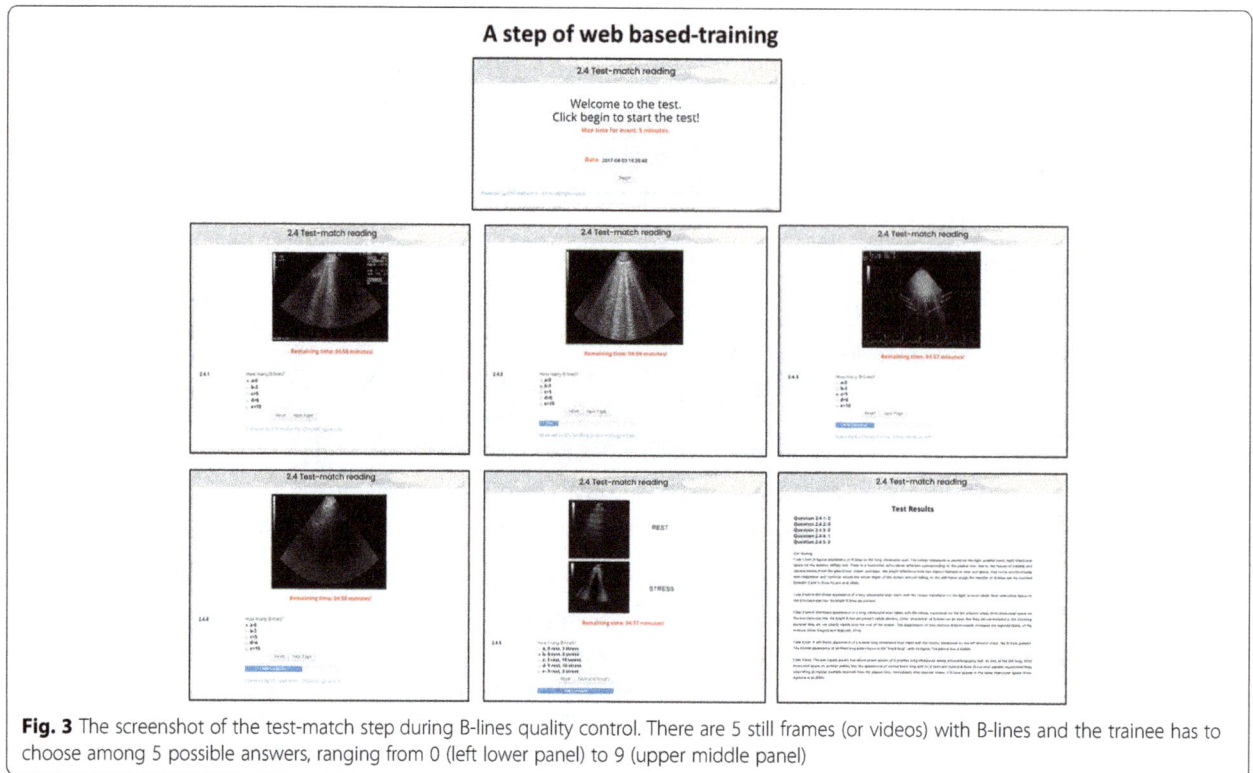

Fig. 3 The screenshot of the test-match step during B-lines quality control. There are 5 still frames (or videos) with B-lines and the trainee has to choose among 5 possible answers, ranging from 0 (left lower panel) to 9 (upper middle panel)

Statistical analysis

Each reader was evaluated against the gold standard of reference standard reading for assessment of individual accuracy (in %). The intra-class correlation coefficient was calculated, for each reader, in the whole series of 20 paired measurements made by the peripheral reader and the reference reader. Intra-observer agreement was tested in 20 peripheral readers who volunteered to repeat the measurement session after at least 3 months from the first reading. A p value < 0.05 was considered significant.

Results

Of the initial 60 readers who started, 53 were B-lines naive (without previous exposure to B-lines). All 60 readers were successfully accredited (Fig. 4): 26 (43%) on first, 24 (40%) on second, and 10 (17%) on third attempt. The 53 B-lines naive scored similarly to the 7 B-lines expert on first attempt (90 versus 95%, p = NS). Compared to the step-1 of quality control for regional wall motion abnormalities [6], the mean reading time per attempt was shorter (17 ± 3 vs 29 ± 12 min, p < .01), the first attempt success rate was higher (43 vs 28%, p < 0.01), and the drop-out of readers smaller (0 vs 28%, p < .01). The average diagnostic accuracy of the 60 accredited readers was 95%. Considering the final attempt of the 60 readers, the Spearman correlation coefficient between the expert reference reading and the reading of each peripheral reader

was very high (R = 0.95, p < .0001). In the 20 peripheral readers who repeated the test a second time at least 3 months after accreditation, the Spearman correlation coefficient was also very high (R = 0.97, p < .0001).

Discussion

A user-friendly web-based learning is highly effective for training B-lines also for echocardiographers without previous exposure to B-lines. After a limited learning effort, the accuracy of B-lines reading is comparable between very experienced and freshly trained readers. B-lines with 4-site simplified scan of the lung has a very high success rate in acquisition and analysis. It has been embedded as an integral part of dual imaging SE adopted as the core protocol in SE2020 for all forms of physical and pharmacological stress for all patients, from coronary artery disease to heart failure.

Comparison with previous studies

The American College of Chest Physicians has defined the knowledge and technical elements required for competence in lung ultrasound [18]. There have been a number of prior lung ultrasound education papers, showing that a limited training of a few hours can improve the capability of execution and interpretation of LUS even in medical students without previous exposure to ultrasound [19, 20]. In the present study we are dealing with a specific and limited aspect of LUS of special

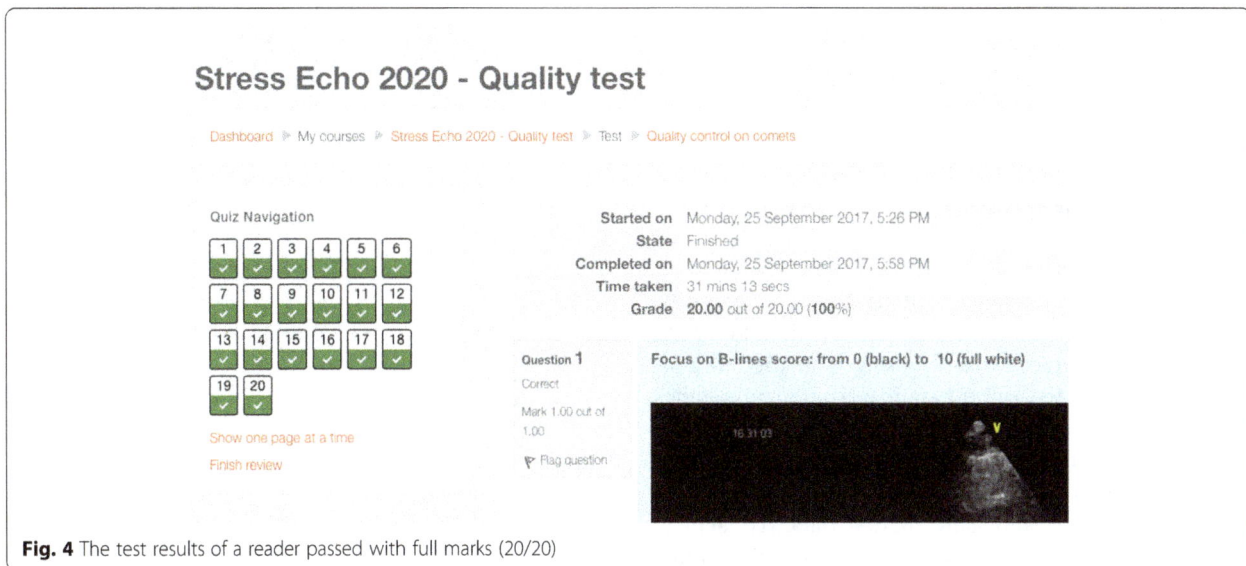

Stress Echo 2020 - Quality test

Dashboard ► My courses ► Stress Echo 2020 - Quality test ► Test ► Quality control on comets

Quiz Navigation

1	2	3	4	5	6
7	8	9	10	11	12
13	14	15	16	17	18
19	20

Show one page at a time

Finish review

Started on   Monday, 25 September 2017, 5:26 PM
State   Finished
Completed on   Monday, 25 September 2017, 5:58 PM
Time taken   31 mins 13 secs
Grade   20.00 out of 20.00 (100%)

Question 1

Correct

Mark 1.00 out of 1.00

⚑ Flag question

Focus on B-lines score: from 0 (black) to 10 (full white)

Fig. 4 The test results of a reader passed with full marks (20/20)

interest for cardiologists, i.e. the detection of B-lines. There is a lack of a specific training and certification pathway in cardiology, and as a result training and performance of LUS varies widely among different institutions. An approach similar to the one adopted in the present study was developed in Pisa for centers recruiting in the LUST study [21]. However, this study differs from the previous one under some aspects: first, it was focused on LUS-SE, not on resting LUS; the adopted scan scheme was the simplified 4-site scan, easier to do, to teach and to learn than the previously adopted 28-site scan; and the quality control procedures required some prior reading and slide presentation to facilitate a standardized learning [9].

Our findings are consistent with a large body of literature showing that stable web applications are increasingly used for improving medical image interpretation skills regardless of time and space and without the need for expensive imaging equipment or a patient to scan [22]. With the adopted web-based approach, the educational path is standardized, shared, and - after validation and refinement - prospectively available in open source, and exploitable for scientific purposes and clinical education. The use of enabling technologies makes the accreditation process faster, smoother and cheaper, and coupled with the open-source platform grants an unprecedented opportunity for continuing education, also fostered by endorsement and governance by the scientific society supporting the study.

Study limitations
We focused on the assessment of B-lines, which is a particularly simple aspect of LUS diagnosis [10, 11]. Similar harmonization and accreditation issues are present for other aspects of SE diagnosis. Separate and parallel training

modules are currently under construction within the framework of "SE 2020" to cover the entire spectrum of key aspects of SE diagnosis, from coronary flow velocity reserve to left ventricular volumes and pulmonary hemodynamics [3].

A key aspect in the evaluation of SE results is the adoption of an undisputed diagnostic "gold standard". The lack of a universally acceptable gold standard makes the assessment of reading performance difficult. From the library of images arriving from all the world and stored in our data bank, we selected cases meeting the conditions of unanimous reading of the two most experienced readers from the reference lab. This is a far from perfect gold standard, yet a reasonable, and perhaps the only possible, one.

We restricted our validation phase to participants in the SE2020 study, who had a substantial reading experience and certification in RWMA as a prerequisite. This reader pool may have been especially knowledgeable and motivated, thereby justifying the excellent learning results. However, 53 of them were B-lines naive, and therefore probably the selection criteria of our readers did not affect the generalizability of results.

We adopted a simplified 4-site scan for acquisition of B-lines at rest and during stress. This approach introduces a substantial abbreviation compared to other protocols such as the 28-region scan originally adopted in the Pisa laboratory in the first application of LUS in heart failure patients [23] and also recommended by an international consensus in 2012 [24]. Over the years, simplified 8-zone and 4-zone lung imaging protocols were proposed [25, 26], with comparable information between the 2 protocols as shown by Platz et al. [25]. Scali et al. showed that the simplified 4-site scan allows to complete the assessment of B-lines in 20 s (instead of the 3 min required by the 28- region scan). There is a linear, close correlation between the 28-site and the 4-site B-lines score [16]. Therefore, there is no significant loss of information when going from 28- to 4-site scan, but a substantial simplification and time saving, vital for SE imaging, when there are so many things to see and so little time available.

Clinical implications

B-lines are a useful adjunct to mainstream SE based on RWMA [27, 28], but its impact may be limited by the relatively few centers currently using it in their routine SE practice, and the lack of standardization in acquisition, scoring and reporting [29]. After a web-based module and certification, the approach is better harmonized and the accumulation of clinical practice also allows the rapid growth of scientifically unique data. To achieve this goal, simplification is essential, and the 4-site simplified scan is ideal for LUS rest and stress testing.

However, the SE technique does not tolerate improvisation, and an accurate standardization of terminology, standards of execution, and interpretation criteria is required before a center is allowed to enter its experience in the common data bank. Similarly to what has been said for meta-analysis [30], multicenter SE studies are like a bouillabaisse: no matter how much seafood (or recruiting centers) is added, one tainted fish (an unreliable center generating inconsistent reading) will spoil the pot.

Conclusion

Web-based learning is highly effective for teaching and harmonizing B-lines reading, with an enormous saving of time and resources versus the conventional hands-on approach of teaching and learning ultrasound techniques. Echocardiographers without previous experience with B-lines learn quickly.

Abbreviations
CAD: Coronary artery disease; LUS: Lung Ultrasound; RWMA: Regional wall motion abnormalities; SE: Stress echocardiography; TE: Transthoracic echocardiography

Acknowledgments
The study was partially funded with the project Aging of the National Research Council.
On behalf of the Stress Echo 2020 Study Group of the Italian Society of Cardiovascular Echography (as per December 20, 2017). Eugenio Picano[1], Maria Grazia Andreassi[1], Clara Carpeggiani[1], Michele De Nes[1], Marco Paterni[1], Lorenza Pratali[1], Quirino Ciampi[2], Bruno Villari[2], Eduardo Bossone[3], Rodolfo Citro[3], Francesco Ferrara[3], Paolo Colonna[4], Marco Fabio Costantino[5], Lauro Cortigiani[6], Antonello D'Andrea[7-1], Claudio Dodi[8], Nicola Gaibazzi[9], Maurizio Galderisi[10], Andrea Barbieri[11], Ines Monte[12], Fabio Mori[13], Iacopo Olivotto[13], Barbara Reisenhofer [14], Federica Re[15], Fausto Rigo[16], Maria Chiara Scali[17,41], Sergio Severino[7-2], Paolo Trambaiolo[19], Miguel Amor[20], Jorge Lowenstein[21], Pablo Martin Merlo[21], Clarissa Borguezan Daros[22], José Luis de Castro e Silva Pretto[23], Marcelo H. Miglioranza[24], Marco A.R. Torres[25], Daniel Quesada Chaves[26], Melissa Rodriguez Israel[26], Iana Simova[27], Albert Varga [28], Gergely Agoston [28], Attila Palinkas [28], Jelena Čelutkienė[29], Jaroslaw D. Kasprzak[30], Karina Wierzbowska-Drabik[30], Ana Djordjevic-Dikic[31], Branko Beleslin [31], Milica Dekleva[32], Aleksandar N. Neskovic[33], Ivan Stankovic[33], Angela Zagatina[34],

Giovanni di Salvo[35], Julio E. Perez [36], Ana Camarozano [37], Anca Corciu[38], Alla Boshchenko[39], Fabio Lattanzi[40], Carlos Cotrim[41], Paula Fazendas[42], Maciej Haberka[43], Bozena Sobkowicz[44], Wojciech Kosmala [45], Tomasz Witkowski[45], Piotr Gosciniak [46], Alessandro Salustri [47], Hugo Rodriguez Zanella[48], Alexandra Nikolic[49], Suzana Gligorova [50], Madalina-Loredana Urluescu [51], Maria Fiorino [52], Giuseppina Novo[53], Tamara Preradovic-Kovacevic[54], Miodrag Ostojic[33, 54], Dario Gregori[55].
[1]Institute of Clinical Physiology, National Research Council, Pisa; [2]Cardiology Division, Fatebenefratelli Hospital, Benevento, Italy; [3]Cardiology Department and Echocardiography Lab, University Hospital "San Giovanni di Dio e Ruggi d'Aragona", Salerno, Italy; [4]Cardiology Hospital, Policlinico of Bari, Italy; [5]Cardiology Department, San Carlo Hospital, Potenza, Italy; [6]Cardiology Department, San Luca Hospital, Lucca, Italy; [7]Cardiology Department, Monaldi Hospital, Second University of Naples, Italy; [8]Casa di Cura Figlie di San Camillo, Cremona, Italy; [9]Cardiology Department, Parma University Hospital, Italy; [10]Department of Advanced Biomedical Sciences, Federico II University Hospital, Naples, Italy; [11]Cardiology Department, Modena University Hospital, Modena, Italy; [12]Cardio-Thorax-Vascular Department, Echocardiography lab, "Policlinico Vittorio Emanuele", Catania University, Italy; [13]Cardiology Department, Careggi Hospital, Florence, Italy; [14]Cardiology Division, Pontedera-Volterra Hospital, ASL Toscana 3 Nord-Ovest, Italy; [15]Cardiology Department, San Camillo-Forlanini Hospital, Roma, Italy; [16]Cardiology Department, Ospedale dell'Angelo Mestre-Venice, Italy; [17]Cardiology Department, Nottola Hospital, Siena, and Cardiothoracic Department, University of Pisa, Italy; [18]Cardiology Department, Ospedale Santa Maria Incoronata dell' Olmo, Cava de' Tirreni, Salerno, Italy; [19]Department of Cardiology, Sandro Pertini Hospital, Rome, Italy; [20]Cardiology Department, Ramos Mejia Hospital, Buenos Aires, Argentina; [21]Cardiodiagnosticos, Investigaciones Medicas, Buenos Aires, Argentina; [22]Cardiology Division, Hospital San José, Criciuma, Brasil; [23]Hospital Sao Vicente de Paulo e Hospital de Cidade, Passo Fundo, Brasil; [24]Cardiology Institute of Rio Grande do Sul, Porto Alegre, Brasil; [25]Hospital de Clinicas de Porto Alegre - Universidade Federal do Rio Grande do Sul, Porto Alegre, Brasil; [26]Hospital San Vicente de Paul, Heredia, Costa Rica; [27]Acibadem City Clinic Cardiovascular Center, University Hospital, Sofia, Bulgaria; [28]Institute of Family Medicine, University of Szeged, and Department of Internal Medicine, Elisabeth Hospital, Hodmezovasarhely, Hungary; [29]Centre of Cardiology and Angiology, Vilnius University Hospital Santaros Klinikos, Faculty of Medicine, Vilnius University, State Research Institute for Innovative Medicine, Vilnius, Lithuania; [30]Chair of Cardiology, Bieganski Hospital, Medical University, Lodz Poland; [31]Cardiology Clinic, Clinical Center of Serbia, Medical School, University of Belgrade, Serbia; [32]Clinical Hospital Zvezdara Belgrade, Serbia; [33]Department of Cardiology, Clinical Hospital Center Zemun, Faculty of Medicine, University of Belgrade, Serbia; [34]Cardiology Department, University Clinic, Saint Petersburg, Russian Federation; [35]Pediatric Cardiology Department, Brompton Hospital, London, UK, Division of Cardiology; [36]Washington University School of Medicine, Barnes-Jewish Hospital, St. Louis, Missouri, USA; [37]Hospital de Clinicas UFPR, Medicine Department, Federal University of Paraná, Curitiba, Brasil; [38]Department of Cardiology, IRCCS Policlinico San Donato Clinic, Milan, Italy; [39]Cardiology Research Institute, Tomsk National Tomsk National Research Medical Center of Russian Academy of Sciences; [40]Cardiothoracic Department, University of Pisa, Italy; [41]Heart Center, Hospital da Cruz Vermelha, Lisbon, and Medical School of University of Algarve, Faro, Portugal; [42]Cardiology Department, Hospital Garcia de Orta, Almada, Portugal; [43]Department of Cardiology, School of Health Sciences, Medical University of Silesia, Katowice, Poland; [44]Department of Cardiology, Medical University of Białystok, Poland; [45]Department of Cardiology, Wroclaw Medical University, Wroclaw, Poland; [46]Department of Cardiology, Provincial Hospital, Szczecin, Poland; [47]Hamad Medical Corporation, Heart Hospital, Doha, Qatar; [48]Instituto Nacional de Cardiologia Ignacio Chavez, Mexico City, Mexico; [49]Institute for Cardiovascular Diseases Dedinje, Belgrade, Serbia; [50]Cardiology Division Ospedale Casilino, Roma Italy; [51]Cardiology Department, County Hospital Sibiu, Invasive and Non-Invasive Center for Cardiac and Vascular Pathology in Adults - CVASIC Sibiu, Faculty of Medicine Sibiu, Romania; [52]Cardiology Division Ospedale Civico Di Cristina Benfratelli Palermo; [53]Cardiology Division, University Hospital, Palermo, Italy; [54]University Clinical Center, Banja Luka, Republic of Srpska, Bosnia and Herzegovina; [55]Department of Biostatistics, University of Padua, Padua, Italy.

Funding
Institutional funding from CNR Institute of Clinical Physiology.

Authors' contributions

EP is the study chairman, designed the protocol, organized the content of web-based training and drafted the manuscript; QC is the principal investigator of SE2020, helped to organize the structure of training, contributed to developing the web-based training, critically revised the manuscript for an intellectually important contribution and approved the submitted version; McS is the project leader of B-lines subproject in SE2020; MdN is the computer scientist who developed the website (SE 2020) and the web-based training material; MP is the computer scientist who organized and governed the quality control access, results, and data analysis; all other authors contributed to study design, undertook the quality control up to certification, are active members of SE 2020 consortium and critically revised the manuscript for an intellectually important contribution and approved the submitted version. RC and PC also coordinated the involvement of SIECVI (Società Italiana di Ecocardiografia e Cardiovascular Imaging). CC is responsible for data quality control and reader's certification.

Consent for publication

All the authors have read and approved the manuscript and accorded the consent for pubblication.

Competing interests

The authors declare that they have no competing interest.

Author details

[1]CNR, Institute of Clinical Physiology, Biomedicine Department, Pisa, Italy. [2]Cardiology Division, Fatebenefratelli Hospital, Benevento, Italy. [3]Cardiology Department and Echocardiography Lab, University Hospital "San Giovanni di Dio e Ruggi d'Aragona", Salerno, Italy. [4]Cardiology Hospital, Policlinico of Bari, Bari, Italy. [5]Cardiology Department, San Carlo Hospital, Potenza, Italy. [6]Cardiology Department, San Luca Hospital, Lucca, Italy. [7]Cardiology Department, Echocardiography Lab, Monaldi Hospital, Second University of Naples, Naples, Italy. [8]Casa di Cura Figlie di San Camillo, Cremona, Italy. [9]Cardiology Department, Parma University Hospital, Parma, Italy. [10]Department of Advanced Biomedical Sciences, Federico II University Hospital, Naples, Italy. [11]Cardiology Department, Modena University Hospital, Modena, Italy. [12]Cardio-Thorax-Vascular Department, Echocardiography lab, Policlinico Vittorio Emanuele, University of Catania, Catania, Italy. [13]Cardiology Department, Careggi Hospital, Florence, Italy. [14]Cardiology Division, Pontedera-Volterra Hospital, ASL Toscana 3 Nord-Ovest, Florence, Italy. [15]Cardiology Department, San Camillo-Forlanini Hospital, Rome, Italy. [16]Cardiology Department, Ospedale dell'Angelo Mestre-Venice, Venice, Italy. [17]Cardiology Department, Nottola Hospital, Siena, Italy. [18]Cardiology Department, Ospedale santa Maria Incoronata dell'Olmo, cava de' Tirreni, Salerno, Italy. [19]Department of Cardiology, Sandro Pertini Hospital, Rome, Italy. [20]Cardiology Department, Ramos Mejia Hospital, Buenos Aires, Argentina. [21]Cardiodiagnosticos, Investigaciones Medicas, Buenos Aires, Argentina. [22]Cardiology Division, Hospital San José, Criciuma, Brasília, Brazil. [23]Hospital Sao Vicente de Paulo e Hospital de Cidade, Passo Fundo, Brazil. [24]Cardiology Institute of Rio Grande do Sul, Porto Alegre, Brazil. [25]Hospital de Clinicas de Porto Alegre - Universidade Federal do Rio Grande do Sul, Porto Alegre, Brazil. [26]Hospital San Vicente de Paul, Heredia, Costa Rica. [27]Acibadem City Clinic Cardiovascular Center, University Hospital, Sofia, Bulgaria. [28]Institute of Family Medicine, University of Szeged, Szeged, Hungary. [29]Centre of Cardiology and Angiology, Vilnius University Hospital Santaros Klinikos, Faculty of Medicine, Vilnius University, State Research Institute for Innovative Medicine, Vilnius, Lithuania. [30]Chair of Cardiology, Bieganski Hospital, Medical University, Lodz, Poland. [31]Cardiology Clinic, Clinical Center of Serbia, Medical School, University of Belgrade, Belgrade, Serbia. [32]Clinical Hospital Zvezdara Belgrade, Belgrade, Serbia. [33]Department of Cardiology, Clinical Hospital Center Zemun, Faculty of Medicine, University of Belgrade, Belgrade, Serbia. [34]Cardiology Department, University Hospital, Saint Petersburg, Russian Federation. [35]Pediatric Cardiology Department, Brompton Hospital, London, UK. [36]Washington University School of Medicine, Barnes-Jewish Hospital, St. Louis, MO, USA. [37]Hospital de Clinicas UFPR, Medicine Department, Federal University of Paranà, Curitiba, Brazil. [38]Department of Cardiology, IRCCS Policlinico San Donato Clinic, Milan, Italy. [39]Cardiology Research Institute, Tomsk National Research Medical Center of Russian Academy of Sciences, Tomsk, Russia. [40]Cardiothoracic Department, University of Pisa, Pisa, Italy. [41]Heart Center, Hospital da Cruz Vermelha, Lisbon and Medical School of University of Algarve, Faro, Portugal. [42]Cardiology Department, Hospital Garcia de Orta, Almada, Portugal. [43]Department of Cardiology, School of Health Sciences, Medical University of Silesia, Katowice, Poland. [44]Department of Cardiology, Medical University of Białystok, Białystok, Poland. [45]Department of Cardiology, Wroclaw Medical University, Wroclaw, Poland. [46]Department of Cardiology, Provincial Hospital, Szczecin, Poland. [47]Hamad Medical Corporation, Heart Hospital, Doha, Qatar. [48]Instituto Nacional de Cardiologia Ignacio Chavez, Mexico City, Mexico. [49]Institute for Cardiovascular Diseases, Dedinje, Belgrade, Italy. [50]Cardiology Division Ospedale Casilino, Rome, Italy. [51]Cardiology Department, County Hospital Sibiu, Invasive and Non-Invasive Center for Cardiac and Vascular Pathology in Adults - CVASIC Sibiu, Faculty of Medicine, Sibiu, Romania. [52]Cardiology Division Ospedale Civico Di Cristina Benfratelli, Palermo, Italy. [53]Cardiology Division, University Hospital, Palermo, Italy. [54]University Clinical Center, Banja Luka, Republic of Srpska, Bosnia and Herzegovina.

References

1. Pellikka PA, Nagueh SF, Elhendy AA, Kuehl CA, Sawada SG. American Society of Echocardiography recommendations for performance, interpretation, and application of stress echocardiography. J Am Soc Echocardiogr. 2007;20:1021–4.
2. Sicari R, Nihoyannopoulos P, Evangelista A, Kasprzak J, Lancellotti P, Poldermans D. European Association of Echocardiography Stress echocardiography expert consensus statement: European Association of Echocardiography (EAE) (a registered branch of the ESC). Eur J Echocardiogr. 2008;9:415–37.
3. Picano E, Ciampi Q, Citro R, et al. Stress echo 2020 : The international Stress Echo study in ischemic and non-ischemic heart disease Cardiov Ultras 2017 ; Jan 18 15 (1): 3. DOI: https://doi.org/10.1186/s12947-016-0092-1
4. Gottdiener JS, Bednarz J, Devereux R, Gardin J, Klein A, Manning WJ, et al. American Society of Echocardiography. American Society of Echocardiography recommendations for use of echocardiography in clinical trials. J Am Soc Echocardiogr. 2004;17:1086–119.
5. Galderisi M, Henein MY, D' hooge J, Sicari R, Badano LP, Zamorano JL, Roelandt J. Recommendations of the European Association of Echocardiography. How to use echo-Doppler in clinical trials: different modalities for different purposes. Eur J Echocardiogr. 2011;12:339–53.
6. Feinstein AR. Diagnostic and spectral markers. Philadelphia: Clinical epidemiology. Saunders; 1985. p. 597–631.
7. Picano E, Landi P, Bolognese L, Chiarandà G, Chiarella F, Seveso G, et al. Prognostic value of dipyridamole echocardiography early after uncomplicated myocardial infarction: a large-scale, multicenter trial. The EPIC study group. Am J Med. 1993;95:608–18.
8. Picano E, Mathias W Jr, Pingitore A, Bigi R, Previtali M. Safety and tolerability of dobutamine-atropine stress echocardiography: a prospective, multicentre study. Echo Dobutamine international cooperative study group. Lancet. 1994;344:1190–2.
9. Ciampi Q, Picano E, Paterni M, Daros CB, Simova I, de Castro e Silva Pretto JL, D'Andrea A, Scali MC, Gaibazzi N, Severino S, Djordjevic-Dikic A, Kasprzak J, Zagatina A, Varga A, Lowenstein J, Merlo P, Amor M, Celeutkiene J, Perez JE, Di Salvo G, Galderisi M, Mori F, Costantino MF, Massa L, Dekleva M, Chavez D Q, Trambaiolo P, Citro R, Colonna P, Rigo F, Torres MAR, Monte I, Stankovic I, Neskovic A, Cortigiani L, Re F, Dodi C, D'Andrea A, Villari B, Arystan A, De Nes M, Carpeggiani C, on behalf of Stress Echo 2020. Quality control of regional wall motion analysis in stress Echo 2020. Int J Cardiol 2017;249479 - 485.
10. Picano E, Frassi F, Agricola E, Gligorova S, Gargani L, Mottola G. Ultrasound lung comets: a clinically useful sign of extravascular lung water. J Am Soc Echocardiogr. 2006;19:356–63.
11. Picano E, Pellikka PA. Ultrasound of extravascular lung water: a new standard for pulmonary congestion. Eur Heart J. 2016;37:2097–104.
12. Agricola E, Picano E, Oppizzi M, Pisani M, Zangrillo A, Margonato A. Assessment of stress-induced pulmonary interstitial edema by chest ultrasound during exercise echocardiography and its correlation with left ventricular function. J Am Soc Echocardiogr. 2006;19:457–63.
13. Scali MC, Cortigiani L, Simionuc A, Gregori D, Marzilli M, Picano E. The added value of exercise-echocardiography in heart failure patients: assessing dynamic changes in extravascular lung water. Eur J Heart Failure. 2017;19:1468–78.
14. Simonovic D, Coiro S, Carluccio E, Girerd N, Deljanic-Ilic M, Ambrosio G. Exercise elicits dynamic changes in extravascular lung water and

hemodynamic congestion in heart failure patients with preserved ejection fraction. Research letter. Eur J Heart Fail. 2018;21. https://doi.org/10.1002/ejhf.1228. [Epub ahead of print]

15. Lancellotti P, Pellikka PA, Budts W, Chaudhry FA, Donal E, Dulgheru R, Edvardsen T, Garbi M, Ha JW, Kane GC, Kreeger J, Mertens L, Pibarot P, Picano E, Ryan T, Tsutsui JM, Varga A. The clinical use of stress echocardiography in non-ischaemic heart disease: recommendations from the European Association of Cardiovascular Imaging and the American Society of Echocardiography. Eur Heart J Cardiovasc Imaging. 2016;17:1191–229.

16. Scali MC, Zagatina A, Simova I, Zhuravskaya N, Ciampi Q, Paterni M, Marzilli M, Carpeggiani C. Picano E. B-lines with Lung Ultrasound: the optimal scan technique at rest and during stress Ultrasound Med Biol. 2017;43:2558–66.

17. Picano E, Scali MC, Ciampi Q, Lichtenstein D. Lung ultrasound for the cardiologist. JACC imaging. 2018;12:381–90.

18. Mayo PH, Beaulieu Y, Doelken P, et al. American College of Chest Physicians/La Société de Réanimation de Langue Française statement on competence in critical care ultrasonography. Chest. 2009;135:1050–60.

19. Beaulieu Y, Laprise R, Drolet P, Thivierge RL, Serri K, Albert M, Lamontagne A, Belliveau M, Denault AY, Patenaude JV. Bedside ultrasound training using web-based e-learning and simulation early in the curriculum of residents. Critical Ultrasound Journal. 2015;7:1.

20. Sun Lim J, Lee S, Ho Do H, Ho Oh K. Can Limited Education of Lung Ultrasound Be Conducted to Medical Students Properly? A Pilot Study BioMed Research International Volume 2017, Article ID 8147075, 6 pages doi https://doi.org/10.1155/2017/8147075

21. Gargani L, Sicari R, Raciti M, Serasini L, Passera M, Torino C, Letachowicz K, Ekart R, Fliser D, Covic A, Balafa O, Stavroulopoulos A, Massy ZA, Fiaccadori E, Caiazza A, Bachelet T, Slotki I, Shavit L, Martinez-Castelao A, Coudert-Krier MJ, Rossignol P, Kraemer TD, Hannedouche T, Panichi V, Wiecek A, Pontoriero G, Sarafidis P, Klinger M, Hojs R, Seiler-Mußler S, Lizzi F, Onofriescu M, Zarzoulas F, Tripepi R, Mallamaci F, Tripepi G, Picano E, London GM, Zoccali C. Efficacy of a remote web-based lung ultrasound training for nephrologists and cardiologists: a LUST trial sub-project. Nephrology Dialysis Transplantation. 2016;31:1982–8.

22. Lindseth F, Hallan ML, Tonnessen MS, Smistad E, Vapenstad C. MIIP: a web-based platform for medical image interpretation training and evaluation focusing on ultrasound. Proceedings Volume 10138, Medical Imaging 2017: Imaging Informatics for healthcare Research and Applications; 10138W; doi: 10.117/12.2254158.

23. Jambrik Z, Monti S, Coppola V, Agricola E, Mottola G, Picano E. Usefulness of ultrasound lung comets as a nonradiologic sign of extravascular lung water. Am J Cardiol. 2004;93:1265–70.

24. Volpicelli G, Elbarbary M, Blaivas M, et al. International Liaison Committee on Lung Ultrasound for International Consensus Conference on Lung Ultrasound International evidence-based recommendations for point-of-care lung ultrasound. Intensive Care Med. 2012;38:577–91.

25. Platz E, Pivetta E, Merz AA, Peck J, Rivero J, Cheng S. Impact of device selection and clip duration on lung ultrasound assessment in patients with heart failure. Am J Emerg Med. 2015;33:1552–6.

26. Ohman J, Harjola VP, Karjalainen P, Lassus J. Assessment of early treatment response by rapid cardiothoracic ultrasound in acute heart failure: cardiac filling pressures, pulmonary congestion and mortality. Eur Heart J Acute Cardiovasc Care. 2018;7:311–20.

27. Picano E, Scali MC. The lung water cascade in heart failure. Echocardiography. 2017;34:1503–7.

28. Picano E, Scali MC. Stress echo, carotid arteries and more: its versatility for our imaging times. Editorial comment JACC img. 2017; https://doi.org/10.1016/j.jcmg.2017.01.023.

29. Picano E, Pellikka PA. Stress echo applications beyond coronary artery disease. Eur Heart J. 2014;35:1033–40.

30. Messerli FH. Meta-analysis and bouillabaisse. Ann Intern Med. 1996;125:519.

21

Assessment of left ventricular systolic and diastolic abnormalities in patients with hypertrophic cardiomyopathy using real-time three-dimensional echocardiography and two-dimensional speckle tracking imaging

Xin Huang[1†], Yan Yue[2†], Yinmeng Wang[3], Yujiao Deng[4], Lu Liu[1], Yanqi Di[1], Shasha Sun[1], Deyou Chen[5], Li Fan[1] and Jian Cao[1*] (iD)

Abstract

Background: Conventional echocardiography is not sensitive enough to assess left ventricular (LV) dysfunction in hypertrophic cardiomyopathy (HCM) patients. This research attempts to find a new ultrasonic technology to better assess LV diastolic function, systolic function, and myocardial longitudinal and circumferential systolic strain of segments with different thicknesses in HCM patients.

Methods: This study included 50 patients with HCM and 40 healthy subjects as controls. The peak early and late mitral annulus diastolic velocities at six loci (E_a' and A_a', respectively) and the E_a'/A_a' ratio were measured using real-time tri-plane echocardiography and quantitative tissue velocity imaging (RT-3PE-QTVI). The mean value of E_a' at six loci (E_m') was obtained for the calculation of E/E_m' ratio. The LV end-diastolic volume (LVEDV), LV end-systolic volume (LVESV), LV stroke volume (LVSV), and LV ejection fraction (LVEF) were measured using real-time three-dimensional echocardiography (RT-3DE). LV myocardial longitudinal peak systolic strain (LPSS) and circumferential peak systolic strain (CPSS) in the apical-middle-basal segments (LPSS_api, LPSS_mid, LPSS_bas; CPSS_api, CPSS_mid, and CPSS_bas, respectively) were obtained using a software for two-dimensional speckle tracking imaging (2D-STI). According to the different segmental thicknesses (STs) in each HCM patient, the values (LPSS and CPSS) of all the myocardial segments were categorized into three groups and the respective averages were computed.

Results: The E_a', A_a', and, E_a'/A_a' ratio in HCM patients were lower than those in the controls (all $p < 0.001$), while the E/E_m' ratio in HCM patients was higher than that in the controls ($p < 0.001$). The LVEDV, LVSV, and LVEF were significantly lower in HCM patients than in controls (all $p < 0.001$). In HCM patients, the LPSS_api, LPSS_mid, LPSS_bas, CPSS_api, CPSS_mid, and CPSS_bas and the LPSS and CPSS of LV segments with different thicknesses were all significantly reduced (all $p < 0.001$).

(Continued on next page)

---

* Correspondence: calvin301@163.com
†Xin Huang and Yan Yue contributed equally to this work.
[1]Department of cardiology, Nanlou Division, Chinese PLA General Hospital, National Clinical Research Center for Geriatric Diseases, Beijing 100853, China
Full list of author information is available at the end of the article

(Continued from previous page)

Conclusions: In HCM patients, myocardial dysfunction was widespread not only in the obviously hypertrophic segments but also in the non-hypertrophic segments; the LV systolic and diastolic functions were damaged, even with a normal LVEF. LV diastolic dysfunction, systolic dysfunction, and myocardial deformation impairment in HCM patients can be sensitively revealed by RT-3PE-QTVI, RT-3DE, and 2D-STI.

Keywords: Hypertrophic cardiomyopathy, Left ventricular, Real-time tri-plane echocardiography and quantitative tissue velocity imaging, Real-time three-dimensional, Two-dimensional speckle tracking imaging, Systolic functions, Diastolic functions

Background

Hypertrophic cardiomyopathy (HCM) is an autosomal dominant genetic disease caused by a genetic mutation in the myocardial sarcomere gene, and is characterized by myocardial hypertrophy, interstitial fibrosis, myocyte disarray, and asymmetrical left ventricular (LV) hypertrophy [1, 2]. Conventional echocardiography has been used to diagnose diastolic dysfunction, which is characterized by impaired left ventricular relaxation with increased stiffness of the left ventricle and diminished filling rates in HCM patients. However, systolic dysfunction cannot be easily determined using conventional methods. Therefore, we often describe systolic function as normal or hyperdynamic in HCM patients, depending on normal or supernormal LV ejection fraction (LVEF). HCM patients often experience symptoms such as breathlessness, fatigue, and reduced exercise capacity [3]. Previously, it was believed that diastolic dysfunction is the predominant cause of these symptoms. However, molecular studies have confirmed that in HCM, cardiac contractile dysfunction occurs before myocardial hypertrophy [4, 5]. Further, several studies have shown that the contractile force of the cardiac myocytes is impaired, despite the apparently normal or enhanced LVEF observed on conventional echocardiography [6, 7]. Therefore, it is important to evaluate the cardiac function of HCM patients using some novel techniques. We designed this study with the aim of quantifying systolic dysfunction and myocardial deformation impairment in HCM patients using real-time three-dimensional echocardiography (RT-3DE) and two-dimensional speckle tracking imaging (2D-STI). Furthermore, LV diastolic function can be evaluated easily and quickly by measuring the mitral valve flow spectrum, but some patients in the pseudonormalization spectrum cannot be clearly assessed by traditional ultrasound technology. Therefore, in this study, measurement of diastolic velocity at six loci in mitral annulus using real-time tri-plane echocardiography and quantitative tissue velocity imaging (3PE-QTVI) was designed for the evaluation of LV diastolic function.

Methods

Study population

The study population included 50 patients with non-obstructive HCM, and they were consecutively selected. These patients had undergone clinical and echocardiographic evaluations at our hospital between October 2016 and November 2017. The inclusion criteria [8] were as follows: (1) A 2D ultrasound showing asymmetric hypertrophy in the LV walls; (2) septum/posterior wall ratio ≥ 1.5; and (3) inter-ventricular septum thickness ≥ 1.5 mm. The exclusion criteria were as follows: (1) ventricular hypertrophy caused by simple apical HCM; (2) resting pressure gradient of the LV outflow tract ≥30 mmHg; (3) end-stage HCM (LVEF < 50%); (4) history of invasive septal reduction therapy (septal myomectomy or alcohol septal ablation); (5) organic (degenerative or rheumatic) valvular disease; (6) myocardial ischemia noted during noninvasive investigation, suggesting coronary artery disease; and (7) prior history of myocardial infarction or myocarditis. According to the segmental thickness (ST) in the diastole, all the segments of HCM patients were divided into three groups: HCM-A group (ST < 12 mm; 227 segments), HCM-B group (ST, 12–15 mm; 281 segments), and HCM-C group (ST > 15 mm; 392 segments). For the healthy control group, 40 age- and gender-matched participants were selected from the same time frame based on the following conditions: (1) normal results on physical examination, echocardiography, electrocardiography (ECG), and biochemistry tests and (2) no coronary artery disease, hypertension, valvular disease, arrhythmia, and systemic disease.

Prepared apparatus

Conventional echocardiography and 2D-STI were performed in all participants, using the Vivid 7-dimension ultrasound machine and an M3S probe. The 3PE-QTVI and RT-3DE examinations were performed using a 3 V probe.

Standard ultrasound examination

The LV end-diastolic diameter (LVDd), LV end-systolic diameter (LVDs), LV posterior wall thickness (LVPWT), inter-ventricular septal thickness (IVST), and left atrial end-systolic dimension (LADs) were measured along the LV long-axis view. The IVST/LVPWT ratio was calculated. The pulsed wave sampling volume was placed under the tips of the mitral valve leaflets from the apical four-chamber view. The peak early and late mitral inflow diastolic velocities (E and A, respectively) were measured using pulse Doppler, and the E/A ratio was calculated.

3PE-QTVI examination

During 3PE-QTVI, LV apical (long-axis and four- and two-chamber) views were obtained synchronously in cardiac cycles. The sampling volume was placed at six loci in the mitral annulus, namely, anterior septum, anterior wall, anterolateral wall, inferolateral wall, inferior wall, and inferior septum. The peak early and late mitral annulus diastolic velocity (E_a' and A_a', respectively) and E_a'/A_a' ratio were measured by 3PE-QTVI. The mean value of E_a' at the six loci (E_m') was obtained for the calculation of E/E_m'.

RT-3DE examination

RT-3DE full volume images were acquired during an end-expiratory breath-hold using a wide-angle acquisition mode in which four wedge-shaped subvolumes were obtained from four consecutive cardiac cycles with the acquisition triggered to the R wave of the ECG; subsequently, these datasets were stored and transferred to a computer for offline analysis. LV end-diastolic volume (LVEDV), LV end-systolic volume (LVESV), LV stroke volume (LVSV), and LVEF were calculated using a four-dimensional LV analysis software.

2D-STI examination

High frame rate images of the LV long-axis, four- and two-chamber, and short-axis views of the basal, middle, and apical segments were obtained, respectively. Three consecutive cardiac cycles were acquired in each view and saved in a cine-loop format for offline analysis supported by a digitized software package. The software package automatically tracked the changes in the width of the region of interest, which was adjusted, as required, to fit the wall thickness. The automatic algorithm obtained an 18-segment model and provided the longitudinal peak systolic strain (LPSS) and circumferential peak systolic strain (CPSS) for each segment. Subsequently, the average LPSS and CPSS values of basal, middle, and apical segments (LPSS-bas, LPSS-mid, LPSS-api; CPSS-bas, CPSS-mid, and CPSS-api, respectively) were calculated. The values (LPSS and CPSS) of all the myocardial segments for each HCM patient were categorized into three groups (HCM-A, HCM-B, and HCM-C) according to the ST, and subsequently, the average was computed.

The aforementioned ultrasound parameters were measured according to the American Society of Echocardiography guidelines and requirements [9].

Statistical analysis

Data analysis was performed using the Statistical Package for the Social Sciences software (SPSS, Version 19.0). The results are presented as mean ± standard deviation. The normality test was used to compare continuous variables, and the one-way analysis of variance was used to compare the echocardiographic values in HCM patients and the control group. Continuous variables obtained from different groups were compared using the Fisher's least significant difference test. All the p values were two-sided, and $p < 0.05$ was considered statistically significant.

Results

General information

The clinical characteristics of HCM patients and the control group are shown in Table 1. Both the groups were well matched with respect to age and gender. No statistical differences were observed in the body surface area, heart rate, and blood pressure between the two groups (all $p > 0.05$).

Conventional echocardiographic parameters

The IVST, LVPWT, septum/posterior wall ratio, and LADs were significantly higher in HCM patients than in the control group (all $p < 0.001$), whereas LVDd and LVDs were significantly lower in HCM patients than in the control group (all $p < 0.001$). Transmitral Doppler measurements showed no significant difference between the peak E, peak A, and E/A in HCM patients and those in the control group (all $p > 0.05$) (Table 1).

3PE-QTVI parameters

In this study, E_a', A_a', and E_a'/A_a' ratio at the six loci in the mitral annulus in HCM patients were lower than those in the control group, whereas the E/E_m' ratio in HCM patients was higher than that in the control group; all the differences were statistically significant (all $p < 0.001$) (Table 2; Fig. 1).

RT-3DE parameters

RT-3DE showed that LVEDV, LVSV, and LVEF were significantly lower in HCM patients than in the control group (all $p < 0.001$), although LVEF was within the normal range (LVEF $> 50\%$) (Table 3; Fig. 2).

Table 1 Clinical characteristics and conventional echocardiographic parameters in HCM patients versus control group

	HCM patients (N = 50)	Control group (N = 40)	p value
Age(years)	46.67 ± 11.09	43.93 ± 8.17	0.195
Gender			
Male	30 (60%)	24 (60%)	
Female	20 (40%)	16 (40%)	
HR(beats/min)	70.51 ± 9.62	68.43 ± 11.95	0.362
BSA(m^2)	1.72 ± 0.15	1.70 ± 0.21	0.612
SBP(mmHg)	124.63 ± 13.05	120.59 ± 9.67	0.106
DBP(mmHg)	78.32 ± 11.57	74.81 ± 9.07	0.119
IVST (mm)	25.33 ± 7.11	9.32 ± 1.35	< 0.001
LVPWT (mm)	14.25 ± 3.15	8.84 ± 1.11	< 0.001
septum/posterior wall ratio	1.86 ± 0.69	1.05 ± 0.10	< 0.001
LVDd (mm)	40.83 ± 4.87	44.16 ± 2.44	< 0.001
LVDs (mm)	23.32 ± 4.09	27.81 ± 1.64	< 0.001
LADs	40.91 ± 0.83	31.85 ± 1.95	< 0.001
E (cm/sec)	79.04 ± 3.26	80.36 ± 3.07	0.053
A (cm/sec)	71.05 ± 2.89	69.89 ± 2.65	0.052
E /A ratio	1.12 ± 0.39	1.15 ± 0.29	0.675

HR heart rate, *BSA* body surface area, *SBP* systolic blood pressure, *DBP* diastolic blood pressure, *IVST* inter-ventricular septal thickness, *LVDd* left ventricular end-diastolic diameter, *LVDs* left ventricular end-systolic diameter, *LVPWT* left ventricular posterior wall thickness, *LADs* left atrium end-systolic dimension. E: mitral inflow peak velocity in early diastole; A: mitral inflow peak velocity in late diastole. Values are expressed as the mean ± SD

2D-STI parameters

A gradual increase in the amplitudes of LPSS and CPSS was observed from the basal segment to the apex in the control group. However, in HCM patients, this regular pattern was not evident, and LPSS$_{-bas}$, LPSS$_{-mid}$, LPSS$_{-api}$, CPSS$_{-bas}$, CPSS$_{-mid}$, and CPSS$_{-api}$ decreased significantly (all $p < 0.001$) (Table 4; Figs. 3 and 4). LPSS and CPSS of the LV myocardial segments in HCM-A, HCM-B, and HCM-C groups were all reduced significantly compared with those in the control group (all $p < 0.001$), and there was a statistically significant difference between LPSS and CPSS of the LV myocardial segments among HCM-A, HCM-B, and HCM-C groups (all $p < 0.001$); a decreased amount of strain correlated with the myocardial thickness grade (Table 5). There was a statistically significant difference in the thickness of the myocardium among HCM-B, HCM-C groups and the control group (all $p < 0.001$); there was no significant difference in the thickness of the myocardium between HCM-A and the control group.

Discussion

Owing to the complexity of a three-dimensional cardiac structure, helical ventricular myocardial band (HVMB) is considered to be a critical cornerstone in understanding cardiac function. The HVMB comprises a helical component, namely an apical vortex

(oblique descending and ascending segments that cross each other at 60° angles en-route to forming) and a basal loop (containing both left and right transverse sides) [10]. During ventricular contraction, all the components coordinate synergistically to achieve myocardial longitudinal shortening, circumferential narrowing or compression, radial thickening, and twisting in favor of ejection. Because of mutation in the genes encoding the sarcomeric protein of the cardiac contractile apparatus, a series of characteristic pathological changes occur in HCM patients. This study aimed to quantify the effects of the pathological changes on the LV systolic and diastolic functions in HCM patients.

Evaluation of LV diastolic function in HCM patients by 3PE-QTVI

The Moderate reduction of diastolic function, usually showing E/A ratio > 1, is due a pseudonormalized phenomenon, which is difficult to distinguish from normal cardiac function. In this study, E and A were not significantly different between HCM patients and the control group, and the E/A ratio was > 1, which means that the mitral valve orifice flow spectrum may not truly reflect the changes in the diastolic function in patients with HCM.

The present study reported that the measurement of early and late mitral annulus diastolic velocity can reflect changes in relaxation and compliance of the left

Table 2 RT-3PE-QTVI parameters in HCM patients versus control group

	HCM patients (N = 50)	Control group (N = 40)	p value
E_a' (cm/sec)			
AS	3.35 ± 1.15	8.14 ± 2.23	< 0.001
AN	3.58 ± 1.25	8.87 ± 1.81	< 0.001
AL	4.24 ± 1.50	9.25 ± 1.80	< 0.001
IL	3.88 ± 1.44	10.26 ± 2.01	< 0.001
IN	3.51 ± 1.46	9.18 ± 1.57	< 0.001
IS	3.44 ± 1.42	8.20 ± 1.31	< 0.001
A_a' (cm/sec)			
AS	5.12 ± 1.84	6.48 ± 0.87	< 0.001
AN	5.22 ± 1.20	7.08 ± 0.56	< 0.001
AL	5.93 ± 1.43	7.21 ± 0.65	< 0.001
IL	6.02 ± 1.58	7.59 ± 1.13	< 0.001
IN	5.68 ± 1.46	7.80 ± 1.32	< 0.001
IS	5.10 ± 1.27	6.63 ± 0.68	< 0.001
E_a' / A_a'			
AS	0.71 ± 0.26	1.27 ± 0.43	< 0.001
AN	0.69 ± 0.20	1.24 ± 0.18	< 0.001
AL	0.74 ± 0.28	1.29 ± 0.23	< 0.001
IL	0.63 ± 0.22	1.45 ± 0.33	< 0.001
IN	0.63 ± 0.25	1.21 ± 0.29	< 0.001
IS	0.69 ± 0.18	1.26 ± 0.32	< 0.001
E/E_m' ratio	21.47 ± 5.36	10.01 ± 3.94	< 0.001

E_a' early diastolic velocity of mitral annulus, A_a' late-diastolic velocity of mitral annulus, E mitral inflow peak velocity in early diastole, E_m' mean value of E_a' at six loci in mitral annulus, AS anterior septum, AN anterior wall, AL anterolateral wall, IL inferolateral wall, IN inferior wall, IS inferior septum. Values are expressed as the mean ± SD

Table 3 RT-3DE parameters in HCM patients versus control group

	HCM patients (N = 50)	Control group (N = 40)	p value
LVEDV(ml)	70.12 ± 13.91	85.59 ± 14.94	< 0.001
LVESV (ml)	31.09 ± 6.02	29.46 ± 5.47	0.187
LVSV (ml)	39.94 ± 10.67	56.25 ± 11.68	< 0.001
LVEF(%)	57.17 ± 4.15	65.13 ± 2.95	< 0.001

LVEDV left ventricular end-diastolic volume, LVESV left ventricular end-systolic volume, LVSV left ventricular stroke volume, LVEF left ventricular ejection fraction. Values are expressed as the mean ± SD

cardiac cycle and susceptibility to heart rate and breathing. In this study, E_a', A_a', and E_a'/A_a' ratio in HCM patients were lower than those in the control group. The results showed that relaxation and compliance of the left ventricle were impaired. In addition, the E/E_m' ratio reflects LV end-diastolic pressure (LVEDP). The E/E_m' ratio in HCM patients significantly increased compared with that in the control group, indicating that LVEDP was significantly higher in HCM patients. When the myocardium of the left ventricle (main pumping chamber) is of abnormal thickness, the myocardial stiffness increases and compliance decreases, which results in increase in LV filling pressure. Long-term restriction of left atrial to ventricular blood filling may lead to left atrial enlargement. Left atrial dilation negatively affects patient condition and prognosis and may lead to atrial fibrillation, heart failure, sudden death, and other cardiovascular events [11, 12].

Evaluation of LV pumping function in HCM patients by RT-3DE

RT-3DE can overcomes the limitations of 2D echocardiography by demonstrating a 3D ventricular shape at different time phases and depicting the whole extent of the ventricular endocardium. In this study, LVEDV, LVSV, and LVEF measured by RT-3DE were observed to have significantly reduced in HCM patients compared with those in the control group, although LVEF

ventricle, independent of the cardiac load [3]. In this study, 3PE-QTVI was used for detection. By obtaining three orthogonal views from a 60° angle synchronously, this technology overcomes the limitations of conventional QTVI, such as display of only one view in each

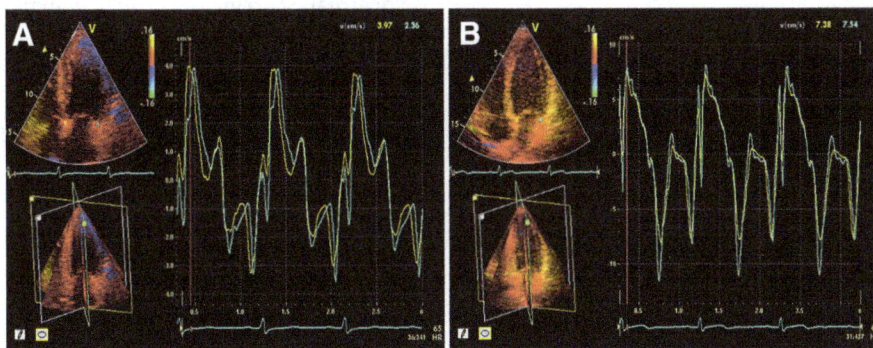

Fig 1. The peak early and late mitral annulus diastolic velocities (Ea' and Aa', respectively) at apical four-chamber view were measured using real-time tri-plane echocardiography and quantitative tissue velocity imaging. Ea' and Aa' are significantly lower in HCM patients than in control group

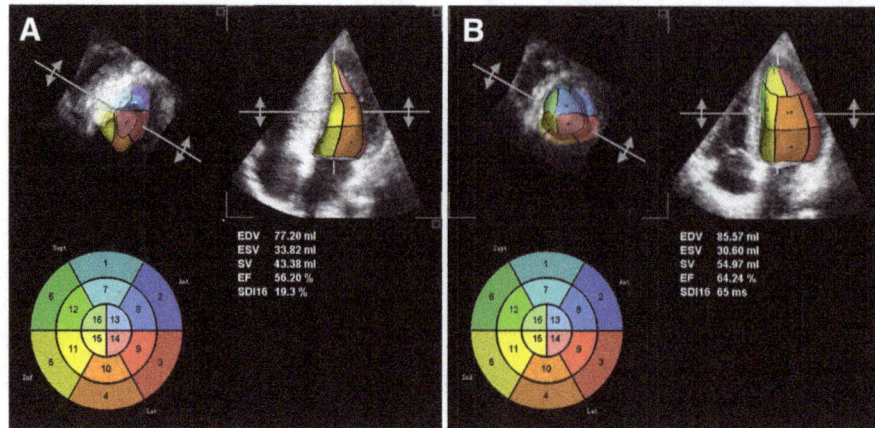

Fig 2. Left ventricular (LV) global shell maps by real-time three-dimensional echocardiography full volume image are shown. Left ventricle is seen as a "wedge-shape" in HCM patients. LV end-diastolic volume (LVEDV), end-systolic volume (LVESV), ejection fraction (LVEF) were significantly lower in HCM patients than in control group

was in the normal range (LVEF > 50%). Ejection fraction, depending on the percentage of stroke volume in LVEDV, mainly reflects changes in the cardiac cavity dimensions and volume, and is obviously affected by cardiac preload and afterload. The hypertrophic myocardium and papillary muscles protrude into the chamber [13], and reduce LV dimensions and volume, which is seen as a wedge- or spade-shaped ventricular cavity in HCM patients. Therefore, LVEF cannot completely reflect the cardiac stroke volume, especially in HCM patients with obviously decreased LV dimension and volume. Merely applying the parameter to evaluate LV systolic function can cause errors or bias [14, 15]. This study showed that LVSV had significantly decreased, although LVEF was in the normal range (LVEF > 50%). Hence, the LVSV may objectively and sensitively reveal the impairment of LV systolic function in HCM patients, despite a normal LVEF. We have previously demonstrated that symptoms such as syncope, palpitation, breathlessness, and exercise

limitation are closely related to diastolic dysfunction. In this study, we considered that those symptoms could also be indicative of reduced LVSV.

Evaluation of LV myocardial deformation in HCM patients by 2D-STI

In this study, LPSS and CPSS values in apical-middle-basal segments showed a regular pattern in the control group. The amplitudes of LPSS and CPSS increased gradually from the basal segment to the apical segment in the control group. However, this regularity was not evident in HCM patients. The LV LPSS and CPSS values of the basal, middle, and apical segments decreased significantly. This indicated that the LV myocardial systolic function was impaired in HCM patients. This impairment of the LV myocardial systolic function could be caused by the following factors: (1) HCM is characterized by abnormal hypertrophy in the cardiomyocytes, increased collagen, and interstitial fibrosis, and even macroscopically visible myocardial scarring [1, 16]; (2) hypertrophic myocardium and myofibrillar disarray are also considered pathological hallmarks of HCM, these are distributed unevenly and arranged irregularly in the form of swirls or clusters [1, 2, 16]; and (3) microvascular dysfunction occurs in HCM, which features myocardial/vascular ratio imbalance (decrease in myocardial capillary density), coronary artery wall thickening, and development of myocardial ischemia [17, 18].

Furthermore, in this study, LPSS and CPSS of the LV myocardial segments with different thicknesses were reduced significantly in HCM patients, even the normal thickness of the HCM-A group was significantly lower than that of the control group, but there

Table 4 STI results of longitudinal and circumferential strain in HCM patients versus control group

	HCM patients (N = 50)	Control group (N = 40)	p value
LPSS-bas	−13.91 ± 5.17	−21.67 ± 3.50	< 0.001
LPSS-mid	−12.59 ± 5.83	−22.02 ± 3.06	< 0.001
LPSS-api	−14.76 ± 6.84	−24.58 ± 3.96	< 0.001
CPSS-bas	−16.99 ± 6.19	−22.13 ± 4.86	< 0.001
CPSS-mid	−15.85 ± 5.34	−23.45 ± 3.70	< 0.001
CPSS-api	−16.24 ± 4.58	−28.32 ± 4.15	< 0.001

LPSS longitudinal peak systolic strain, *CPSS* circumferential peak systolic strain. Values are expressed as the mean ± SD

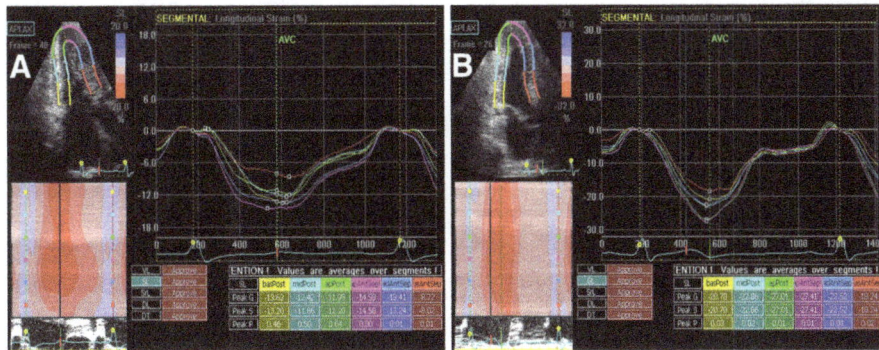

Fig 3. Two-dimensional speckle tracking images in left ventricular apical long-axis view are shown. Left ventricular longitudinal peak systolic strain in HCM patients is significantly lower than in control group

was no significant difference in the thickness of the myocardium between HCM-A and the normal control group. Further, the decreased amount of strain correlated with the myocardial thickness grade. Thus, the myocardial systolic dysfunction not only in the obvious hypertrophic segments but also in the non-hypertrophic segments suggested that myocardial systolic dysfunction in HCM patients may precede myocardial hypertrophy. This result is consistent with the results reported in previous studies [15]. Therefore, myocardial systolic dysfunction may occur first and the hypertrophy could be a compensatory response. The more obvious the magnitude of hypertrophy, the more serious is the impairment of myocardial strain. Just as demonstrated by Urbano-Moral et al. [19], the extent of hypertrophy is the primary factor altering myocardial mechanics. For HCM patients, the degree of myocardial hypertrophy is one of the parameters evaluated during regular follow-ups, and this study suggests that this evaluation may be important for assessing myocardial function, predicting the progress of the disease, and guiding therapy in clinical practice.

Limitations

Several limitations of this study must be considered. First, because the sample size was rather small, the results obtained from this study may not be statistically strong. Second, evaluation by RT-3DE and 2D-STI was significantly dependent on the quality of image. The assessments were feasible in patients with sufficient images quality. Some situations such as poor acoustic window (resulting in poor images) of cardiac patients with arrhythmia and examiner's subjective experience could have affected the accuracy and reliability of the data. In this study, the patients with poor images or arrhythmia were ruled out. Third, LVEF of HCM group is significantly lower than that of control group, even though it is within normal range. That can be a basic difference between two groups of this study, and consequently affect the other results comparing two groups. HCM group of this study may be patients with systolic dysfunction as well as diastolic dysfunction. Finally, a bias existed in different echocardiographic software packages from various ultrasound machine vendors, which may have affected the measurement repeatability and accuracy within acceptable limits.

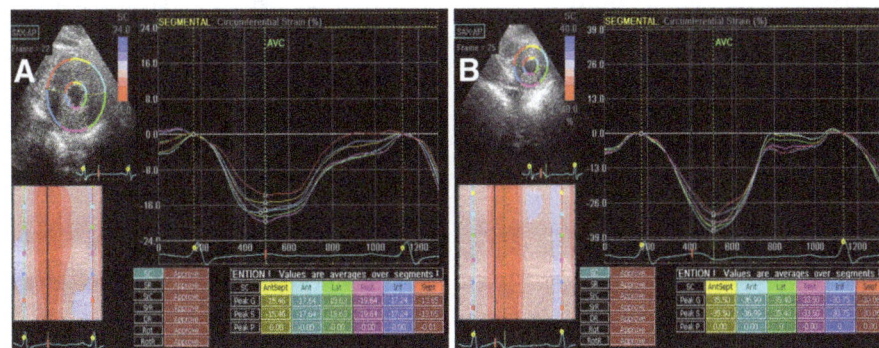

Fig 4. Two-dimensional speckle tracking images in left ventricular short-axis view at the apical level are shown. Left ventricular circumferential peak systolic strain is significantly lower in HCM patients than in control group

Table 5 STI results of the peak systolic longitudinal and circumferential strain in different segmental thickness(ST) groups in HCM patients and control group

	HCM-A (ST<12 mm, 227segments)	HCM-B (ST:12–15 mm, 281segments)	HCM-C (ST>15 mm, 392 segments)	Control group (720 segments)
ST	9.45 ± 1.25	13.39 ± 1.21[*#]	17.53 ± 1.84[*#&]	9.37 ± 1.18
LPSS	−17.79 ± 3.75[*]	− 13.51 ± 4.02[*#]	−10.03 ± 3.17[*#&]	−22.89 ± 3.41
CPSS	−19.83 ± 4.07[*]	− 16.19 ± 5.71[*#]	−13.32 ± 4.39[*#&]	−24.61 ± 3.52

Values are expressed as the mean ± SD
[*]$p < 0.001$ vs. Control group' segment
[#]$p < 0.001$ vs. HCM-A group (ST < 12 mm)
[&]$p < 0.001$ vs. HCM-B group (ST:12 mm − 15 mm)

Conclusions

This study shows that widespread myocardial dysfunction occurred not only in the obvious hypertrophic segments but also in the non-hypertrophic segments. The more obvious the magnitude of hypertrophy, the more serious is the impairment of myocardial strain. The LV systolic and diastolic functions were damaged; however, the LVEF in HCM patients was in the normal range. The LV diastolic dysfunction, systolic dysfunction, and myocardial deformation impairment in HCM patients can be early, objectively, and sensitively revealed by RT-3PE-QTVI, RT-3DE, and 2D-STI.

Abbreviations

2D-STI: Two-dimensional speckle tracking imaging; 3PE-QTVI: Real-time tri-plane echocardiography and quantitative tissue velocity imaging; A: The peak late mitral annulus diastolic velocities; A_a': The peak late mitral annulus diastolic velocities at six loci; CPSS: Circumferential peak systolic strain; $CPSS_{api}$: Circumferential peak systolic strain in the apical segments; $CPSS_{bas}$: Circumferential peak systolic strain in the basal segments; $CPSS_{mid}$: Circumferential peak systolic strain in the middle segments; E: The peak early mitral annulus diastolic velocities; E_a': The peak early mitral annulus diastolic velocities at six loci; E_m': The mean value of E_a' at six loci; HCM: Hypertrophic cardiomyopathy; HCM-A: Segmental thickness < 12 mm; HCM-B: Segmental thickness: 12–15 mm; HCM-C: Segmental thickness > 15 mm; HVMB: Helical ventricular myocardial band; IVST: Inter-ventricular septal thickness; LADs: Left atrial end-systolic dimension; LPSS: Longitudinal peak systolic strain; $LPSS_{api}$: Longitudinal peak systolic strain in the apical segments; $LPSS_{bas}$: Longitudinal peak systolic strain in the basal segments; $LPSS_{mid}$: Longitudinal peak systolic strain in the middle segments; LV: Left ventricular; LVDd: Left ventricular end-diastolic diameter; LVDs: Left ventricular end-systolic diameter; LVEDP: Left ventricular end-diastolic pressure; LVEDV: Left ventricular end-diastolic volume; LVEF: Left ventricular ejection fraction; LVESV: Left ventricular end-systolic volume; LVPWT: Left ventricular posterior wall thickness; LVSV: Left ventricular stroke volume; RT-3DE: real-time three-dimensional echocardiography; ST: Segmental thickness

Authors' contributions

XH and YY as the co-first author, JC as the corresponding author: they designed this study and analyzed and interpreted the patient data, drafted the manuscript, control and guarantee that all aspects of the work were investigated and resolved. YW, YD, LL, YD, SS, DC, and LF were responsible for acquisition of data, analysis and interpretation of data, revising the manuscript, and they control and guarantee that all aspects of the work were investigated and resolved. All authors read and approved the final manuscript.

Consent for publication

All the authors contributed substantially to the project and agreed for sending the manuscript to *Cardiovascular Ultrasound*. There is no competing interest and the data are available.

Competing interests

The authors declare that they have no conflict of interests.

Author details

[1]Department of cardiology, Nanlou Division, Chinese PLA General Hospital, National Clinical Research Center for Geriatric Diseases, Beijing 100853, China. [2]Department of medical administration, Chinese PLA General Hospital, Beijing 100853, China. [3]Department of Respiration, Clifford Hospital, Guangzhou 511495, China. [4]Department of Ultrasound, Chinese PLA General Hospital, Beijing 100853, China. [5]Department of Outpatient, Chinese PLA General Hospital, Beijing 100853, China.

References

1. Marian AJ, Braunwald E. Hypertrophic cardiomyopathy: genetics, pathogenesis, clinical manifestations, diagnosis, and therapy. Circ Res. 2017; 121(7):749–70.
2. Kocovski L, Fernandes J. Sudden cardiac death: a modern pathology approach to hypertrophic cardiomyopathy. Arch Pathol Lab Med. 2015; 139(3):413–6.
3. Abozguia K, Nallur-Shivu G, Phan TT, Ahmed I, Kalra R, Weaver RA, et al. Left ventricular strain and untwist in hypertrophic cardiomyopathy: relation to exercise capacity. Am Heart J. 2010;159(5):825–32.
4. Pislaru C, Anagnostopoulos PC, Seward JB, Greenleaf JF, Belohlavek M. Higher myocardial strain rates during isovolumic relaxation phase than during ejection characterize acutely ischemic myocardium. J Am Coll Cardiol. 2002;40(8):1487–94.
5. Rust EM, Albayya FP, Metzger JM. Identification of a contractile deficit in adult cardiac myocytes expressing hypertrophic cardiomyopathy-associated mutant troponin T proteins. J Clin Invest. 1999;103(10):1459–67.
6. Ozawa K, Funabashi N, Takaoka H, Kamata T, Kanaeda A, Saito M, et al. Characteristic myocardial strain identified in hypertrophic cardiomyopathy subjects with preserved left ventricular ejection fraction using a novel multi-layer transthoracic echocardiography technique. Int J Cardiol. 2015;184:237–43.
7. Marian AJ. Pathogenesis of diverse clinical and pathological phenotypes in hypertrophic cardiomyopathy. Lancet. 2000;355(9197):58–60.
8. Gersh BJ, Maron BJ, Bonow RO, Dearani JA, Fifer MA, Link MS, et al. 2011 ACCF/AHA Guideline for the Diagnosis and Treatment of Hypertrophic Cardiomyopathy: a report of the American College of Cardiology Foundation/American Heart Association Task Force on Practice Guidelines. Developed in collaboration with the American Association for Thoracic Surgery, American Society of Echocardiography, American Society of Nuclear Cardiology, Heart Failure Society of America, Heart Rhythm Society, Society for Cardiovascular Angiography and Interventions, and Society of Thoracic Surgeons. J Am Coll Cardiol. 2011;58(25):e212–60.
9. Lang RM, Bierig M, Devereux RB, Flachskampf FA, Foster E, Pellikka PA, et al. Recommendations for chamber quantification: a report from the American Society of Echocardiography's guidelines and standards committee and the chamber quantification writing group, developed in conjunction with the European Association of Echocardiography, a branch of the European Society of Cardiology. J Am Soc Echocardiogr. 2005;18(12):1440–63.
10. Buckberg G. The helical ventricular myocardial band during standard echocardiography: a structure-function relationship. Echocardiography. 2015;32(2):199–204.

11. Parato VM, Antoncecchi V, Sozzi F, Marazia S, Zito A, Maiello M, et al. Echocardiographic diagnosis of the different phenotypes of hypertrophic cardiomyopathy. Cardiovasc Ultrasound. 2016;14(1):30.

12. Graca B, Ferreira MJ, Donato P, Castelo-Branco M, Caseiro-Alves F. Cardiovascular magnetic resonance imaging assessment of diastolic dysfunction in a population without heart disease: a gender-based study. Eur Radiol. 2014;24(1):52–9.

13. Zhang HJ, Wang H, Sun T, Lu MJ, Xu N, Wu WC, et al. Assessment of left ventricular twist mechanics by speckle tracking echocardiography reveals association between LV twist and myocardial fibrosis in patients with hypertrophic cardiomyopathy. Int J Cardiovasc Imaging. 2014;30(8):1539–48.

14. Yoshikawa H, Suzuki M, Hashimoto G, Kusunose Y, Otsuka T, Nakamura M, et al. Midwall ejection fraction for assessing systolic performance of the hypertrophic left ventricle. Cardiovasc Ultrasound. 2012;10:45.

15. Liu L, Tuo S, Zhang J, Zuo L, Liu F, Hao L, et al. Reduction of left ventricular longitudinal global and segmental systolic functions in patients with hypertrophic cardiomyopathy: study of two-dimensional tissue motion annular displacement. Exp Ther Med. 2014;7(6):1457–64.

16. Villa AD, Sammut E, Zarinabad N, Carr-White G, Lee J, Bettencourt N, et al. Microvascular ischemia in hypertrophic cardiomyopathy: new insights from high-resolution combined quantification of perfusion and late gadolinium enhancement. J Cardiovasc Magn Reson. 2016;18:4.

17. Sciagra R, Calabretta R, Cipollini F, Passeri A, Castello A, Cecchi F, et al. Myocardial blood flow and left ventricular functional reserve in hypertrophic cardiomyopathy: a (13)NH3 gated PET study. Eur J Nucl Med Mol Imaging. 2017;44(5):866–75.

18. Kao YC, Lee MF, Mao CT, Chen WS, Yang NI, Cherng WJ, et al. Differences of left ventricular systolic deformation in hypertensive patients with and without apical hypertrophic cardiomyopathy. Cardiovasc Ultrasound. 2013;11:40.

19. Urbano-Moral JA, Rowin EJ, Maron MS, Crean A, Pandian NG. Investigation of global and regional myocardial mechanics with 3-dimensional speckle tracking echocardiography and relations to hypertrophy and fibrosis in hypertrophic cardiomyopathy. Circ Cardiovasc Imaging. 2014;7(1):11–9.

22

Reproducibility of Transcranial Doppler ultrasound in the middle cerebral artery

Jakub Kaczynski[1*], Rachel Home[2], Karen Shields[3], Matthew Walters[4], William Whiteley[5], Joanna Wardlaw[5] and David E. Newby[1]

Abstract

Background: Transcranial Doppler ultrasound remains the only imaging modality that is capable of real-time measurements of blood flow velocity and microembolic signals in the cerebral circulation. We here assessed the repeatability and reproducibility of transcranial Doppler ultrasound in healthy volunteers and patients with symptomatic carotid artery stenosis.

Methods: Between March and August 2017, we recruited 20 healthy volunteers and 20 patients with symptomatic carotid artery stenosis. In a quiet temperature-controlled room, two 1-h transcranial Doppler measurements of blood flow velocities and microembolic signals were performed sequentially on the same day (within-day repeatability) and a third 7–14 days later (between-day reproducibility). Levels of agreement were assessed by interclass correlation co-efficient.

Results: In healthy volunteers (31±9 years, 11 male), within-day repeatability of Doppler measurements were 0.880 (95% CI 0.726–0.950) for peak velocity, 0.867 (95% CI 0.700–0.945) for mean velocity, and 0.887 (95% CI 0.741–0.953) for end-diastolic velocity. Between-day reproducibility was similar but lower: 0.777 (95% CI 0.526–0.905), 0.795 (95% CI 0.558–0.913), and 0.674 (95% CI 0.349–0.856) respectively. In patients (72±11 years, 11 male), within-day repeatability of Doppler measurements were higher: 0.926 (95% CI 0.826–0.970) for peak velocity, 0.922 (95% CI 0.817–0.968) for mean velocity, and 0.868 (95% CI 0.701–0.945) for end-diastolic velocity. Similarly, between-day reproducibility revealed lower values: 0.800 (95% CI 0.567–0.915), 0.786 (95% CI 0.542–0.909), and 0.778 (95% CI 0.527–0.905) respectively. In both cohorts, the intra-observer Bland Altman analysis demonstrated acceptable mean measurement differences and limits of agreement between series of middle cerebral artery velocity measurements with very few outliers. In patients, the carotid stenoses were 30–40% ($n = 9$), 40–50% ($n = 6$), 50–70% ($n = 3$) and > 70% ($n = 2$).
No spontaneous embolisation was detected in either of the groups.

Conclusions: Transcranial Doppler generates reproducible data regarding the middle cerebral artery velocities. However, larger studies are needed to validate its clinical applicability.

Keywords: Transcranial Doppler, Microembolic signals, Carotid artery stenosis, Ischaemic stroke

---

* Correspondence: jakub.kaczynski@ed.ac.uk
[1]British Heart Foundation Centre for Cardiovascular Science, University of Edinburgh, Chancellor's Building, 49 Little France Crescent, Edinburgh EH16 4SA, UK
Full list of author information is available at the end of the article

Background

Ischaemic stroke remains a major global cause of disability and death that is associated with an enormous social and economic burden [1]. Up to 25% of ischaemic strokes are caused by atherosclerosis of the internal carotid artery [2, 3]. Carotid atherosclerosis is a complex disease that is characterised by the deposition of luminal atheroma that may rupture, thrombose and embolise [2]. The resulting thromboembolism can lead to a stroke or transient ischaemic attack (TIA) [4].

Transcranial Doppler is a well established real-time imaging modality that evaluates cerebral blood flow velocity and detects microembolic signals in patients who suffer from cerebral or retinal ischaemia [5]. Microembolic signals in symptomatic carotid artery stenosis are associated with an increased risk of a recurrent ipsilateral focal ischaemia [6–14] and and correlate with a greater number of magnetic resonance imaging detectable cerebral infarcts when compared with patients free from microembolism [15–18]. The intraoperative transcranial Doppler has enabled clinicians to lower the rate of the most serious post carotid endarterectomy complication such as thromboembolic stroke from 4 to 0.2% through detection of the middle cerebral artery flow cessation due to the intraluminal carotid artery thrombosis [19, 20]. Whereas, transcranial Doppler directed infusion of Dextran 40 has in some centres successfully erased the rate of postoperative thromboembolic cerebral ischaemia from 2.7 to 0% [8, 21]. Despite these benefits from transcranial Doppler, routine use has not been advocated amongst vascular specialists.

Although multiple studies have been conducted on flow velocities in basal cerebral arteries in both healthy volunteers and patients [22–33], reproducibility data are limited to a hand full of reports. These include four articles involving healthy subjects [34–37] and one study that recruited patients with clinical diagnosis of ischaemic stroke ($n = 3$) or TIA ($n = 7$) but provided no information regarding the clinical type of neurovascular event or underlying carotid artery stenosis [5]. In contrast, published data on microembolic signals detection in patients with symptomatic carotid artery stenosis includes systematic reviews, meta-analyses [38–41] international multicenter reproducibility studies that have described the reproducibility of transcranial Doppler as sufficient for clinical use [10, 42, 43].

Our objective was to assess the intra-observer repeatability and reproducibility of transcranial Doppler for velocimetry measurements and microemboli detection in healthy volunteers and patients with symptomatic carotid artery stenosis that could form the basis for our future study investigating reliable identification of a vulnerable carotid plaque.

Methods

Study design

This was an observational investigative study. The study was approved by the local Research Ethics Committee (16/SS/0217), and written consent was obtained from all participants. The research protocol is available on ClinicalTrial.gov (ID NCT 03050567).

Study population

Cohorts ($n = 20$ per cohort) of healthy volunteers and patients with symptomatic carotid artery stenosis were recruited between March–August 2017. Among the patient group, five patients that were excluded due to an absent temporal window, were subsequently replaced. Healthy volunteers were > 18 years old and had no previous history of cerebrovascular disease. Patients with evidence of an acute neurovascular syndrome (stroke, TIA, retinal ischaemia) due to carotid artery disease were recruited from the acute neurovascular clinics at Edinburgh Royal Infirmary within a maximum of 14 days of symptom onset. The inclusion criteria were the symptomatic cerebrovascular event (stroke, TIA or amaurosis fugax) and radiological confirmation of carotid artery stenosis of > 30%. This included patients scheduled for carotid endarterectomy (> 50% for men and > 70% for women, by North American Symptomatic Carotid Endarterectomy Trial criteria) or treated conservatively with an optimal medical therapy (if patient declined surgical intervention or is outside surgical criteria for carotid endarterectomy) [3].

Study protocol

All subjects underwent clinical evaluation prior to participation. In the patient group, this included assessment of relevant carotid Doppler ultrasound and brain imaging investigations (computed tomography or magnetic resonance imaging). In both cohorts, three 1-h transcranial Doppler measurements were performed by the same examiner over two study visits. During the first study visit, two examinations were performed separated by 1 h (Fig. 1). The final (third) examination was obtained on a separate study visit within 14 days of the first examination (Fig. 1).

Transcranial Doppler ultrasound

All examinations were performed in a semi-recumbent position in a quiet temperature-controlled room. The middle cerebral artery was identified through the temporal window and the sample volume adjusted to obtain a stable visually and acoustically optimal signal. In healthy subjects, the side of the middle cerebral artery insonation was randomly allocated. In patients with symptomatic carotid artery stenosis, transcranial Doppler was performed on the symptomatic middle cerebral artery (ipsilateral to the index event). A head frame (Marc 600 Spencer Technologies, USA) was fitted to reduce motion and to secure a constant angle of the middle cerebral artery insonation depth at 40–65 mm from the skull surface. All recordings were made using the ST^3 Transcranial Doppler Ultrasound System (Spencer Technologies, USA) with a 2-MHz transducer. Emboli were identified using characteristic short audible sound (range 10–100 ms, intensity threshold above 7 dB) and spectral appearance using the International Consensus Group microembolus identification criteria and assisted by an automated Embolus Detection Software (Spencer Technologies, USA) [44]. The Doppler wave forms were reassessed to exclude artefact and confirm the presence of true emboli. The mean of maximal, mean and end-diastolic flow velocities were determined from the mean of measurements obtained over ten cardiac cycles.

Statistical analysis

Continuous variables were expressed as mean ± standard deviation for normally distributed data, and categorical variables were expressed as total and percentage. To quantify intra-observer repeatability and reproducibility of imaging measurements, the intra-class correlation co-efficient (ICC) was calculated and Bland-Altman analysis undertaken. Statistical significance was taken as a two-sided $P < 0.05$. Statistical analyses were performed with the use of IBM SPSS Statistics for Mac, version 23 (Armonk, New York, IBM Corp, USA).

Results

All participants tolerated transcranial Doppler examinations well and completed all assessments.

Healthy volunteers

In total, 60 transcranial Doppler assessments were performed on 20 healthy volunteers who had a mean age of 31±9 years, and 11 were male. All subjects had the temporal window available, and the mean middle cerebral artery insonation depth was 51 mm (Table 1) with peak velocities averaging around 70–85 cm/s (Table 1).

Overall, the ICC for both repeatability and reproducibility in healthy volunteers group revealed a good reliability (ICC 0.75–0.90) with wider confidence intervals obtained for the peak and mean reproducibility values when compared with the repeatability measurements (Table 2). An intra-observer Bland Altman analysis demonstrated acceptable mean measurement differences and limits of agreement between series of middle cerebral artery velocity measurements with very few outliers (Figs. 2 and 3). As expected no microembolic signals were detected.

Table 1 Summary of the middle cerebral artery blood flow velocity and insonation depth in healthy volunteers and patients

Healthy Volunteers			
Velocity (cm/s)	Examination 1	Examination 2	Examination 3
Peak	75.70 ± 23.91	72.00 ± 20.28	82.75 ± 19.93
Mean	49.95 ± 15.30	47.05 ± 12.85	52.60 ± 11.73
Diastolic	34.70 ± 11.28	29.50 ± 10.65	35.45 ± 8.40
MCA depth (mm)	51.75 ± 2.65	51.75 ± 2.94	51.20 ± 2.93
Patients			
Velocity (cm/s)	Examination 1	Examination 2	Examination 3
Peak	73.70 ± 18.94	73.10 ± 16.62	71.20 ± 17.62
Mean	45.40 ± 11.79	45.20 ± 10.83	43.50 ± 9.96
Diastolic	27.30 ± 8.90	27.10 ± 8.14	25.60 ± 6.57
MCA depth (mm)	51.40 ± 5.33	51.55 ± 5.21	51.65 ± 5.24

Data are presented as mean ± standard deviation. MCA, middle cerebral artery

Patients

Patients had a mean age of 72±11 years, and 11 were men (Table 3). Presenting diagnosis included 18 transient ischaemic attacks (11 cerebral, 7 ocular) and 2 cases of ischaemic stroke. The degree of stenoses measured by Duplex ultrasound scan were: 30–40% ($n = 9$), 40–50% ($n = 6$), 50–70% ($n = 3$) and > 70% ($n = 2$). Five patients (4 females, 1 male) had an absent acoustic temporal window. The mean middle cerebral artery insonation depth was 51 mm (Table 1) and peak cerebral artery

Table 2 Summary of ICC velocity values for repeatability and reproducibility assessments in healthy volunteers and patients

Healthy Volunteers		
Repeatability (Exam 1 vs Exam 2)	ICC	95% CI
Peak	0.880	0.726–0.950
Mean	0.867	0.700–0.945
End-diastolic	0.887	0.741–0.953
Reproducibility (Visit 1 vs Visit 2)	ICC	95% CI
Peak	0.777	0.526–0.905
Mean	0.795	0.558–0.913
End-diastolic	0.674	0.349–0.856
Patients		
Repeatability (Exam 1 vs Exam 2)	ICC	95% CI
Peak	0.926	0.826–0.970
Mean	0.922	0.817–0.968
End-diastolic	0.868	0.701–0.945
Reproducibility (Visit 1 vs Visit 2)	ICC	95% CI
Peak	0.800	0.567–0.915
Mean	0.786	0.542–0.909
End-diastolic	0.778	0.527–0.905

Date are reported as mean with 95% limits of agreement for assessments

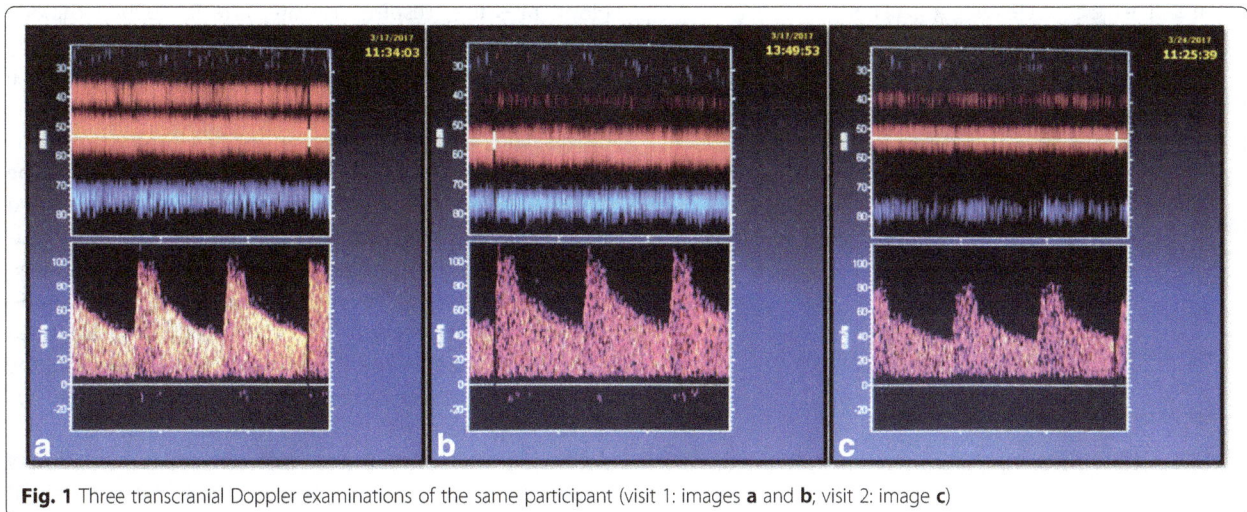

Fig. 1 Three transcranial Doppler examinations of the same participant (visit 1: images **a** and **b**; visit 2: image **c**)

blood flow velocities were 70–75 cm/s (Table 1). The overall intra-observer ICC for repeatability and reproducibility displayed at least good (ICC 0.75–0.90) agreement that reached an excellent agreement (ICC > 0.90) for the peak and mean repeatability velocity values (Table 2). Similarly, wider confidence intervals were found for the peak and mean reproducibility values when compared with the repeatability assessments. The Bland Altman plots showed acceptable mean measurement differences and limits of agreement between series of middle cerebral artery velocity measurements with very few outliers (Figs. 4 and 5). No microembolic signals were detected during transcranial Doppler assessments.

Discussion

In this study, we have demonstrated that transcranial Doppler generates reproducible data regarding the velocity measurements. Transcranial Doppler utilises an acoustic temporal bone window through which the

ultrasound beam can focus on the middle cerebral artery, which receives 80% of an ipsilateral internal carotid artery inflow [27]. The obtained middle cerebral artery insonation depth in both cohorts reflects published data [10, 45, 46].

In general, the success of transcranial Doppler imaging diminishes with an older age due to an increased temporal bone thickness that impairs the transmission of ultrasound waves through the skull [47, 48]. This has been observed primarily in approximately 10% of non-Caucasian elderly female participants [49]. However, others report temporal window failure in almost third of examined subjects [50].

Multiple studies described substantially different normal reference velocity values of cerebral arteries blood flow [22, 24, 25, 27, 29, 31] but the most frequently quoted normal middle cerebral artery velocity under resting condition ranges from 35 to 90 cm/sec with a mean of 60 cm/sec [29]. Our velocity values mirror the results published by others, except for the lower mean

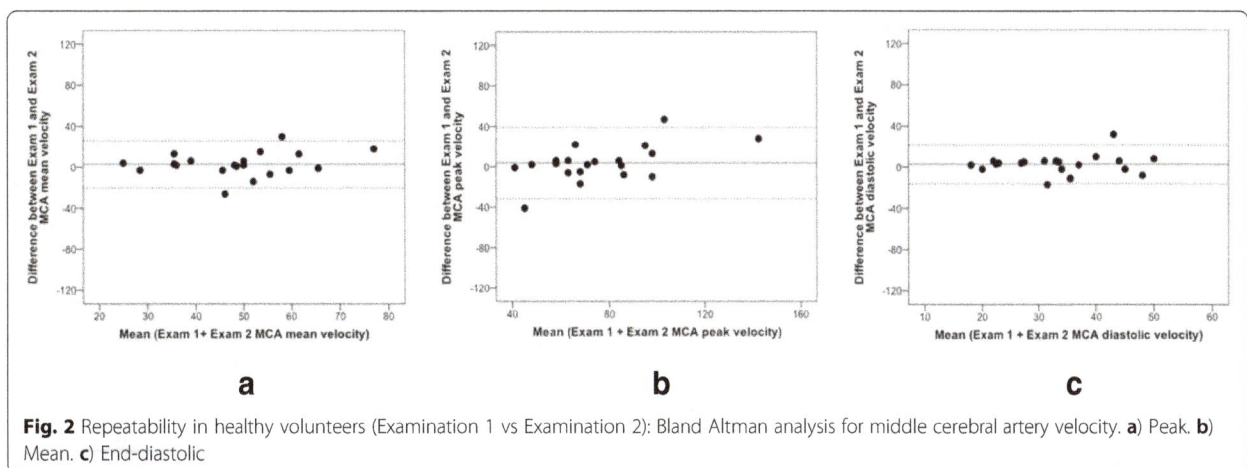

Fig. 2 Repeatability in healthy volunteers (Examination 1 vs Examination 2): Bland Altman analysis for middle cerebral artery velocity. **a**) Peak. **b**) Mean. **c**) End-diastolic

Table 3 Baseline characteristics of patients

Characteristics	n (%) Total = 20
Demographics	
Age, years	72±10.6
Male	11 (55)
Vital signs	
Systolic BP	146.6 ±27.3
Diastolic BP	77.4±11.0
Heart rate/min	70.15 ±14.89
Smoker status	
Current smoker	2 (10)
Former smoker	12 (60)
Never smoked	6 (30)
Presenting diagnosis	
Cerebral TIA	9 (45)
Ocular TIA	7 (35)
Stroke	2 (10)
Duplex scan severity of stenosis (%)	
30–40%	9 (45)
4–50%	6 (30)
50–70%	3 (15)
> 70%	2 (10)
Duration between index event and 1st transcranial Doppler (days)	11.6±2.4
Relevant medical history	
Hypertension	15 (75)
Hypercholesterolemia	20 (100)
Diabetes Mellitus	3 (15)
Ischaemic Heart Disease	4 (20)
Peripheral Vascular Disease	1 (5)
TIA	4 (20)
Stroke	3 (15)
Chronic Obstructive Pulmonary Disease	3 (15)
Baseline medication therapy	
Antiplatelet	18 (90)
Anticoagulant	2 (10)
Statin	20 (100)
Beta-blocker	4 (20)
Angiotensin-converting enzyme inhibitor	7 (35)

Data are presented as mean (standard deviation) or as percentage (%) where appropriate

diastolic middle cerebral artery velocity. However, this could be explained by various physiological and technical factors that can affect velocity readings. First, physiological cardiovascular changes such as heart rate,

blood pressure, respiratory rate, arterial carbon dioxide tension alter middle cerebral artery blood flow on a daily basis [51, 52]. Second, psychological factors (emotional state, fatigue) by influencing the above physiological cardiovascular autonomic responses can impact on the cerebral blood flow [51]. Unsurprisingly, changes in the cerebral metabolism due to cognitive activation also affect the middle cerebral artery blood flow. Some authors demonstrated that arithmetic activity produced very similar values to the resting blood flow values, whereas higher levels of arithmetic difficulty produced smaller changes in the blood flow [53]. Therefore, the above factors could have potentially influenced the obtained velocity values.

The main technical aspect that can impact on velocity measurement is the angle of insonation that is obtained between the middle cerebral artery and ultrasound beam [5, 34]. However, this is more relevant when large acoustic window such as the foramen of magnum is used, because it permits significant angle variation [34]. Fortunately, small temporal window with a sharp angle of insonation (0°-30°) that is relatively stable minimises any influence on obtained velocities values [5]. Hence, the maximum error has been estimated to be less than 15% [34, 35]. Finally, individual variability of the middle cerebral artery size, length and tortuosity are also contributing to the scattering of the velocity measurements [27, 29, 37].

In general, cerebral flow velocity decreases with age in a bimodal pattern with a first decline above the age of 40 years and a further reduction above 60 years of age [22, 26, 27, 54]. Unsurprisingly, our data demonstrate similar results with lower velocity values in patients cohort when compared with the healthy volunteers. Overall the obtained ICC values in our study represent a good repeatability and reproducibility in both cohorts. However, the peak and mean ICC repeatability values recorded in patients group reached an excellent agreement (ICC > 0.90). In both cohorts, the peak and mean ICC reproducibility values decrease with wider confidence intervals when compared to the repeatability values. This likely reflects the combination of technical variation and biological variation which will be much greater when measurements are conducted on separate days rather than within a day. For example, this could include probe displacement from the original middle cerebral artery segment that was sampled during the first study visit. This may also reflect the well described anatomical variability of the circle of Willis including diameter discrepancy of the individual parts of the middle cerebral artery [27, 29]. In effect, an over or under-estimated velocity values can be reported depending on the diameter of an insonated artery. The slightly higher ICC values obtained in the patients group could be explained by the lower

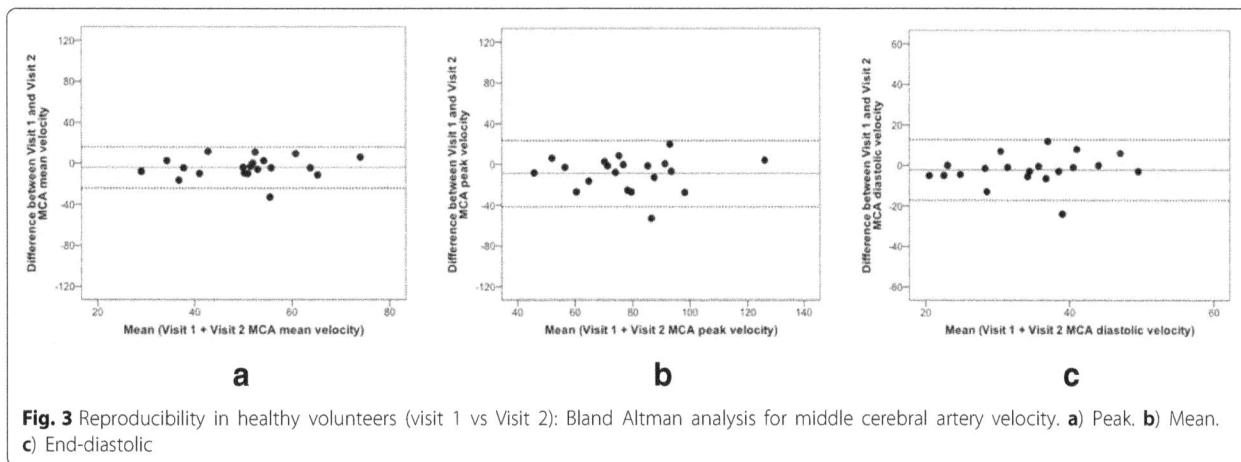

Fig. 3 Reproducibility in healthy volunteers (visit 1 vs Visit 2): Bland Altman analysis for middle cerebral artery velocity. **a)** Peak. **b)** Mean. **c)** End-diastolic

range of physiological fluctuations and more consistent velocity measurements [28].

Finally, the equipment characterists such as head frame that supports the transducers could account for some differnces in velocity values. In our study we have used a professional head frame system (Marc 600 Spencer Technologies, USA) that minimises the motion and maintains a constant angle of insonation of the middle cerebral artery. Interestingly, no single reproducibility study on velocity measurements described any form of secure fixation of transducers during the examinations [5, 34–37]. Similarly, systematic reviews and meta-analyses on microembolic signals detection provide no information on any head-frame systems used by individual studies [38–41]. This raises many questions regarding the methodological aspects of these studies that have been conducted more than 20 years ago.

Although our data regarding transcranial Doppler velocities measurements echoes other researchers findings, it should be interpreted with caution owing to many methodological limitations of the published analyses including a limited number of reproducibility studies

that contain small sample size and variable imaging protocols. Furthermore, evidence for the transcranial Doppler criteria to predict the degree of intracranial arteries stenoses remains inconclusive and controversial [18]. Several studies failed to demonstrate reproducible data on specific cut-off points for the velocities values with the percentage of stenosis [30, 32, 33, 55–57]. Some authors have proposed middle cerebral artery velocity of > 80 cm/sec as a criterion for stenosis [57], whereas others used velocities > 100 cm/sec when diagnosing stenosing lesions [54]. In contrast, some researchers have highlighted the importance of additional measurements such as side-to-side differences in velocities (> 30%) or increase in velocity (> 50%) along with the assessment of collateral flow using temporary manual occlusions of the common carotid artery [30, 32]. However, one must remember potential pitfalls with such approach because high velocities in collateral circulation can indicate different diameters of the middle cerebral arteries on two sides [30]. In effect, high blood flow velocities may be caused simply by the smaller diameter of MCA despite otherwise normal anatomy [33]. Finally, the largest study (The

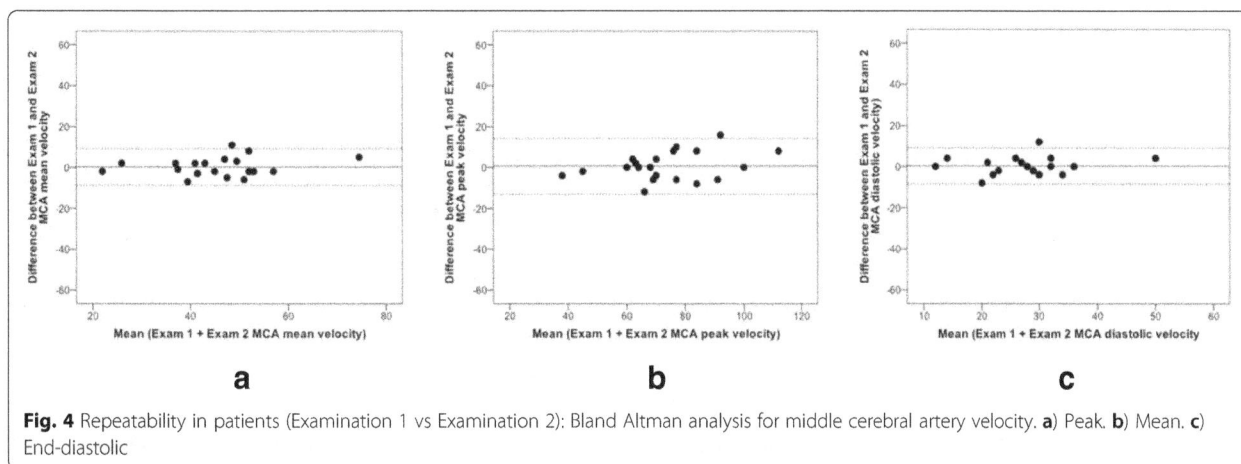

Fig. 4 Repeatability in patients (Examination 1 vs Examination 2): Bland Altman analysis for middle cerebral artery velocity. **a)** Peak. **b)** Mean. **c)** End-diastolic

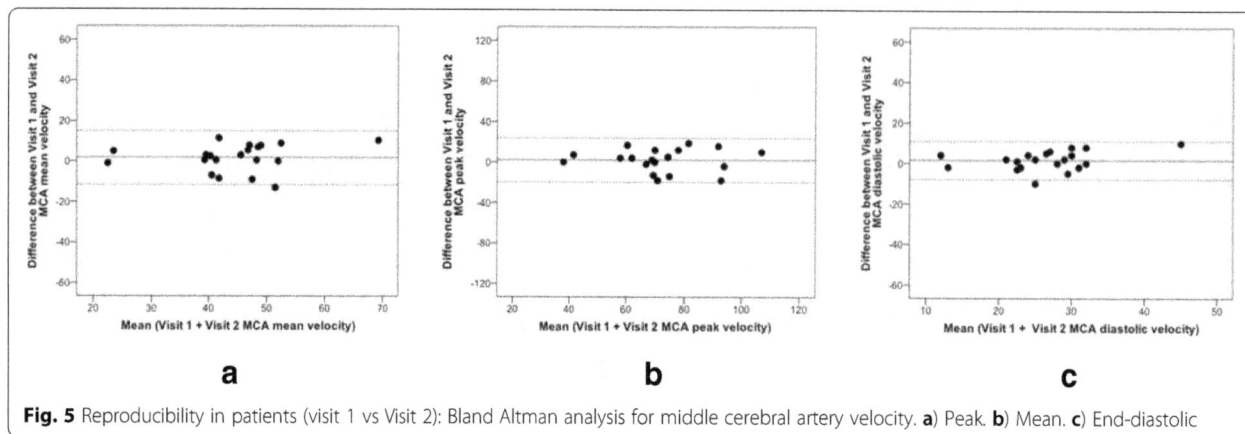

Fig. 5 Reproducibility in patients (visit 1 vs Visit 2): Bland Altman analysis for middle cerebral artery velocity. **a**) Peak. **b**) Mean. **c**) End-diastolic

Stroke Outcomes and Neuroimaging of Intracranial Atherosclerosis (SONIA) Trial) that attempted to validate transcranial Doppler findings with magnetic resonance angiography against the standard cerebral digital subtraction angiography regarding the identification of intracranial arterial disease revealed disappointingly low results of positive predictive values for transcranial Doppler (36%) and magnetic resonance angiography (59%) [55]. In effect, the transcranial Doppler's clinical applicability regarding the abnormal velocity values assessment remains limited.

Despite complete 1-h transcranial Doppler assessments performed in our study, the lack of microembolic signals in patients with symptomatic carotid artery stenosis was disappointing. The reported incidence varied from 12 to 100% in individual studies [40, 58, 59]. Nevertheless, considerable differences regarding criteria for microembolic signals detection, timing after stroke, duration of monitoring and antithrombotic agents used have been identified among many studies [10, 40, 58]. Consequently, the majority of published data described microembolic signals in about 30–40% of individuals with symptomatic carotid artery stenosis when transcranial Doppler was performed for 1 h [39, 40, 59, 60].

Still, there are several potential explanations for the absent embolisation. Thromboembolism is a dynamic and random process with a generally reported low frequency of microembolic signals during 1-h long examination [60, 61]. Although 1-h long transcranial Doppler evaluation time is recommended for patients with symptomatic carotid artery stenosis, longer assessments increase the chances of successful emboli detection [60]. This was demonstrated by ambulatory recordings (greater than 5 h) with portable transcranial Doppler equipment that has yield greater number of microembolic signals when compared with the traditional 60 min approach [62, 63]. However, at present, an ambulatory transcranial Doppler recording remains primarily a research tool due to lack of a robust equipment.

Another possible explanation refers to the severity of carotid artery stenosis and plaque morphology. Microembolic signals are more common in patients with the higher degree of carotid artery stenosis, which in turn is associated with specific carotid plaque features reported histologically such as ulceration, intraplaque haemorrhage and surface thrombus [11, 18, 39, 49, 59, 64, 65]. These high-risk plaque features are more likely to lead to the development of stroke because they produce larger emboli that consist of thrombi [59]. Whereas, small embolic particles comprising of fibrin and platelets aggregates that lodge in small arteriolar branches, may be lysed by endogenous protective haemostatic defences, hence clinically may represent TIA [59]. The majority of our patients had a non-surgical grade of carotid artery stenosis and presented with TIA. Therefore, these factors could be potentially responsible for no detectable microembolic signals.

The various components of microembolic signals responds differently to treatment [39]. For example, antiplatelet agents are more effective for emboli originating from the symptomatic carotid artery stenosis, and reduce the rate of microembolic signals [11, 12]. On the other hand, anticoagulants deal more effectively with microembolic signals from a cardiac source [11, 39]. The majority of participants (90%) in our study have been on an antiplatelet agent at the time of the first transcranial Doppler assessment, and this could represent another potential confounder. Finally, microembolic signals are more likely to be detected within the first week after the index event, and in patients with recent stroke rather than with TIA [66]. Again, we have performed transcranial Doppler as soon as possible, but due to various logistic factors, only two patients had transcranial Doppler within seven days from their index event.

The main limitations of this study are the small sample size, and single-centre design. However, the main purpose of the study was to demonstrate reproducibility of the transcranial Doppler and this was achieved. At present, transcranial Doppler remains underutilised in clinical practice due to lack of human expertise, time-consuming recordings with the need for a continuous visual and audible evaluation [13, 60]. Furthermore, unsolved technical and methodological limitations of transcranial Doppler regarding the velocity assessments restrict its clinical applicability. However, its use during carotid surgery has shown that the clinical use of this non-invasive, non-ionising, portable and safe technique could be extended to vascular surgery specialists as part of the routine perioperative strategy that could reduce the risk of neurovascular events even further [20].

Conclusions

Our findings indicate that transcranial Doppler provides reproducible data on middle cerebral artery velocities. However, these findings should be interpreted with caution for the many technical and methodological limitations that the transcranial Doppler still presents. Larger studies with the colour transcranial Doppler may enable delivery of a robust data on velocity assessments along with the quantification of intracranial stenoses.

Abbreviations
ICC: Intra-Class Correlation; SD: Standard Deviation; TIA: Transient Ischaemic Attack

Acknowledgements
We acknowledge the support of staff of the Clinical Research Facility at Royal Infirmary of Edinburgh.

Funding
This study was funded by the Princess Margaret Research Development Fellowship.

Authors' contributions
JK: study design, data collection, analysis, interpretation, drafting and revising the manuscript. RH: study design, data analysis and interpretation. KS: study design, acquisition of data, analysis and interpretation. MW: drafting and critical revision of the manuscript. WW: study design, data analysis, interpretation, drafting and revising the manuscript. JW: study design, data analysis, interpretation, drafting and revising the manuscript. DN: study design, data analysis, interpretation, drafting and revising the manuscript. All authors have read and approved the final version of the manuscript.

Authors' information
JK: Clinical Research Fellow presently supported by the British Heart Foundation Clinical Research Fellowship (FS/17/50/33061). RH: Medical student at University of Edinburgh. KS: Vascular technologist specialised in the transcranial Doppler imaging at Queen Elizabeth University Hospital in Glasgow. MW: Professor of Clinical Pharmacology, Head of the Undergraduate Medical School University of Glasgow and Director of Scottish Stroke Research Network. WW: MRC Clinician Scientist & Honorary Consultant Neurologist at Royal Infirmary of Edinburgh. JW: Head of Edinburgh Imaging, Director of Brain Research Imaging Centre, Honorary Consultant Neuroradiologist at Royal Infirmary of Edinburgh. DEN: British Heart Foundation John Wheatley Chair of Cardiology, Consultant Cardiologist at Royal Infirmary of Edinburgh.

Consent for publication
Not applicable.

Competing interests
The authors declare that they have no competing interests to declare.

Author details
[1]British Heart Foundation Centre for Cardiovascular Science, University of Edinburgh, Chancellor's Building, 49 Little France Crescent, Edinburgh EH16 4SA, UK. [2]College of Medicine and Veterinary Medicine, University of Edinburgh, 47 Little France Crescent, Edinburgh EH16 4TJ, UK. [3]Stroke Unit, Queen Elizabeth University Hospital, 1345 Govan Road, Glasgow G51 4TF, UK. [4]College of Medical, Veterinary and Life Sciences, Wolfson Medical School Building, University of Glasgow, University Avenue, Glasgow G12 8QQ, UK. [5]Royal Infirmary of Edinburgh, 51 Little France Crescent, Old Dalkeith Road, Edinburgh EH16 4SA, UK.

References
1. Naylor AR. Why is the management of asymptomatic carotid disease so controversial? Surgeon. 2015;13:34–43.
2. Vavra AK, Eskandari MK. Treatment options for symptomatic carotid stenosis: timing and approach. Surgeon. 2015;13:44–51.
3. Writing G, Naylor AR, Ricco JB, de Borst GJ, Debus S, de Haro J, Halliday A, Hamilton G, Kakisis J, Kakkos S, Lepidi S, Markus HS, McCabe DJ, Roy J, Sillesen H, van den Berg JC, Vermassen F, Esvs Guidelines C, Kolh P, Chakfe N, Hinchliffe RJ, Koncar I, Lindholt JS, Vega de Ceniga M, Verzini F, Esvs Guideline R, Archie J, Bellmunt S, Chaudhuri A, Koelemay M, et al. Editor's Choice - Management of Atherosclerotic Carotid and Vertebral Artery Disease: 2017 clinical practice guidelines of the European Society for Vascular Surgery (ESVS). Eur J Vasc Endovasc Surg. 2018;55:3–81.
4. Valton L, Larrue V, le Traon AP, Massabuau P, Géraud G. Microembolic signals and risk of early recurrence in patients with stroke or transient ischemic attack. Stroke. 1998;29:2125–8.
5. Totaro R, Marini C, Cannarsa C, Prencipe M. Reproducibility of transcranial Dopplersonography: a validation study. Ultrasound Med Biol. 1992;18:173–7.
6. Markus HS. Transcranial Doppler detection of circulating cerebral emboli. A review Stroke. 1993;24:1246–50.
7. Grotta JC, Alexandrov AV: Preventing Stroke. 2001.
8. Lennard N, Smith J, Dumville J, Abbott R, Evans DH, London NJ, Bell PR, Naylor AR. Prevention of postoperative thrombotic stroke after carotid endarterectomy: the role of transcranial Doppler ultrasound. J Vasc Surg. 1997;26:579–84.
9. Abbott AL, Chambers BR, Stork JL, Levi CR, Bladin CF, Donnan GA. Embolic signals and prediction of ipsilateral stroke or transient ischemic attack in asymptomatic carotid stenosis: a multicenter prospective cohort study. Stroke. 2005;36:1128–33.
10. Markus HS, Ackerstaff R, Babikian V, Bladin C, Droste D, Grosset D, Levi C, Russell D, Siebler M, Tegeler C. Intercenter agreement in reading Doppler embolic signals. Stroke. 1997;28:1307–10.
11. Markus HS, Droste DW, Kaps M, Larrue V, Lees KR, Siebler M, Ringelstein EB. Dual antiplatelet therapy with clopidogrel and aspirin in symptomatic carotid stenosis evaluated using Doppler embolic signal detection. Circulation. 2005;111:2233–40.
12. Imray CH, Tiivas CA. Are some strokes preventable? The potential role of transcranial doppler in transient ischaemic attacks of carotid origin. The Lancet Neurology. 2005;4:580–6.
13. Spence JD. Transcranial Doppler monitoring for microemboli: a marker of a high-risk carotid plaque. Semin Vasc Surg. 2017;30:62–6.

14. Abbott AL, Levi CR, Stork JL, Donnan GA, Chambers BR. Timing of clinically significant microembolism after carotid endarterectomy. Cerebrovasc Dis. 2007;23:362-7.

15. Sarkar S, Ghosh S, Ghosh SK, Collier A. Role of transcranial Doppler ultrasonography in stroke. Postgrad Med J. 2007;83:683-9.

16. Kimura K, Minematsu K, Koga M, Arakawa R, Yasaka M, Yamagami H, Nagatsuka K, Naritomi H, Yamaguchi T. Microembolic signals and diffusion-weighted MR imaging abnormalities in acute ischemic stroke. Am J Neuroradiol. 2001;22:1037-42.

17. Wolf O, Heider P, Heinz M, Poppert H, Sander D, Greil O, Weiss W, Hanke M, Eckstein H-H. Microembolic signals detected by transcranial Doppler sonography during carotid endarterectomy and correlation with serial diffusion-weighted imaging. Stroke. 2004;35:e373-5.

18. Babikian VL, Feldmann E, Wechsler LR, Newell DW, Gomez CR, Bogdahn U, Caplan LR, Spencer MP, Tegeler C, Ringelstein EB. Transcranial Doppler ultrasonography: year 2000 update. J Neuroimaging. 2000;10:101-15.

19. Lennard N, Smith JL, Gaunt ME, Abbott RJ, London NJ, Bell PR, Naylor AR. A policy of quality control assessment helps to reduce the risk of intraoperative stroke during carotid endarterectomy. Eur J Vasc Endovasc Surg. 1999;17:234-40.

20. Naylor AR, Hayes PD, Allroggen H, Lennard N, Gaunt ME, Thompson MM, London NJ, Bell PR. Reducing the risk of carotid surgery: a 7-year audit of the role of monitoring and quality control assessment. J Vasc Surg. 2000;32:750-9.

21. Lennard NS, Vijayasekar C, Tiivas C, Chan CW, Higman DJ, Imray CH. Control of emboli in patients with recurrent or crescendo transient ischaemic attacks using preoperative transcranial Doppler-directed dextran therapy. Br J Surg. 2003;90:166-70.

22. Demirkaya S, Uluc K, Bek S, Vural O. Normal blood flow velocities of basal cerebral arteries decrease with advancing age: a transcranial Doppler sonography study. Tohoku J Exp Med. 2008;214:145-9.

23. Aaslid R, Markwalder T-M, Nornes H. Noninvasive transcranial Doppler ultrasound recording of flow velocity in basal cerebral arteries. J Neurosurg. 1982;57:769-74.

24. Arnolds BJ, von GM R, Transcranial Dopplersonography. Examination technique and normal reference values. Ultrasound Med Biol. 1986;12:115-23.

25. Krejza J, Mariak Z, Walecki J, Szydlik P, Lewko J, Ustymowicz A. Transcranial color Doppler sonography of basal cerebral arteries in 182 healthy subjects: age and sex variability and normal reference values for blood flow parameters. AJR Am J Roentgenol. 1999;172:213-8.

26. Hennerici M, Rautenberg W, Sitzer G, Schwartz A. Transcranial Doppler ultrasound for the assessment of intracranial arterial flow velocity--part 1. Examination technique and normal values. Surg Neurol. 1987;27:439-48.

27. Ringelstein EB, Kahlscheuer B, Niggemeyer E, Otis SM. Transcranial Doppler sonography: anatomical landmarks and normal velocity values. Ultrasound Med Biol. 1990;16:745-61.

28. Venkatesh B, Shen Q, Lipman J. Continuous measurement of cerebral blood flow velocity using transcranial Doppler reveals significant moment-to-moment variability of data in healthy volunteers and in patients with subarachnoid hemorrhage. Crit Care Med. 2002;30:563-9.

29. Lindegaard K-F, Lundar T, Wiberg J, Sjøberg D, Aaslid R, Nornes H. Variations in middle cerebral artery blood flow investigated with noninvasive transcranial blood velocity measurements. Stroke. 1987;18:1025-30.

30. Lindegaard K-F, Bakke SJ, Grolimund P, Aaslid R, Huber P, Nornes H. Assessment of intracranial hemodynamics in carotid artery disease by transcranial Doppler ultrasound. J Neurosurg. 1985;63:890-8.

31. Grolimund P, Seiler RW. Age dependence of the flow velocity in the basal cerebral arteries--a transcranial Doppler ultrasound study. Ultrasound Med Biol. 1988;14:191-8.

32. Niederkorn K, Myers LG, Nunn CL, Ball MR, McKinney WM. Three-dimensional transcranial Doppler blood flow mapping in patients with cerebrovascular disorders. Stroke. 1988;19:1335-44.

33. Ley Pozo J, Bernd Ringelstein E. Noninvasive detection of occlusive disease of the carotid siphon and middle cerebral artery. Ann Neurol. 1990;28:640-7.

34. Maeda H, Etani H, Handa N, Tagaya M, Oku N, Kim B-H, Naka M, Kinoshita N, Nukada T, Fukunaga R. A validation study on the reproducibility of transcranial Doppler velocimetry. Ultrasound Med Biol. 1990;16:9-14.

35. McMahon CJ, McDermott P, Horsfall D, Selvarajah JR, King AT, Vail A. The reproducibility of transcranial Doppler middle cerebral artery velocity measurements: implications for clinical practice. Br J Neurosurg. 2007;21:21-7.

36. Shen Q, Stuart J, Venkatesh B, Wallace J, Lipman J. Inter observer variability of the transcranial Doppler ultrasound technique: impact of lack of practice on the accuracy of measurement. J Clin Monit Comput. 1999;15:179-84.

37. Baumgartner RW, Mathis J, Sturzenegger M, Mattle HP. A validation study on the intraobserver reproducibility of transcranial color-coded duplex sonography velocity measurements. Ultrasound Med Biol. 1994;20:233-7.

38. Best LM, Webb AC, Gurusamy KS, Cheng SF, Richards T. Transcranial Doppler ultrasound detection of microemboli as a predictor of cerebral events in patients with symptomatic and asymptomatic carotid disease: a systematic review and meta-analysis. Eur J Vasc Endovasc Surg. 2016;52:565-80.

39. King A, Markus HS. Doppler embolic signals in cerebrovascular disease and prediction of stroke risk: a systematic review and meta-analysis. Stroke. 2009;40:3711-7.

40. Ritter MA, Dittrich R, Thoenissen N, Ringelstein EB, Nabavi DG. Prevalence and prognostic impact of microembolic signals in arterial sources of embolism. A systematic review of the literature. J Neurol. 2008;255:953-61.

41. Udesh R, Natarajan P, Thiagarajan K, Wechsler LR, Crammond DJ, Balzer JR, Thirumala PD. Transcranial Doppler monitoring in carotid Endarterectomy: a systematic review and meta-analysis. J Ultrasound Med. 2017;36:621-30.

42. Markus H, Bland JM, Rose G, Sitzer M, Siebler M. How good is intercenter agreement in the identification of embolic signals in carotid artery disease? Stroke. 1996;27:1249-52.

43. Cullinane M, Reid G, Dittrich R, Kaposzta Z, Ackerstaff R, Babikian V, Droste DW, Grossett D, Siebler M, Valton L, Markus HS. Evaluation of new online automated embolic signal detection algorithm, including comparison with panel of international experts. Stroke. 2000;31:1335-41.

44. Ringelstein EB, Droste DW, Babikian VL, Evans DH, Grosset DG, Kaps M, Markus HS, Russell D, Siebler M. Consensus on microembolus detection by TCD. Stroke. 1998;29:725-9.

45. Alexandrov AV, Sloan MA, Tegeler CH, Newell DN, Lumsden A, Garami Z, Levy CR, Wong LK, Douville C, Kaps M. Practice standards for transcranial Doppler (TCD) ultrasound. Part II. Clinical indications and expected outcomes. Journal of Neuroimaging. 2012;22:215-24.

46. Alexandrov AV, Sloan MA, Wong LK, Douville C, Razumovsky AY, Koroshetz WJ, Kaps M, Tegeler CH. Practice standards for transcranial Doppler ultrasound: part I—test performance. J Neuroimaging. 2007;17:11-8.

47. Itoh T, Matsumoto M, Handa N, Maeda H, Hougaku H, Hashimoto H, Etani H, Tsukamoto Y, Kamada T. Rate of successful recording of blood flow signals in the middle cerebral artery using transcranial Doppler sonography. Stroke. 1993;24:1192-5.

48. Wijnhoud AD, Franckena M, van der Lugt A, Koudstaal PJ, Dippel ED. Inadequate acoustical temporal bone window in patients with a transient ischemic attack or minor stroke: role of skull thickness and bone density. Ultrasound Med Biol. 2008;34:923-9.

49. Markus HS. Transcranial Doppler ultrasound. Br Med Bull. 2000;56:378-88.

50. Marinoni M, Ginanneschi A, Forleo P, Amaducci L. Technical limits in transcranial Doppler recording: Inadquate acoustic windows. Ultrasound Med Biol. 1997;23:1275-7.

51. Stroobant N, Vingerhoets G. Test-retest reliability of functional transcranial Doppler ultrasonography. Ultrasound Med Biol. 2001;27:509-14.

52. Vingerhoets G, Stroobant N. Lateralization of cerebral blood flow velocity changes during cognitive tasks. A simultaneous bilateral transcranial Doppler study. Stroke. 1999;30:2152-8.

53. Vingerhoets G, Stroobant N. Reliability and validity of day-to-day blood flow velocity reactivity in a single subject: an fTCD study. Ultrasound Med Biol. 2002;28:197-202.

54. Bragoni M, Feldmann E. Transcranial Doppler indices of intracranial hemodynamics. Neurosonology Boston: Mosby. 1996:129-40.

55. Feldmann E, Wilterdink JL, Kosinski A, Lynn M, Chimowitz MI, Sarafin J, Smith HH, Nichols F, Rogg J, Cloft HJ, Wechsler L, Saver J, Levine SR, Tegeler C, Adams R, Sloan M, Stroke O. Neuroimaging of intracranial atherosclerosis trial I: the stroke outcomes and neuroimaging of intracranial atherosclerosis (SONIA) trial. Neurology. 2007;68:2099-106.

56. Lindegaard K-F, Bakke SJ, Aaslid R, Nornes H. Doppler diagnosis of intracranial artery occlusive disorders. J Neurol Neurosurg Psychiatry. 1986;49:510-8.

57. Rorick MB, Nichols FT, Adams RJ. Transcranial Doppler correlation with angiography in detection of intracranial stenosis. Stroke. 1994;25:1931-4.

58. Markus HS, Harrison MJ. Microembolic signal detection using ultrasound. Stroke. 1995;26:1517–9.
59. Stork JL, Kimura K, Levi CR, Chambers BR, Abbott AL, Donnan GA. Source of microembolic signals in patients with high-grade carotid stenosis. Stroke. 2002;33:2014–8.
60. Markus H. Monitoring embolism in real time. Circulation. 2000;102:826–8.
61. Dittrich R, Ritter MA, Droste DW. Microembolus detection by transcranial doppler sonography. Eur J Ultrasound. 2002;16:21–30.
62. Mackinnon AD, Aaslid R, Markus HS. Ambulatory transcranial Doppler cerebral embolic signal detection in symptomatic and asymptomatic carotid stenosis. Stroke. 2005;36:1726–30.
63. Mackinnon AD, Aaslid R, Markus HS. Long-term ambulatory monitoring for cerebral emboli using transcranial Doppler ultrasound. Stroke. 2004;35:73–8.
64. Sitzer M, Muller W, Siebler M, Hort W, Kniemeyer HW, Jancke L, Steinmetz H. Plaque ulceration and lumen thrombus are the main sources of cerebral microemboli in high-grade internal carotid artery stenosis. Stroke. 1995;26:1231–3.
65. Verhoeven B, de Vries J, Pasterkamp G, Ackerstaff R, Schoneveld AH, Velema E, de Kleijn D, Moll FL. Carotid atherosclerotic plaque characteristics are associated with microembolization during carotid endarterectomy and procedural outcome. Stroke. 2005;36:1735–40.
66. Azarpazhooh MR, Chambers BR. Clinical application of transcranial Doppler monitoring for embolic signals. J Clin Neurosci. 2006;13:799–810.

23

Layer-specific strain analysis in patients with suspected stable angina pectoris and apparently normal left ventricular wall motion

Mustafa Adem Yılmaztepe[*] and Fatih Mehmet Uçar

Abstract

Background: Non-invasive imaging tests are widely used in the evaluation of stable angina pectoris (SAP). Despite these tests, non-significant coronary lesions are not a rare finding in patients undergoing elective coronary angiography (CAG). Two-dimensional (2D) speckle tracking global longitudinal strain (GLS) imaging is a more sensitive and accurate technique for measuring LV function than conventional 2D methods. Layer-specific strain analysis is a relatively new method that provides endocardial and epicardial myocardial layer assessment. The aim of the present study was to evaluate longitudinal layer-specific strain (LSS) imaging in patients with suspected SAP.

Methods: Patients who underwent CAG for SAP were retrospectively screened. A total of 79 patients with no history of heart disease and wall motion abnormalities were included in the study. Forty-three patients with coronary lesions > 70% constituted the coronary artery disease (CAD) group and 36 patients without significant CAD constituted the control group. Layer-specific GLS transmural, endocardium, and epicardium values (GLS-trans, GLS-endo, and GLS-epi, respectively) were compared between the groups.

Results: Patients in the CAD group had significantly lower GLS values in all layers (GLS-trans: -18.2 + 2.4% vs -22.2 + 2.2% $p < .001$; GLS-endo: -20.8 + 2.8% vs -25.3 + 2.6%, $p < .001$; GLS-epi: 15.9 + 2.4% vs -19.5 + 1.9%, $p < .001$). Multivariate adjustment demonstrated GLS-trans as the only independent predictor of CAD [OR:0.472, CI (0.326–0.684), $p < .001$]. Additionally, the GLS values were all lower in myocardial perfusion scintigraphy (MPS) true-positive patients compared with MPS false-positive patients (GLS-trans: -17.7 ± 2.4 vs. -21.9 ± 2.4%, $p < .001$; GLS-endo: -20.2 ± 2.9% vs -24.9 ± 2.9%, $P < .001$; GLS-epi: 15.4 ± 2.6% vs. -19.2 ± 1.8%, $P < .001$).

Conclusion: Resting layer-specific strain as assessed by 2D speckle tracking analysis demonstrated that GLS values were reduced in all layers of myocardium with SAP and with no wall motion abnormalities. LSS analysis can improve the identification of patients with significant CAD but further prospective larger scale studies are needed to put forth the incremental value of LSS analysis over transmural GLS.

Keywords: Coronary artery disease, Left ventricle function, Echocardiography, 2D speckle tracking, Layer specific strain

* Correspondence: mayilmaztepe@yahoo.com
Department of Cardiology, School of Medicine, Trakya University, 22030
Edirne, Turkey

Background

Coronary artery disease is one of the major causes of mortality and morbidity. Noninvasive imaging techniques (NIIT) are recommended in the diagnosis and risk stratification of patients with suspected stable angina pectoris (SAP) [1]. Resting transthoracic echocardiography is one of the leading tests used in the evaluation of patients with stable CAD. However, despite critical CAD, many patients do not exhibit wall motion abnormalities with resting conventional echocardiography when structural heart disease and history of prior myocardial infarction do not exist. In addition to TTE, exercise electrocardiography (ECG), myocardial perfusion scintigraphy (MPS), or stress echocardiography are widely used. Exercise ECG is the most widely available technique but has the lowest sensitivity and specificity. Nuclear imaging tests are chosen for providing high diagnostic accuracy but the major limitations are radiation exposure and lesser availability [2]. Dobutamine stress echocardiography is also a low cost and widely available technique without radiation exposure, it has a high sensitivity and specificity similar to nuclear perfusion scintigraphy, but the need of expertise limits its use [3]. Despite NIIT, nonsignificant coronary lesions are not a rare finding in patients undergoing elective coronary angiography. In a recently published study, the rate of significant CAD in elective coronary angiograms was 38% [4].

Myocardial strain analysis by two dimensional speckle tracking echocardiography (2D STE) has a higher diagnostic accuracy in detecting left ventricular dysfunction. Recently published studies revealed lower values of deformation in patients with acute coronary syndrome, diabetes mellitus [5], hypertension [1], and SAP [6–12]. In addition to global longitudinal strain (GLS), layer-specific strain (LSS) analysis provides the assessment of each myocardial layer separately. Strain analysis of longitudinal endocardial layer can give more accurate data about LV function and early signs of ischemia because endocardium is more susceptible to ischemia.

The aim of the present study was to evaluate layer-specific GLS in patients with suspected SAP and normal left ventricular wall motion.

Methods

Patients who underwent diagnostic coronary angiography for SAP between January 2016 and January 2017 were screened from the electronic database. Patients with previous myocardial infarction, acute coronary syndrome, a history of coronary intervention or coronary artery bypass graft surgery, moderate-to-severe valvular disease, heart failure, segmental wall motion abnormalities, atrial fibrillation, reduced ejection fraction, and with malignancy were all excluded.

Echocardiographic images were assessed for suitability by an experienced cardiologist who was blinded to the other imaging results of the patients. All of the echocardiographic images were obtained using Vivid 7 Dimension or Vivid S70 systems (GE Healthcare, Horton, Norway) and imported to the EchoPAC workstation. Recordings with poor image quality that did not qualify for speckle tracking strain analysis were excluded. A total of 79 patients with good quality 2D echocardiographic images suitable for strain analysis, whose resting echocardiographic examination was performed within 1 week of the diagnostic coronary angiography were included in the study.

Conventional echocardiographic measurements were performed in accordance with the guidelines [13]. Biplane left ventricle ejection fraction was calculated using the modified Simpson method. End-systolic and end-diastolic diameters, and septal and posterior wall thickness were measured from the parasternal long axis view using M-mode. The diameter of the left atrium was measured using M-mode from the parasternal long view.

Two-dimensional speckle tracking strain analysis was performed by an experienced cardiologist according to the guidelines [14] from the recorded 2D grayscale images using Echopac software, without clinical knowledge of the patients. Cine-loop recorded, three beats of 2D images from 3 apical views (apical 2 chamber, 4 chamber and apical long axis views) with frame rates of 50–80 frames/s were accepted as suitable for strain analysis. In each view, regions of interests were outlined by defining one point on each side of the mitral annulus and one point at the apex. Then, the software automatically traced the borders of the LV myocardium; manual adjustments were made if necessary. Images with poor tracking quality and with more than one untrackable segments were excluded. After manual adjustments, the software calculated strain values in each view. End-systole was defined as aortic valve closure in the apical long axis view. A 17-segment bull's eye view was formed after processing all three apical views. GLS-trans, endocardial, and epicardial values (GLS-trans, GLS-endo, and GLS-epi, respectively) were calculated automatically by the software. Regional longitudinal strain (RLS) was also calculated for all layers, based on the 17 segment model according to the perfusion territories of 3 major coronary arteries by averaging all segments peak strain values within each territory [15].

Intra-observer reliability was assessed by re-analyzing the images of 15 patients 30 days after the first analysis by the same operator. Inter-observer reliability assessment was performed by comparing the measurements of 15 randomly chosen patients, performed by another operator.

Coronary angiographic images were evaluated by an experienced cardiologist who was blinded to patients' data. Lesions $\geq 70\%$ stenosis were accepted as critical stenosis. Patients with significant coronary artery disease were classified as the CAD group, and those without significant CAD were classified as the control group.

The study was conducted in accordance with Declaration of Helsinki and was approved by the local ethics committee.

Statistical analysis

Statistical analysis was performed using IBM SPSS version 22 (IBM SPSS Statistics for Windows, Armonk, NY, IBM Corp). Categorical variables are expressed as numbers and percentages and continuous variables are expressed as mean ± standard deviation. The Kolmogorov-Smirnov test was used to assess the distribution of variables. Continuous variables were compared using the independent samples t-test or Mann-Whitney U test. Categorical values were compared using the Chi-square (χ^2) test or Fisher's exact test. The areas under the Receiver operating characteristics (ROC) curves and their area under the curve (AUC) were constructed for layer-specific GLS and RLS. Inter- and intra-observer reliability were evaluated using Bland-Altman analysis and intra-class correlation. A value of $P < .05$ was accepted as significant.

Results

In total, 79 patients suspected of having stable coronary artery disease were included in the study; 36 without significant CAD (control group) and 43 patients with significant CAD (CAD group). The clinical data of the of the study population are given in Table 1. The ratio of female patients was higher in the control group [$n = 24$ (66.7%) vs. $n = 11$ (25.6%), $P < .001$]. There were no differences between the groups in terms of HT, DM, hyperlipidemia [16], and body mass index (BMI). Twelve (33.3%) of the patients in the control group had MPS, and 20 (46.5%) of the patients in the CAD group had MPS before CAG ($p = 0.235$). Most (83.4%) of the patients in the CAD group had LAD lesions.

Conventional echocardiographic measures and strain values are presented in Table 2. Layer-specific strain measurements were all lower in the CAD group (GLS-trans: $-18.2 \pm 2.4\%$ vs. $-22.2 \pm 2.2\%$, $P < .001$; GLS-endo: $-20.8 \pm 2.8\%$ vs. $-25.3 \pm 2.6\%$, $P < .001$; GLS-epi: $-15.9 \pm 2.4\%$ vs. $-19.5 \pm 1.9\%$, $P < .001$) (Table 2). A comparison of the difference between GLS-endo and GLS-epi revealed a lesser amount of difference in the CAD group (GLS-endo-epi, 5.0 ± 1.1 vs. 5.7 ± 1.2, $P = .007$). RLS values are given in Table 3, all layers in major coronary artery territories demonstrated significantly lower deformation values in patients with significant stenosis.

ROC curves were constructed for layer-specific GLS in patients with CAD (Fig. 1). The diagnostic performance of GLS-trans, GLS-endo and GLS-epi were all significant. The cut-off values for GLS-trans, GLS-endo and GLS-epi were -19.3%, -23.4% and -17.3%, respectively (Table 4).

Table 1 Clinical and angiographical characteristic of the patients

	CAD $n = 43$	Control $n = 36$	P
Demographic data and risk factors			
Age	60.4 ± 9.8	56.4 ± 8.1	.072
Male	32 (74.4%)	12 (33.3%)	<.001
Female	11 (25.6%)	24 (66.7%)	
HT	38 (88.4%)	32 (88.9%)	.943
DM	16 (37.2%)	10 (27, 8%)	.374
HL	30 (69.8%)	20 (55.6%)	.192
BMI, kg/m^2	28.3 ± 5.0	29.7 ± 4.8	.252
MPS	20 (46.5%)	12 (33.3%)	.235
Coronary angiographic parameters			
One Vessel Disease	16	–	
Two Vessel Disease	14	–	
Three vessel disease	13	–	
LMCA	3	–	
LAD	36	–	
Cx	22	–	
RCA	25	–	

BMI Body-mass index, *CAD* Coronary artery disease, *Cx* Circumflex artery, *DM* Diabetes Mellitus, *HL* Hyperlipidemia, *HT* Hypertension, *LAD* Left anterior descending artery, *LMCA* Left main coronary artery, *MPS* Myocardial perfusion scintigraphy, *RCA* Right coronary Artery

After multivariate adjustment (age, sex, BMI, HT, DM, GLS-endo, GLS-epi and GLS transmural) GLS-trans was found as the only independent predictor of CAD [OR:0.472, CI (0.326–0.684), $p < .001$]. ROC curves for layer-specific RLS were shown in Fig. 2 and the analysis of

Table 2 Conventional echocardiographic parameters and longitudinal strain values

	CAD $n = 43$	Control $n = 36$	P
Echocardiogphic parameters			
LV EF, %	65.4 ± 5.3	66.4 ± 4.8	.426
LV EDD, mm	47.5 ± 4.8	47.9 ± 5.1	.737
LV ESD, mm	30.7 ± 4.8	30.9 ± 4.4	.933
LV mass, g/m^2	98.7 ± 18.5	92.0 ± 22.5	.115
LA diameter, mm	38.7 ± 3.7	37.1 ± 2.9	.030
E/e'	8.7 ± 1.7	8.2 ± 1.4	.413
2D Global longitudinal strain (GLS) parameters			
GLS transmural, %	−18.2 ± 2.4	−22.2 ± 2.2	<.001
GLS endocardium, %	−20.8 ± 2.8	−25.3 ± 2.6	<.001
GLS epicardium, %	−15.9 ± 2.4	−19.5 ± 1.9	<.001
GLS endo-epi	5.0 ± 1.1	5.7 ± 1.2	.007

CAD Coronary artery disease, *EDD* End-diastolic diameter, *EF* Ejection fraction, *ESD* End-systolic diameter, *E* Pulsed wave transmitral early diastolic velocity, *e'* Early myocardial diastolic velocity, *GLS* Global longitudinal strain, *LA* Left atrium, *LV* Left ventricle

Table 3 Regional longitudinal strain values

	CAD	Control	P
LAD			
RLS transmural, %	−18.1 ± 2.4	−22.4 ± 2.7	<.001
RLS endocardium,%	−22.1 ± 3.3	−26.7 ± 3.5	<.001
RLS epicardium, %	−15.2 ± 2.4	− 19.2 ± 2.3	<.001
Cx			
RLS transmural, %	−16.6 ± 3.2	−21.2 ± 2.8	<.001
RLS endocardium,%	−18.8 ± 3.4	−24.2 ± 3.3	<.001
RLS epicardium, %	−14.8 ± 3.1	−19.0 ± 2.5	<.001
RCA		.	
RLS transmural, %	−19.2 ± 3.0	−22.7 ± 3.1	<.001
RLS endocardium,%	−21.3 ± 3.2	−25.0 ± 3.2	<.001
RLS epicardium, %	−17.7 ± 2.9	−20.8 ± 2.8	0.001

CAD Coronary artery disease, *Cx* Circumflex artery, *LAD* Left anterior descending artery, *RCA* Right coronary artery, *RLS* Regional longitudinal strain

the curves with AUC were presented in Table 5. RLS$_{LAD}$ and RLS$_{Cx}$ had better predictive power for the detection of significant stenosis in the coronary artery supplying the associated territory, there were no differences between layers in terms of predictive value. (Table 5).

Patients with MPS were grouped as MPS true-positive and MPS false-positive. A comparison of these two groups demonstrated lower strain values in all layers in the true-positive MPS group (GLS-trans: − 17.7 ± 2.4 vs. -21.9 ± 2.4%, *P* < .001; GLS-endo: − 20.2 ± 2.9% vs. -24.9 ± 2.9%, *P* < .001; GLS-epi: 15.4 ± 2.6% vs. -19.2 ± 1.8%, *P* < .001) (Table 6). Layer- specific strain analysis was compared between the

sexes in both groups. There were no significant differences in terms of GLS between the sexes in both groups (Table 7).

Intra-class correlation and Bland-Altman analysis (Fig. 3) was used for the evaluation of intra- and inter-observer variability. Intra-observer reliability, as assessed by inter-class correlation coefficients for GLS-trans, GLS-endo, and GLS-epi were 0.957 (95% CI: 0.876–0.985), 0.937 (95% CI: 0.822–0.978), and 0.945 (95% CI: 0.844–0.990), respectively. Inter-observer reliability, as assessed by inter-class correlation coefficients for GLS-trans, GLS-endo, and GLS-epi were 0.950 (95% CI: 0.857–0.983), 0.920 (95% CI: 0.779–0.972), and 0.951 (95% CI: 0.860–0.983), respectively.

Discussion

The current study demonstrated that GLS was significantly reduced in patients with stable CAD. LSS analysis revealed that all myocardial layers were affected in patients with significant CAD.

Evaluation of left ventricular function and wall motion analysis with conventional 2D echocardiography mostly fails to provide additional information, particularly when there is no history of prior myocardial infarction or structural heart disease. 2D speckle tracking strain analysis is a semi-automated technique that is more sensitive and accurate in measuring LV function than conventional 2D methods. Recently published studies demonstrated that longitudinal myocardial strain imaging with 2D speckle tracking had a diagnostic and prognostic value in patients with acute coronary syndromes [7, 17], and it has also been demonstrated as an independent predictor of significant CAD in patients with SAP [11]. Liou et al. [18]

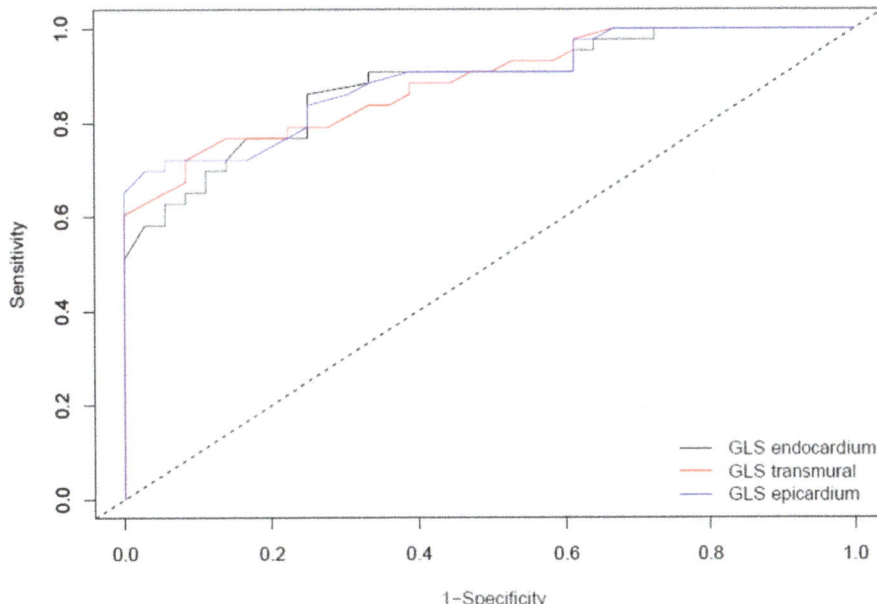

Fig. 1 Receiver operating curves demonstrating value of layer-specific GLS for the diagnosis of CAD. Legends: GLS = Global longitudinal strain

Table 4 Analysis of receiver operating characteristic curves and cut-off values for layer-specific global longitudinal strain

	AUC (95% CI)	Cut-off value	Sensitivity	Specifity	P-value
GLS transmural	0.891 (0.823–0.954)	−19.3%	69.8%	97.2%	<.001
GLS endocardium	0.881 (0.808–0.905)	−23.4%	86.0%	75.0%	<.001
GLS epicardium	0.885 (0.815–0.955)	−17.3%	72.1%	91.7%	<.001

GLS Global longitudinal strain

claimed that GLS could be an early marker of CAD in symptomatic patients. Stankovic et al. [5] demonstrated that strain imaging was superior to visual assessment in the detection of LAD stenosis. In line with these studies, we also demonstrated reduced transmural GLS in patients with significant CAD.

Although studies have been published showing the efficacy of GLS in detecting LV dysfunction with resting TTE examination [5, 12, 19], there are limited data about LSS imaging in stable CAD. LSS analysis allows us to assess each layer of the myocardium separately. Longitudinal endocardial strain is expected to be the most sensitive parameter for detecting significant CAD because ischemia initially affects the endocardium, indicating that LSS could provide additional information in patients suspected SAP. Multi-layer strain imaging has been assessed in patients with non-ST elevation acute coronary syndromes and the results indicated that it could be useful in identifying patients with significant CAD [6, 20]. The correlation of fractional flow reserve (FFR) values and regional LSS was investigated in a retrospective study in patients with SAP [21]. The results demonstrated lower transmural and endocardial longitudinal strain values in lesions with FFR < 0.75. A recently published study assessed LSS in patients with reversible ischemia using MPS [22]. In conclusion, the study revealed that all layers of the myocardium were affected in patients with significant CAD and claimed that both GLS and LSS could increase the diagnostic accuracy of single-photon emission computed tomography (SPECT) imaging. Similarly, in the present study we also investigated patients who underwent elective coronary

angiography with suspected SAP. Our results were also in agreement with the study by Hagemann et al. [22], demonstrating that transmural, endocardial, and epicardial longitudinal strain (LS) values were all lower in patients with CAD compared with the control group. Additionally, in the current study, patients with true-positive and false-positive MPS were also compared and in line with the above-mentioned study, strain values were lower in all layers in patients with true-positive MPS (Table 6) [22]. Although it's hard to draw a definite conclusion with this limited number of patients, these results also imply that 2D strain imaging might improve the diagnostic value of SPECT imaging, however, further prospective studies are needed.

Since endocardial thickening and shortening with systole is greater than epicardial changes, the deformation rate normally decreases from endocardium to epicardium [23–25]. In the current study, in parallel with the abovementioned studies, the gradient in strain values from endocardium to epicardium was apparent in both groups, whereas it was significantly lower in patients with significant CAD, indicating a higher reduction in the endocardial layer (Table 2).

In patients with CAD, ischemia extends from endocardium to epicardium. Initially subendocardial area is affected and endocardial LS deteriorates before epicardial LS abnormalities become apparent [21]. In line with other studies, the present study demonstrated that, in addition to endocardial and transmural LS, epicardial LS values had also reduced in CAD patients [6, 22, 26]. It should be noted that although the deformation among the layers of the myocardium is heterogeneous, it's not independent

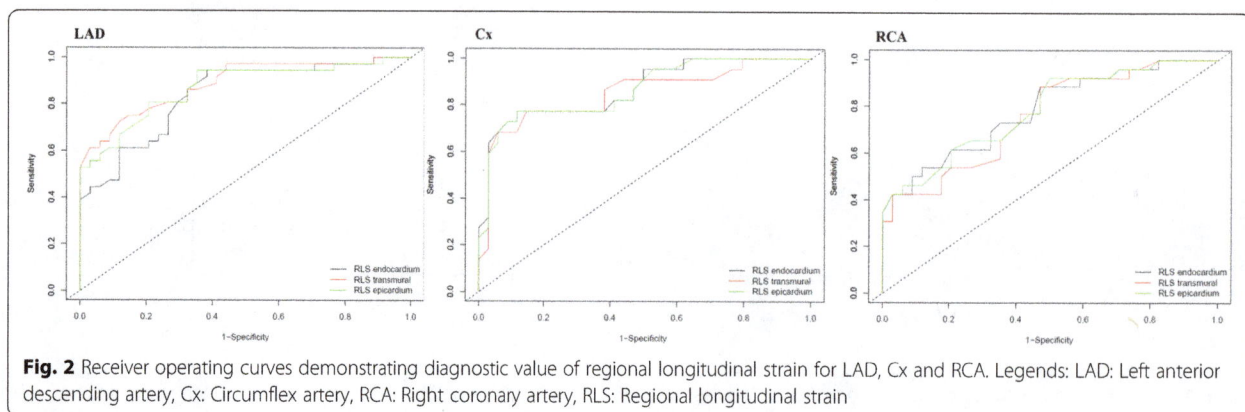

Fig. 2 Receiver operating curves demonstrating diagnostic value of regional longitudinal strain for LAD, Cx and RCA. Legends: LAD: Left anterior descending artery, Cx: Circumflex artery, RCA: Right coronary artery, RLS: Regional longitudinal strain

Table 5 Analysis of receiver operating characteristic curves for layer-specific regional longitudinal strain

	AUC (95%CI)	P-value
RLS$_{LAD}$ transmural	0.871 (0.787–0.954)	<.001
RLS$_{LAD}$ endocardium	0.839 (0.746–0.931)	<.001
RLS$_{LAD}$ epicardium	0.885 (0.808–0.962)	<.001
RLS$_{Cx}$ transmural	0.862 (0.762–0.964)	<.001
RLS$_{Cx}$ endocardium	0.866 (0.767–0.966)	<.001
RLS$_{Cx}$ epicardium	0.848 (0.736–0.961)	<.001
RLS$_{RCA}$ transmural	0.783 (0.667–0.899)	<.001
RLS$_{RCA}$ endocardium	0.784 (0.667–0.900)	<.001
RLS$_{RCA}$ epicardium	0.758 (0.636–0.880)	0.003

Cx Circumflex artery, LAD Left anterior descending artery, RCA Right coronary artery, RLS Regional longitudinal strain

Table 7 Global lonigtudinal strain in female vs male patients

Control Group

Variable	Female n = 24	Male n = 12	P
GLS transmural, %	− 22.5 ± 2.4	− 21.6 ± 1.8	.235
GLS endocardium, %	− 25.6 ± 2.8	−24.6 ± 2.1	.284
GLS epicardium, %	− 19.9 ± 2.0	− 19.1 ± 1.6	.250

Coronary Artery Disease Group

Variable	Female n = 11	Male n = 32	P
GLS transmural, %	− 18.5 ± 2.6	− 18.1 ± 2.4	.664
GLS endocardium, %	− 21.0 ± 3.2	− 20.8 ± 2.8	.790
GLS epicardium, %	− 15.9 ± 2.9	− 15.9 ± 2.3	.949

GLS Global longitudinal strain

from each other. Despite layered structure, the structural integrity of myocardium causes any deformation in one layer to affect the adjacent tissue. The deformation of one layer consists of active function of the layer and passive function from the adjacent layer. Furthermore, CAD severity and lack of collaterals, particularly in the presence of occluded coronary arteries, affect the extend of ischemia from endocardium to epicardium.

Although the ROC curve analysis demonstrated that transmural, endocardial and epicardial GLS had a value in the diagnosis of significant CAD (Fig. 1.), after multivariable regression analysis, only transmural GLS stayed independently associated with CAD. In contrast to the present study, endocardial layer was independently associated with CAD in the studies by Sarvari et al. [26] and Zhang et al. [6]. Additionally, as distinct from these studies, Hagemann et al. [22] claimed that epicardial and mid-myocardial GLS were better predictors of CAD.

Layer-specific RLS was also assessed in addition to GLS. Since CAD causes segmental wall motion abnormalities, RLS analysis sounds reasonable but there's limited data. Liu et al. [20] demonstrated that endocardial GLS and RLS$_{LAD}$ had higher accuracy in identifying LAD stenosis. In the current study, ROC curves for LAD, Cx and RCA territories demonstrated that transmural, endocardial and epicardial LS had diagnostic value but RLS$_{LAD}$ and RLS$_{Cx}$ had better discriminative power than RLS$_{RCA}$ (Fig. 2) On the contrary, due to lack of segmental reference values, and higher inter-vendor variabilities, guidelines do not

Table 6 Layer specific GLS values in myocardial perfusion true positive vs false positive patients

Variable	MPS true positive n = 20	MPS false positive n = 12	P
GLS transmural, %	−17.7 ± 2.4	−21.9 ± 2.4	<.001
GLS endocardium, %	−20.2 ± 2.9	−24.9 ± 2.9	<.001
GLS epicardium, %	−15.4 ± 2.6	−19.2 ± 1.8	<.001

GLS Global longitudinal strain, MPS Myocardial perfusion scintigraphy

recommend strict RLS analysis [13, 27]. The mismatch between RLS and the specific territory of diseased coronary artery can be explained by the anatomical changes in the course of coronary arteries, and microvascular connections causing zones of dual arterial perfusion. Furthermore, it has also been shown that remote areas not supplied by stenotic coronary arteries had also lower strain values than control subjects [20].

Normal values for GLS and LSS have not been standardized yet. Inter-vendor variability, age and sex related changes in strain values are the main factors preventing the determination of cut-off value. It's recommended to use the same software and vendor-specific normal reference values for interpretation [28, 29]. Marwick et al. [30] used the same vendor as we did and demonstrated an average GLS of − 18.6 ± 0.1%. Takidiki et al. assessed normal range of 2D LS and compared three vendors (− 21.3 ± 2.1% vs − 18.9 ± 2.5% vs − 19.9 ± 2.4, p < .001). Recently three studies, using the same vendor as we used, were published investigating the normal values of longitudinal LSS [23–25]. Nakata et al. [24] defined the normal values for transmural, endocardial and epicardial GLS as − 20.0 ± 2.0%, − 23.1 ± 2.3% and − 17.6 ± 1.9%, respectively, whereas the values found by Alcidi et al. for all layers were − 22.7 ± 1.8%, − 25.4 ± 2.1% and − 21.1 ± 1.8%, respectively. Shi et al. [23] also identified similar values for all layers (− 21.3 ± 2.9%, − 24.3 ± 3.1%, and − 18.9 ± 2.8%, respectively). In aggreement with these studies the cut-off values for GLS-trans, GLS-endo and GLS-epi were similar to the normal values abovementioned (− 19.3%, − 23.4% and − 17.3%, respectively).

There are numerous factors such as age, sex, DM, and HT that can affect longitudinal strain. Tadic et al. [31] demonstrated that patients with non-complicated DM and HT also had impaired LV longitudinal strain. In the present study, the rates of DM and HT were similar in both groups. However, the ratio of female patients was higher in the normal coronary angiography group, similar

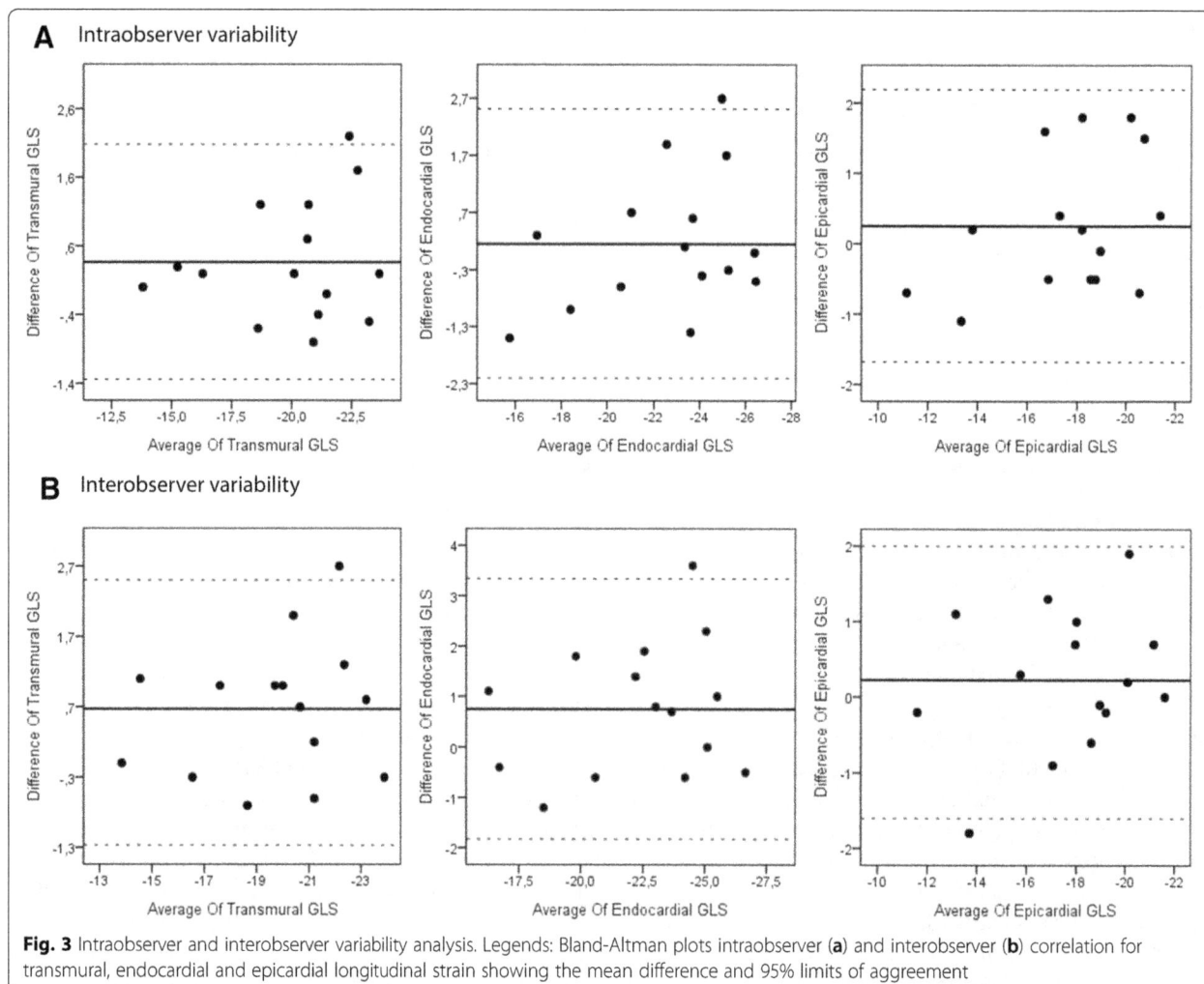

Fig. 3 Intraobserver and interobserver variability analysis. Legends: Bland-Altman plots intraobserver (**a**) and interobserver (**b**) correlation for transmural, endocardial and epicardial longitudinal strain showing the mean difference and 95% limits of aggreement

to previous studies. In the study by Sorenson et al. [11], the rate of male patients was 75% vs. 35% in patients with and without significant CAD, respectively. Previous studies have reported different results about the effect of sex on LSS parameters. Nakata et al. [24] and Shi et al. [23] demonstrated that female patients tended to have higher strain values compared with men, whereas Alcidi et al. [25] could not show a sex-specific difference. Although the results of the studies are conflicting, this difference can be attributed as a confounding factor. However, when we analyzed both groups separately in terms of sex and GLS, the results demonstrated that strain values did not differ between the sexes (Table 7).

Limitations

The present study has several limitations. First, the retrospective nature of this study may have caused a loss of data and selection bias. Secondly, this is a small-scale study with a limited number of patients. As in all studies based on echocardiography, image quality and operator experience have a great effect on proper analysis.

Randomized, prospective, multicenter, larger scale studies powerful enough to assess the effect of all confounding factors are needed to overcome these limitations.

Conclusion

Resting layer-specific LS as assessed by 2D speckle tracking analysis demonstrated that GLS values were reduced in all layers of the myocardium in patients with SAP and with no wall motion abnormalities. These results indicate that GLS can improve the identification of patients with significant CAD but further studies are needed to put forth the incremental value of LSS analysis over transmural GLS.

Abbreviations
2D STE: Two dimensional speckle tracking echocardiography; AUC: Area under the curve; CAD: Coronary artery disease; Cx: Circumflex artery; DM: Diabetes Mellitus; ECG: Electrocardiography; GLS: Global longitudinal strain; HT: Hypertension; LAD: Left anterior descending artery; LS: Longitudinal strain; LSS: Layer-specific strain; MPS: Myocardial perfusion scintigraphy; NIIT: Noninvasive imaging techniques; RCA: Right coronary artery; RLS: Regional longitudinal strain; ROC: Receiver operating characteristics; SAP: Stable angina pektoris; TTE: Transthoracic echocardiography

Authors' contributions

MAY, FMU conducted the patients' enrolment, data collection and echocardiographic imaging. Both authors read and approved the final manuscript.

Consent for publication

Not applicable.

Competing interests

The authors declare that they have no competing interests.

References

1. Task Force M, Montalescot G, Sechtem U, Achenbach S, Andreotti F, Arden C, Budaj A, Bugiardini R, Crea F, Cuisset T, et al. 2013 ESC guidelines on the management of stable coronary artery disease: the task force on the management of stable coronary artery disease of the European Society of Cardiology. Eur Heart J. 2013;34(38):2949–3003.
2. Buechel RR, Kaufmann BA, Tobler D, Wild D, Zellweger MJ. Non-invasive nuclear myocardial perfusion imaging improves the diagnostic yield of invasive coronary angiography. Eur Heart J Cardiovasc Imaging. 2015;16(8):842–7.
3. Sicari R, Cortigiani L. The clinical use of stress echocardiography in ischemic heart disease. Cardiovasc Ultrasound. 2017;15(1):7.
4. Patel MR, Peterson ED, Dai D, Brennan JM, Redberg RF, Anderson HV, Brindis RG, Douglas PS. Low diagnostic yield of elective coronary angiography. N Engl J Med. 2010;362(10):886–95.
5. Stankovic I, Putnikovic B, Cvjetan R, Milicevic P, Panic M, Kalezic-Radmili T, Mandaric T, Vidakovic R, Cvorovic V, Neskovic AN. Visual assessment vs. strain imaging for the detection of critical stenosis of the left anterior descending coronary artery in patients without a history of myocardial infarction. Eur Heart J Cardiovasc Imaging. 2015;16(4):402–9.
6. Zhang L, Wu WC, Ma H, Wang H. Usefulness of layer-specific strain for identifying complex CAD and predicting the severity of coronary lesions in patients with non-ST-segment elevation acute coronary syndrome: compared with syntax score. Int J Cardiol. 2016;223:1045–52.
7. Caspar T, Samet H, Ohana M, Germain P, El Ghannudi S, Talha S, Morel O, Ohlmann P. Longitudinal 2D strain can help diagnose coronary artery disease in patients with suspected non-ST-elevation acute coronary syndrome but apparent normal global and segmental systolic function. Int J Cardiol. 2017;236:91–4.
8. Bendary A, Tawfeek W, Mahros M, Salem M. The predictive value of global longitudinal strain on clinical outcome in patients with ST-segment elevation myocardial infarction and preserved systolic function. Echocardiography. 2018;35(7):915–21.
9. Zuo H, Yan J, Zeng H, Li W, Li P, Liu Z, Cui G, Lv J, Wang D, Wang H. Diagnostic power of longitudinal strain at rest for the detection of obstructive coronary artery disease in patients with type 2 diabetes mellitus. Ultrasound Med Biol. 2015;41(1):89–98.
10. Huang H, Ruan Q, Lin M, Yan L, Huang C, Fu L. Investigation on left ventricular multi-directional deformation in patients of hypertension with different LVEF. Cardiovasc Ultrasound. 2017;15(1):14.
11. Biering-Sorensen T, Hoffmann S, Mogelvang R, Zeeberg Iversen A, Galatius S, Fritz-Hansen T, Bech J, Jensen JS. Myocardial strain analysis by 2-dimensional speckle tracking echocardiography improves diagnostics of coronary artery stenosis in stable angina pectoris. Circ Cardiovasc Imaging. 2014;7(1):58–65.
12. Moustafa S, Elrabat K, Swailem F, Galal A. The correlation between speckle tracking echocardiography and coronary artery disease in patients with suspected stable angina pectoris. Indian Heart J. 2018;70(3):379–86.
13. Lang RM, Badano LP, Mor-Avi V, Afilalo J, Armstrong A, Ernande L, Flachskampf FA, Foster E, Goldstein SA, Kuznetsova T, et al. Recommendations for cardiac chamber quantification by echocardiography in adults: an update from the American Society of Echocardiography and the European Association of Cardiovascular Imaging. Eur Heart J Cardiovasc Imaging. 2015;16(3):233–70.
14. Voigt JU, Pedrizzetti G, Lysyansky P, Marwick TH, Houle H, Baumann R, Pedri S, Ito Y, Abe Y, Metz S, et al. Definitions for a common standard for 2D speckle tracking echocardiography: consensus document of the EACVI/ASE/ industry task force to standardize deformation imaging. Eur Heart J Cardiovasc Imaging. 2015;16(1):1–11.
15. Cerqueira MD, Weissman NJ, Dilsizian V, Jacobs AK, Kaul S, Laskey WK, Pennell DJ, Rumberger JA, Ryan T, Verani MS, et al. Standardized myocardial segmentation and nomenclature for tomographic imaging of the heart. A statement for healthcare professionals from the cardiac imaging Committee of the Council on clinical cardiology of the American Heart Association. Circulation. 2002;105(4):539–42.
16. Trobs M, Achenbach S, Plank PM, Marwan M, Rother J, Klinghammer L, Blachutzik F, Schlundt C. Predictors of technical failure in Transradial coronary angiography and intervention. Am J Cardiol. 2017;120(9):1508–13.
17. Meimoun P, Abouth S, Clerc J, Elmkies F, Martis S, Luycx-Bore A, Boulanger J. Usefulness of two-dimensional longitudinal strain pattern to predict left ventricular recovery and in-hospital complications after acute anterior myocardial infarction treated successfully by primary angioplasty. J Am Soc Echocardiogr. 2015;28(11):1366–75.
18. Liou K, Negishi K, Ho S, Russell EA, Cranney G, Ooi SY. Detection of obstructive coronary artery disease using peak systolic global longitudinal strain derived by two-dimensional speckle-tracking: a systematic review and meta-analysis. J Am Soc Echocardiogr. 2016;29(8):724–35 e724.
19. Hubbard RT, Arciniegas Calle MC, Barros-Gomes S, Kukuzke JA, Pellikka PA, Gulati R, Villarraga HR. 2-dimensional speckle tracking echocardiography predicts severe coronary artery disease in women with normal left ventricular function: a case-control study. BMC Cardiovasc Disord. 2017;17(1):231.
20. Liu C, Li J, Ren M, Wang ZZ, Li ZY, Gao F, Tian JW. Multilayer longitudinal strain at rest may help to predict significant stenosis of the left anterior descending coronary artery in patients with suspected non-ST-elevation acute coronary syndrome. Int J Cardiovasc Imaging. 2016;32(12):1675–85.
21. Nishi T, Funabashi N, Ozawa K, Takahara M, Fujimoto Y, Kamata T, Kobayashi Y. Resting multilayer 2D speckle-tracking transthoracic echocardiography for the detection of clinically stable myocardial ischemic segments confirmed by invasive fractional flow reserve. Part 1: vessel-by-vessel analysis. Int J Cardiol. 2016;218:324–32.
22. Hagemann CE, Hoffmann S, Olsen FJ, Jorgensen PG, Fritz-Hansen T, Jensen JS, Biering-Sorensen T. Layer-specific global longitudinal strain reveals impaired cardiac function in patients with reversible ischemia. Echocardiography. 2018;35(5):632–42.
23. Shi J, Pan C, Kong D, Cheng L, Shu X. Left ventricular longitudinal and circumferential layer-specific myocardial strains and their determinants in healthy subjects. Echocardiography. 2016;33(4):510–8.
24. Nagata Y, Wu VC, Otsuji Y, Takeuchi M. Normal range of myocardial layer-specific strain using two-dimensional speckle tracking echocardiography. PLoS One. 2017;12(6):e0180584.
25. Alcidi GM, Esposito R, Evola V, Santoro C, Lembo M, Sorrentino R, Lo Iudice F, Borgia F, Novo G, Trimarco B, et al. Normal reference values of multilayer longitudinal strain according to age decades in a healthy population: A single-centre experience. Eur Heart J Cardiovasc Imaging. 2017;jex306. https://doi.org/10.1093/ehjci/jex306.
26. Sarvari SI, Haugaa KH, Zahid W, Bendz B, Aakhus S, Aaberge L, Edvardsen T. Layer-specific quantification of myocardial deformation by strain echocardiography may reveal significant CAD in patients with non-ST-segment elevation acute coronary syndrome. JACC Cardiovasc Imaging. 2013;6(5):535–44.
27. Takeuchi M, Wu VC. Application of left ventricular strain to patients with coronary artery disease. Curr Opin Cardiol. 2018;33(5):464–9.
28. Dohi K, Sugiura E, Ito M. Utility of strain-echocardiography in current clinical practice. J Echocardiogr. 2016;14(2):61–70.
29. Farsalinos KE, Daraban AM, Unlu S, Thomas JD, Badano LP, Voigt JU. Head-to-head comparison of global longitudinal strain measurements among nine different vendors: the EACVI/ASE inter-vendor comparison study. J Am Soc Echocardiogr. 2015;28(10):1171–81 e1172.
30. Marwick TH, Leano RL, Brown J, Sun JP, Hoffmann R, Lysyansky P, Becker M, Thomas JD. Myocardial strain measurement with 2-dimensional speckle-tracking echocardiography: definition of normal range. JACC Cardiovasc Imaging. 2009;2(1):80–4.
31. Tadic M, Cuspidi C, Vukomanovic V, Ilic S, Obert P, Kocijancic V, Celic V. Layer-specific deformation of the left ventricle in uncomplicated patients with type 2 diabetes and arterial hypertension. Arch Cardiovasc Dis. 2018;111(1):17–24.

24

The new clinical standard of integrated quadruple stress echocardiography with ABCD protocol

Eugenio Picano[1]* (iD), Quirino Ciampi[2], Karina Wierzbowska-Drabik[3], Mădălina-Loredana Urluescu[4], Doralisa Morrone[5] and Clara Carpeggiani[1]

Abstract

Background: The detection of regional wall motion abnormalities is the cornerstone of stress echocardiography. Today, stress echo shows increasing trends of utilization due to growing concerns for radiation risk, higher cost and stronger environmental impact of competing techniques. However, it has also limitations: underused ability to identify factors of clinical vulnerability outside coronary artery stenosis; operator-dependence; low positivity rate in contemporary populations; intermediate risk associated with a negative test; limited value of wall motion beyond coronary artery disease. Nevertheless, stress echo has potential to adapt to a changing environment and overcome its current limitations.

Integrated-quadruple stress-echo: Four parameters now converge conceptually, logistically, and methodologically in the Integrated Quadruple (IQ)-stress echo. They are: 1- regional wall motion abnormalities; 2-B-lines measured by lung ultrasound; 3-left ventricular contractile reserve assessed as the stress/rest ratio of force (systolic arterial pressure by cuff sphygmomanometer/end-systolic volume from 2D); 4- coronary flow velocity reserve on left anterior descending coronary artery (with color-Doppler guided pulsed wave Doppler). IQ-Stress echo allows a synoptic functional assessment of epicardial coronary artery stenosis (wall motion), lung water (B-lines), myocardial function (left ventricular contractile reserve) and coronary small vessels (coronary flow velocity reserve in mid or distal left anterior descending artery). In "ABCD" protocol, A stands for Asynergy (ischemic vs non-ischemic heart); B for B-lines (wet vs dry lung); C for Contractile reserve (weak vs strong heart); D for Doppler flowmetry (warm vs cold heart, since the hyperemic blood flow increases the local temperature of the myocardium). From the technical (acquisition/analysis) viewpoint and required training, B-lines are the kindergarten, left ventricular contractile reserve the primary (for acquisition) and secondary (for analysis) school, wall motion the university, and coronary flow velocity reserve the PhD program of stress echo.

Conclusion: Stress echo is changing. As an old landline telephone with only one function, yesterday stress echo used one sign (regional wall motion abnormalities) for one patient with coronary artery disease. As a versatile smart-phone with multiple applications, stress echo today uses many signs for different pathophysiological and clinical targets. Large scale effectiveness studies are now in progress in the Stress Echo2020 project with the omnivorous "ABCD" protocol.

Keywords: B-lines, Coronary flow reserve, Echocardiography, Force, Left ventricular contractility, Lung water, Stress echocardiography, Wall motion abnormalities

* Correspondence: picano@ifc.cnr.it; eugenio.picano@ifc.cnr.it
[1]Institute of Clinical Physiology, National Council Research, Via Giuseppe Moruzzi 1, 56124 Pisa, Italy
Full list of author information is available at the end of the article

Background

Utilization trends of stress echo

Stress echocardiography (SE) is since decades an established technique for coronary artery disease (CAD) detection and risk stratification [1], with a recognized position in expert recommendations of scientific societies [2, 3] and general cardiology guidelines [4, 5]. In recent years, the new cost-conscious and radiation-conscious climate was the main driver of the observed reduction in myocardial stress scintigraphy and simultaneous growth of SE [6]. In Australia, from 2002 to 2013 the rate of SE use increased 4-fold [7]. In the same time period, the use of other established stress techniques such as stress myocardial scintigraphy remained stable or declined (Fig. 1). In privately insured US patients younger than 65 years, the use of SE increased by 27% from 2005 to 2012 [8]. In Mayo Clinic, the use of myocardial scintigraphy showed a 20-fold rise from 1990 to 1999, but since 2000 SE was introduced and in 2012 the relative utilization rate was 5 SE to 1 scintigraphy [9]. In Ontario, Canada, from 2011 to 2014 the utilization rate of stress scintigraphy decreased at a mean annual rate of - 1.3%, whereas SE in the same period increased at a mean annual rate of + 65.8% [10].

The increased use of SE brings with it an increased risk of inappropriateness [11]. Inappropriate testing is a waste of public health money and also lowers the diagnostic and prognostic value of SE [11–13]. Three indications, account for 79% of all inappropriate testing: symptomatic patients with low pre-test probability of CAD having an interpretable ECG and ability to exercise, asymptomatic patients who had undergone angioplasty less than 2 years before, and asymptomatic patients with low risk [11–14].

SE and the road to sustainability

The prescription of a single individual cardiac stress imaging test has a large economic, environmental and public health impact since around 10 million stress cardiac imaging test are performed each year in USA only. Small economic wastes, environmental footprint, individual risks of the single inappropriate test multiplied by millions per year represent an avoidable burden for the society and the planet, and a significant population risk [14].

The direct cost of a stress myocardial scintigraphy is 2- to 4- fold higher than SE (5). The difference further widens if we include - as we should - indirect costs due to environmental impact on planet and long-tem costs due to cancer [15].

The environmental impact of a single cardiovascular magnetic resonance or myocardial perfusion scintigraphy is 5- to 100-times higher than that of a SE on human health, ecosystem effects and resource use. One ton of CO_2 emissions costs 50 US dollars in indirect costs, including contribution to climate change and ozone layer destruction. One echocardiogram produces about 2 kg of CO_2 and a 3 Tesla magnetic resonance imaging produces 200 to 300 kg of CO_2 [16, 17].

The radiation dose of a single myocardial scintigraphy ranges from 200 to 4000 chest x-rays, whereas there is no radiation exposure for SE or magnetic resonance. In terms of population burden, the almost 8 million stress myocardial scintigraphy scans per year in the USA translate into a population risk of about 8 thousand new cancers in the lifetime [18], which represent also an extra-cost of around 50,000 US dollars per cancer [17].

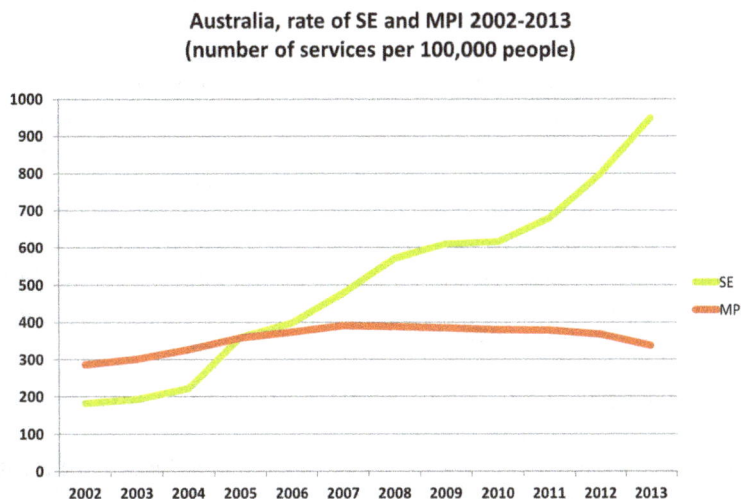

Fig. 1 Utilization trends of stress echo. The utilization trends of stress echo compared to myocardial stress scintigraphy in Australia, years 2002–2012 (redrawn from Fonseca et al., ref. [10])

It is therefore not only important the value, but also the cost and the risk of what we are doing in the cardiac imaging lab. In the cost-benefit balance, the cost must include the long-term environmental burden, not only the direct cost. In the risk-benefit balance, the risk must include the long-term cancer risk, not only the acute risks of stress or contrast injection [19]. This obvious concept was a game-changer in the last 15 years [14]. Until 2004, almost no cardiologist knew the radiation doses and risks of what he or she was doing to the patient [20]. Today, mainstream cardiology prescribes that good training should create a culture of respect for radiation hazard and a commitment to minimize exposure and maximize protection [21] .

In this changing scenario, SE plays a key role as the most cost-effective gatekeeper to coronary angiography and ischemia-driven revascularization, associated with fewer downstream coronary angiographies and subsequent risk of adverse events, as shown by a recent meta-analysis including 30 randomized trials on 33,356 patients with low risk acute coronary syndromes or suspected CAD [22]. The strategy centered on functional imaging with SE for prognostic stratification minimizes the radiation exposure associated with an anatomy-first approach by CT coronary angiography complemented by functional testing with scintigraphy, which frequently reaches cumulative exposures in the range of 5000 chest X-rays per patient and sometimes per exam as shown in the Radio-EVINCI international trial [23]. Compared in a randomized manner to exercise-ECG in a low-to- moderate risk population with suspected CAD, a strategy based on upfront SE led to a 20% reduction of costs, due to the combined effects of a reduction in downstream testing, emergency visits and duration of hospital stay [24]. Therefore, a systematic use of SE cuts the costs of downstream testing, deflates the volumes of myocardial scintigraphies, reduces the need for noninvasive and invasive coronary angiography, and puts a substantial barrier, also in medico-legal terms, to the shortcut to anatomy-driven, prognostically futile and inappropriate coronary revascularizations [25]. The optimized and versatile use of SE is an effective way for primary prevention of cancer through the reduction of inappropriate and unjustified use of ionizing testing and therapies [26]. After 25 years of follow-up, 26% of those with positive SE (compared to 17% of patients with negative SE) will die of cancer, and this happens more frequently in patients exposed to higher levels of ionizing testing and therapies [27].We should always minimize the avoidable long-term damage of tomorrow when treating the cardiac patient today, exactly as the oncologists should minimize the prognosis-limiting future cardiac damage when treating cancer with radiotherapy and chemotherapy. A comprehensive risk-benefit analysis should include the

chances of long-term damage decades down the line in organs other than those targeted by the primary therapeutic effort.

The limitations of contemporary SE
In spite of its unsurpassed strengths which make it a dominant technique due to low cost, absence of radiation, environmental friendly nature and versatility coupled with universal availability, SE has important weaknesses that restrict its use and value.

The stenotico-centric approach to CAD diagnosis
The vulnerabilities of the patient with CAD and/or heart failure (HF) are multiple and complex, and RWMA is not helpful to capture factors independent from coronary artery stenosis. For any given coronary stenosis or even in the absence of it, the clinical vulnerability to adverse events is more likely in presence of coronary microcirculation abnormalities, alveolar-capillary membrane distress determining increased extravascular lung water, and myocardial scar or fibrosis of the left ventricle (LV) limiting the global contractile reserve [28].

Subjectivity of reading
The operator-dependence can be minimized - not abolished - by expert training and adoption of conservative reading criteria, with credentialing via standardized web-based training and certification [29]. Reading harmonization is made easier in the era of connectivity and a second-opinion obtained in real time by senior readers via web and smart-phones [30] can substantially improve the standards of the laboratory, whereas the clinical help of quantitative advanced technologies remains unsettled during stress [2, 3].

The low positivity rate of RWMA
The changing profile of patients referred for CAD has dramatically reduced the rate of positive tests based on RWMA, dropped from 70% in the early eighties to < 10% in the first decade of the new millennium [31]. This is due to the higher percentage of patients referred to SE under anti-ischemic therapy, with atypical or absent symptoms and low pre-test probability of disease [31]. The predictive value of the test depends upon the prevalence of the disease in the population under study. The application of SE to a population with 10% prevalence of disease implies that a positive test is associated with a probability of < 50% of having the disease (the so-called "false positive paradox").

The intermediate risk associated with a negative test for RWMA
The risk associated with a negative test is intermediate, not low, and significantly higher than that associated

with the negativity of a myocardial perfusion stress test. A recent meta-analysis on 36 studies with 14, 506 patients with known or suspected CAD showed that the hard-event rate (cardiac death and myocardial infarction) in patients with a negative SE for RWMA is still 1.77% per year, which is not so low [32].

The limited value of RWMA outside CAD
The population of patients arriving to the SE lab is changing, with a greater percentage of patients with HF, valvular heart disease, adult congenital heart disease, pulmonary hypertension, extreme physiology [33]. In these patients RWMA have little to offer, and the versatility of the technique is largely underused in patients who would certainly benefit from a more comprehensive approach.

Quadruple imaging IQ-SE: the ABCD protocol
In order to overcome the main limitations of SE based only on RWMA, a new standard of practice has been proposed merging four different parameters with different pathophysiological targets (Fig. 2). In the ABCD protocol, A stands for asynergy and targets a critical epicardial artery stenosis through RWMA; B for B-lines and evaluates pulmonary interstitial edema; C for left ventricular contractile reserve (LVCR) and assesses global myocardial function; and D for Doppler which offers insight into coronary microcirculatory function with coronary flow velocity reserve (CFVR). The main conceptual, methodological and clinical features of the 4 key parameters are shown in Tables 1 and 2.

The ABCD parameters are conceptually merged, temporally synchronized, and methodologically harmonized in the new standard adopted in SE 2020 study: the Integrated Quadruple (IQ)-SE [34].

The technical challenges are not much greater than that posed by imaging and assessment of RWMA alone. Some of the new parameters are faster to image and simpler to measure than the old ones. The acquisition of diagnostic images is the simplest for B-lines, simple with LVCR, not-so-simple for RWMA and more difficult for CFVR. The image analysis is the simplest for B-lines and CFVR, not-so-simple for LVCR and more difficult for RWMA. All in all, integrating the required training for image acquisition and analysis, B-lines can be considered the kindergarten, LVCR the primary (for acquisition) or secondary (for analysis) school, RWMA the university, and CFVR the PhD course of the SE *cursus studiorum*.

A for regional wall motion asynergy: ischemic or non-ischemic heart
The conceptual meaning
The cardinal sign of transient myocardial ischemia is a stress-induced regional asynergy (also called dyssynergy) in its three degrees: hypokinesia (reduction of systolic motion and thickening); akinesia (absence of systolic thickening and motion); and dyskinesia (paradoxical systolic movement and systolic thinning) [1]. The absence of RWMA identifies a non-ischemic heart (Fig. 3, first row); its presence an ischemic heart (Fig. 4, first row). Ischemia is required for RWMA, but even under ideal imaging conditions RWMA can occur without ischemia (for instance in left bundle branch block or pacemaker stimulation from the right ventricle or myocardial fibrosis in non-ischemic dilated cardiomyopathy), and ischemia (or even infarction) can occur without RWMA. In fact, the detection of RWMA requires a critical ischemic mass of at least 20% of transmural wall thickness and about 5% of the total myocardial mass. Therefore,

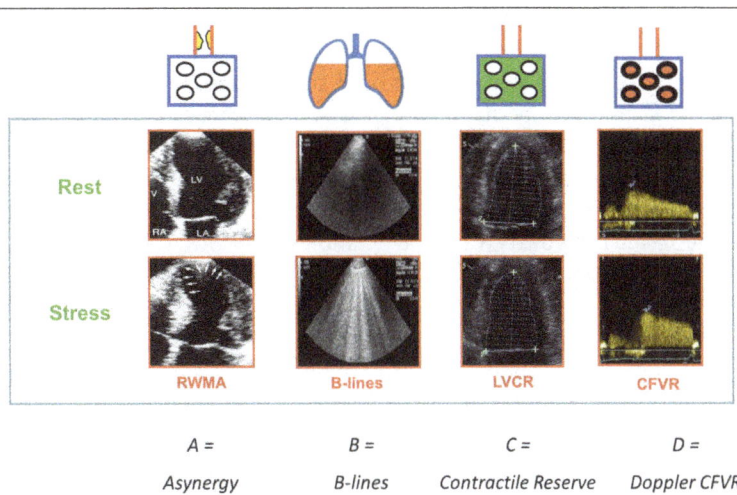

Fig. 2 The targets of integrated quadruple imaging stress echo. The 4 patho-physiological targets of IQ-SE: epicardial coronary artery stenosis (with RWMA); lung water (with B-lines); myocardial function (with LVCR); small vessels (with CFVR)

Table 1 The pathophysiological and methodological basis of the IQ-SE protocol

	RWMA	B-lines	LVCR	CFVR
ABCD protocol	A, Asynergy	B, B-lines	C, Contractility	D, Doppler
Target	Epicardial Coronary Stenosis	Lung	Myocardium	LAD stenosis and small vessels
Variable	Ischemia	Water	Force	Flow reserve
Echocardiography	2D	LUS	2-D	PWD
Best projection	4-,3–2 ch	4-site scan	4- and 2-ch	Modified 3-ch
Imaging time	Minutes	Seconds	Seconds	Minutes
Analysis time	Seconds	Seconds	Seconds	Seconds
Feasibility	> 90%	Near 100%	> 95%	> 80%
Evidence	Excellent	Initial	Moderate	Good
Reading	Qualitative	Semi-quantitative	Quantitative	Quantitative
Key parameter	WMSI	B-lines score	ESV	Peak velocity
Abnormal Cut-off	> 1.0	≥ 2.0	< 2.0[a]	< 2.0

[a]< 1.1 in vasodilator stress

relatively milder and more localized forms of ischemia do not leave echocardiographic fingerprints on RWMA [1] .

Pathophysiology
RWMA are linked to stress-induced subendocardial hypoperfusion, usually caused by a critical reduction in coronary flow reserve due to an anatomically and physiologically significant epicardial artery stenosis [1]. A reduction in subendocardial blood flow of 20% produces a 20% decrease in regional wall thickening (mild hypokinesis); a 50% reduction in subendocardial blood flow a 40% reduction in wall thickening (severe hypokinesis); and when subendocardial blood flow is reduced by 80%, akinesia occurs. When the flow reduction is extended to the subepicardial layer, dyskinesia occurs [1].

In viable segments with resting RWMA, stress will normalize function through an increase in flow. This allows to separate viable from necrotic segment, the latter showing no improvement after stress with a fixed wall motion response (akinesis at rest- unchanged after stress). The possibility of recruiting the inotropic reserve might appear paradoxical in the presence of hibernation or stunning. The traditional concept is that a decrease in resting coronary blood flow indicates that coronary vasodilating reserve is exhausted. However, hibernating and stunned segments have some residual coronary vasodilatory reserve, which is mirrored by contractile reserve. The

physiology of myocardium is that of an erectile organ, and in the low flow range the increase in flow is paralleled by an increase in regional function [35].

Methodology
RWMA is summarized in the Wall Motion Scored Index, with a segmental score from 1 = normal/ hyperkinetic to 4 = dyskinetic in a 16- or 17-segment model of the LV (2, 3). Stress values of peak Wall Motion Score Index may range from normal (rest = stress = 1.0) to mild (1.07–1.40), moderate (1.41–1.69), and severe (≥1.70) left ventricular dysfunction, with higher values associated with worse outcome [36].

Clinical evidences
RWMA are more specific (around 90%) but less sensitive (around 80%) than perfusion abnormalities for the detection of CAD, and this is true regardless of the employed stress or imaging technique [2–5]. The ischemic response by RWMA is a strong prognostic predictor of subsequent hard events and death in all patients subsets, from low risk patients with stable angina and preserved baseline left ventricular function to patients with known CAD and previous myocardial infarction [2–5]. The risk stratification can be improved with the combination of RWMA with clinical parameters, if we consider 6 simple items to build a score ranging from zero to 6 which acts as a multiplier of SE risk. The considered items are: age > 65 years; male sex; diabetes; left bundle branch block; anti-anginal therapy at the time of testing; wall motion abnormalities at rest [37]. The hard-event rate of a negative SE increases 20-fold in a negative SE and 100-fold in a positive SE when going from 0 to 1 to 5–6 clinical risk factors.

In patients with reduced resting left ventricular function, an improvement in regional wall motion during SE

Table 2 The prognostic potential of the IQ-SE protocol

	Very Low risk	Very High risk
RWMA	Absent	Present
LUS	A-lines	B-lines
LVCR	Preserved	Reduced
CFVR-LAD	Preserved	Reduced
Risk for major events	< 0.5% per year	> 10% per year

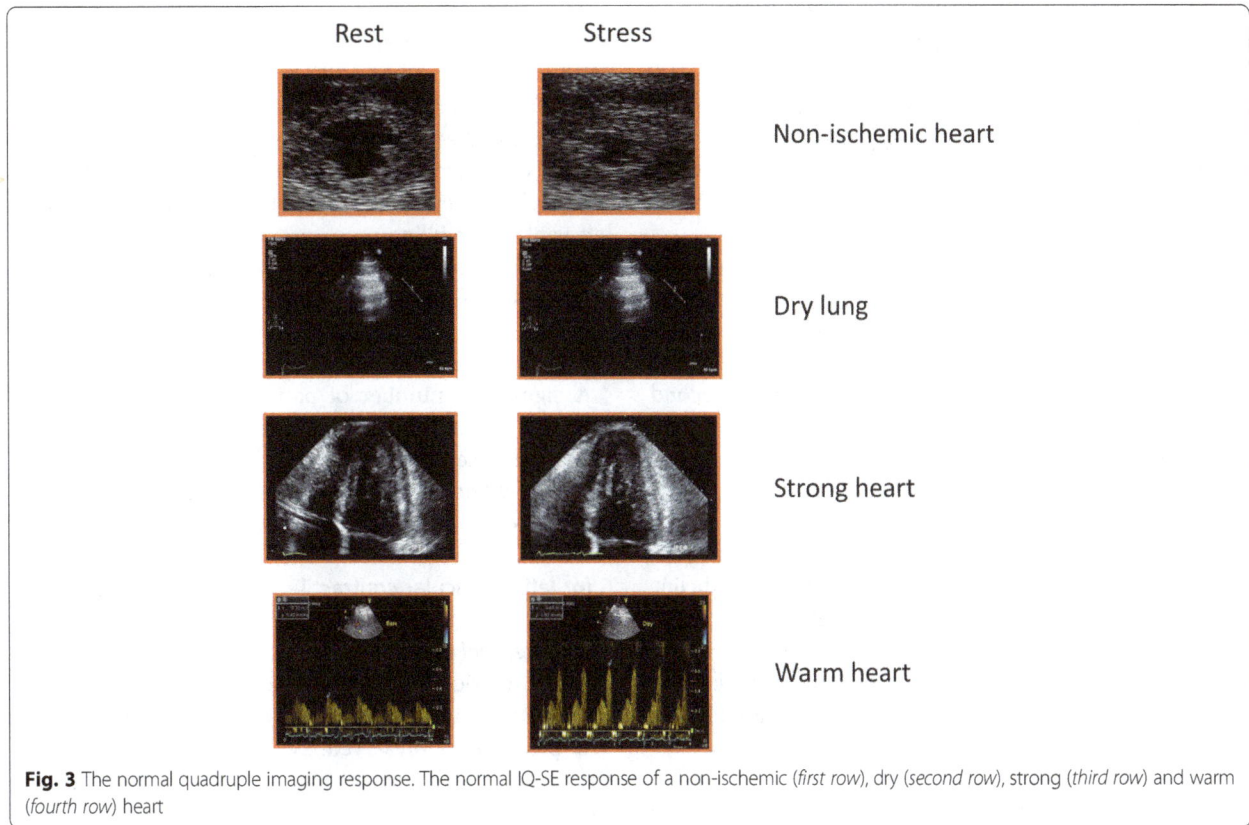

Fig. 3 The normal quadruple imaging response. The normal IQ-SE response of a non-ischemic (*first row*), dry (*second row*), strong (*third row*) and warm (*fourth row*) heart

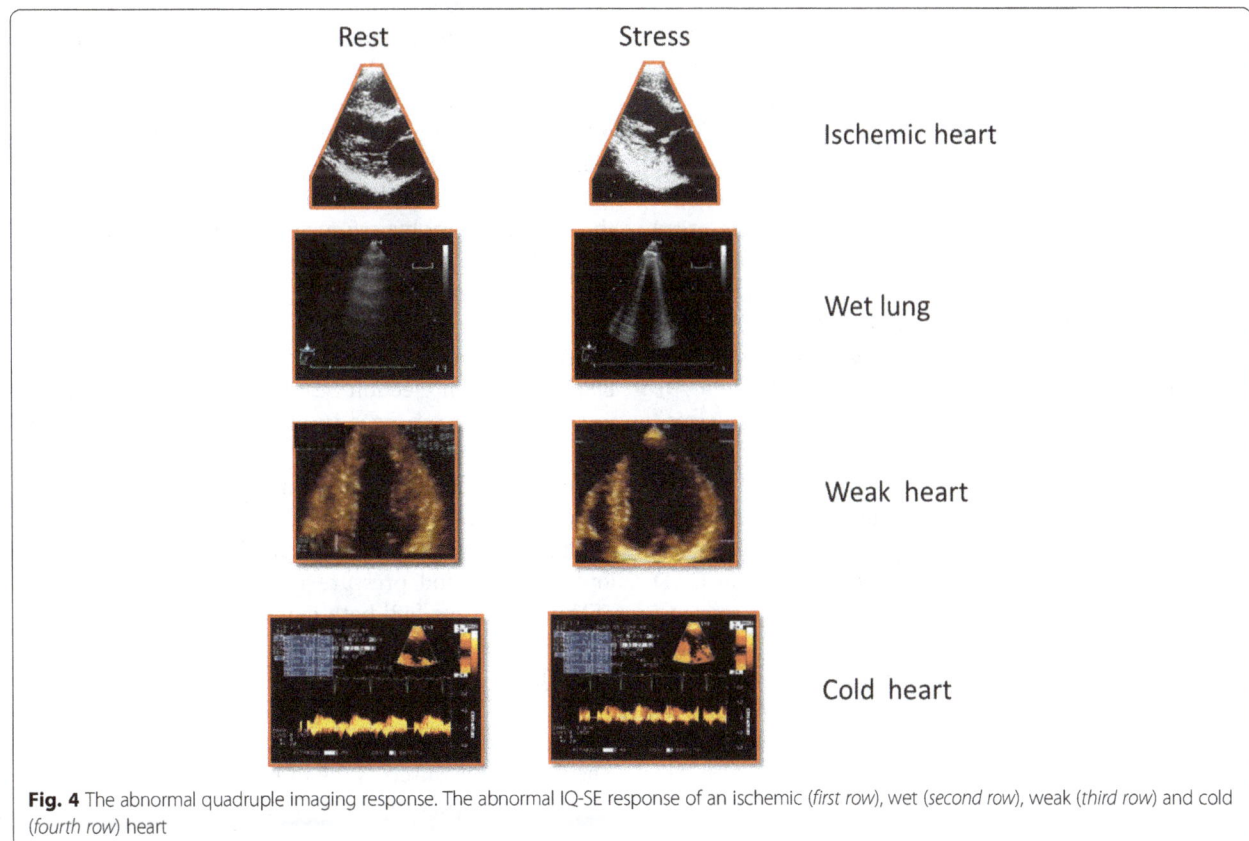

Fig. 4 The abnormal quadruple imaging response. The abnormal IQ-SE response of an ischemic (*first row*), wet (*second row*), weak (*third row*) and cold (*fourth row*) heart

("viability response") is associated with a better survival in different groups of patients: early after acute transmural myocardial infarction, chronic ischemic CAD, non-ischemic dilated cardiomyopathy on medical therapy [2–5] or treated with cardiac resynchronization therapy [38].

B for B-lines: wet or dry lung
The conceptual meaning
The normal A-profile (normal lung sliding with A-lines) detected with lung ultrasound (LUS) identifies a relatively dry lung (Fig. 3, second row) with < 500 mL of extravascular lung water. The B-profile (normal lung sliding and B-lines increasing during stress) a wet lung (Fig. 4, second row) with abnormal accumulation of extravascular lung water [39].

Pathophysiology
The B-profile with normal lung sliding and B-lines provides a unique way to evaluate semi-quantitatively subclinical pulmonary congestion which heralds impending acute HF and cannot be assessed reliably with standard approaches of measuring weight gain, pulmonary crackles on lung auscultation, or Kerley B-lines on chest X-rays [40].

Methodology
LUS focused on B-lines usually starts within 5 s of the end of exercise, or antidote administration in pharmacological stress. The 4-site simplified scan requires on average 20 s, and is equally accurate than the more time-consuming 28-site scan previously adopted [41]. Scanning is performed on the anterior and lateral hemithoraces, from midaxillary to mid-clavicular lines on the third intercostal space. Each site is scored from 0 (A-lines) to 10 (white lung of coalescing B-lines). The cumulative score range is from 0 to 40, with delta (Δ, stress- rest) values < 2 considered normal. The intra- and inter-observer variability are < 5 and < 10% respectively. An increase of B-lines during stress ≥2 is significant (abnormal). Stress B-lines values may range from normal dry lung (rest = stress = 0–1), or wet lung with mild (2–5), moderate (6–9), and severe (≥10) accumulation of extravascular lung water.

Clinical evidences
B-lines during stress are detectable in the majority of patients with HF and either reduced [42] and preserved ejection fraction (EF) [43], and may also appear in CAD patients during physical or pharmacological stress [44]. Their appearance or worsening during stress is associated with higher resting levels of cardiac natriuretic peptides, lower anaerobic threshold during spiroergometry testing, and a worse outcome, with higher mortality and rate of re-hospitalization for acute decompensated HF [44]. In patients with CAD, stress B-lines are associated with extensive RWMA but may occur also in patients

with normal left ventricular function and normal coronary arteries, in presence of severe mitral regurgitation, systolic blood pressure > 200 mmHg or increased systolic pulmonary artery pressure due to diastolic dysfunction [44]. Rest and especially (further upstream) stress B-lines are an early event in the pre-symptomatic "lung water cascade" of events eventually leading from increase in left ventricular filling pressures to pulmonary congestion and clinical decompensation. They might eventually become a specific marker of cardiac origin of dyspnea in the same way as a RWMA is today considered a highly specific marker of ischemic origin of chest pain [45].

A significant number of patients can show B-lines at rest and during stress due to interstitial lung disease. However, these fibrotic ("dry") B- lines do not change with exercise, differently from watery ("wet") B-lines which increase with exercise and decrease with diuretics [44].

C for left ventricular contractile reserve: weak or strong heart
The conceptual meaning
The left ventricular force (also called elastance) is a measure of the intrinsic contractile state of the ventricle [46]. The presence of preserved LVCR during SE identifies a strong heart with higher values of peak stress force and smaller LV end-systolic volume (ESV) than baseline (Fig. 3, third row). An abnormal LVCR is associated with a weak heart with lower peak values of force and larger LV ESV at peak stress than baseline (Fig. 4, third row). LVCR contains information on left ventricular volumes and systolic blood pressure missed by RWMA, and on the other side RWMA gives an information on subendocardial layer perfusion missed by LVCR, which is usually normal in presence of localized hypoperfusion, also for the compensatory hyperfunction of non-ischemic regions or layers. The heart can be ischemic but strong, and non-ischemic yet weak.

Pathophysiology
Differently from ejection fraction (EF), LVCR is not (or less) affected by changes in preload, afterload and heart rate. The conventional definition of contractile reserve by ≥5 points increase in EF only in 40% of cases agrees with LVCR defined by force [47]. Force definition incorporates two well recognized prognostic markers, since low systolic blood pressure response and increased LV ESV during stress [48] both determine a blunted force response and have been separately associated with increased mortality.

Methodology
The force is measured as the ratio of end-systolic pressure (by cuff sphygmomanometer)/ESV (by 2D echocardiography). The calculation of ESV by 2D echocardiography is

a relatively precise measurement, with > 90% measurements within 10% difference, and a substantially lower inter-observer variability of ESV than end-diastolic volume [49, 50]. LVCR is the peak stress/rest ratio of left ventricular force. LVCR values during dobutamine or exercise stress may range from normal (> 2.0) to mild (1.5–2.0), moderate (1.01–1.49), and severe (≤1.0) dysfunction. Values are shifted towards lower values (abnormal < 1.1) for vasodilator stresses [47].

Clinical evidences

LVCR is highly feasible during all forms of stress: exercise [51], pacing [52], dobutamine [53] and dipyridamole [54]. In patients with stable angina and normal resting left ventricular function, LVCR reduction during dipyridamole stress showed a 86% sensitivity and 87% specificity for the detection of angiographically assessed CAD [55]. When outcome is the gold standard, LVCR reduction outperforms RWMA, Δ-WMSI and Δ-EF in predicting adverse events including death [53, 56, 57]. In absence of RWMA, an impaired LVCR is more often present with underlying critical CAD and/ or myocardial scar in brain-dead marginal heart donors who underwent autoptic verification after stress [54].

D for Doppler flowmetry in coronary flow velocity reserve: warm or cold heart

The conceptual meaning

The increase in coronary blood flow during hyperemia can be conceptually associated with changes in the local myocardial temperature. Experimental and clinical studies show that a decrease in blood flow leads to a drop of regional myocardial temperature, and an increase leads to the immediate appearance of warm spots detectable by a noninvasive thermogram [58]. Therefore the presence of a preserved CFVR identifies a warm heart (Fig. 3, fourth row), whereas an abnormal (reduced) CFVR is associated with a cold heart (Fig. 4, fourth row).

Pathophysiology

CFVR can be impaired in presence of a physiologically significant epicardial artery stenosis and in this case is usually - but not always - accompanied by RWMA [33]. A blunted CFVR often occurs with normal coronary arteries in absence of RWMA, in presence of an altered coronary microcirculation, as it can be found for instance in non-ischemic dilated cardiomyopathy, hypertrophic cardiomyopathy, HF with normal EF, aortic stenosis, acute rejection of transplanted heart and several other conditions [3, 33].

Methodology

Noninvasively assessed CFVR obtained from TTE is tightly correlated with invasively assessed coronary flow

reserve [59]. Acquisition of pulsed-wave Doppler of coronary flow velocity on LAD is performed at baseline and peak stress, usually just before RWMA and LVCR. It is the least feasible and the more technically demanding of the new parameters: it can be obtained in over 90% of patients on mid-distal LAD, but requires state-of-the art technology and dedicated training. Once properly acquired, it is easy to measure and has simple, stress-independent prognostic cut-offs (abnormal values < 2.0). Although most data have been obtained with vasodilator stress [59], which is by far technically easier and therefore more popular for assessing CFVR, similar data can be obtained with dobutamine [60] and with semi-supine exercise stress [61] . Stress values may range from normal (> 2.0) to mild (1.7–2.0), moderate (1.41–1.69), and severe (≤1.40) dysfunction [59].

Clinical evidences

In patients with suspected CAD, CFVR has high sensitivity but limited specificity for CAD detection and only targets the left anterior descending coronary artery, which limits the diagnostic usefulness [59] . The main interest in CFVR is therefore for risk stratification. Patients with negative SE identified on the basis of absence of RWMA can be reclassified as at intermediate risk if a reduced CFVR is present. A reduced CFVR predicts a higher mortality, is not affected - differently from RWMA [62] - by concomitant anti-anginal therapy [63] and has additional and independent prognostic value over RWMA in different patients' subsets, including stable coronary artery disease [63], non-ischemic dilated cardiomyopathy [64], hypertrophic cardiomyopathy [65], and asymptomatic moderate-to-severe aortic stenosis with normal EF and normal coronary arteries [66]. The prognostic information is incremental over that provided by myocardial perfusion scintigraphy in patients with suspected CAD [67].

Risk stratification of SE results beyond regional wall motion abnormalities

The integration of 4 different variables into a single one-stop shop expands the risk stratification potential of SE. The current approach to risk stratification is based on presence or absence of RWMA (Fig. 5, upper row). This approach is the only possible evidence-based strategy today [4, 5] but clearly under-uses the unique versatility of SE when dual and triple imaging are applied. In 103 patients with HF and reduced EF studied with dual (RWMA+B-lines) imaging, during a median follow-up of 8 months new major events occurred in 36% of patients without exercise-induced RWMA with moderate-to-severe B-lines, and only in 5% of those with absent or mild stress B-lines [42]. In 91 patients with HF due to idiopathic dilated cardiomyopathy studied with dual (RWMA+LVCR)

Risk stratification beyond regional wall motion abnormalities

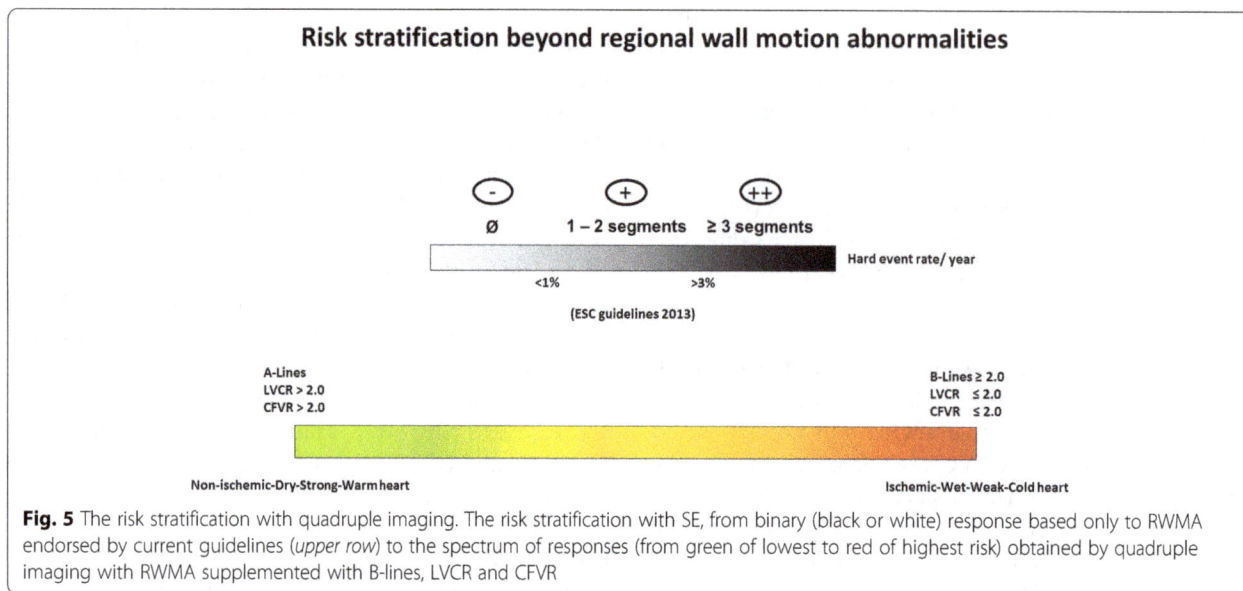

Fig. 5 The risk stratification with quadruple imaging. The risk stratification with SE, from binary (black or white) response based only to RWMA endorsed by current guidelines (*upper row*) to the spectrum of responses (from green of lowest to red of highest risk) obtained by quadruple imaging with RWMA supplemented with B-lines, LVCR and CFVR

imaging, event rate at 18 months was 4% in patients with, and 37% in patients without preserved LVCR [53]. In 4313 patients with known or suspected stable CAD studied with dual (RWMA+ CFVR) imaging, the 4-year mortality associated with a negative test for RWMA was 3% in patients with preserved CFVR and 12% in those with reduced CFVR [68]. In 375 diabetic patients without dipyridamole-induced RWMA and studied with triple imaging (RWMA+ LVCR+CFVR), the rate of hard events at 3-year follow-up was 3% in patients with both normal CFVR and LVCR, 5-fold higher in patients with abnormality of either CFVR or LVCR, and 9-fold higher in patients with both abnormal CFVR and LVCR [69]. The black and white risk stratification becomes color-coded with a spectrum of responses (from benign all-negative green-code to malignant all-positive red-code) (Fig. 5, lower row).

The ABCD protocol in diastolic stress echocardiography

A specific and challenging aspect for SE is the diagnosis of diastolic dysfunction. Diastolic SE is useful in patients with unexplained shortness of breath, exertional fatigue or poor exercise capacity, with normal left ventricular ejection fraction, high cardiac natriuretic peptides, especially in presence of cardiovascular risk factors (advanced age, arterial systemic hypertension, diabetes mellitus, obesity, sedentary lifestyle) and structural alterations of resting TTE such as left atrial volume index dilation and left ventricular hypertrophy. SE is currently recommended in patients falling in the normal or gray zone of diastolic function at rest, as determined by an integration of several parameters: mitral velocities (E, E wave deceleration time, A and E/A ratio), mitral annular velocity (e'), E/e' ratio, peak velocity of tricuspid regurgitant jet and left atrial volume index [70]. During exercise, tricuspid regurgitant jet

velocity and E/e' are considered the most valuable parameters, and their increase suggests the presence of pulmonary hemodynamic congestion and increased LV filling pressures indicative of diastolic dysfunction during stress [71] .

Recent data suggest that the current approach based mainly on tricuspid regurgitant jet velocity and E/e' can suffer from substantial feasibility and accuracy problems [50, 72]. Other parameters may be more feasible and possibly more useful during stress, such as acceleration time of pulmonary flow and B-lines. Acceleration time is measured as the time interval between onset of systolic flow to peak flow, and the normal value is > 105 ms [73]. It decreases with increases in pulmonary artery mean and systolic pressures [74]. The initial clinical experience demonstrates a substantially higher feasibility of acceleration time compared to tricuspid regurgitant jet velocity during stress [75]. Experimental data suggest that the presence and progression of HF with preserved EF is accompanied by shortening of acceleration time and increase of B-lines [76].

Therefore, the ABCD protocol has potential to be applied also in diastolic SE, since the regional wall motion abnormalities (A) must be ruled out in the initial evaluation with SE to screen the origin of dyspnea due to ischemia or mitral regurgitation or left ventricular outflow tract obstruction. B-lines can be present as a hallmark of the cardiogenic origin of dyspnea and have a specific, attractive potential in this specific application [43]. Left ventricular contractile reserve (C) can be useful to detect a subclinical occult systolic dysfunction in a subset of these patients [77]. D might be helpful for a more comprehensive pathophysiological and prognostic assessment of these patients, who are known to have a reduced coronary flow reserve associated with a worse outcome [78]. In addition to the core ABCD protocol, new parameters can be added. E for E/e' and end-diastolic volume to identify a limited diastolic volume reserve and reduced LV compliance during stress, with higher E/e' values for lower end-diastolic volumes compared to normals [79]. F for tricuspid regurgitant or pulmonary systolic forward Flow, possibly complementing each other for assessing pulmonary hypertension. The standard ABCD protocol may become ABCDEF protocol for diastolic SE, but prospective validation of this working hypothesis is needed at this point.

Conclusion

With the ABCD protocol, IQ-SE separates ischemic hearts with RWMA from non-ischemic hearts without RWMA; dry lungs with A-lines from wet lungs with B-profile; strong hearts with normal LVCR and reduced ESV from weak hearts with blunted LVCR and dilated ESV; and warm hearts with preserved CFVR from cold hearts with reduced CFVR. The new BCD parameters need minimal extra-imaging and extra-analysis time, but the potential benefits are extraordinary, since IQ-SE gains versatility and objectivity, increases the positivity rate, expands the domain of application of SE from CAD to HF patients, and improves the risk stratification potential. The annual hard-event rate of a test with quadruple negativity (non-ischemic, dry, strong and warm heart) is substantially lower than that associated with a test with quadruple positivity (ischemic, wet, weak and cold heart). All possible combinations of intermediate responses can be found in between the highest risk (quadruple positivity) and lowest risk (quadruple negativity) pattern [34].

In addition to the universal IQ-SE protocol, other parameters can be added in special subsets. As it is not possible to assess all variables during stress in all patients, the parameters of potential interest should be prioritized for the individual patient on the basis of the perceived importance of each [33]. Priority will be given to right ventricular function in patients with repaired tetralogy of Fallot, to pulmonary hemodynamics in patients with primary or secondary pulmonary hypertension, to valve gradients and regurgitation in patients with valvular heart disease [80], and to intraventricular gradients in patients with HCM [33, 71].

The old landline telephone with a single sign (RWMA) for one patient with known or suspected CAD [81] is now a versatile smart-phone with multiple applications, and can be tailored in the individual patient according to clinical needs. Large scale effectiveness studies with IQ-SE are now under way with the Stress Echo 2020 project [82], and will hopefully provide the evidence needed for large scale acceptance of the omnivorous

(with all variables) and ubiquitous (for all patients) "ABCD" protocol.

Abbreviations
CAD: Coronary artery disease; CFVR: Coronary flow velocity reserve; EF: Ejection fraction; ESV: End-systolic volume; HF: Heart failure; IQ-SE: Integrated quadruple stress echocardiography; LUS: Lung ultrasound; LV: Left ventricle; LVCR: Left ventricular contractile reserve; RWMA: Regional wall motion abnormalities; SE: Stress echocardiography

Acknowledgements
The technical assistance of Michele De Nes, informatic technician of Pisa Institute of Clinical Physiology of National Research Council, was highly appreciated.

Funding
The study was made possible by The Ageing project funding of the Italian national Research Council (P001328).

Authors' contributions
EP drafted the manuscript, and all authors revised it for critically intellectual content. All authors read and approved the final manuscript.

Consent for publication
Not applicable

Competing interests
The Authors declare that they have no competing interests.

Author details
[1]Institute of Clinical Physiology, National Council Research, Via Giuseppe Moruzzi 1, 56124 Pisa, Italy. [2]Fatebenefratelli Hospital of Benevento, Viale Principe di Napoli, 12, 82100 Benevento, Italy. [3]Department of Cardiology, Medical University of Lodz, Bieganski Hospital, Ul Kniaziewicza 1/5, 91-347 Lodz, Poland. [4]CVASIC Research Center Sibiu, "Lucian Blaga" University of Sibiu, Sibiu, Romania. [5]Cardiothoracic department, Cisanello Hospital, University of Pisa, Pisa, Italy.

References
1. Picano E. Stress echocardiography. From pathophysiological toy to diagnostic tool. Point of view. Circulation. 1992;85:1604–12.
2. Pellikka PA, Nagueh SF, Elhendy AA, et al. American Society of Echocardiography recommendations for performance, interpretation, and application of stress echocardiography. J Am Soc Echocardiogr. 2007;20:1021–4.
3. Sicari R, Nihoyannopoulos P, Evangelista A, Kasprzak J, Lancellotti P, Poldermans D, on behalf of the European Association of Echocardiography, et al. Stress echocardiography expert consensus statement. European Association of Echocardiography (EAE) (a registered branch of the ESC). Eur J Echocardiogr. 2008;9:415–37.
4. Montalescot G, Sechtem U, Achenbach S, Andreotti F, Arden C, Budaj A, et al. 2013 ESC guidelines on the management of stable coronary artery disease: the task force on the management of stable coronary artery disease of the European Society of Cardiology. Eur Heart J. 2013;34:2949–3003.
5. Wolk MJ, Bailey SR, Doherty JU, Douglas PS, Hendel RC, Kramer CM, American College of Cardiology Foundation Appropriate Use Criteria Task Force, et al. ACCF/AHA/ASE/ASNC/HFSA/HRS/SCAI/SCCT/SCMR/STS 2013

multimodality appropriate use criteria for the detection and risk assessment of stable ischemic heart disease: a report of the American College of Cardiology Foundation Appropriate Use Criteria Task Force, American Heart Association, American Society of Echocardiography, American Society of Nuclear Cardiology, Heart Failure Society of America, Heart Rhythm Society, Society for Cardiovascular Angiography and Interventions, Society of Cardiovascular Computed Tomography, Society for Cardiovascular Magnetic Resonance, and Society of Thoracic Surgeons. J Am Coll Cardiol. 2014;63:380–406.

6. Picano E. Stress echocardiography: a historical perspective. Special article. Am J Med. 2003;114:126–30.

7. Fonseca R, Otahal P, Wiggins N, Marwick TH. Growth and geographical variation in the use of cardiac imaging in Australia. Int Med J. 2015;45:1115–25.

8. Kini V, McCarthy FH, Dayoub E, Bradley SM, Masoudi FA, Ho PM, et al. Cardiac stress test trends among US patients younger than 65 years, 2005-2012. JAMA Cardiol. 2016;1:1038–42.

9. Jouini H, Askew JW, Crusan DJ, Miller TD, Gibbons RJ. Temporal trends of single-photon emission computed tomography myocardial perfusion imaging in patients without prior coronary artery disease: a 22-year experience at a tertiary academic medical center. Am Heart J. 2016;176:127–33.

10. Roifman I, Wijeysundera HC, Austin PC, Maclagan NC, Rezai MR, Wright GA, et al. Temporal trends in the utilization of noninvasive diagnostic tests for coronary artery disease in Ontario between 2008 and 2014: a population-based study. Can J Cardiol. 2017;33:279–82.

11. Picano E, Pasanisi E, Brown J, Marwick TH. A gatekeeper for the gatekeeper: inappropriate referrals to stress echocardiography. Am Heart J. 2007;154:285–90.

12. Gibbons RJ, Miller TD, Hodge D, et al. Application of appropriateness criteria to stress single-photon emission tomography sestamibi studies and stress echocardiograms in an academic medical center. J Am Coll Cardiol. 2008;51:1283–9.

13. Cortigiani L, Bigi R, Bovenzi F, Molinaro S, Picano E, Sicari R. Prognostic implication of appropriateness criteria for pharmacologic stress echocardiography performed in an outpatient clinic. Circ Cardiovasc Imaging. 2012;5:298–305.

14. Picano E. Sustainability of medical imaging. Education and debate. BMJ. 2004;328:578–80.

15. Picano E. Economic and biological costs of cardiac imaging. Cardiovasc Ultrasound. 2005;3:13.

16. Marwick TH, Buonocore J. Environmental impact of cardiac imaging tests for the diagnosis of coronary artery disease. Heart. 2011;97:1128–31.

17. Braga L, Vinci B, Leo CG, Picano E. The true cost of cardiovascular imaging: focusing on downstream, indirect, and environmental costs. Cardiovasc Ultrasound. 2013;17:11.

18. Berrington de Gonzalez A, Kim KP, Smith-Bindman R, Mc Areavey D. Myocardial perfusion scans: projected population cancer risks from current levels of use in the United States. Circulation. 2010;122:2403–10.

19. Varga A, Garcia MA, Picano E, International Stress Echo Complication Registry. Safety of stress echocardiography (from the international stress Echo complication registry). Am J Cardiol. 2006;98:541–3.

20. Correia MJ, Hellies A, Andreassi MG, Ghelarducci B, Picano E. Lack of radiological awareness among physicians working in a tertiary care cardiological Centre. Int J Cardiol. 2005;103:307–11.

21. Hirschfield JW, Ferrari VA, Bengel FM, et al. 2018 ACC/HRS/NASCI/SCAI/SCCT Expert consensus document on optimal use of ionizing radiation in cardiovascular imaging. Best practices for safety and effectiveness, part 2 - radiological equipment operation, dose-sparing methodologies, patient and medical personnel protection. JACC. 2018;71:2829–55.

22. Siontis GC, Mavridis D, Greenwood JP, Coles B, Nikolakopoulou A, Jüni P, Windecker S. Outcomes of non-invasive diagnostic modalities for the detection of coronary artery disease: network meta-analysis of diagnostic randomised controlled trials. BMJ. 2018;360:k504.

23. Carpeggiani C, Picano E, Brambilla M, Michelassi C, Knuuti J, Kauffmann P, Underwood RS, Neglia D, For the EVINCI investigators. Variability of radiation doses of cardiac imaging tests:the RADIO-EVINCI substudy (radiation dose subproject of the EVINCI study). BMC Cardiovasc Disord. 2017;17:63.

24. Gurunathan S, Kostas Z, Akhtar M, Asrar A, Mehta V, Karogiannis N, Vamvakidou A, Khattar R, Senior R. Cost-effectiveness of a management strategy based on exercise echocardiography versus exercise electrocardiography in patients presenting with suspected angina during long term follow up: a randomized study. Int J Cardiol. 2018;259:1–7.

25. Carpeggiani C, Marraccini P, Morales MA, Prediletto R, Landi P, Picano E. Inappropriateness of cardiovascular radiological imaging testing; a tertiary care referral center study. PLoS One. 2013;8:e81161.

26. Picano E, Vañó E, Rehani MM, Cuocolo A, Mont L, Bodi V, et al. The appropriate and justified use of medical radiation in cardiovascular imaging: a position document of the ESC associations of cardiovascular imaging, percutaneous cardiovascular interventions and electrophysiology. Eur Heart J. 2014;35:665–72.

27. Carpeggiani C, Landi P, Michelassi C, Andreassi MG, Sicari R, Picano E. Stress echo positivity predicts cardiac death. J Am Heart Assoc. 2017;6:e007104.

28. Picano E, Scali MC. Stress echo, carotid arteries and more: its versatility for our imaging times. JACC Cardiovasc Imaging. 2018;11:181–3.

29. Ciampi Q, Picano E, Paterni M, Daros CB, Simova I, de Castro e Silva Pretto JL, on behalf of stress Echo 2020, et al. Quality control of regional wall motion analysis in stress Echo 2020. Int J Cardiol. 2017;249:479–85.

30. Scali MC, Bellagamba CA, Ciampi Q, Simova I, de Castro e Silva Pretto JL, Djordjevic-Dikic A, Dodi C, Cortigiani L, Zagatina A, Trambaiolo P, Torres MA, Citro R, Colonna P, Paterni M, Picano E. Stress echocardiography with smartphone: real-time remote reading for regional wall motion. Int J Cardiovasc Imaging. 2017;33:1731–6.

31. Carpeggiani C, Landi P, Michelassi C, Sicari R, Picano E. The declining frequency of inducible myocardial ischemia during stress echocardiography over 27 consecutive years (1983-2009). Int J Cardiol. 2016;224:57–61.

32. Smulders MW, Jaarsma C, Nelemans PJ, Bekkers SCAM, Bucerius J, Leiner T, et al. Comparison of the prognostic value of negative non-invasive cardiac investigations in patients with suspected or known coronary artery disease– a meta-analysis. Eur Heart J Cardiovasc Imaging. 2017;18:980–7.

33. Picano E, Pellikka PA. Stress echo applications beyond coronary artery disease. Eur Heart J. 2014;35:1033–40.

34. Picano E, Morrone D, Scali MC, Huqi A, Coviello K, Ciampi Q. Integrated quadruple stress echocardiography. Minerva Cardioangiol. 2018; https://doi.org/10.23736/S0026-4725.18.04691-1. [Epub ahead of print]

35. Torres MA, Picano E, Parodi G, Sicari R, Veglia F, Giorgetti A, Marzullo P, Parodi O. The flow-functional relationship in patients with chronic coronary artery disease and reduced regional function: a positron emission tomography and two-dimensional echocardiography study with coronary vasodilator stress. J Am Coll Cardiol. 1997;30:65–70.

36. Severi S, Picano E, Michelassi C, Lattanzi F, Landi P, Distante A, L'Abbate A. Diagnostic and prognostic value of dipyridamole echocardiography in patients with suspected coronary artery disease: comparison with exercise electrocardiography. Circulation. 1994;89:1160–73.

37. Cortigiani L, Carpeggiani C, Sicari R, Michelassi C, Bovenzi F, Picano E. Simple six-item risk score improves risk prediction capability of stress echocardiography. Heart. 2010;104:760–6.

38. Ciampi Q, Carpeggiani C, Michelassi C, Villari B, Picano E. Left ventricular contractile reserve as a predictor of response to cardiac resynchronization therapy in heart failure: a systematic review and a meta-analysis. BMC Cardiovasc Disord. 2017;17:223.

39. Picano E, Frassi F, Agricola E, Gligorova S, Gargani L, Mottola G. Ultrasound lung comets: a clinically useful sign of extravascular lung water. J Am Soc Echocardiogr. 2006;19:356–63.

40. Picano E, Pellikka PA. Ultrasound of extravascular lung water: a new standard for pulmonary congestion. Eur Heart J. 2016;14:2091–104.

41. Scali MC, Zagatina A, Simova I, Zhuravskaya N, Ciampi Q, Paterni M, Marzilli M, Carpeggiani C, Picano E. B-lines with Lung Ultrasound: the optimal scan technique at rest and during stress. Ultrasound Med Biol. 2017;43:2558–63.

42. Scali MC, Cortigiani L, Simionuc A, Gregori D, Marzilli M, Picano E. The added value of exercise-echocardiography in heart failure patients: assessing dynamic changes in extravascular lung water. Eur J Heart Fail. 2017;19:1468–78.

43. Simonovic D, Coiro S, Carluccio E, Girerd N, Deljanic-Ilic M, Ambrosio G. Exercise elicits dynamic changes in extravascular lung water and hemodynamic congestion in heart failure patients with preserved ejection fraction. Research letter. Eur J Heart Fail. 2018;21. https://doi.org/10.1002/ejhf.1228. Epub ahead of print.

44. Picano E, Scali MC, Ciampi Q, Lichtenstein D. Lung ultrasound for the cardiologist. JACC Imaging. 2018;12:381–90.

45. Picano E, Scali MC. The lung water cascade. Echocardiography. 2017;34:1503–7.

46. Bombardini T. Myocardial contractility in the echo lab: molecular, cellular and pathophysiological basis. Cardiovasc Ultrasound. 2005;8:3–27.

47. Bombardini T, Zoppè M, Ciampi Q, Cortigiani L, Agricola E, Salvadori S, Loni T, Pratali L, Picano E. Myocardial contractility in the stress echo lab: from pathophysiological toy to clinical tool. Cardiovasc Ultrasound. 2013;18:11–41.

48. Thurakhia MP, Mc Manus DD, Wholey MA, Schiller NB. Increase in end-systolic volume after exercise independently predicts mortality in patients with coronary heart disease: data from the heart and soul study. Eur Heart J. 2009;30:2478–84.

49. Crowley AL, Yow E, Barnhart HX, Daubert MA, Bigelow R, Sullivan DC. Critical review of current approaches for echocardiographic reproducibility and reliability assessment in clinical research. J Am Soc Echocardiogr. 2016;29:1144–54.

50. Obokata M, Kane GC, Reddy YN, Olson TP, Melenovsky V, Borlaug BA. Role of Diastolic Stress Testing in the Evaluation for Heart Failure With Preserved Ejection Fraction: A Simultaneous Invasive-Echocardiographic Study. Circulation. 2017;135:825–38. https://doi.org/10.1161/CIRCULATIONAHA.116.024822. Epub 2016 Dec 30

51. Bombardini T, Correia MJ, Cicerone C, Agricola E, Ripoli A, Picano E. Force-frequency relationship in the echo lab: a non invasive assessment of Bowditch Treppe? J Am Soc Echo. 2003;17:832–41.

52. Bombardini T, Agrusta M, Natsvlishvili N, Solimene F, Papp R, Coltorti F, Varga A, Mottola G, Picano E. Noninvasive assessment of left ventricular contractility by pacemaker stress echocardiography. Eur J Heart Fail. 2005;7:173–81.

53. Grosu A, Bombardini T, Senni M, Duino V, Gori M, Picano E. End-systolic pressure/volume relationship during dobutamine stress echo: a prognostically useful non-invasive index of left ventricular contractility. Eur Heart J. 2005;26:2404–12.

54. Leone O, Gherardi S, Targa L, Pasanisi E, Mikus P, Tanganelli P, Arpesella G, Picano E, Bombardini T. Stress echocardiography as a gatekeeper to donation in aged marginal donor hearts: anatomic and pathologic correlations of abnormal stress echocardiography results. J Heart Lung Transplant. 2009;28:1141–9.

55. Bombardini T, Gherardi S, Marraccini P, Schlueter MC, Sicari R, Picano E. The incremental diagnostic value of coronary flow reserve and left ventricular elastance during high-dose dipyridamole stress echocardiography in patients with normal wall motion at rest. Int J Cardiol. 2013;168:1683–4.

56. Cortigiani L, Bombardini T, Corbisiero A, Mazzoni A, Bovenzi F, Picano E. The additive prognostic value of end-systolic pressure-volume relationship in diabetic patients with negative Dobutamine stress echocardiography by wall motion criteria. Heart. 2009;95:1429–35.

57. Matsumoto K, Tanaka H, Onishi A, Motoji Y, Tatsumi K, Sawa T, et al. Bi-ventricular contractile reserve offers an incremental prognostic value for patients with dilated cardiomyopathy. Eur Heart J Cardiovasc Imaging. 2015;16:1213–23.

58. Robicsek F, Masters TN, Svenson RH, Daniel WG, Daugherty HK, Cook JW, Selle JG. The application of thermography in the study of coronary blood flow. Surgery. 1978;84:858–64.

59. Rigo F. Coronary flow reserve in stress-echo lab. From pathophysiologic toy to diagnostic tool. Cardiovasc Ultrasound. 2005;3:8.

60. Lowenstein JA, Caniggia C, Rousse G, Amor M, Sánchez ME, Alasia D, et al. Coronary flow velocity reserve during pharmacologic stress echocardiography with normal contractility adds important prognostic value in diabetic and nondiabetic patients. J Am Soc Echocardiogr. 2014;27:1113–9.

61. Zagatina A, Zhuravskaya N. The additive prognostic value of coronary flow velocity reserve during exercise echocardiography. Eur Heart J Cardiovasc Imaging. 2017;18:1179–84.

62. Sicari R, Cortigiani L, Bigi R, Landi P, Raciti M, Picano E. The prognostic value of pharmacologic stress echo is affected by concomitant anti-ischemic therapy at the time of testing. Circulation. 2004;109:1428–31.

63. Sicari R, Rigo F, Gherardi S, Galderisi M, Cortigiani L, Picano E. The prognostic value of Doppler echocardiographic-derived coronary flow reserve is not affected by concomitant antiischemic therapy at the time of testing. Am Heart J. 2008;156:573–9.

64. Rigo F, Gherardi S, Galderisi M, Pratali L, Cortigiani L, Sicari R, Picano E. The prognostic impact of coronary flow reserve assessed by Doppler echocardiography in non-ischemic dilated cardiomyopathy. Eur Heart J. 2006;27:1319–23.

65. Cortigiani L, Rigo F, Gherardi S, Galderisi M, Sicari R, Picano E. Prognostic implications of coronary flow reserve in left anterior descending coronary artery in hypertrophic cardiomyopathy. Am J Cardiol. 2008;102:926–32.

66. Banovic M, Vujisic-Tesic B, Brkovic V, Petrovic M, Nedeljkovic I, Popovic D, et al. Prognostic value of coronary flow reserve in asymptomatic moderate or severe aortic stenosis with preserved ejection fraction and nonobstructed coronary arteries. Echocardiography. 2014;31:428–33.

67. Gan LM, Svedlund S, Wittfeldt A, Eklund C, Gao S, Matejka G, et al. Incremental value of transthoracic Doppler echocardiography-assessed coronary flow reserve in patients with suspected myocardial ischemia undergoing myocardial perfusion scintigraphy. J Am Heart Assoc. 2017;18:6. https://doi.org/10.1161/JAHA.116.004875.

68. Cortigiani L, Rigo F, Gherardi S, Bovenzi F, Molinaro S, Picano E, et al. Coronary flow reserve during dipyridamole stress echocardiography predicts mortality. JACC Cardiovasc Imaging. 2012;5:1079–85.

69. Cortigiani L, Huqi A, Ciampi Q, Bombardini T, Bovenzi F, Picano E. Integration of wall motion, coronary flow velocity and left ventricular contractile reserve in a single test: prognostic value of vasodilator stress echocardiography in diabetic patients. J Am Soc Echocardiogr. 2018;31:692–701.

70. Nagueh SF, Smiseth OA, Appleton CP, Byrd BF 3rd, Dokainish H, Edvardsen T, et al. Recommendations for the Evaluation of Left Ventricular Diastolic Function by Echocardiography: An Update from the American Society of Echocardiography and the European Association of Cardiovascular Imaging. J Am Soc Echocardiogr. 2016;29:277–314. https://doi.org/10.1016/j.echo.2016.01.011.

71. Lancellotti P, Pellikka PA, Budts W, Chaudhry FA, Donal E, Dulgheru R, et al. The clinical use of stress echocardiography in non-ischaemic heart disease: recommendations from the European Association of Cardiovascular Imaging and the American Society of Echocardiography. Eur Heart J Cardiovasc Imaging. 2016;17:1191–229.

72. Sharifov OF, Schiros CG, Aban I, Denney TS, Gupta H. Diagnostic Accuracy of Tissue Doppler Index E/e' for Evaluating LeftVentricular Filling Pressure and Diastolic Dysfunction/Heart Failure With Preserved Ejection Fraction: A Systematic Review and Meta-Analysis. J Am Heart Assoc. 2016;5 https://doi.org/10.1161/JAHA.115.002530.

73. Kitabatake A, Inoue M, Asao M, Masuyama T, Tanouchi J, Morita T, et al. Noninvasive evaluation of pulmonary hypertension by a pulsed Doppler technique. Circulation. 1983;68:302–9.

74. Wang YC, Huang CH, Tu YK. Pulmonary hypertension and pulmonary artery acceleration time: a systematic review and meta-analysis. J Am Soc Echocardiogr. 2018;31:201–10.

75. Wierzbowska-Drabik K , Picano E, Bossone E, Ciampi Q, Lipiec P, Kasprzak JD. Tricuspid Regurgitant Velocity and Pulmonary Flow Acceleration Time for estimating Pulmonary Pressure during Exercise Stress Echocardiography. EHJ - Cardiov Imag 2018; December suppl (abstract).

76. Villalba-Orero M, López-Olañeta MM, González-López E, Padrón-Barthe L, García-Prieto J, Wai T, et al. Lung ultrasound as a translational approach for non-invasive assessment of heart failure with reduced or preserved ejection fraction in mice. Cardiovasc Res. 2017;113:1113–23.

77. Biering-Sørensen T, Santos M, Rivero J, McCullough SD, West E, Opotowsky AR, et al. Left ventricular deformation at rest predicts exercise-induced elevation in pulmonary artery wedge pressure in patients with unexplained dyspnoea. Eur J Heart Fail. 2017;19:101–10. https://doi.org/10.1002/ejhf.659. Epub 2016 Nov 22

78. Taqueti VR, Solomon SD, Shah AM, Desai AS, Groarke JD, Osborne MT, et al. Coronary microvascular dysfunction and future risk of heart failure with preserved ejection fraction. Eur Heart J. 2018;39:840–9. https://doi.org/10.1093/eurheartj/ehx721.

79. Shimiaie J, Sherez J, Aviram G, Megidish R, Viskin S, Halkin A, et al. Determinants of effort intolerance in patients with heart failure. JACC Heart Failure. 2015;3:803–14.

80. Picano E, Pibarot P, Lancellotti P, Monin JL, Bonow RO. The emerging role of exercise testing and stress echocardiography in valvular heart disease. J Am Coll Cardiol. 2009;54:2251–60.

81. Sicari R, Cortigiani L. The clinical use of stress echocardiography in ischemic heart disease. Cardiovasc Ultrasound. 2017;15:7. (review)

82. Picano E, Ciampi Q, Citro R, D'Andrea A, Scali MC, Cortigiani L, et al. Stress echo 2020: The international stress Echo study in ischemic and non-ischemic heart disease. Cardiovasc Ultrasound. 2017;15(1):3. https://doi.org/10.1186/s12947-016-0092-1.

Comparison of mitral annulus geometry between patients with ischemic and non-ischemic functional mitral regurgitation: implications for transcatheter mitral valve implantation

Background

In Europe, mitral regurgitation (MR) represents the second most frequent heart valve disease after aortic valve stenosis [1]. Among patients with moderate and severe MR, 30% are affected by functional MR (FMR) with high prevalence of the ischemic etiology [2]. Despite clinical indication, 49% of patients with MR are denied for surgery due to advanced age, reduced ejection fraction or multiple comorbidities [3] and, among them, the vast majority is represented by patients with FMR [4]. In the last decade, percutaneous transcatheter procedures, simulating surgical techniques, have been developed to extend the therapeutic options for high surgical risk patients with MR. Among them, transcatheter mitral valve replacement (TMVR) represents the newest option [5–7].

Mitral valve (MV) geometry quantification is of paramount importance for the success of TMVR, and transthoracic (TTE) three-dimensional echocardiography (3DE) represents a useful tool to select the patients with the highest likelihood of uncomplicated implant [8]. It has been previously reported that MV geometry may differ in ischemic and non-ischemic FMR. In patients with ischemic MR (IMR), regional wall motion abnormalities and left ventricular [9] remodeling are more often associated with mitral annulus (MA) asymmetric dilatation [10]. Conversely, in non-ischemic MR (nIMR) global LV remodeling leads to symmetric MA dilatation [11]. Yet, MV geometry in FMR has been mainly compared to organic MR, and only few small echocardiographic studies analyzed MV geometry differentiating between IMR and nIMR [10–13]. However, none of them provided MA geometry characterization framed to pre-procedural screening for TMVR [8].

The aim of this study was to asses MV geometry in patients with FMR that would potentially benefit of TMVR, focusing on the comparison of MA geometry between IMR and nIMR patients in two key moments of the cardiac cycle —mid-systole and early-diastole.

Methods

Study population

Using the electronical database of the echocardiography laboratory of the department of cardiac, thoracic and vascular sciences of the University of Padua, 94 patients with severe FMR and complete transthoracic echocardiography performed between November 2010 and March 2018, have been retrospectively selected. Inclusion criteria were: age > 18 years; severe FMR according to current guidelines [14]; availability of good quality 3D data sets of both the left ventricle (LV) and the MV. We excluded patients with organic MR, mitral stenosis, aortic stenosis, more than moderate aortic regurgitation, or those with valve prostheses. Each patient was assigned to the IMR or nIMR subgroup according to his/her clinical history and the documentation of presence/absence

of significant coronary artery diseases. The study was approved by the University of Padua Ethics Committee (protocol no. 70299).

Mitral valve analysis software package validation

Two sub-studies were carried on to validate the software package used to quantitate MV geometry (4D Auto MVQ, GE Vingmed Ultrasound AS, Horten, Norway). First, the same operator (P.A.) performed the quantitative analysis of the MV in a blinded fashion, and after a time interval of one month form each other, using the same TTE data sets and both the new and a previously validated [15, 16] (4D MV Analysis; Tomtec Imaging Systems, Unterschleissheim, Germany) software packages. Second, 3D TTE and transesophageal (TEE) echocardiographic MV data sets were analyzed using the same software package for MV quantitative analysis (4D Auto MVQ, GE Vingmed Ultrasound AS, Horten, Norway) by the same operator (P.A.) in a blinded fashion, after a time interval of one week.

Echocardiography and quantitative image analysis

All transthoracic examinations were performed using a commercially available Vivid E9 system (GE Vingmed Ultrasound AS, Horten, Norway) equipped with a 4 V probe for 3DE acquisitions according to a standardized protocol. Image analysis was performed on a dedicated workstation equipped with a commercially available software package for offline analysis of 3D datasets (EchoPac 2.02). Quantitation of LV volumes and ejection fraction (LVEF) was performed using 4D Auto-LVQ software [17] (GE Vingmed Ultrasound AS, Horten, Norway). Left atrium (LA) maximum volume was measured using the biplane disk summation method, at LV end-systole [18]. MR severity and conventional MV geometry parameters —antero-posterior (AP) and commissural (CC) diameters, tenting height and tenting area— were assessed according to current recommendations [14]. 3D MA analysis was performed on dedicated datasets by a single experienced observer (P.A.), using a new, commercially available, software package (4D Auto MVQ, GE Vingmed Ultrasound AS, Horten, Norway), in two moments of the cardiac cycle: early-diastole and mid-systole. Firstly, two time points were identified in the way that the selected frame of the analysis was midway among them. For mid-systolic analysis, the two time-points were early-systole (the frame after MV closure) and end-systole (the frame before MV begins to open). For early diastolic analysis, after identification of early-diastolic frame (first frame when MV start to open), the two time-points were placed 8 frames before and after the selected early-diastolic frame. The two orthogonal planes were adjusted to visualize the commissural and longitudinal view of MV (the longitudinal plane intersected the MV at the level of

A2 and P2 scallops). For initialization, anatomic landmarks have to be added at the level of MA in the longitudinal view (posterior, P; anterior, A; leaflets coaptation point, Coap; and aortic valve, Ao) and commissural view (MA1 and MA2). The software package automatically created a 3D model of the MV in the selected frame which could eventually be edited manually, if needed (Fig. 1). Automatic quantitative parameters of the MV geometry were: MA 3D area; MA 2D area (projected 2D area at the level of the best fit plane); MA perimeter; MA AP diameter, as the distance between the two landmarks A and P; MA anterolateral-posteromedial diameter (ALPM), as the longest diameter of MA perpendicular to AP diameter; sphericity index (as the ratio between AP and ALPM diameters); MA CC diameter, as the distance between the two commissure; MA inter-trigonal distance, measured between the two automatically identified trigons; MA height, as the distance between the lowest and the highest points of MA; the non-planimetry angle, that assesses the saddle shape of MA; mitral-aortic angle, as the angle between the aortic valve and the MA (along the AP direction) planes; anterior and posterior leaflets area and length, MV tenting height, tenting area and tenting volume.

Statistical analysis

The normal distribution of the variables was checked using the Kolmogorov-Smirnov test. Continuous data were presented as mean ± standard deviation (SD) or Median (25°-75°) and categorical variables as absolute numbers and percentages, as appropriate. In the validation study, we used Pearson or Spearman correlation to test the relationships between TTE mid-systolic MA parameters, measured using the two software packages,

and mid-systolic and early-diastolic parameters obtained from TTE and TEE data sets in the same patient. In addition, Bland–Altman plots were used to assess the mean difference and the limits of agreement between them. Paired t test or Wilcoxon rank test were used, as appropriate, for comparing the MV dimension obtained by TTE and TEE data set in the same patient.

Variables were compared between IMR and nIMR patients using the unpaired t or the Mann-Whitney tests, as appropriate. Chi-square was used to compare the categorical variables. A paired t test or Wilcoxon signed rank test was used to compare systolic and diastolic dimensions within the same subgroups, as appropriate. Percentage change of the systo-diastolic measurements was also calculated.

Data analyses was performed using SPSS version 20.0 (SPSS, Inc., Chicago, IL) and GraphPad Prism V 7 (GraphPad Software, La Jolla, NY). Differences among variables were considered significant at p value < 0.05.

Results

Validation study

The TTE validation cohort included 30 patients (15 with IMR; 22 men; mean age 64 ± 2 year) with good image quality. The temporal resolution of the 3D dataset for MV quantification was 35 ± 3 volumes per second (vps). Close correlations and good agreements were found between the measurements obtained with the two software packages (Figs. 2 and 3).

The TEE validation cohort included 15 patients (8 with IMR; 14 men; mean age 63 ± 15 year). As expected, both image quality (excellent quality in 75%

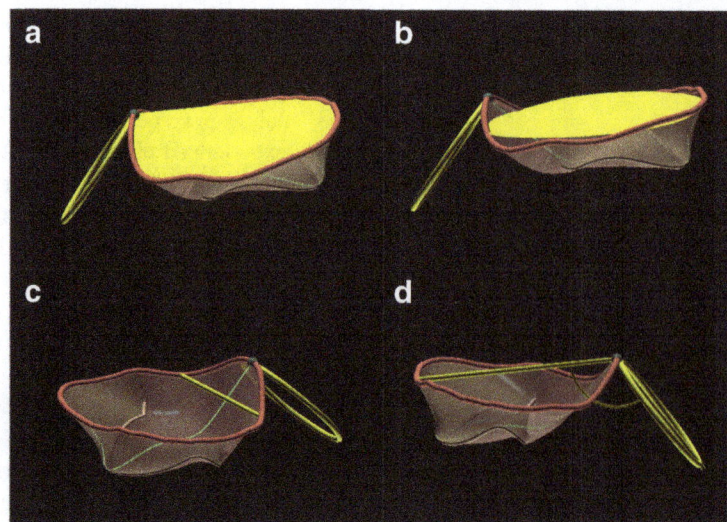

Fig. 1 Mitral annulus parameters automatically analyzed at mid-systolic frame. Legend: Panel **a** 3D mitral annulus area, **b** mitral annulus area at the best fit plane, **c** Inter-trigonal distance, **d** Aorto-Mitral angle

Comparison of mitral annulus geometry between patients with ischemic and non-ischemic functional mitral...

225

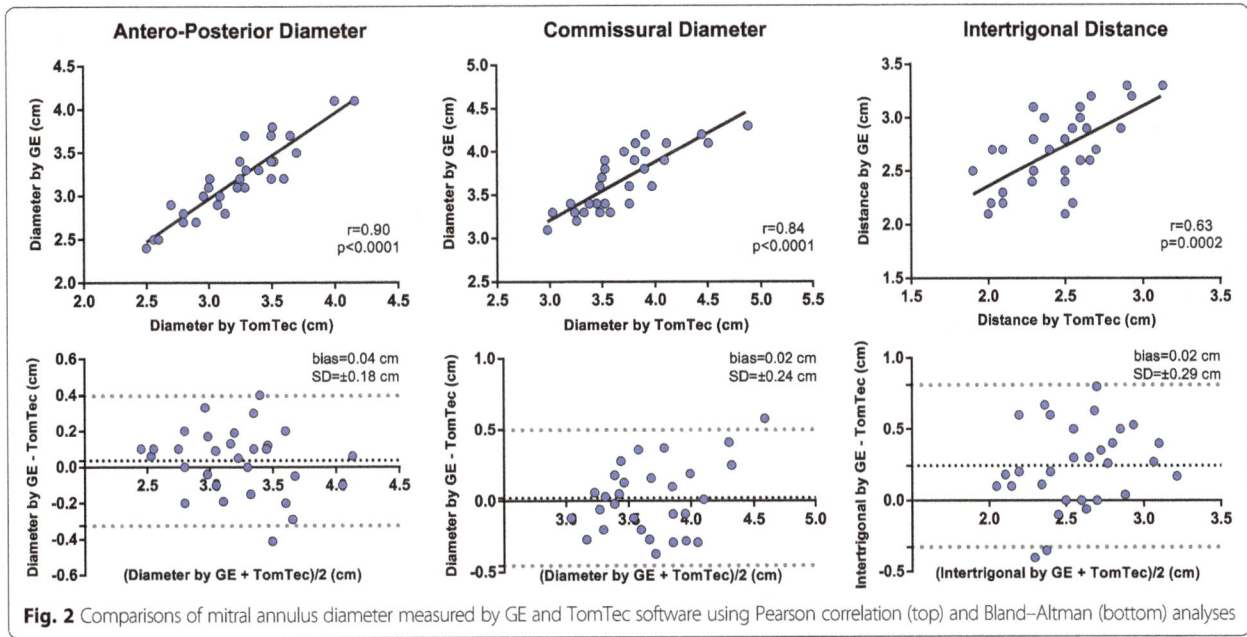

Fig. 2 Comparisons of mitral annulus diameter measured by GE and TomTec software using Pearson correlation (top) and Bland–Altman (bottom) analyses

versus 25%, respectively, $p = 0.009$) and temporal resolution (34 ± 15 vps versus 29 ± 10 vps, respectively, $p < 0.05$) were higher for TEE than TTE data sets. The mean time lapse between TTE and TEE data set acquisitions was 1(0–6) day.

Measurements obtained from TEE data sets resulted in slightly larger area, perimeter and AP diameter (Table 1). However, there was a close correlation between the two techniques and the differences were not clinically relevant. Among linear dimension, ALPM, commissural diameter and diastolic inter-trigonal distance are the most similar in TEE and TTE data sets, while tenting area, tenting volume and non-planar showed the largest differences (Table 1).

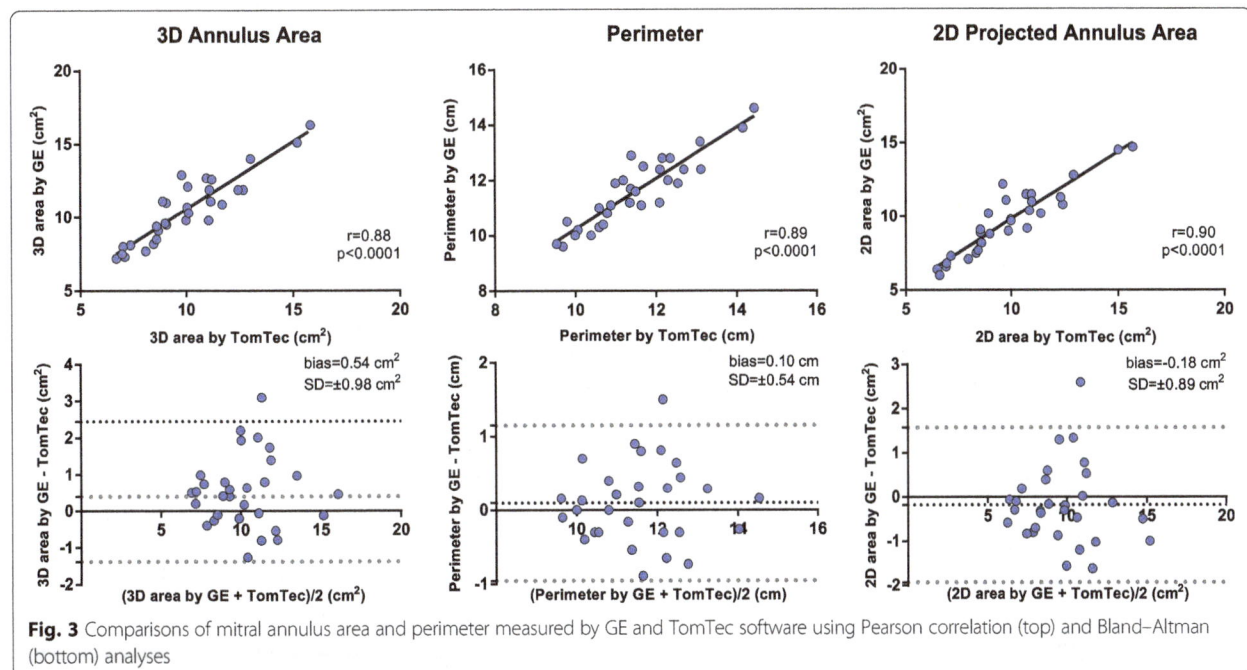

Fig. 3 Comparisons of mitral annulus area and perimeter measured by GE and TomTec software using Pearson correlation (top) and Bland–Altman (bottom) analyses

Table 1 Comparison of mitral annulus parameter among transthoracic and transoesophageal data sets

	Transthoracic N = 15	Transoesophageal N = 15	p	r
Diastolic dimension				
Annulus area (3D) (cm²)	11.5 ± 3.1	12.4 ± 3.2	0.031	0.879**
Annulus best fit plane (cm²)	10.6 ± 3.0	11.7 ± 3.1	0.016	0.869**
Annulus perimeter (cm)	12.1 ± 1.7	12.6 ± 1.6	0.036	0.883**
AP diameter (cm)	3.5 ± 0.5	3.8 ± 0.5	0.012	0.799**
ALPM diameter (cm)	3.7 ± 0.5	3.8 ± 0.5	0.342	0.840**
Commissural diameter (cm)	3.7 ± 0.4	3.8 ± 0.5	0.231	0.777**
Itertrigonal distance (cm)	2.8 ± 0.3	3.0 ± 0.4	0.094	0.715**
Sphericity index	0.9 ± 0.1	1.0 ± 0.1	0.150	0.157
Annulus height (mm)	7.3 ± 1.7	6.8 ± 1.6	0.343	0.559*
Non planar angle	156 ± 13	152 ± 11	0.314	0.474
Mitro-aortic angle	131 ± 8	125 ± 10	0.039	0.418
Systolic dimension				
Annulus area (3D) (cm²)	10.2 ± 2.6	11.0 ± 2.6	0.006	0.936**
Annulus best fit plane (cm²)	9.3 ± 2.5	10.2 ± 2.5	0.001	0.959**
Annulus perimeter (cm)	11.4 ± 1.5	11.8 ± 1.4	0.010	0.943**
AP diameter (cm)	3.2 ± 0.4	3.4 ± 0.6	0.002	0.624* ᵖ
ALPM diameter (cm)	3.6 ± 0.5	3.6 ± 0.4	0.329	0.857**
Commissural diameter (cm)	3.5 ± 0.4	3.6 ± 0.4	0.151	0.889**
Itertrigonal distance (cm)	2.6 ± 0.4	3.0 ± 0.4	0.000	0.830**
Sphericity index	0.9 ± 0.1	0.9 ± 0.1	0.062	0.321ᵖ
Annulus height (mm)	7.0 ± 1.3	7.0 ± 1.4	0.910	0.300
Non planar angle (°)	153 ± 10	153 ± 9	0.893	0.240
Aorto-mitral angle (°)	139 ± 10	129 ± 8	0.005	0.367
Tenting height (mm)	10.3 ± 2.0	7.2 ± 3.6	0.02	- 0.108
Tenting area (cm²)	2.3 ± 0.6	2.3 ± 0.7	0.934	0.542*
Tenting volume (mL)	4.2 ± 1.3	4.1 ± 1.5	0.742	0.747**

Data are expressed as Mean ± Standard Deviation
Abbreviations: ALPM anterolateral-posteromedial, AP antero-posterior diameter
* for correlation with p < 0.05; ** for correlation with p < 0.001; ᵖ evaluated with Sperman's correlation

Comparison of mitral annulus geometry between ischemic and non-ischemic mitral regurgitation

We enrolled 94 patients, 41 (43,6%) with IMR and 53 (56,4%) with nIMR. Patients with IMR were more frequently male and had a higher incidence of hypertension, diabetes and dyslipidemia (Table 2). The severity of MR was comparable between the two groups (Table 3). Although patients in both groups showed severe LV dilatation and dysfunction, patients with IMR had a higher LVEF (31 (26–38)% versus 28 (22–32)%, p = 0.030) and LV wall motion score index (2.1 ± 0.3 versus 1.9 ± 0.6, p = 0.021) (Table 3).

Temporal resolution of the 3D dataset dedicated for MV quantification was higher in IMR than in nIMR

patients (33 ± 14 vps versus 40 ± 16 vps, p = 0.023). All data sets had enough good quality for the quantitative analysis. The image quality was graded excellent in 47 patients (50%), good in 32 (34%), and fair in 15 (16%) and it was comparable between IMR and nIMR patients (p = 0.634).

Using conventional two-dimensional echocardiography MV geometry parameters, patients with nIMR showed larger AP diameter both in diastole (41 ± 7 mm in nIMR versus 38 ± 6 mm in IMR, p = 0.029) and in systole (37 ± 6 mm in nIMR versus 34 ± 4 mm in IMR, p = 0.024). Conversely, CC diameter (43 ± 8 mm in nIMR versus 39 ± 9 mm in IMR, p = 0.088), tenting height (9 ± 3 mm in nIMR versus 8.5 ± 3 mm in IMR, p = 0.180)

Table 2 Demographics and clinical characteristics

	Ischemic mitral regurgitation $N = 41$	Non ischemic mitral regurgitation $N = 53$	p
Age (years)	69 (63–75)	64 (55–72)	0.081
Men (%)	*35 (85)*	*35 (66)*	*0.033*
Body surface area (m²)	1.8 (1.7–1.9)	1.9 (1.7–2.0)	0.374
Heart rate (bpm)	71 (59–85)	75 (65–86)	0.237
Systolic blood pressure (mmHg)	110 (100–120)	100 (95–115)	0.340
Diastolic blood pressure(mmHg)	65 (60–71)	65 (60–70)	0.233
Hypertension	*32 (80%)*	*25 (48.1%)*	*0.002*
Diabetes	*15 (37.5%)*	*8 (15.4%)*	*0.015*
Dyslipidemia	*30 (75%)*	*22 (42.3%)*	*0.002*
Smokers	23 (57.5%)	24 (46.2%)	0.280
Resynchronization therapy	8 (20%)	17 (32.7%)	0.175

Data are expressed as Median (25°-75°) or Number (%). Italicized values highlight statistically significant differences

and tenting area (1.9 ± 0.7 cm² in nIMR versus 1.7 ± 0.6 cm² in IMR, $p = 0.189$) were similar between the two groups.

At 3DE analysis, both subgroups had similar diastolic geometry of MA, even though all MA dimensions were slightly larger in nIMR. nIMR patients showed larger mid-systolic 3D area and perimeter of the MA with longer leaflets. However, the area of the annulus at the best fit plane, and all diameters (AP, CC, ALPM diameter and trans-trigonal distance) did not differ between IMR and nIMR patients. Tenting height and area did not differ between IMR and nIMR patients, whereas tenting volume, annulus height and aorto-mitral angle were larger in nIMR patients (Table 4).

Table 3 Echocardiography characteristics

	Ischemic mitral regurgitation $N = 41$	Non ischemic mitral regurgitation $N = 53$	p
MR Vena contracta (mm)	7 (6–8)	7 (6–8)	0.658
MR PISA radius (mm)	7 (6–8)	8 (7–9)	0.138
MR EROA (mm2)	2 (2–3)	2.1(2–3)	0.421
MR R Vol (mL)	38 (28–58)	38.5 (29–47.7)	0.803
sPAP	47 (35–56)	44 (35–49)	0.211
TR severity	Trivial 6 (11.3%)	Trivial 6 (15.4%)	0.753
	Mild 29 (54.7%)	Mild 20 (51.3%)	
	Moderate11 (20.8%)	Moderate10 (25.6%)	
	Severe 7 (13.2%)	Severe3 (7.7%)	
AR severity	None 25 (49%)	None 25 (65%)	0.437
	Trivial 13 (25%)	Trivial 6 (15%)	
	Mild 12 (23.5%)	Mild 9 (22.5%)	
	Moderate 1 (2%)	Moderate 0 (0%)	
LV EDV (ml/m²)	134 (114–153)	143 (116–178)	0.078
LV ESV (mL/m²)	96 (68–109)	105 (78–135)	0.075
Ejection Fraction (%)	*31 (26–38)*	*28 (22–32)*	*0.030*
Indexed LA volume (mL/m2)	*60 (51–68)*	*70 (53–91)*	*0.031*

Data are expressed as Median (25°-75°) or Number (%)
Abbreviations: *AR* aortic regurgitation, *EROA* effective regurgitant orifice area, *LA* left atrial, *LV EDV* left ventricular end-diastolic volume, *LV ESV* left ventricular end-systolic volume, *MR* mitral regurgitation, *PISA* proximal isovelocity surface area, *R Vol* regurgitant volume, *sPAP* systolic pulmonary artery pressure, *TR* tricuspid regurgitation. Italicized values highlight statistically significant differences

Table 4 Three-dimensional mitral valve dimension

	Ischemic mitral regurgitation $N=41$	Non ischemic mitral regurgitation $N=53$	p
Diastolic dimension			
Annulus area (3D) (cm²)	10.7 ± 2.5[a]	11.6 ± 2.7[a]	0.124
Annulus best fit plane (cm²)	9.9 ± 2.3[a]	10.7 ± 2.5[a]	0.135
Annulus perimeter (cm)	11.7 ± 1.4[a]	12.2 ± 1.4[a]	0.111
AP diameter (cm)	3.3 ± 0.4[a]	3.5 ± 0.5[a]	0.072
ALPM diameter (cm)	3.6 ± 0.4[a]	3.8 ± 0.5[a]	0.129
Commissural diameter(cm)	3.6 ± 0.4	3.7 ± 0.4	0.300
Itertrigonal distance (cm)	2.7 ± 0.4[a]	2.8 ± 0.3[a]	0.374
Annulus height (mm)	6.3 ± 1.7[a]	6.8 ± 1.7[a]	0.144
Sphericity index	0.9 ± 0.1[a]	0.9 ± 0.1[a]	0.963
Non planar angle (°)	156 ± 11[a]	153 ± 10[a]	0.232
Anterior leaflet area (cm²)	7.5 ± 1.6[a]	8.0 ± 1.6[a]	0.142
Posterior leaflet area (cm²)	7.2 ± 2.3[a]	7.5 ± 2.1[a]	0.413
Anterior leaflet length (cm)	2.9 ± 0.4	3.3 ± 0.9[a]	0.102
Posterior leaflet length (cm)	1.6 ± 0.4[a]	1.7 ± 0.6[a]	0.319
Aorto-mitral angle (°)	131 ± 9[a]	135 ± 11[a]	0.115
Systolic dimension			
Annulus area (3D) (cm²)	*9.8 ± 2.3*	*10.8 ± 2.7*	*0.046*
Annulus best fit plane (cm²)	9 ± 2.1	9.9 ± 2.5	0.063
Annulus perimeter (cm)	*11.2 ± 1.3*	*11.8 ± 1.5*	*0.048*
AP diameter (cm)	3.1 ± 0.4	3.2 ± 0.5	0.063
ALPM diameter (cm)	3.5 ± 0.4	3.7 ± 0.5	0.065
Commissural diameter(cm)	3.5 ± 0.4	3.7 ± 0.4	0.130
Itertrigonal distance (cm)	2.5 ± 0.3	2.7 ± 0.3	0.051
Annulus height (mm)	*6.7 ± 1.6*	*7.5 ± 1.9*	*0.047*
Sphericity index	0.9 ± 0.08	0.9 ± 0.1	0.598
Non planar angle (°)	153 ± 11	150 ± 10	0.268
Anterior leaflet area (cm²)	*6.5 ± 1.6*	*7.4 ± 1.7*	*0.006*
Posterior leaflet area (cm²)	*5.7 ± 1.7*	*6.5 ± 1.9*	*0.049*
Anterior leaflet length (cm)	*2.8 ± 0.6*	*3 ± 0.4*	*0.022*
Posterior leaflet length (cm)	*1.3 ± 0.4*	*1.5 ± 0.8*	*0.022*
Aorto-mitral angle (°)	*135 ± 10*	*141 ± 11*	*0.011*
Tenting height (mm)	9.3 ± 2.6	10.3 ± 2.8	0.082
Tenting area (cm²)	2.2 ± 0.7	2.4 ± 0.8	0.141
Tenting volume (mL)	*4 ± 1.7*	*4.7 ± 1.7*	*0.047*

Data are expressed as Mean ± Standard Deviation
Abbreviations: ALPM anterolateral-posteromedial, AP antero.posterior diameter
Italicized values highlight statistically significant differences
[a]Statistical difference vs systolic dimension

Mitral annulus dynamics

In both groups, MA significantly reduced its dimensions in systole (except for the CC diameter) with similar percentage change of the measurement in both groups ($p > 0.05$) (Tables 4 and 5). During systole, the MA mitral-aortic angle flattens, while the non-planarity angle becomes more acute.

Discussion

In the present study, we used 3D TTE to compare MA geometry in patients with severe ischemic and non-ischemic FMR, who are potential candidates for TMVR.

The main findings of our study were in patients with FMR: i, diastolic MA geometry is similar in both nIMR

Table 5 Fractional changes of the mitral annulus parameters between diastole and systole

	Ischemic mitral regurgitation N = 41	Non ischemic mitral regurgitation N = 53	p
MA area (3D) fraction (%)	-6 (-11.7 — -1.8)	-4.3 (-9.8 — -1.3)	> 0.05
MA best fit plane fraction (%)	-6.3 (-13 — -4)	-6.7 (-11.4 — -1.8)	> 0.05
MA perimeter fraction (%)	-3.2 (-5.8 — -0.4)	-2.1 (-4.6 — -0.8)	> 0.05
AP diameter fraction (%)	-7.4 (-11.4 — -2.4)	-5.9 (-11.2 — -1.3)	> 0.05
ALPM diameter fraction (%)	-2.9 (-6.9 — 0.0)	0.0 (-7.3 — 0.0)	> 0.05
CC diameter fraction (%)	-2.6 (-5.5 — 2.9)	0.0 (-4.7 — 2.7)	> 0.05
TT distance fraction (%)	-4.8 (-12.4 — 0.0)	-3.1 (-10 — 3.8)	> 0.05
Non planar angle fraction (%)	-2 (-6.3 — 2.5)	-2.4 (-5.6 — 2)	> 0.05
Aorto-mitral angle fraction (%)	3.7 (-2.5 — 8.4)	3.4 (0–8.4)	> 0.05

Data are expressed as Median (25°-75°)
Abbreviations: *ALPM* anterolateral-posteromedial, *AP* antero-posterior diameter, *CC* commissural, *MA* mitral annulus, *TT*, trans-trigonal

and IMR patients; ii, systolic MV geometry significantly differs between the groups.

Validation study

Multimodality imaging represents the gold standard for planning transcatheter mitral valve procedures, TEE and multi-slice computed tomography (MSCT) playing the major role [19]. Due to longer survival of patients with chronic heart diseases and progressive aging of the general population, the number of patients who could benefit of TMVR is likely to increase, and 3DTTE will be of paramount importance as a screening tool for the analysis of MV geometry. Previous clinical studies assessing MA geometry used 3DTEE data sets [20, 21] to obtain adequate spatial and temporal resolution for quantitative analysis of the MV. However, the progressive improvement of 3DE technology allows to obtain better and better quality 3DE data sets with TTE, too. Moreover, feasibility and cost/effectiveness considerations suggest that TTE approach would be better suited to screen potential candidates to TMVR. Accordingly, we decided to explore the use of 3DTTE data sets perform quantitative analysis of the MV in patients with FMR. In our patients, MA dimensions obtained from TTE datasets were similar to those obtained with the 3D TEE approach in the validation study.

Comparison of mitral annulus dimension between ischemic and non-ischemic mitral regurgitation

We focused our study on patients with FMR because they represent the main potential target of new TMVR. The few previous studies that analyzed the possible differences between IMR and nIMR [10–13] included a limited number of patients and were focused only on MA size (annulus area and diameters), without any information about the MV geometry (MA area at the best fit plane, mitro-aortic angle, length of the anterior leaflet) which are crucial to select patients for TMVR [19].

In this study, we reported all MV anatomical and geometrical features that should be assessed before TMVR [8, 22] and demonstrated that patients with severe IMR and nIMR have similar, symmetrical, diastolic (maximal) MA dimension. The 3D MA area obtained from our patients were comparable with the maximum MA surface area reported by Veronesi et al. [12] in a smaller group of patients using TTE 3DE datasets. Our results are also in agreement with those reported by Daimon et al. [10] who showed that diastolic MA diameters did not differ among IMR and nIMR. However, the actual MA sizes in our patients were slightly larger than in their cohorts. This finding could be partially explained by the different time point selected for the analysis (mid-diastolic phase, compared to early-diastole in our study).

While in our study mid-systolic 3D annulus area and perimeter are significantly larger in patients with nIMR, MA area at the best fit plane and MA diameter were similar. It has been suggested that the projected 3D MA area at the level of the best fit plane is the most reliable parameter of MA geometry to be used for planning TMVR compared to the saddle-shaped 3D area [22]. Though, our MA area at the best fit plane resulted smaller than the mean projected MA area measured in a recent MSCT study [23] on 32 patients with FMR of different etiologies and severity, it is already known that 3DE can underestimate measurement compared with MSCT due to its suboptimal lateral resolution in the coronal plane [24].

A new D-shaped MA segmentation developed by Blanke et al. [25], with the truncation of anterior saddle horn at the level of inter-trigonal line, has been used to select candidates to Tiara [5], Tendyne [7] and Intrepid [6] valve implants. This method was also recently applied by Mak et al. [26] using 3D TEE with comparable results, but it is unclear at this early stage of TMVR experience whether this is the best parameter to size the prosthesis for TMVR interventions [27].

Left ventricular out flow tract (LVOT) obstruction is a possible complication related to TMVR that can be predicted during procedure planning because it is related to the design of the prosthesis and patient anatomy (interventricular septal dimension, LV size, aorto-mitral angle, anterior leaflet length). 3DE allows the measurement of both the aorto-mitral angle (the angle between the aortic valve and the MA along the AP direction) and anterior leaflet length. None of the previous MSCT nor the 3DE studies reported these parameters in patients considered for TMVR. In our study we found that nIMR group presented significantly wider aorto-mitral angle that balance the potential higher risk of LVOT obstruction due to longer and larger anterior leaflets in these patients.

Mitral annulus dynamics

MA is dynamic structure characterized by contraction and expansion phase during cardiac cycle [12, 28]. These changes, although less pronounced than in normal subjects, have been reported also in patients with IMR [20, 29] and nIMR [12]. We found that in patients with severe FMR, MA is significantly smaller in mid-systole compared to early diastolic phase. This findings underline the necessity of a multiphasic MA assessment to select patients for TMVR [8], but the few investigations that analyzed MA dimension in moderate or severe FMR (potentially candidates for TMVR), reported only the measurement in one phase of the cardiac cycle [12, 13].

Implications for trans-catheter mitral valve selection

TMVR represents a promising option for patients with severe FMR, and assessment of MA dimension and geometry is of paramount importance to size the device and also to plan future development of new prostheses. We found that, patients with IMR and nIMR have similar MA geometry, supporting the concept that there is no need of different prosthesis sizing according to etiology of the FMR. However, we found that nIMR patients had significantly larger and longer anterior mitral leaflet, that could increase the risk of LVOT obstruction. Therefore, for nIMR patients it could be more appropriate to select a device that has an anterior hook to fix the anterior leaflet of the native MV. On the other hand, nIMR patients showed a wider aorto-mitral angle that could counterbalance the higher risk of LVOT obstruction carried by longer anterior leaflet. Probably, this sub-group of patients would be eligible also for devices that have larger protrusion or flaring into LV.

The significant change of MA during the cardiac cycle, also preserved in patients with severe FMR, stresses the need to evaluate accurately the smallest MA dimension in order to reduce the risk of excessive stress of the prosthesis frame by MA.

Study limitations

We acknowledge several limitations of our study. First, to obtain all the measurements needed to plan TMVR from 3DE data sets, we used a new MV software package that was not previously validated. To overcome this limitation, we compared the measurements obtained with the new software package with those obtained from the same data sets using a validated software [16] with a close correlations and good agreement. However, we did not compare our measurement with MSCT, which represents the current gold standard to select patients for TMVR.

Secondly, currently available 3DE software packages allow MV dynamic analysis only during the systolic phase of the cardiac cycle. While mid-systole could be defined by the operator according to MV opening and closure or automatically by the software (as mid-way between R and T waves on the ECG tracing), early-diastole has to be manually identified by the operator with an increased possibility of errors. Current literature reports contradicting data about the moment when MA reaches its maximum and minimum sizes, however the importance of definition of maximum MA dimension is of paramount importance for accurate device's sizing and emphasizes the need of multiphasic annular measurement.

Conclusion

The reported MA geometry in a relatively large group of patients with severe FMR, potentially candidates for TMVR, represents useful information for transcatheter MV prosthesis design and patient selection. Patients with ischemic and non-ischemic aetiologies of FMR have similar maximum dimensions, yet systolic differences between the two groups should be taken into account to tailor prosthesis's selection.

Abbreviations

3DE: Three-dimensional echocardiography; ALPM: Anterolateral-posteromedial; AP: Antero-posterior; CC: Commissural; FMR: Functional mitral regurgitation; IMR: Ischemic MR; LA: Left atrium; LV: Left ventricle/ventricular; LVEF: Ejection fraction; LVOT: Left ventricular outflow tract; MA: Mitral annulus; MR: Mitral regurgitation; MSCT: Multi-slice computed tomography; MV: Mitral valve; nIMR: Non-ischemic mitral regurgitation; TMVR: Transcatheter mitral valve replacement; TEE: Transesophageal echocardiography; TTE: Transthoracic echocardiography; VPS: Volumes per second

Authors' contributions

All authors have contributed significantly to the submitted work: LPB: study design, critical revision of the first draft and final approval of the manuscript; PA: study design, image acquisition, data analysis, first draft and final approval of the manuscript; BE and NR: data collection, image analysis and final approval of the manuscript; SM and CP: image acquisition and final approval of the manuscript; ACG, DM and SI: critical revision of the first draft and final approval of the manuscript.

Consent for publication

"Not applicable" in this section.

Competing interests

Drs Badano and Muraru are consultants for and have received equipment grants from GE Healthcare (Little Chalfont, United Kingdom) and TomTec Imaging Systems (Unterschleissheim, Germany). The other authors do not have competing interests.

Author details

[1]Department of Cardiac, Thoracic and Vascular Science, University of Padua, Via Giustiniani 2, 35128 Padua, Italy. [2]University of Medicine and Pharmacy "Carol Davila", Bucharest, Romania. [3]Tanta University Hospital, Tanta, Egypt.

References

1. Nkomo VT, Gardin JM, Skelton TN, Gottdiener JS, Scott CG, Enriquez-Sarano M. Burden of valvular heart diseases: a population-based study. Lancet. 2006;368:1005–11.
2. Monteagudo Ruiz JM, Galderisi M, Buonauro A, Badano L, Aruta P, Swaans MJ, et al. Overview of mitral regurgitation in Europe: results from the European registry of mitral regurgitation (EuMiClip). Eur Heart J Cardiovasc Imaging. 2018;19:503–7.
3. Mirabel M, Iung B, Baron G, Messika-Zeitoun D, Detaint D, Vanoverschelde JL, et al. What are the characteristics of patients with severe, symptomatic, mitral regurgitation who are denied surgery? Eur Heart J. 2007;28:1358–65.
4. Goel SS, Bajaj N, Aggarwal B, Gupta S, Poddar KL, Ige M, et al. Prevalence and outcomes of unoperated patients with severe symptomatic mitral regurgitation and heart failure. comprehensive analysis to determine the potential role of MitraClip for this unmet need J Am Coll Cardiol. 2014;63:185–6.
5. Banai S, Verheye S, Cheung A, Schwartz M, Marko A, Lane R, et al. Transapical mitral implantation of the Tiara bioprosthesis. pre-clinical results JACC Cardiovasc Interv. 2014;7:154–62.
6. Bapat V, Rajagopal V, Meduri C, Farivar RS, Walton A, Duffy SJ, et al. Early experience with new Transcatheter mitral valve replacement. J Am Coll Cardiol. 2018;71:12–21.
7. Lutter G, Lozonschi L, Ebner A, Gallo S, Marin Y, Kall C, Missov E, et al. First-in-human off-pump transcatheter mitral valve replacement. JACC Cardiovasc Interv. 2014;7:1077–8.
8. Blanke P, Naoum C, Webb J, Dvir D, Hahn RT, Grayburn P, et al. Multimodality imaging in the context of Transcatheter mitral valve replacement. Establishing Consensus Among Modalities and Disciplines JACC Cardiovasc Imaging. 2015;8:1191–208.
9. Boekstegers P, Hausleiter J, Baldus S, von Bardeleben RS, Beucher H, Butter C, et al. Percutaneous interventional mitral regurgitation treatment using the Mitra-clip system. Clin Res Cardiol. 2014;103:85–96.
10. Daimon M, Saracino G, Gillinov AM, Koyama Y, Fukuda S, Kwan J, et al. Local dysfunction and asymmetrical deformation of mitral annular geometry in ischemic mitral regurgitation: a novel computerized 3D echocardiographic analysis. Echocardiography. 2008;25:414–23.
11. Nagasaki M, Nishimura S, Ohtaki E, Kasegawa H, Matsumura T, Nagayama M, et al. The echocardiographic determinants of functional mitral regurgitation differ in ischemic and non-ischemic cardiomyopathy. Int J Cardiol. 2006;108: 171–6.
12. Veronesi F, Corsi C, Sugeng L, Caiani EG, Weinert L, Mor-Avi V, et al. Quantification of mitral apparatus dynamics in functional and ischemic mitral regurgitation using real-time 3-dimensional echocardiography. J Am Soc Echocardiogr. 2008;21:347–54.
13. Kwan J, Shiota T, Agler DA, Popovic ZB, Qin JX, Gillinov MA, et al. Geometric differences of the mitral apparatus between ischemic and dilated cardiomyopathy with significant mitral regurgitation: real-time three-dimensional echocardiography study. Circulation. 2003;107:1135–40.
14. Lancellotti P, Moura L, Pierard LA, Agricola E, Popescu BA, Tribouilloy C, et al. European Association of Echocardiography recommendations for the assessment of valvular regurgitation. Part 2: mitral and tricuspid regurgitation (native valve disease). Eur J Echocardiogr. 2010;11:307–32.
15. Mihaila S, Muraru D, Piasentini E, Miglioranza MH, Peluso D, Cucchini U, et al. Quantitative analysis of mitral annular geometry and function in healthy volunteers using transthoracic three-dimensional echocardiography. J Am Soc Echocardiogr. 2014;27:846–57.
16. Anwar AM, Soliman OI, Nemes A, Germans T, Krenning BJ, Geleijnse ML, et al. Assessment of mitral annulus size and function by real-time 3-dimensional echocardiography in cardiomyopathy: comparison with magnetic resonance imaging. J Am Soc Echocardiogr. 2007;20:941–8.
17. Muraru D, Cecchetto A, Cucchini U, Zhou X, Lang RM, Romeo G, et al. Intervendor consistency and accuracy of left ventricular volume measurements using three-dimensional echocardiography. J Am Soc Echocardiogr. 2018;31:158–68 e1.
18. Lang RM, Badano LP, Mor-Avi V, Afilalo J, Armstrong A, Ernande L, et al. Recommendations for cardiac chamber quantification by echocardiography in adults: an update from the American Society of Echocardiography and the European Association of Cardiovascular Imaging. Eur Heart J Cardiovasc Imaging. 2015;16:233–70.
19. Mackensen GB, Lee JC, Wang DD, Pearson PJ, Blanke P, Dvir D, et al. Role of echocardiography in Transcatheter mitral valve replacement in native mitral valves and mitral rings. J Am Soc Echocardiogr. 2018;31:475–90.
20. Levack MM, Jassar AS, Shang EK, Vergnat M, Woo YJ, Acker MA, et al. Three-dimensional echocardiographic analysis of mitral annular dynamics: implication for annuloplasty selection. Circulation. 2012;126:S183–8.
21. Flachskampf FA, Chandra S, Gaddipatti A, Levine RA, Weyman AE, Ameling W, et al. Analysis of shape and motion of the mitral annulus in subjects with and without cardiomyopathy by echocardiographic 3-dimensional reconstruction. J Am Soc Echocardiogr. 2000;13:277–87.
22. Theriault-Lauzier P, Mylotte D, Dorfmeister M, Spaziano M, Andalib A, Mamane S, et al. Quantitative multi-slice computed tomography assessment of the mitral valvular complex for transcatheter mitral valve interventions part 1: systematic measurement methodology and inter-observer variability. EuroIntervention. 2016;12:e1011–e20.
23. Theriault-Lauzier P, Dorfmeister M, Mylotte D, Andalib A, Spaziano M, Blanke P, et al. Quantitative multi-slice computed tomography assessment of the mitral valvular complex for transcatheter mitral valve interventions part 2: geometrical measurements in patients with functional mitral regurgitation. EuroIntervention. 2016;12:e1021–e30.
24. Khalique OK, Kodali SK, Paradis JM, Nazif TM, Williams MR, Einstein AJ, et al. Aortic annular sizing using a novel 3-dimensional echocardiographic method: use and comparison with cardiac computed tomography. Circ Cardiovasc Imaging. 2014;7:155–63.
25. Blanke P, Dvir D, Cheung A, Ye J, Levine RA, Precious B, et al. A simplified D-shaped model of the mitral annulus to facilitate CT-based sizing before transcatheter mitral valve implantation. J Cardiovasc Comput Tomogr. 2014; 8:459–67.
26. Mak GJ, Blanke P, Ong K, Naoum C, Thompson CR, Webb JG, et al. Three-dimensional echocardiography compared with computed tomography to determine mitral annulus size before Transcatheter mitral valve implantation. Circ Cardiovasc Imaging. 2016;9:1–9.
27. Khalique OK, Hahn RT. Multimodality imaging in Transcatheter mitral interventions: buzzword or modern age toolbox? Circ Cardiovasc Imaging. 2016;9:1–3.
28. Jiang L, Owais K, Matyal R, Khabbaz KR, Liu DC, Montealegre-Gallegos M, et al. Dynamism of the mitral annulus: a spatial and temporal analysis. J Cardiothorac Vasc Anesth. 2014;28:1191–7.
29. Owais K, Montealegre-Gallegos M, Jeganathan J, Matyal R, Khabbaz KR, Mahmood F. Dynamic changes in the ischemic mitral annulus: implications for ring sizing. Ann Card Anaesth. 2016;19:15–9.

26

Left atrium remodeling predicts late recurrence of paroxysmal atrial fibrillation after second generation cryoballoon ablation

Andreea Motoc[1][*] (iD), Juan-Pablo Abugattas[2], Bram Roosens[1], Esther Scheirlynck[1], Benedicte Heyndrickx[1], Carlo de Asmundis[2], Gian-Battista Chierchia[2], Steven Droogmans[1][†] and Bernard Cosyns[1][†]

Abstract

Background: Atrial fibrillation (AF) is the most common arrhythmia worldwide. Nowadays, AF ablation is a valuable treatment option. It has been shown that the left atrium (LA) diameter is a predictor of AF recurrence after cryoballoon ablation (CBA). Since it does not reflect the true LA size, we compared the role of different LA anatomical parameters using echocardiography for the prediction of AF recurrence after CBA.

Methods: We retrospectively included 209 patients (mean age 56.1 ± 13.6 years, male 62%) with paroxysmal AF undergoing CBA. A transthoracic echocardiography was performed in all patients.

Results: At a mean follow-up of 16.9 ± 6.3 months, AF recurred in 25.4% of the patients. LA anterior - posterior diameter (LAD), LA minimum volume (LAmin) and early AF recurrence were independent predictors of recurrence. Based on receiver operating characteristics, cut – off values for LAD and, LAmin were 41 mm, 23.69 mL, respectively. The negative predictive values for recurrence were 73% and 87.3% respectively. In patients with AF recurrence, a significant proportion (30.2%) showed LA longitudinal remodeling (LA superior – inferior diameter) even though classically measured LAD was normal.

Conclusions: Longitudinal LA remodeling plays an additional role for predicting AF recurrence after CBA, in patients without LAD dilation. Moreover, LAmin had a high negative predictive value and was an independent predictor of AF recurrence. Therefore, a more complete LA anatomical assessment allows a better prediction of AF recurrences after CBA.

Keywords: Atrial fibrillation, Cryoballoon ablation, Left atrium, Echocardiography

Background

Atrial fibrillation (AF) is the most common cardiac arrhythmia, with an increasing frequency worldwide, and it is associated with an elevated risk for stroke, heart failure and mortality. Its prevalence in developed countries is currently estimated to 1.5–2% of the general population [1]. Resinusalisation is one of the main goals in AF patients. Several ablation strategies have proven to be efficient in the treatment of AF [2, 3]. Among them, one of the most promising and effective approaches is the second generation cryoballoon ablation (CBA) (Arctic Front Advance, Medtronic). However, up to 20% of patients experience AF recurrence after CBA [4, 5].

Recent data have shown that an increase of the left atrium (LA) anterior - posterior diameter (LAD) assessed by echocardiography is a powerful predictor of recurrence after CBA [4, 6]. A possible explanation for the recurrence of AF could be the presence of myocardial fibrosis and remodeling of the LA [7]. However, LAD does not reflect the true size of the LA [8, 9]. We hypothesized that a more complete analysis of the LA dimensions could be a

* Correspondence: andreea.motoc@gmail.com
†Steven Droogmans and Bernard Cosyns contributed equally to this work.
[1]Centrum Voor Hart-en Vaatziekten (CHVZ), Department of Cardiology, UZ Brussel, Laarbeeklaan 101, 1090 Brussels, Belgium
Full list of author information is available at the end of the article

better predictor of AF recurrence after CBA. Therefore, we compared the role of different anatomical parameters of the LA measured by echocardiography for predicting the recurrence of AF after CBA.

Methods

Patient characteristics

We retrospectively included 209 patients having undergone CBA for paroxysmal AF in our center from January 2014 to February 2016.

Baseline demographic characteristics can be found in Table 1. CHA_2DS_2-VASc score was calculated according to European Society of Cardiology Guidelines [1].

The study was approved by the local Ethical Committee and was carried out in accordance with the ethical principles for medical research involving human subjects established by Helsinki's Declaration, protecting the privacy of all participants, as well as the confidentiality of their personal information. All patients provided written informed consents.

Transthoracic echocardiography

A comprehensive transthoracic echocardiography (TTE) (using GE Vingmed Ultrasound, Vivid E9, Horten, Norway; Phillips Epiq, Philips, Andover, Massachusetts) was performed in all patients, according to the recommendations [10, 11]. Standard parasternal long and short axis views and apical two-, three - and four - chamber views were available in all patients. Left ventricular (LV) dimensions were measured using M – Mode in the parasternal long axis view. LAD was measured using anatomical M-mode and two – dimensional assessment (2D) in the parasternal long axis view. LA maximum (LAmax) and minimum (LAmin) volumes were measured in two - and four chamber views, using the biplane area-length method (Fig. 1). LA volumes were indexed based on the patient's body surface area. Left atrium superior - inferior diameter was measured in apical two - and four chamber views (Fig. 2). Doppler mitral inflow peak early diastolic (E), peak atrial systolic velocities (A) and deceleration time were measured. Tissue Doppler imaging at the level of the mitral annulus was used to measure peak early diastolic septal and lateral e', as well as peak late diastolic a', corresponding to the P-wave on the electrocardiogram (ECG) [10, 12].

To determine the reproducibility of the LAD, LA superior – inferior diameter, LAmax and LAmin, the measurements were repeated in 20 randomly selected patients by an additional investigator and by the same primary investigator 1 week later. During the repeated analysis, the investigators were blinded to the results of all previous measurements.

Pre-procedural management

The antiarrhythmic drugs (AADs) were discontinued at least 3 days before the procedure, except for amiodarone, which was stopped one month before.

Cryoballon ablation procedure

Our standard ablation procedure has been previously reported in detail [13]. Briefly, after obtaining LA access, through a steerable 15 Fr sheath (FlexCath Advance®, Medtronic©), an inner lumen mapping catheter (ILMC) (Achieve®, Medtronic©) was advanced in each pulmonary vein (PV) ostium and baseline electrical information was gathered. Optimal vessel occlusion was considered as achieved upon selective contrast injection showing total contrast retention with no backflow into the atrium. Once occlusion was documented, cryothermal energy was started for at least 180 s. Usually, the PVs were treated as follows: first, the left superior PV (LSPV), then the left inferior (LIPV), right inferior (RIPV) and right superior (RSPV). PV activity was recorded with the ILMC at a proximal site within the ostium prior to ablation in each vein. If PV potentials (PVPs) were visible during energy delivery, time to isolation was recorded as the time from the start of the cryoenergy application until the PVPs completely disappeared or were dissociated from LA activity. In cases of phrenic nerve palsy (PNP), recovery of diaphragmatic contraction was carefully monitored for 30 min. Further additional cryoenergy applications were not applied if the veins were isolated after the initial freeze. If needed, pacing from the distal and/or proximal coronary sinus was performed to recognise far field atrial signals from PVPs recorded on the mapping catheter. During the whole procedure, activated clotting time was maintained > 250 s. In order to avoid phrenic nerve palsy, diaphragmatic stimulation was achieved by pacing the phrenic nerve during septal pulmonary veins ablations.

Postablation management

Patients were discharged the day after ablation if the clinical status was stable. Following the procedure, all the patients were continuously monitored with ECG telemetry for at least 18 h. Oral anticoagulation was not discontinued for the ablation and continued for at least 2 months following the CHA_2DS_2 - VASc score. During the blanking period (BP), AADs were continued. The decision to continue AADs after the BP or to perform a repeat procedure was taken if a first episode of recurrence of AF occurred.

Follow-up

All the included patients underwent physical examination and a 24 h Holter recording at 1, 3, 6 and 12 months after the ablation. Additional Holter

Table 1 Baseline clinical and demographic characteristics

Characteristic	Study population ($n = 209$)	AF recurrence − ($n = 156$)	AF recurrence + ($n = 53$)	P value
Age (y)	56.1 ± 13.5	55.6 ± 13.5	57.4 ± 13.7	0.335
Male gender (n, %)	130 (62.2)	98(62.8)	32 (60.4)	0.753
Body mass index (kg/m^2)	26.5 ± 4.7	26.3 ± 4.5	27 ± 5.3	0.549
Tobacco use (n, %)	52 (24.8)	35 (28.8)	17(32)	0.281
Hypertension (n, %)	86 (41.1)	59 (37.8)	27 (50.9)	0.094
Diabetes (n, %)	16 (7.7)	9 (5.8)	7 (13.2)	0.079
Dyslipidemia (n, %)	75 (35.9)	55 (35.3)	20 (37.7)	0.747
History of heart failure (n, %)	6 (2.9)	4 (2.6)	2 (3.8)	0.651
Coronary artery disease (n, %)	15 (7.2)	10 (6.4)	5 (9.4)	0.464
History of TIA[a]/CVA[b](n, %)	19 (9.1)	15 (9.6)	4 (7.5)	0.653
Failed drugs before ablation				
Flecainide (n, %)	46 (22)	31(19.8)	15(28.3)	0.177
Propafenone(n, %)	1(0.47)	0 (0)	1(1.8)	0.083
Amiodarone(n, %)	9 (4.3)	6 (3.8)	3 (5.6)	0.555
Sotalol (n, %)	24 (11.4)	16 (10.2)	8 (15)	0.316
Metoprolol (n, %)	2 (0.9)	2 (1.2)	0 (0)	0.412
Bisoprolol (n, %)	78 (37.3)	57 (36.5)	21 (39.6)	0.620
Nebivolol (n, %)	6 (3.8)	5 (3.2)	1 (1.8)	0.632
ACE[c] inhibitors before ablation	26 (12.4)	20 (12.8)	6 (11.3)	0.809
ARBs[d] before ablation	11 (5.2)	9 (5.7)	2 (3.7)	0.592
Prior ablation	39 (18.6)	29 (18.5)	10 (18.8)	0.547
- AVNRT[e]	13 (6.2)	12 (7.7)	1 (1.9)	1.000
- Right atrial flutter	13 (6.2)	8 (5.1)	5 (9.4)	1.000
- AF[f]	11 (5.3)	8 (5.1)	3 (5.7)	1.000
- Other	2 (1.0)	1 (0.6)	1 (1.9)	1.000
CHA$_2$DS$_2$-VASc score	1.3 ± 1.4	1.2 ± 1.3	1.6 ± 1.7	0.134
Oral anticoagulation (n, %)	60 (28.7)	41 (26.3%)	19 (35.8%)	0.552
Aspirin (n, %)	23 (11)	17 (10.9)	6 (11.3)	0.874
Follow-up duration (months)	16.8 ± 6.3	16.9 ± 5.7	16.6 ± 7.7	0.795
Re-do ablation	31 (14.8)	0 (0)	31 (58.4)	–
Medication in BP[g]				
- Flecainide (n, %)	62 (29.6)	42 (26.9)	20 (37.7)	0.122
- Propafenone (n, %)	2 (0.95)	1 (0.64)	1 (1.8)	0.415
- Amiodarone (n, %)	9 (4.3)	6 (3.8)	3 (5.6)	0.561
- Sotalol (n, %)	49 (23.4)	34 (21.8)	15 (28.3)	0.310
- Metoprolol (n, %)	1(0.4)	1(0.6)	0 (0)	0.562
- Bisoprolol (n, %)	111 (53.11)	81 (51.9)	30 (56.6)	0.497
- Nebivolol (n, %)	4 (1.9)	4 (2.5)	0 (0)	0.241
- ACE inhibitors (n, %)	27 (12.9)	21 (13.4)	6 (11.3)	0.710
- ARBs (n, %)	6 (2.8)	6	0	0.150
Medication after BP				
- Flecainide (n, %)	25 (11.9)	17 (10.8)	8 (15)	0.398
- Propafenone (n, %)	2 (0.9)	0 (0)	2 (3.7)	0.060
- Amiodarone (n, %)	6 (2.8)	3 (1.9)	3 (5.6)	0.154

Table 1 Baseline clinical and demographic characteristics *(Continued)*

Characteristic	Study population (n = 209)	AF recurrence – (n = 156)	AF recurrence + (n = 53)	P value
- Sotalol (n, %)	26 (12.4)	18 (11.5)	8 (15)	0.478
- Metoprolol (n, %)	1 (0.4)	1(0.6)	0 (0)	0.562
- Bisoprolol (n, %)	62 (29.6)	50 (23.9)	12 (22.6)	0.211
- Nebivolol (n, %)	6 (2.8)	5 (3.2)	1 (1.8)	0.628
- ACE inhibitors (n, %)	27 (12.9)	21 (13.4)	6 (11.3)	0.710
- ARBs (n, %)	6 (2.8)	6	0	0.150
Recurrence in BP	8 (3.8)	0 (0)	8(15.1)	< 0.001

[a]*TIA* Transient ischaemic attack, [b]*CVA* Cerebrovascular accident, [c]*ACE* inhibitors, angiontensin – converter enzyme inhibitors, [d] *ARBs* angiotensin receptor blockers, [e] *AVNRT* atrioventricular nodal reentry tachycardia, [f]*AF* atrial fibrillation, [g]*BP* blanking period

monitoring was performed if arrhythmic symptoms occurred. All documented AF episodes > 30 s were considered as a recurrence. A BP of 3 months was considered for the study.

Statistical analysis

Continuous variables are expressed as mean ± standard deviation. Categorical variables are expressed as percentages. Comparisons of continuous variables were done with a Student t-test or Mann-Whitney U-test and binomial variables with a chi-square or Fisher test as appropriate. Receiver-operator characteristic (ROC) curves were constructed to evaluate the performance of variables in predicting AF recurrence and to calculate adjusted cut-off values, specificity and sensitivity of the parameters (using Youden's Index) in the prediction of AF recurrence. Freedom from AF recurrence was estimated by Kaplan-Meier method and time-dependent comparisons by the log-rank test. In order to evaluate potential predictors of AF recurrence, a separate Cox proportional hazard model was used. Intraclass correlation coefficient (ICC) was used to determine the intra- and inter - observer variability. The calculated ICCs were judged as follows: 0.50 to 0.74 poor to moderate, 0.75 to 0.92 good and > 0.93 excellent. Statistical significance was considered with a P-value < 0.05. Statistical analyses were conducted using IBM SPSS Statistic for Windows, Version 24.0 (Armonk, NY: IBM Corp.)

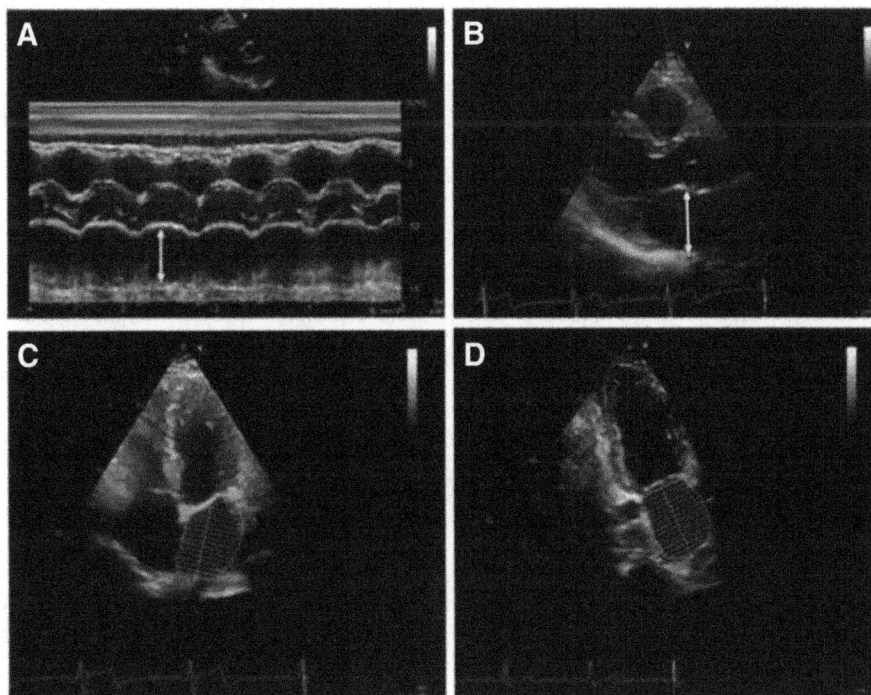

Fig. 1 a. Illustration of the left atrium anterior – posterior diameter measurement in M-Mode, using the parasternal long axis view. **b.** Left atrium anterior – posterior diameter measurement in 2D parasternal long axis view. **c.** Left atrium volume measurement in four – chamber view. **d.** Left atrium volume measurement in two – chamber view

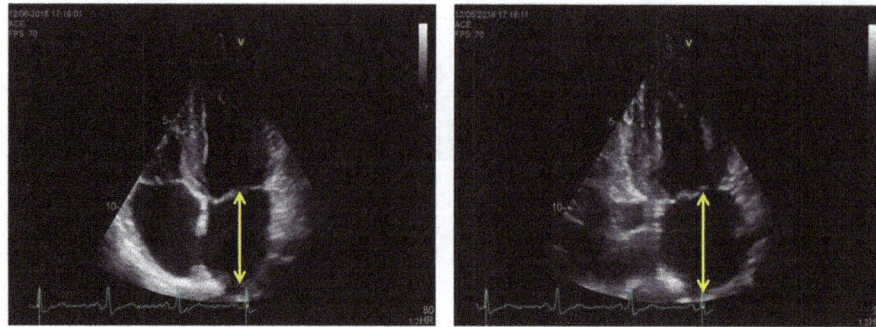

Fig. 2 Left atrium length (superior - inferior diameter) is measured perpendicular from the mid-point of the segment that unifies the hinge points of the mitral leaflets to the roof of the left atrium

Results

At a mean follow – up of 16.8 ± 6.3 months after the BP, 53 (25.4%) patients presented recurrences of AF.

Baseline population characteristics and recurrences

Baseline clinical and demographic characteristics of the study population are listed in Table 1. There was a significant difference between the groups with and without recurrence for patients who presented early AF recurrence.

Echocardiographic characteristics are presented in Table 2. In brief, there was a significant difference in patients with and without recurrence respectively for LV end-diastolic diameter (50.3 ± 7.9 mm vs. 47.2 ± 6.5 mm, $p = 0.013$), LV mass index (83.7 ± 28.4 g/m^2 vs. 76.6 ± 26.3 g/m^2, $p = 0.045$), LAD (42.2 ± 7.2 mm vs. 39 ± 6.1 mm, $p = 0.013$), LAmax (67.3 ± 27.8 mL vs. 57.7 ± 21.2 mL, $p = 0.036$), LAmin (36.7 ± 20.1 mL vs. 27.5 ± 14.9 mL, $p = 0.004$) and LAmin indexed (18.1 ± 9.3 mL/m^2 vs. 14.1 ± 7.4 mL/m^2, $p = 0.007$).

Procedural data

All the patients underwent the procedure with the large 28-mm CBA. At the beginning of the procedure, 203 (97.1%) patients were in sinus rhythm. The mean total procedure and fluoroscopy time were 66.9 ± 20.2 min, respectively 13.8 ± 7.5 min. The mean number of freeze-thaw cycles was 1.2 ± 0.4 in the LSPV, 1.1 ± 0.3 in the LIPV, 1.19 ± 0.44 in the RSPV, 1.2 ± 0.5 in the RIPV. The mean minimal temperatures obtained were -48.7 ± 8.6 °C in LSPV, -48.7 ± 8.6 in LIPV, -49.2 ± 10.8 in RSPV, -46 ± 14.6 in RIPV. There were no significant differences regarding the procedural data between the two groups. Procedural data can be found in Table 3.

Global versus longitudinal LA remodeling and AF recurrences

Fig. 3 illustrates that using only the LAD, with an adjusted cut-off value of 41 mm, led missing up to 30.2%

of AF recurrences. In the patients with recurrence without LAD dilation, a significant number of patients had longitudinal LA remodeling (increased superior – inferior LA diameter, with an adjusted cut-off value of 41 mm).

LA volumes and AF recurrences

Multivariate regression analysis showed that LAD, LAmin and early AF recurrence were independent predictors of AF recurrence after the BP, as illustrated in Table 4.

ROC analysis revealed that for a cut-off value of 23.69 ml for LAmin it was associated with a high sensitivity for predicting AF recurrence after the BP (79.5% sensitivity, 46% specificity). For the above mentioned adjusted cut-off values, LAmin had a high negative predictive values for AF recurrences 87.3% .

In contrast, for LAD, sensitivity and specificity were 56.3% and 66%, respectively, with a lower negative predictive value of 73% compared to LAmin.

Reproducibility

Intraobserver variability was excellent for all the parameters. For LAD the ICC was 0.972, for LA superior – inferior diameter ICC = 0.95, for LAmax ICC = 0.964 and for LAmin ICC = 0.940. Interobserver reliability was good for LAD (ICC = 0.906), LAmax (ICC = 0.907) and LAmin (0.860) and excellent for LA superior – inferior diameter (ICC = 0.96).

Discussion

The main findings of our study are: 1) recurrence of AF after the BP occurred in 25.4% of all subjects with paroxysmal AF. 2) In the group of patients with AF recurrence, longitudinal remodeling (increased superior – inferior LA diameter) was also present in patients with normal LAD. 3) In the global population of patients undergoing CBA, LA minimum volume was an independent predictor of AF recurrences after the BP. These

Table 2 Echocardiographic parameters

Characteristic	Study population ($n = 209$)	AF recurrence − ($n = 156$)	AF recurrence + ($n = 53$)	P value
Heart rate during echocardiography	75.6 ± 14.5	76.3 ± 14.1	75.6 ± 14.5	0.080
Left ventricle				
- LVEF[a], %	54.4 ± 5.2	54.6 ± 4.7	53.8 ± 6.4	0.343
- LV[b] EDD[c], mm	48 ± 7	47.2 ± 6.5	50.3 ± 7.9	0.013
- LV ESD[d], mm	30.4 ± 5.8	30.4 ± 5.9	30.5 ± 5.7	0.939
- IVS$_d$[e], mm	9.5 ± 1.7	9.5 ± 1.78	9.6 ± 1.7	0.763
- PW$_d$[f], mm	9.3 ± 1.6	9.1 ± 1.4	9.6 ± 1.8	0.131
- LV mass, g	140.4 ± 72.8	136.8 ± 70.1	150.9 ± 80	0.073
- LV mass index, g/m^2	78.4 ± 26.9	76.6 ± 26.3	83.7 ± 28.4	0.045
- LV EDV[g], mL	99 ± 32.5	96.4 ± 30.5	109.8 ± 39.6	0.223
- LV ESV[h], mL	46.8 ± 20.8	45.4 ± 20.6	52.4 ± 21.6	0.196
Left atrium				
- LA[i] antero-posterior diameter, mm	39.8 ± 6.5	39 ± 6.1	42.2 ± 7.2	0.013
- LA antero-posterior diameter indexed, mm/m^2	20.4 ± 3.4	20.1 ± 3.3	20.4 ± 3.4	0.182
- LA superior- inferior diameter, mm	48.8 ± 7.6	48.3 ± 7.6	50.3 ± 7.4	0.095
- LA maximum volume, mL	60 ± 23.3	57.7 ± 21.2	67.3 ± 27.8	0.036
- LA maximum volume indexed, ml/m^2	30.4 ± 10.8	29.5 ± 10	33.5 ± 12.6	0.067
- LA minimum volume, mL	29.8 ± 16.8	27.5 ± 14.9	36.7 ± 20.1	0.004
- LA minimum volume indexed, mL/m^2	15.1 ± 8	14.1 ± 7.4	18.1 ± 9.3	0.007
Doppler				
- E- wave velocity, m/s	0.6 ± 0.1	0.6 ± 0.1	0.6 ± 0.1	0.768
- A – wave velocity, m/s	0.5 ± 0.1	0.5 ± 0.1	0.4 ± 0.1	0.405
- E/A (ratio)	1.4 ± 0.5	1.3 ± 0.5	1.4 ± 0.5	0.314
- DTE[j], ms	180.8 ± 44.4	180.2 ± 45.4	182.7 ± 41.6	0.482
- TDI[k] e' septal, cm/s	7.4 ± 2.1	7.3 ± 2	7.8 ± 2.5	0.366
- TDI e' lateral,cm/s	9.4 ± 4.9	9.6 ± 5.3	9 ± 2.8	0.965
- E/e' avg. (ratio)	8.6 ± 2.9	8.7 ± 2.9	8.4 ± 3.2	0.893
- TDI a' septal, cm/s	7.4 ± 2	7.6 ± 2	6.8 ± 2	0.053
- TDI a' lateral, cm/s	8 ± 2.4	8.1 ± 2.4	7.5 ± 2.4	0.111
Mitral regurgitation (n, %)	97 (46.4)	70 (44.8)	27 (50.9)	0.594
- Mild (n, %)	90 (43.1)	64 (41)	26 (49.1)	
- Moderate (n, %)	7 (3.3)	6 (3.8)	1 (1.9)	
Mitral annulus calcification (n, %)	10 (4.8)	7 (4.5)	3 (5.7)	0.677
Aortic regurgitation (mild) (n, %)	24 (11.9)	20 (12.8)	4 (7.5)	0.298
Tricupid regurgitation (n, %)	106 (50.7)	77 (49.3)	29 (54.7)	0.338
- Mild (n, %)	96 (45.9)	70 (44.8)	26 (49)	
- Moderate (n, %)	9 (4.3)	7 (4.4)	2 (3.7)	
- Severe (n, %)	1 (0.4)	0 (0)	1 (1.8)	
TAPSE[l], mm	23.1 ± 4	23 ± 3.7	23.5 ± 4.9	0.253
IVC[m], mm	14.3 ± 4	14.1 ± 3.9	15.1 ± 4.2	0.258
TR[n] gradient, mmHg	24.9 ± 7.5	25.1 ± 7.7	24.1 ± 6.9	0.783

[a]LVEF left ventricle ejection fraction, [b]LV left ventricle, [c]EDD end – diastolic diameter, [d]ESD end – systolic diameter, [e]IVSd Interventricular septum end-diastolic diameter, [f]PWd posterior wall end-diastolic diameter, [g]EDV end – diastolic volume, [h]ESV end – systolic volume, [i]LA left atrium, [j]DTE deceleration time of E – wave, [k]TDI, tissue Doppler imaging, [l]TAPSE tricuspid annulus plane systolic excursion, [m]IVC inferior vena cava, [n]TR tricuspid regurgitation

Table 3 Procedural data

Characteristic	Study population (n = 209)	AF recurrence − (n = 156)	AF recurrence + (n = 53)	P value
Procedural time, min	66.9 ± 20.2	67 ± 20.3	66.5 ± 19.9	0.918
Fluoroscopy time, min	13.8 ± 7.5	13.4 ± 7.2	14.7 ± 8.3	0.452
Freezes in LSPV[a]	1.2 ± 0.4	1.2 ± 0.4	1.2 ± 0.4	0.656
Freezes in LIPV[b]	1.1 ± 0.3	1.1 ± 0.4	1.1 ± 0.3	0.215
Freezes in RSPV[c]	1.1 ± 0.4	1.1 ± 0.4	1.2 ± 0.4	0.086
Freezes in RIPV[d]	1.2 ± 0.5	1.2 ± 0.4	1.2 ± 0.5	0.366
LSPV freeze duration, s	223.6 ± 78.9	224.8 ± 80.5	220 ± 74.6	0.782
LIPV freeze duration, s	208.2 ± 65.5	211.1 ± 69	199.7 ± 53. 7	0.412
RSPV freeze duration, s	208.5 ± 79	206 ± 75	215.9 ± 89.8	0.647
RIPV freeze duration, s	225.4 ± 89.1	223 ± 89.4	232.5 ± 88.8	0.147
Min temp[e] in LSPV, °C	−48.7 ± 8.6	−48.7 ± 9.5	−48.6 ± 5	0.325
Min temp in LIPV, °C	−45.4 ± 8.6	- 45.5 ± 9.5	− 44.9 ± 5.4	0.192
Min temp in RSPV, °C	−49.2 ± 10.8	−49.3 ± 11.9	−47 ± 14.6	0.246
Min temp in RIPV, °C	−46 ± 14.6	− 45.4 ± 16.3	−47.9 ± 6.5	0.698
Pulmonary veins variants	102 (48.8)	79 (50.6)	23 (43.3)	0.347
- Left common ostium	58 (27.8)	42 (26.9)	16 (30.2)	0.647
- Right middle pulmonary vein	29 (13.9)	25 (16.0)	4 (7.5)	0.124
- Right common ostium	8 (3.8)	7 (4.5)	1 (1.9)	0.640
- Other	7 (3.3)	5 (3.2)	2 (3.8)	0.686

[a]*LSPV* left superior pulmonary vein, [b]*LIPV* left inferior pulmonary vein, [c]*RSPV* right superior pulmonary vein, [d]*RIPV* right inferior pulmonary vein, [e]*Min temp*, minimum temperature

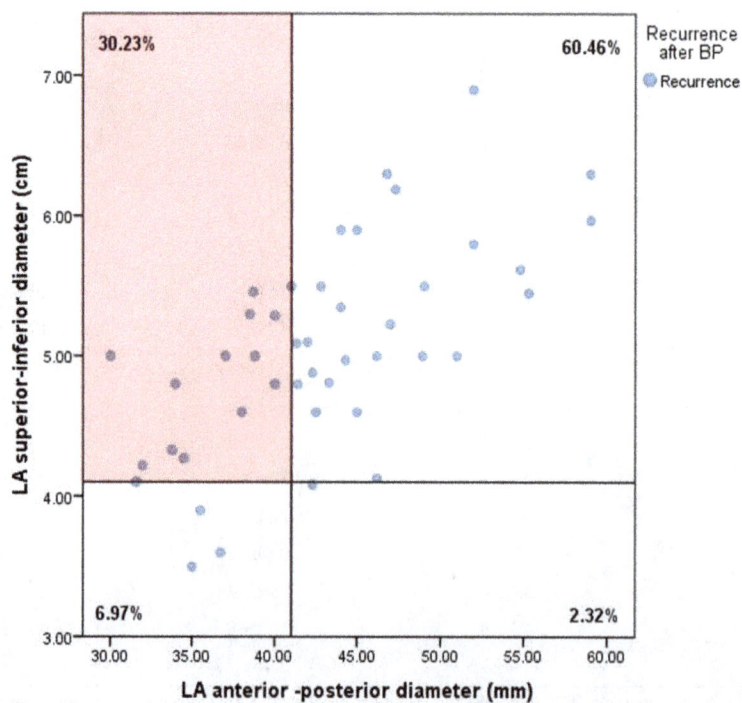

Fig. 3 Proportions of patients with AF recurrences according to the adjusted cut – off values for LA superior – inferior diameter (41 mm) and LA anterior – posterior diameter (41 mm), showing that 30.2% of patients with recurrence had longitudinal remodeling, in the absence of an increased anterior-posterior diameter

Table 4 Predictors of atrial fibrillation recurrence

| Parameters | Univariate analysis | | Multivariate analysis | | | | | |
| | | | Model 1 | | Model 2 | | Model 3 | |
	HR[h] (95% CI[i])	p	HR (95% CI)	p	HR (95% CI)	p	HR (95% CI)	p
AHT[a]	1.608 (0.937–2.762)	0.085	1.675 (0.886 - 3.166)	0.112	1.489 (0.771–2.875)	0.236	1.433 (0.773–2.658)	0.254
DM[b]	2.141 (0.963–4.763)	0.062	1.447 (0.549–3.816)	0.455	1.410 (0.541–3.679)	0.482	1.389 (0.523–3.688)	0.509
Recurrence in BP[c]	4.867 (2.174–10.892)	< 0.001*	4.457 (1.647–12.062)	0.003*	4.990 (1.884–13.215)	0.001*	4.504 (1.830–11.088)	0.001*
LV[d] mass index	1.010 (0.998–1.022)	0.100	1.008 (0.993–1.023)	0.301	1.007 (0.992–1.021)	0.366	1.003 (0.990–1.015)	0.681
LAD[e]	1.017 (1.006–1.028)	0.003*	1.062 (1.010–1.117)	0.018*				
LAmax[f]	1.024 (1.011–1.036)	< 0.001*			1.009 (0.996–1.022)	0.157		
LAmin[g]	1.078 (1.031–1.127)	0.001*					1.016 (1.001–1.031)	0.039*

[a]*AHT* arterial hypertension, [b]*DM* diabetes mellitus, [c]*BP* blanking period, [d]*LV* left ventricle, [e]*LAD* left atrium diameter, [f]*LAmax* left atirum maximum volume, [g]*LAmin* left atrium minimum volume, [h]*HR* hazard ratio; [i]*CI* confidence interval, *p < 0.05

results suggest that AF recurrence after ablation also occurs in the absence of global LA remodeling assessed by LAD.

This study evaluates the role of additional anatomical parameters of the LA using two-dimensional echocardiography for the prediction of recurrence of AF after the BP in patients who have undergone CBA.

The incidence of recurrence of AF after the BP in our study was of 25.4%, which is consistent with results of previous studies. Gerede et al. [6] have reported a rate of recurrence after the BP of 31.3%. In a recent study published by Coutino et al. [5] they showed a rate of recurrence after the BP of 25.2%. Previous studies have shown that the presence of recurrence during the BP is an independent predictor of late AF recurrence, which was also confirmed by our analysis [14, 15].

Previous studies have shown that the enlargement of LAD is an independent predictor of recurrence of AF after the BP, suggesting that the remodeling of the LA is a leading cause for late recurrences of AF [4, 6]. This is consistent with our results that report LAD as a predictor of recurrence of AF after CBA.

However, the remodeling of the LA can occur non-uniformly, correlating with reduced success of different ablation techniques [9, 16] and furthermore, LAD is not considered as representative of LA dimension following the EACVI/ASE recommendations [10, 11] . Our study shows that 30.2% of the patients with a normal LAD, but a dilated superior – inferior diameter presented AF recurrence after the BP. This novel finding suggests that longitudinal remodeling is also involved in AF recurrence after ablation. However, longitudinal LA dilation could also be observed in patients without recurrence and was not significantly predictive for AF recurrence. These data shows that LA remodeling is a spatial process.

Therefore, LA volumes assessment may be a more discriminative parameter of remodeling to predict AF recurrence.

Interestingly, our study showed that LAmin was an independent predictors of AF recurrence after the BP, and that it was associated with a high sensitivity for predicting recurrence for the adjusted cut-off values (79.5%).

Limited data is available regarding the value of LA minimum volume and its prognostic value for different cardiovascular events. LAmin volume was associated with the occurrence of AF in an elderly cohort, as showed by Fatema et al. [17] and it was the most accurate parameter reflecting anatomical remodeling associated with paroxysmal AF in a recent study performed by Schaaf et al. [7]. In several studies, LA minimum volume was associated with diastolic dysfunction starting from incipient stages [18, 19]. However, we did not find a significant difference regarding the diastolic function between the groups with and without recurrence. These findings suggest that LA minimum volume represents a more subtle form of LA remodeling that could also trigger the occurrence of AF recurrence after ablation.

Whether LA minimum volume may have a better prognostic value in predicting late AF recurrences following cryoballoon ablation requires further investigations.

As suggested by Canpolat et al. [20], CBA may have a positive impact on LA reverse remodeling. Since the remodeling is a continuous process, measurements performed at a single moment may not reflect the truth and a temporal trend of the LA volumes should be assessed. However, data regarding LA reverse remodeling is limited and there are no clear definitions for it, therefore it should be evaluated in further studies.

Study limitations

This is a single center retrospective study, therefore results may not be generalized. Larger prospective clinical studies are warranted to confirm our findings. Moreover, the present study addressed the prognostic value of LA anatomy only in paroxysmal AF and cannot be extrapolated to a persistent AF population undergoing CBA.

Future perspectives

As mentioned earlier, it is widely accepted that anatomical remodeling is associated with recurrence of AF after ablation [4, 6, 9, 16, 21, 22]. 2D echocardiography can provide useful information for the detection of patients at risk to develop recurrences of AF, but LA volumes are still based on only two orthogonal planes and related to geometrical assumptions. Our results suggest that LA longitudinal remodeling could play an additional role in the prediction of AF recurrences, as the expansion of the LA can be asymmetrical. Therefore, advanced imaging techniques such as three – dimensional (3D) echocardiography can overcome these limitations and provide more accurate and reproducible LA measurements [23]. Moreover, several studies showed that LA strain could predict recurrence of AF after catheter ablation. Therefore, strain imaging may bring additional information regarding the more subtle structural and functional left atrium remodeling in such patients and could be used for the follow-up assessment of possible reverse atrial remodeling [24–26].

Conclusions

The results of our study showed that LA longitudinal remodeling, assessed by the increase of LA superior – inferior diameter plays an additional role in AF recurrence after CBA. Moreover, LA minimum volume was an independent predictors of AF recurrences after the BP, suggesting that less advanced forms of LA remodeling, not detected by the dilation of LAD can trigger AF recurrences. Further large – scale prospective randomized studies are needed to confirm our results.

Abbreviations

AADs: Antiarrhythmic drugs; AF: Atrial fibrillation; BP: Blanking period; CBA: Cryoballoon ablation; ECG: Electrocardiogram; ICC: Intraclass correlation coefficient; ILMC: Inner lumen mapping catheter; LA: Left atrium; LAD: Left atrium anterior - posterior diameter; LAmax: Left atrium maximum volume; LAmin: Left atrium minimum volume; LIPV: Left inferior pulmonary vein; LSPV: Left superior pulmonary vein; LV: Left ventricle; PNP: Phrenic nerve palsy; PV: Pulmonary vein; PVPs: Pulmonary vein potentials; RIPV: Right inferior pulmonary vein; ROC: Receiver - operator characteristic; RSPV: Right superior pulmonary vein; TTE: Transthoracic echocardiography

Funding

Andreea Motoc received a grant from Centrum Voor Hart - en Vaatziekten as fellow in cardiac imaging.
Juan - Pablo Abugattas received a grant from Centrum Voor Hart - en Vaatziekten as postgraduate fellow in cardiac electrophysiology and pacing.
Gian - Battista Chierchia received compensation for teaching purposes and proctoring from AF solutions, Medtronic.
Carlo de Asmundis received compensation for teaching purposes and proctoring from AF solutions, Medtronic and research grants on behalf of the Heart Rhythm Management center from Biotronik, Medtronic, St Jude Medical - Abbot, Livanova, Boston Scientific, Biosense Webster.

Authors' contributions

All authors contributed equally in analyzing and interpreting the patients' data and writing the manuscript. All authors read and approved the final manuscript.

Consent for publication

Not applicable.

Competing interests

The authors declare that they have no competing interests.

Author details

[1]Centrum Voor Hart-en Vaatziekten (CHVZ), Department of Cardiology, UZ Brussel, Laarbeeklaan 101, 1090 Brussels, Belgium. [2]Heart Rhythm Management Centre, UZ Brussel, Laarbeeklaan 101, 1090 Brussels, Belgium.

References

1. Kirchhof P, et al. 2016 ESC guidelines for the management of atrial fibrillation developed in collaboration with EACTS. Eur Heart J. 2016;37(38): 2893–962.
2. Chen C-F, Gao X-F, Duan X, Chen B, Liu X-H, Xu Y-Z. Comparison of catheter ablation for paroxysmal atrial fibrillation between cryoballoon and radiofrequency: a meta-analysis. J Interv Card Electrophysiol. 2017;48(3):351–66.
3. Garg J, et al. Cryoballon versus Radiofrequency Ablation for Atrial Fibrillation: A Meta-analysis of 16 Clinical Trials. J Atr Fibrillation. 2016;9(3): 1429.
4. Aytemir K, et al. Safety and efficacy outcomes in patients undergoing pulmonary vein isolation with second-generation cryoballoondagger. Eur Eur pacing, arrhythmias, Card Electrophysiol J Work groups Card pacing, arrhythmias, Card Cell Electrophysiol Eur Soc Cardiol. 2015;17(3):379–87.
5. Coutiño H-E, et al. Role of the burden of premature atrial contractions during the blanking period following second-generation cryoballoon ablation in predicting late recurrences of atrial arrhythmias. J Interv Card Electrophysiol. 2017;49(3):329–35.
6. Gerede DM, et al. Prediction of recurrence after cryoballoon ablation therapy in patients with paroxysmal atrial fibrillation. Anatol J Cardiol. 2015; 16(7):482–88.
7. Schaaf M, et al. Left atrial remodelling assessed by 2D and 3D echocardiography identifies paroxysmal atrial fibrillation. Eur Heart J Cardiovasc Imaging. 2017;18(1):46–53.
8. Badano LP, et al. How many patients would be misclassified using M-mode and two-dimensional estimates of left atrial size instead of left atrial volume? A three-dimensional echocardiographic study. J Cardiovasc Med (Hagerstown). 2008;9(5):476–84.
9. Nedios S, et al. Comparison of left atrial dimensions in CT and echocardiography as predictors of long-term success after catheter ablation of atrial fibrillation. J Interv Card Electrophysiol. 2015;43(3):237–44.
10. Lancellotti P, Zamorano JL, Habib G, Badano L. The EACVI Textbook of Echocardiography. Oxford: Oxford University Press; 2016.
11. Lang RM, et al. Recommendations for cardiac chamber quantification by echocardiography in adults: an update from the American Society of Echocardiography and the European Association of Cardiovascular Imaging. Eur Heart J Cardiovasc Imaging. 2015;16(3):233–70.
12. Nagueh SF, et al. Recommendations for the evaluation of left ventricular diastolic function by echocardiography: an update from the American Society of Echocardiography and the European Association of Cardiovascular Imaging. Eur Heart J Cardiovasc Imaging. 2016;17(12):1321–60.
13. De Regibus V, et al. Single freeze strategy with the second- generation cryballoon for atrial fibrillation: a multicenter international retrospective analysis in a large cohort of patients. J Interv Card Electrophysiol. 2017;49(2): 173–80.
14. Ciconte G, et al. Single 3-minute freeze for second-generation cryoballoon ablation: one-year follow-up after pulmonary vein isolation. Hear Rhythm. 2015;12(4):673–80.
15. Evranos B, et al. Predictors of atrial fibrillation recurrence after atrial fibrillation ablation with cryoballoon. Cardiol J. 2013;20(3):294–303.
16. Nedios S, et al. Characteristic changes of volume and three-dimensional structure of the left atrium in different forms of atrial fibrillation: predictive value after ablative treatment. J Interv Card Electrophysiol. 2011;32(2):87–94.
17. Fatema K, et al. Minimum vs. maximum left atrial volume for prediction of first atrial fibrillation or flutter in an elderly cohort: a prospective study. Eur J Echocardiogr. 2009;10(2):282–6.

Left atrium remodeling predicts late recurrence of paroxysmal atrial fibrillation after second generation cryoballoon...

241

18. Russo C, et al. Left atrial minimum volume and reservoir function as correlates of left ventricular diastolic function: impact of left ventricular systolic function. Heart. 2012;98(10):813–20.

19. Yamano M, et al. Impact of left ventricular diastolic property on left atrial function from simultaneous left atrial and ventricular three-dimensional echocardiographic volume measurement. Am J Cardiol. 2017;119(10):1687–93.

20. Canpolat U, Aytemir K, Ozer N, Oto A. The impact of cryoballoon-based catheter ablation on left atrial structural and potential electrical remodeling in patients with paroxysmal atrial fibrillation. J Interv Card Electrophysiol. 2015;44(2):131–9.

21. Evranos B, et al. Increased left atrial pressure predicts recurrence following successful cryoablation for atrial fibrillation with second-generation cryoballoon. J Interv Card Electrophysiol. 2016;46(2):145–51.

22. Neumann T, et al. Cryoballoon ablation of paroxysmal atrial fibrillation: 5-year outcome after single procedure and predictors of success. Eur Eur Pacing, Arrhythmias, Card Electrophysiol J Work Groups Card Pacing, Arrhythmias, Card Cell Electrophysiol Eur Soc Cardiol. 2013;15(8):1143–9.

23. Badano LP, et al. Left Atrial Volumes and Function by Three-Dimensional Echocardiography: Reference Values, Accuracy, Reproducibility, and Comparison With Two-Dimensional Echocardiographic Measurements. Circ. Cardiovasc. Imaging. 2016;9(7)

24. Cameli M, Mandoli GE, Loiacono F, Sparla S, Iardino E, Mondillo S. Left atrial strain: a useful index in atrial fibrillation. Int J Cardiol. 2016;220:208–13.

25. Yasuda R, et al. Left atrial strain is a powerful predictor of atrial fibrillation recurrence after catheter ablation: study of a heterogeneous population with sinus rhythm or atrial fibrillation. Eur Heart J Cardiovasc Imaging. 2015;16(9):1008–14.

26. Sarvari SI, et al. Strain echocardiographic assessment of left atrial function predicts recurrence of atrial fibrillation. Eur Heart J Cardiovasc Imaging. 2016;17(6):660–7.

27

Quantitative analysis of mitral valve morphology in atrial functional mitral regurgitation using real-time 3-dimensional echocardiography atrial functional mitral regurgitation

Tao Cong[1*†] (iD), Jinping Gu[2†], Alex Pui-Wai Lee[3], Zhijuan Shang[1], Yinghui Sun[1], Qiaobing Sun[1], Hong Wei[1], Na Chen[1], Siyao Sun[1] and Tingting Fu[1]

Abstract

Background: Atrial fibrillation (AF) can result in atrial functional mitral regurgitation (MR), but the mechanism remains controversial. Few data about the relationship between the 3-dimensional morphology of the MV and the degree of MR in AF exist.

Methods: Real-time 3-dimensional transesophageal echocardiography (3D-TEE) of the MV was acquired in 168 patients with AF (57.7% persistent AF), including 25 (14.9%) patients with moderate to severe MR (the MR+ group) and 25 patients without AF as controls. The 3-dimensional geometry of the MV apparatus was acquired using dedicated quantification software.

Results: Compared with the group of patients with no or mild MR (the MR- group) and the controls, the MR+ group had a larger left atrium (LA), a more dilated mitral annulus (MA), a reduced annular height to commissural width ratio (AHCWR), indicating flattening of the annular saddle shape, and greater leaflet surfaces and tethering. MR severity was correlated with the MA area ($r^2 = 0.43$, $P < 0.01$) and the annulus circumference ($r^2 = 0.38$, P < 0.01). A logistic regression analysis indicated that the MA area (OR: 1.02, 95% CI: 1.01–1.03, P < 0.01), AHCWR (OR: 0.24, 95% CI: 0.14–0.35, $P = 0.04$) and MV tenting volume (OR: 3.24, 95% CI: 1.16–9.08, $P = 0.03$) were independent predictors of MR severity in AF patients.

Conclusions: The mechanisms of "atrial functional MR" are complex and include dilation of the MA, flattening of the annular saddle shape and greater leaflet tethering.

Keywords: Atrial fibrillation, Mitral regurgitation, Three-dimensional transesophageal echocardiography

Background

The MV apparatus consists of several components: the LA, MA, mitral leaflets, chordae tendineae, papillary muscles, and left ventricle (LV). Dysfunction of any one of these components can lead to MR. MR can be classified according to the presence of mitral leaflet disease (organic MR) or only secondary involvement of the leaflets (functional MR) [1] and can also be categorized according to Carpentier's classification as normal (Type I), excessive (Type II), or restrictive (Type III) according to the motion of the MV [2]. Among these types of MR, normal leaflet motion MR is less common than the other types and almost exclusively results from organic leaflet disease [1]. However, AF may lead to Type I MR, even though the mechanism remains controversial. Most reports have suggested that AF causes functional Type I MR through atrial remodeling that leads to MA dilation [3–5]. However, it cannot be determined at present whether combinations of other structural MV abnormalities

* Correspondence: congtao1975@163.com
†Tao Cong and Jinping Gu contributed equally to this work.
[1]Department of Cardiology, The First Affiliated Hospital of Dalian Medical University, Dalian 116000, Liaoning, China
Full list of author information is available at the end of the article

occur in AF patients with MR (e.g., changes in MA geometry or the size of the MV leaflets). An understanding of these mechanisms may provide more detailed information for surgeons for planning the surgical treatment of AF in patients with severe MR [6].

With the development of 3D-TEE, high-resolution imaging and quantification of the morphology of the entire mitral apparatus have become feasible [7–10]. 3D-TEE studies of MV geometry have led to a new understanding of the pathogenesis of functional MR. [11, 12] Few data exist on the relationship between the 3D morphology of the MV and the degree of MR in AF, which is a common cause of functional MR. [3, 13] Therefore, we undertook a 3D-TEE study in patients with AF to investigate the relationship between 3D MV morphology and clinically moderate to severe MR.

Methods

Patient selection

We retrospectively screened 321 patients with AF out of 472 patients who underwent transthoracic echocardiography (TTE) and 3D-TEE on the same day due to clinical indications between June 2014 and May 2016 (Fig. 1). The study population consisted of consecutive patients with symptom improvement or drug-refractory AF, including

persistent or paroxysmal AF,they all fit the indications of ablation according to the guideline [14].We performed 3D-TEE to exclude left atrial thrombi and collected images of MR and 3D images of the MV. AF patients were excluded from the study if they had organic heart disease (including rheumatic heart disease, coronary heart disease, congenital heart disease, MV prolapse, moderate to severe MA or MV calcification according to the echocardiographic calcification score [15] or MV surgery, etc.), Patients with a left ventricular ejection fraction (LVEF) < 50% were excluded to avoid including patients whose MR might be due to ventricular dysfunction. AF was classified according to the clinical characteristics into two types: paroxysmal AF (self-terminating, lasting for < 7 days) and persistent AF (lasting ≥7 days or terminated by intervention). We enrolled sex-, age-, and body surface area-matched patients with no AF and MR from the remaining cohort.

Echocardiography

At first, using TTE, we obtained routine parameters, including left ventricular end diastolic diameter (LVEDD), left ventricular end systolic diameter (LVESD) and left atrial anterior posterior diameter (LAAPD), using an iE Elite system (Philips Healthcare, Andover, MA, USA). The LV volume and LVEF were calculated using a modified version of

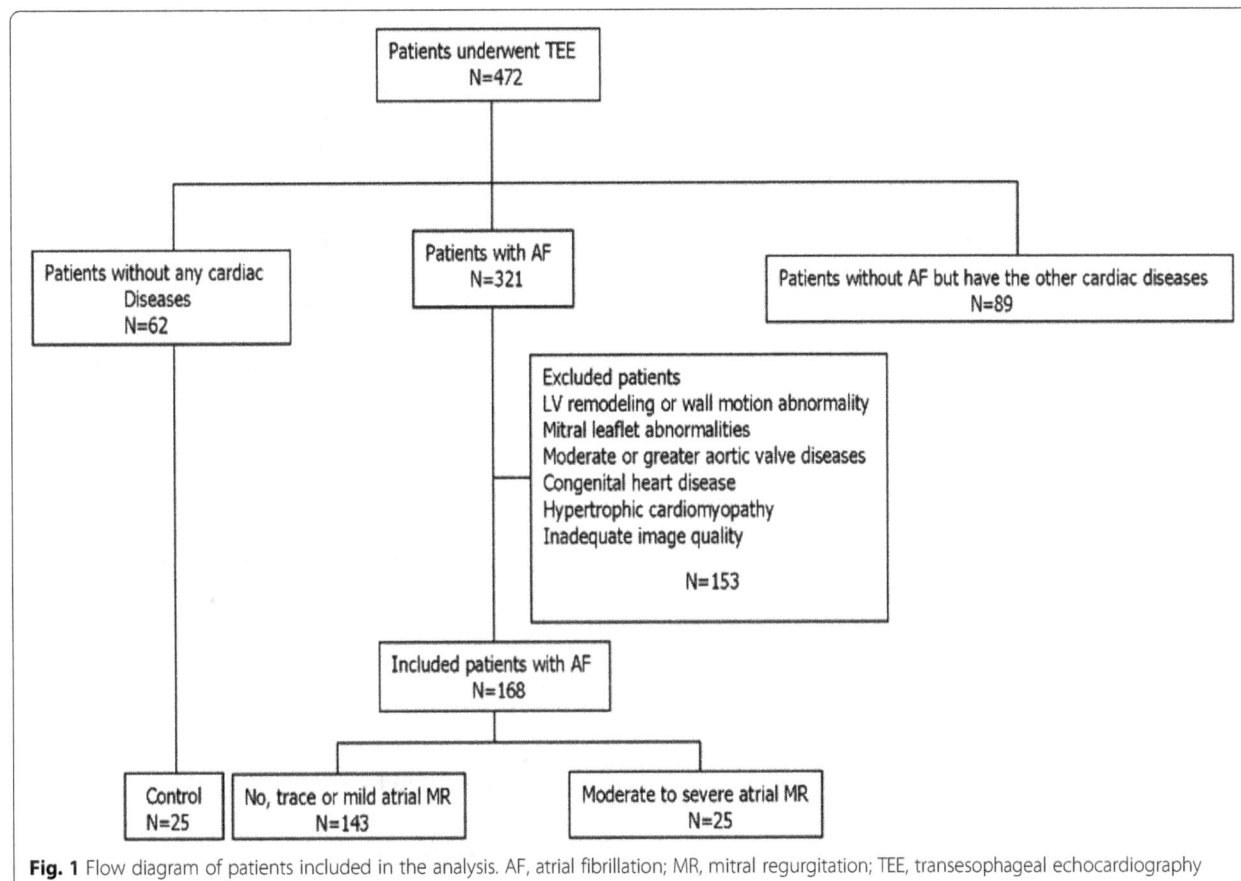

Fig. 1 Flow diagram of patients included in the analysis. AF, atrial fibrillation; MR, mitral regurgitation; TEE, transesophageal echocardiography

Simpson's method. LA volume was defined as the largest LA volume just before the MV opening and was measured from an apical view using the biplane method of discs. Diastolic function was described with in terms of the E/E' ratio, where E was measured using pulsed Doppler of the mitral inflow from the four-chamber view, and E' was the average of the septal and lateral MA diastolic velocities using tissue Doppler imaging. For the patients with AF, the above data were measured during an index beat, which was the beat after the nearly equal preceding and prepreceding intervals [16]. 3D-TEE of the MV was performed using a fully sampled matrix transducer (X7-2 t). Zoomed 3D images of the mitral apparatus, including the annulus, leaflets, and aortic valve were acquired. The region of interest was adjusted to the smallest volume to obtain higher frame rates (> 8). For patients with sinus rhythm, the 3D images were recorded with multiple cardiac beats (2–4 beats), and for patients with AF, 3D data were acquired from the index beat, as described above. The images were acquired carefully to ensure optimal image quality without stitching artifacts. Under the color Doppler model, the maximum regurgitation jet area (RJA) and the effective regurgitation orifice (ERO) were obtained, and the ERO was used to assess the severity of MR [17, 18]. The MR color jet area was measured based on mosaic signals in the apical 4-chamber, apical 2-chamber, and apical long-axis views, and the color Doppler scale and Nyquist limit were set to 50–70 cm/s. The ERO of the MR was quantified using the proximal isovelocity surface area method [19]. Moderate to severe MR was defined by the presence of following criteria: ERO ≥ 0.3 cm^2 (MR+). Mild MR was defined by the presence of the following criteria: ERO < 0.3 cm^2 (MR-). In addition, supportive parameters, including RJA, continuous wave Doppler jet configuration, pulsed wave Doppler transmitral flow, and pulmonary venous flow were examined in an integrative approach for evaluating MR severity, as previously recommended [19]. In addition, the patients with no or trace MR for whom the ERO could not be obtained were also included in the MR- group.

Quantitative assessment of the mitral apparatus

Images were analyzed offline by an investigator. The quantitative morphological analysis of the mitral valve was performed using dedicated software (QLAB MVQ, Philips 9.1 version) [20]. The images were presented in 4 quadrants, including 3 orthogonal planes, each representing an anatomic plane derived from the 3D data, and a volume-rendered view. The end-systolic frame, immediately before aortic valve closure, was tagged in the cine-loop sequence. The image was oriented by adjusting the rotation of the image data in the orthogonal planes thus ensuring that the mitral valve was bisected by the 2 long-axis planes and that the short-axis plane was parallel to the plane of

the valve. Initially, the 4 major annulus reference points were tagged in the appropriate planes. The annulus shape was then manually outlined by defining intermediate reference points in 18 radial planes (i.e., 36 reference points) that were rotated around the long axis. The mitral valve was then segmented to map the leaflet contour and coaptation by manually tracing the leaflets in multiple parallel long-axis planes spanning the valve from commissure to commissure (6 trace points per centimeter). Finally, the reconstructed mitral valve apparatus was displayed, and the parameters were automatically generated. Parameters describing the annular geometry included anteroposterior diameter (APD), commissural width (the distance between the posteromedial and anterolateral horns of the annulus, CW), height (the maximal vertical distance between the highest and lowest annular points AH), projected area (AA) and circumference (AC). The ratio of annular height-to-commissural width (AHCWR) was computed as an indicator of annular saddle-shaped nonplanarity. We studied the 3D leaflet surface topography by assessing the leaflet area [including anterior leaflet (AL) and posterior leaflet (PL) area]and tenting volume (Fig. 2).

Statistical analysis

Continuous variables are expressed as the mean ± SD, and categorical variables are expressed as absolute values and percentages. Normal distribution of the continuous parameters was verified using the Kolmogorov–Smirnov test and compared using one-way analysis of variance (ANOVA) with post-test Bonferroni correction. Categorical variables were compared using the Chi-squared test or Fisher's exact test where indicated. All tests were two-sided, and statistical significance was defined as $P < 0.05$. Correlations between continuous variables were explored using Pearson analysis. Variables with a P-value less than 0.1 between patients of the MR+ and MR- groups were included in a multivariable logistic regression analysis using stepwise forward elimination to identify factors with independent associations with the severity of MR (duration of AF, LA volume, E/E', annulus area, annulus circumference, annulus CW, AHCWR, AL surface area, PL surface area and leaflet tenting volume). To evaluate the reliability of 3D echocardiographic results, intra-observer and inter-observer variability was assessed. 15 subjects were randomly chosen for that analysis, The intraclass correlation coefficient (ICC) was calculated.

Results

Study population and baseline characteristics

Complete datasets were available for 168 patients with AF (paroxysmal AF: 95, 56.5%). We divided the patients into 2 groups according to the severity of MR (MR+ and

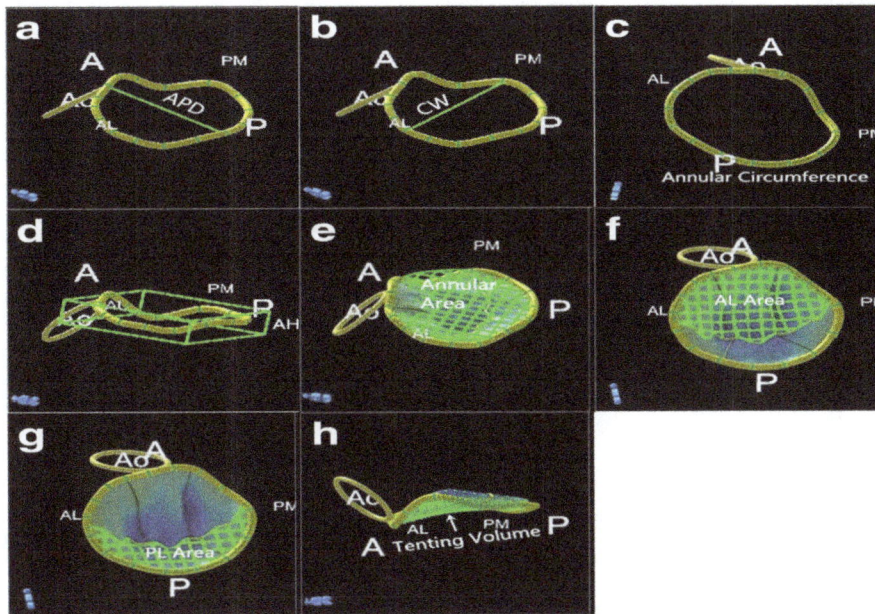

Fig. 2 Parameters of 3-dimensional geometry of the mitral valve. A, Anteroposterior diameter (APD). B, Commissural width (CW). C, Annular circumference. D, Annular height (AH). E, Annular area on the projection plane. F and G, Areas of the exposed anterior leaflet (AL) and posterior leaflet (PL) surfaces. H, Leaflet tenting volume

MR- groups). Twenty-five patients with moderate to severe MR according to the standard were included in the MR+ group, while other patients with no, trace or mild regurgitation were included in the MR- group. Twenty-five patients with no AF and MR were included in the controls. The clinical characteristics of the three groups are listed in Table 1. Patients in the MR+ group, when compared to those in the MR- group, had a longer duration of AF (4.9 ± 0.5 VS 4.3 ± 1.0 years, $P < 0.01$), and there was no significant difference in the types of AF between the two groups (paroxysmal AF: 12 [48.8%] vs. 83 [58.2%], $P = 0.12$).

TTE findings

The TTE measurements are shown in Table 2. As expected by design, in the MR+ group, patients had increased LA volume compared with patients in the MR- group and controls (MR+ 98 ± 22 ml vs. MR- 81 ± 18 ml, $P < 0.01$; both $P < 0.01$ vs. controls 57 ± 5 ml). The E/E′ ratio was significantly elevated in the MR+ group, whereas it

Table 1 Baseline characteristics

variable	Control (n = 25)	Patients with AF (n = 168)		p
		MR- Group (143)	MR+ Group (n = 25)	
Age, years	66 ± 7	62 ± 6	66 ± 7	0.20
Women, n (%)	12(48.9)	68(47.8)	11(46.9)	0.96
Body surface area, m^2	1.88 ± 0.16	1.92 ± 0.18	1.87 ± 0.15	0.22
Paroxysmal AF, n (%)		83(58.2%)	12(48.8%)	0.12
Duration of AF, years		4.3 ± 1.0	4.9 ± 0.5[#]	<0.01
History of Hypertension, n (%)	14 (56%)	90 (58%)	16 (64%)	0.55
History of Diabetes Mellitus, n (%)	5 (20%)	32 (21%)	4 (16%)	0.6
Status during echocardiography				
Sinus rhythm, n (%)	25(100%)	36(25.1%)*	8(30.4%)*	<0.01
Heart rate, (beats/min)	84 ± 17	89 ± 16	92 ± 12	0.46
Systolic blood pressure, mmHg	128 ± 13	134 ± 12	132 ± 16	0.86
Diastolic blood pressure, mmHg	68 ± 9	77 ± 10	73 ± 8	0.59

*$P < 0.01$ vs. controls, #$P < 0.01$ vs. MR-Group

Table 2 Measurements on Transthoracic Echocardiography

variable	Control (n = 25)	Patients with AF (n = 168)		P
		MR- Group (143)	MR+ Group (n = 25)	
LV end-diastolic diameter, mm	44 ± 2	46 ± 4	46 ± 3	0.17
LV end-systolic diameter, mm	30 ± 2	30 ± 3	31 ± 3	0.31
LV end-diastolic volume, ml	85 ± 8	87 ± 11	89 ± 12	0.20
LV end-systolic volume, ml	30 ± 4	32 ± 5	31 ± 5	0.30
LV ejection fraction, %	64 ± 5	64 ± 4	64 ± 2	0.66
LA anterior-posterior Diameter, mm	34 ± 2	39 ± 5*	41 ± 4*	<0.01
LA volume, ml	57 ± 5	81 ± 18*	98 ± 22*,#	<0.01
E/E'	8.0 ± 0.9	8.2 ± 0.8	9.2 ± 1.2*#	<0.01
Mitral regurgitation severity				
Regurgitation area, cm^2		1.84 ± 0.52	4.37 ± 0.68#	<0.01
EROA, cm^2		0.18 ± 0.07	0.47 ± 0.07#	<0.01

LV left ventricle, LA left atrium, EROA effective regurgitant orifice area. *P <0.01 vs. controls, #P<0.01 vs. MR-Group

was comparable in the MR- group and controls (MR+ 9.2 ± 1.2 vs. MR- 8.2 ± 0.8, P < 0.01; MR+ vs. controls 8.0 ± 0.9, P < 0.01). The ERO of the MR+ group was also larger than that of the MR- group (0.47 ± 0.07 cm^2 vs. 0.18 ± 0.07 cm^2, P < 0.01).

3D mitral valve geometry
Annulus
Compared with those in the MR- group and controls, patients in the MR+ group had A dilated MA with a significantly increased annulus area, circumference and commissural width. Commonly, the mitral annulus adopts a non-planar saddle shape [21–23] with elevation of the anterior and posterior annular segments, and the low points of the saddle are close to the lateral and medial commissures. In this study, the average AHCWR value of

patients in the MR+ group was significantly lower than that of patients in the MR- group and controls (MR+ 15 ± 5% vs. MR- 17 ± 4%, P < 0.05; both P < 0.05 vs. controls 19.4 ± 4.3%), indicating the progressive flattening of the mitral annulus (Table 3) in patients with AF with moderate to severe MR.

Leaflet
Compared with those in the MR- group and controls, the leaflet surface area (anterior: MR+ 6.81 ± 1.91 cm^2 vs. MR- 5.34 ± 1.81 cm^2 P < 0.01, MR+ vs. controls 5.38 ± 0.99 cm^2, P < 0.01; posterior: MR+ 6.14 ± 1.30 cm^2 vs. MR- 5.41 ± 1.49 cm^2, P = 0.02) and tenting volume of the mitral valve (MR+ 2.67 ± 1.07 ml vs. MR- 1.72 ± 0.89 ml, P < 0.01, MR+ vs. controls 1.72 ± 0.73 ml, P < 0.01) were significantly higher in patients in the MR+ group (Fig. 3).

Table 3 Three-Dimensional Mitral Valve Geometry

variable	Control (n = 25)	Patients with AF (n = 168)		P
		MR- Group (143)	MR+ Group (n = 25)	
Annulus				
Area cm^2	8.86 ± 1.03	9.53 ± 1.42*	12.66 ± 0.85*#	<0.01
Circumference mm	108 ± 9	115 ± 8*	134 ± 13*#	<0.01
Anteroposterior diameter mm	30.6 ± 2.4	32.0 ± 20.4	32.9 ± 20.4	0.90
Commissural width mm	36.3 ± 2.3	38.3 ± 3.0*	41.0 ± 3.8*#	<0.01
High mm	7.6 ± 2.0	6.3 ± 1.5*	6.2 ± 2.2*	<0.01
AHCWR %	19.4 ± 4.3	17.3 ± 4.4†	15.2 ± 5.1*‡	<0.01
Leaflet				
Anterior leaflet surface area cm^2	5.38 ± 0.99	5.34 ± 1.81	6.81 ± 1.91*#	<0.01
Posterior leaflet surface area cm^2	5.96 ± 1.37	5.41 ± 1.49	6.14 ± 1.30‡	0.03
MV tenting volume ml	1.72 ± 0.73	1.72 ± 0.89	2.67 ± 1.07*#	<0.01

AHCWR annular height-to-commissural width ratio, MV mitral valve
†P <0.05 vs. controls, ‡P <0.05 vs. MR-Group. *P <0.01 vs. controls, #P <0.01 vs. MR-Group

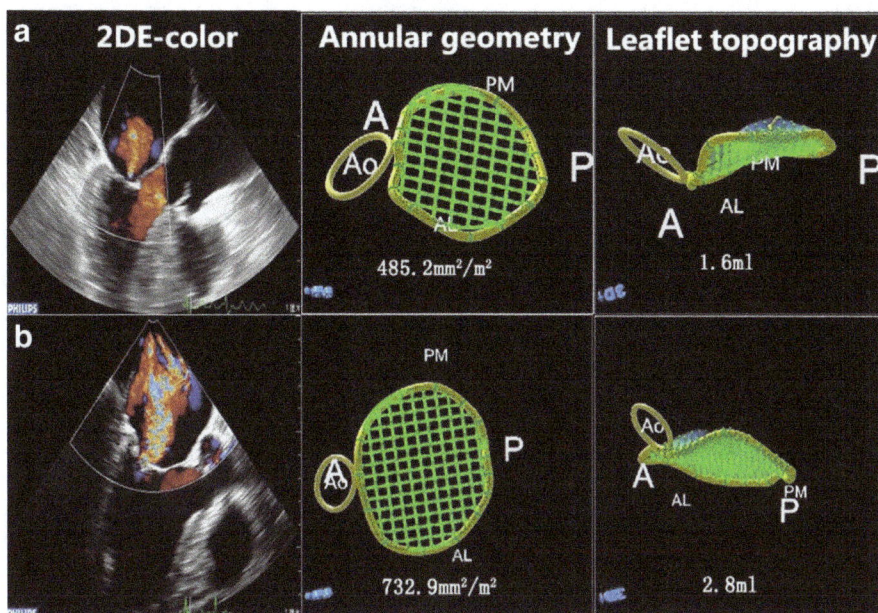

Fig. 3 Differences in the MV morphology between mild and severe atrial functional MR in patients with AF. A, Example of mild atrial MR with the annular area and leaflet tenting volume. B, Example of severe atrial functional MR with enlargement of the annular area and leaflet tenting volume

3D mitral valve morphology is associated with MR severity

Structural deformation of the mitral valve increased with increasing MR severity in patients with AF. Larger EROs were found to be associated with greater annular area ($r^2 = 0.48$, $P < 0.01$; Fig. 4) and annular circumference ($r^2 = 0.38$, $P < 0.01$; Fig. 5).

To identify independent factors associated with MR severity in patients with AF, stepwise logistic regression analysis was performed; variables found to be significant or of borderline significance by univariate analysis ($P \leq 0.10$), including duration of AF, LA volume, E/E', AA, AC, annulus CW, AHCWR, AL surface area, PL surface area and leaflet tenting volume, were included in the equation. The AA (OR: 1.02, 95% CI: 1.01–1.03, $P < 0.01$), AHCWR (OR: 0.24, 95% CI: 0.14–0.35, $P = 0.04$) and MV tenting volume (OR: 3.24, 95% CI: 1.16–9.08, $P = 0.03$) were found to be independent risk factors affecting the severity of MR.

Reproducibility of the MV parameters

Intraobserver ICC for AA, AC, APD, CW and AH were 0.91 (95% CI, 69–98%), 0.84 (95% CI, 46–96%), 0.88 (95% CI, 58–97%), 0.86 (95% CI, 55–96%), 0.97 (95% CI, 86–99%), Intraobserver ICC for AL surface area, PL

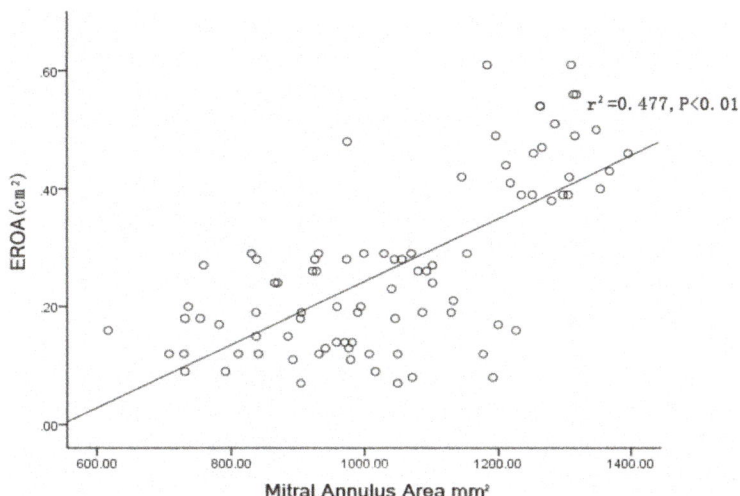

Fig. 4 Correlation of the effective regurgitation orifice area (EROA) with the mitral annulus area

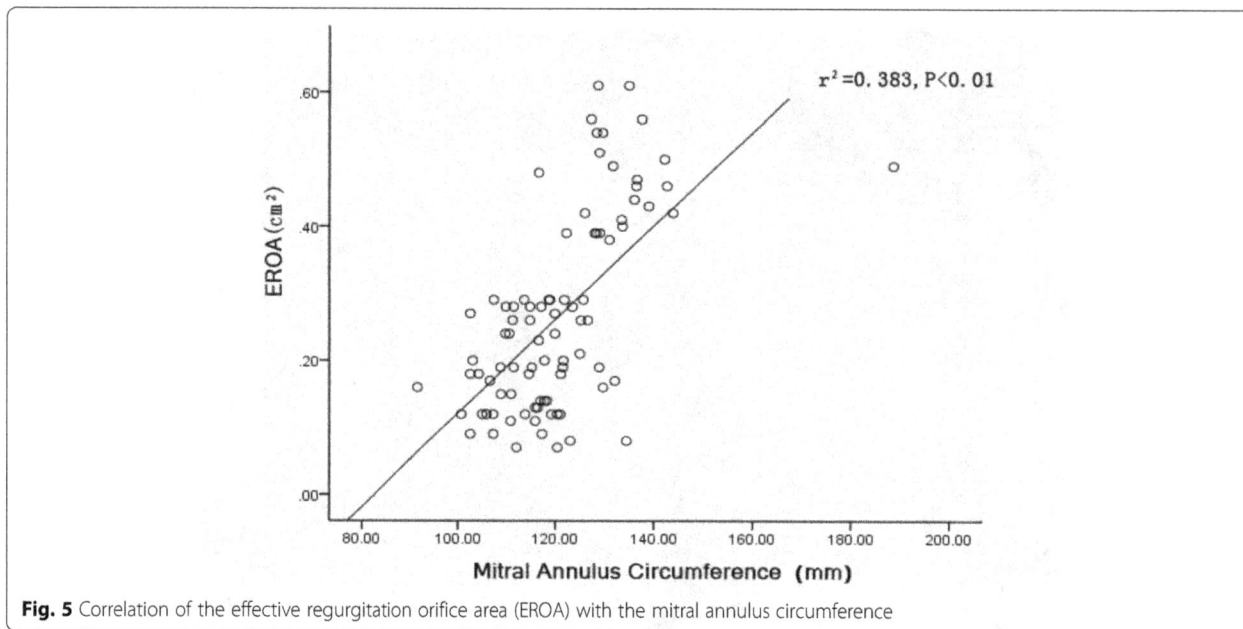

Fig. 5 Correlation of the effective regurgitation orifice area (EROA) with the mitral annulus circumference

surface area and MV tenting volume were 0.95 (95% CI, 81–99%), 0.87 (95% CI, 57–97%), 0.91 (95% CI, 70–98%). Interobserver ICC for AA, AC, APD, CW and AH were 0.79 (95% CI, 34–94%), 0.90 (95% CI, 64–98%), 0.92 (95% CI, 71–98%), 0.86 (95% CI, 54–96%), 0.87 (95% CI, 57–97%), Interobserver ICC for AL surface area, PL surface area and MV tenting volume were 0.81 (95% CI, 18–95%), 0.95 (95% CI, 81–99%), 0.92 (95% CI, 74–98%).

Discussion

The results of our study indicated the following: (1) long-lasting AF including paroxysmal AF causes atrial functional MR; (2) atrial functional MR has multiple deterioration factors, including LA enlargement, morphological changes of the mitral apparatus, and MA dilatation; and (3) flattening of the annular saddle shape and leaflet tethering are independent factors for determining the severity of atrial functional MR.

In our study, 15.0% of AF patients exhibited moderate or severe MR. These results are in accordance with previous studies [3, 4, 10]. Gertz et al. reported severe MR in 6.5% of AF patients, and MR was alleviated in patients with sinus rhythm after cardioversion [3]. Another study indicated that the incidence of moderate and severe MR were higher in AF patients (66% vs 6%) [13]. However, the findings from other studies were not consistent with these results; Otsuji or Zhou et al. [24, 25] thought that isolated AF may not lead to severe MR. Combining our findings with those of previous studies, we propose that AF may be a cause of moderate to significant MR rather than simply a concurrent finding. As noted by Gertz et al., this can be called atrial functional MR.

Pathophysiology of atrial functional MR

Using 3D-TEE, we were able to evaluate the possible pathophysiological mechanism underlying atrial functional MR. Previous studies have indicated that the mechanism of MR include LA enlargement and MA dilatation. In recent years, some scholars have studied the mechanism of atrial functional MR using 3D-TEE [12, 26, 27]; in addition to the changes described above, they also found geometric changes of the MA and the insufficient leaflet remodeling to annular dilatation. However, the subjects of the studies were patients with persistent AF, and few researchers have focused on mitral leaflet adaptations in patients with moderate to significant atrial functional MR. In our study, both paroxysmal AF and persistent AF were included to investigate whether or not paroxysmal AF could also result in atrial functional MR. In addition, although 3D-TEE was used to analyze changes in the size and MA geometrical morphology in AF patients with moderate to severe MR, we also attempted to determine the role of mitral leaflet adaptation changes in the genesis of MR.

In our study, there was no significant difference in the incidence of paroxysmal AF between the two studied groups, but the duration of AF was longer in MR+ group. Patients in the MR+ group had a larger LA, MA circumference and projection area, in addition to the observed changes in 3D MA geometry. The surrogate of annular saddle-shaped non-planarity, AHCWR, was reduced, representing a progressive flattening of the mitral annulus. This result was confirmed by another study [26], in which the author appraised the morphology and function of the MV in patients with atrial functional MR and found that the MA area, MA area fraction, nonplanarity angle, and posterior mitral leaflet angle were independent determinants of the EROA of MR. It has been postulated that the saddle shape of the annulus in systole may provide a configuration that is more capable of withstanding the stresses imposed by left ventricular pressure [11, 19], and Salgo et al. [28] demonstrated that optimal leaflet stress reductions occur with AHCWR values in the range of 15 to 20%; however, when AHCWR falls to 15%, the MA becomes more flattened, and leaflet stress increases markedly. In our study, AHCWR was found to be an independent factor leading to moderate or severe MR. Therefore, we suggest that in addition to MA dilation, flattening of the mitral annulus is also involved in the mechanism of atrial functional MR.

Interestingly, we also found that the surface area of both mitral leaflets and valvular tenting volume were significantly greater in the MR+ group. This is the phenomenon of "valvular deformation". The first sign is enlargement of the MV area, which can be considered mitral adaptation, and has been observed in patients with LV remodeling and MA dilatation in ischemic or dilated cardiomyopathy [11]. Our results showed that the MV may have the capacity to adapt by enlargement to some extent in response to mechanical stretching from MA dilatation caused by LA remodeling. However, if the extent of MA dilation is beyond the limits of leaflet adaptation, then leaflet coaptation will be insufficient, and atrial functional MR may occur. The second sign is MV tenting, which is often present in left ventricular dysfunction [29]. In our study, the MV tenting volume was found to be an independent factor affecting MR severity, consistent with the findings of Yiu et al. [30] that the major determinant of the ERO in functional MR was mitral deformation (i.e., systolic valvular tenting, which was measured as the valvular tenting area using 2D echocardiography); the subjects in their study were patients with left ventricular dysfunction, which was different from our study. In our study, although the systolic function of the LV was normal, dilation of the MA also resulted in an increase in the distance between the papillary muscle (PM) heads and the MA. We observed an increase in valvular tenting volume using 3D echocardiography, which illustrates the above mentioned changes. Subsequent tethering restricts systolic closure motion of the MV leaflets [31]. Tenting is characterized by insufficient systolic leaflet body displacement towards the annulus, with coaptation limited to the leaflet tips [32], resulting in functional MR.

In the present study, the E/E' ratio was higher in the MR+ group indicating that the LA pressure was increased in patients with moderate or severe functional MR, and this may be one of the important mechanisms leading to functional MR. As with another study, the author described that elevated LA pressure was a key determinant of functional MR in both patients with preserved and reduced LVEF [33]. However, in patients with MR, the E/E' ratio is generally increased due to increased flow across the regurgitant valve. It has been reported that LV filling pressures were not predictable by the E/E' ratio in subjects with MR and preserved LV function [34]. Therefore, further studies are needed to confirm the value of the E/E' ratio in patients with functional mitral regulation.

Clinical significance

Epidemiological data show that the incidence of AF gradually increases with advancing age [35], and Gertz et al. found a 6.4% incidence rate of functional MR in patients initially presenting with AF [3]. Therefore, the prevalence of atrial functional MV will increase progressively. It is generally believed that MR instigates atrial and annular remodeling in a vicious cycle and that the latter will lead to worsening MR and eventual heart failure with disease progression [1]. Therefore, atrial functional MR will become increasingly important in the future. Our findings have important implications for understanding the mechanism of atrial functional MR and the options for treatment. The main causes of atrial functional MR are the remodeling of the left atrium and the MA. The primary purpose of treatment is to reverse the remodeling of the left atrium and the MA in order to maintain sinus rhythm. Experiments have demonstrated the effectiveness of this treatment [3]. Furthermore, because the MV tenting volume independently aggravated the atrial functional MR, repair strategies should aim to restore effective leaflet coaptation by reducing the MA area and leaflet tethering at the PM, such as by simultaneous annuloplasty and chordal cutting. Several smaller studies have shown that this treatment can improve the prognosis of patients [36, 37]. On the other hand, apically directed leaflet tethering is the predominant mechanism of MR, and the risk of recurrence of MR after undersized annuloplasty is increased [38].

Study limitations

This was a cross-sectional study; therefore, our study suffered from the typical limitations of a cross-sectional analysis. The number of patients in the study was limited; therefore, our study should be considered a hypothesis-generating study. Our study included patients with paroxysmal and persistent AF, and although our results failed to show the different effects of the two types of fibrillation on MR, in theory, the effect of persistent AF on the atrium and mitral annulus was greater and was also confirmed by the experiment [3]. The reason for this result may be the limited numbers of patients included in our study. Due to the older version of the analysis software used, we failed to analyze the dynamic changes in the MA.

Conclusions

Our findings suggest that some patients with AF will develop moderate to severe MR (atrial functional MR). The mechanism of atrial functional MR involves multiple factors; in particular, MA dilatation, flattening of the annular saddle shape and leaflet tethering are the most influential factors affecting deterioration.

Abbreviations
3D-TEE: 3 dimensional transesophageal echocardiography; AF: Atrial fibrillation; AH: Annular height; AHCWR: Annular height to commissural width ratio; ANOVA: Analysis of variance; APD: Anteroposterior diameter; CW: Commissural width; ERO: Effective regurgitation orifice; EROA: Effective regurgitation orifice area; LA: Left atrium; LAAPD: Left atrial anterior posterior diameter; LV: Left ventricle; LVEDD: Left ventricular end diastolic diameter; LVEF: Left ventricular ejection fraction; LVESD: Left ventricular end systolic diameter; MA: Mitral annulus; MR: Mitral regurgitation; MV: Mitral valve; PM: Papillary muscle; RJA: Regurgitation jet area; TTE: Transthoracic echocardiography

Authors' contributions
TC, JG and AP-WL analyzed the patients' data. TC and JG were major contributors in writing the manuscript. ZS, YS, HW, QS, NC, SS and TF performed the echo cardiography examination. All authors read and approved the final manuscript.

Consent for publication
All of the authors agree to submit this paper for publication.

Competing interests
The authors declare that they have no competing interest.

Author details
[1]Department of Cardiology, The First Affiliated Hospital of Dalian Medical University, Dalian 116000, Liaoning, China. [2]Department of Intensive Care Unit, The Second Affiliated Hospital of Dalian Medical University, Liaoning, China. [3]Division of Cardiology, Department of Medicine and Therapeutics, The Prince of Wales Hospital of Chinese University of Hong Kong, Hong Kong, China.

References
1. Enriquez-Sarano M, Akins CW, Vahanian A. Mitral regurgitation. Lancet. 2009;373:1382–94.
2. Carpentier A, Chauvaud S, Fabiani JN, Deloche A, Relland J, Lessana A, D'Allaines C, Blondeau P, Piwnica A, Dubost C. Reconstructive surgery of mitral valve incompetence: ten-year appraisal. J Thorac Cardiovasc Surg. 1980;79:338–48.
3. Gertz ZM, Raina A, Saghy L, Zado ES, Callans DJ, Marchlinski FE, Keane MG, Silvestry FE. Evidence of atrial functional mitral regurgitation due to atrial fibrillation: reversal with arrhythmia control. J Am Coll Cardiol. 2011;58:1474–81.
4. Tanimoto M, Pai RG. Effect of isolated left atrial enlargement on mitral annular size and valve competence. Am J Cardiol. 1996;77:769–74.
5. Kihara T, Gillinov AM, Takasaki K, Fukuda S, Song JM, Shiota M, Shiota T. Mitral regurgitation associated with mitral annular dilation in patients with lone atrial fibrillation: an echocardiographic study. Echocardiography. 2009;26:885–9.
6. Vohra HA, Whistance RN, Magan A, et al. Mitral valve repair for severe mitral regurgitation secondary to lone atrial fibrillation. European journal of cardio-thoracic surgery : official journal of the European Association for Cardio-thoracic Surgery. 2012;42:634–7.
7. Vohra HA, Whistance RN, Magan A, Sadeque SA, Livesey SA. Live 3-dimensional transesophageal echocardiography initial experience using the fully-sampled matrix array probe. J Am Coll Cardiol. 2008;52:446–9.
8. Maffessanti F, Marsan NA, Tamborini G, Sugeng L, Caiani EG, Gripari P, Alamanni F, Jeevanandam V, Lang RM, Pepi M. Quantitative analysis of mitral valve apparatus in mitral valve prolapse before and after annuloplasty: a three-dimensional intraoperative transesophageal study. Journal of the American Society of Echocardiography : official publication of the American Society of Echocardiography. 2011;24:405–13.
9. Chandra S, Salgo IS, Sugeng L, Weinert L, Tsang W, Takeuchi M, Spencer KT, O'Connor A, Cardinale M, Settlemier S, Mor-Avi V, Lang RM. Characterization of degenerative mitral valve disease using morphologic analysis of real-time three-dimensional echocardiographic images: objective insight into complexity and planning of mitral valve repair. Circulation Cardiovascular imaging. 2011;4:24–32.
10. Lee AP, Hsiung MC, Salgo IS, Fang F, Xie JM, Zhang YC, Lin QS, Looi JL, Wan S, Wong RH, Underwood MJ, Sun JP, Yin WH, Wei J, Tsai SK, Yu CM. Quantitative analysis of mitral valve morphology in mitral valve prolapse with real-time 3-dimensional echocardiography: importance of annular saddle shape in the pathogenesis of mitral regurgitation. Circulation. 2013;127:832–41.
11. Chaput M, Handschumacher MD, Tournoux F, Hua L, Guerrero JL, Vlahakes GJ, Levine RA. Mitral leaflet adaptation to ventricular remodeling: occurrence and adequacy in patients with functional mitral regurgitation. Circulation. 2008;118:845–52.
12. Ring L, Dutka DP, Wells FC, Fynn SP, Shapiro LM, Rana BS. Mechanisms of atrial mitral regurgitation: insights using 3d transoesophageal echo. Eur Heart J Cardiovasc Imaging. 2014;15:500–8.
13. Sharma S, Lardizabal J, Monterroso M, Bhambi N, Sharma R, Sandhu R, Singh S. Clinically unrecognized mitral regurgitation is prevalent in lone atrial fibrillation. World J Cardiol. 2012;4:183–7.
14. January CT, Wann LS, Alpert JS, Calkins H, Cigarroa JE, Cleveland JC Jr, Conti JB, Ellinor PT, Ezekowitz MD, Field ME, Murray KT, Sacco RL, Stevenson WG, Tchou PJ, Tracy CM, Yancy CW. 2014 AHA/ACC/HRS guideline for the management of patients with atrial fibrillation: a report of the American College of Cardiology/American Heart Association Task Force on Practice Guidelines and the Heart Rhythm Society. J Am Coll Cardiol. 2014;64:e1–e76.
15. Movva R, Murthy K, Romero-Corral A, Seetha Rammohan HR, Fumo P, Pressman GS. Calcification of the mitral valve and annulus: systematic evaluation of effects on valve anatomy and function. Journal of the American Society of Echocardiography : official publication of the American Society of Echocardiography. 2013;26:1135–42.
16. Tabata T, Grimm RA, Greenberg NL, Agler DA, Mowrey KA, Wallick DW, Zhang Y, Zhuang S, Mazgalev TN, Thomas JD. Assessment of lv systolic function in atrial fibrillation using an index of preceding cardiac cycles. Am J Physiol Heart Circ Physiol. 2001;281:H573–80.
17. Castello R, Lenzen P, Aguirre F, Labovitz A. Variability in the quantitation of mitral regurgitation by doppler color flow mapping: comparison of transthoracic and transesophageal studies. J Am Coll Cardiol. 1992;20:433–8.
18. Castello R, Lenzen P, Aguirre F, Labovitz AJ. Quantitation of mitral regurgitation by transesophageal echocardiography with doppler color flow mapping: correlation with cardiac catheterization. J Am Coll Cardiol. 1992;19:1516–21.
19. Zoghbi WA, Enriquez-Sarano M, Foster EI. Recommendations for evaluation of the severity of native valvular regurgitation with two-dimensional and doppler echocardiography. Journal of the American Society of Echocardiography : official publication of the American Society of Echocardiography. 2003;16:777–802.
20. Jin CN, Salgo IS, Schneider RJ. Using anatomic intelligence to localize mitral valve prolapse on three-dimensional echocardiography. Journal of the American Society of Echocardiography : official publication of the American Society of Echocardiography. 2016;29:938–45.
21. Levine RA, Handschumacher MD, Sanfilippo AJ, Hagege AA, Harrigan P, Marshall JE, Weyman AE. Three-dimensional echocardiographic reconstruction of the mitral valve, with implications for the diagnosis of mitral valve prolapse. Circulation. 1989;80:589–98.
22. Kopuz C, Erk K, Baris YS. Morphometry of the fibrous ring of the mitral valve. Annals of anatomy = Anatomischer Anzeiger : official organ of the Anatomische Gesellschaft. 1995;177:151–4.
23. Levine RA, Triulzi MO, Harrigan P, Weyman AE. The relationship of mitral annular shape to the diagnosis of mitral valve prolapse. Circulation. 1987;75:756–67.
24. Otsuji Y, Kumanohoso T, Yoshifuku S. Isolated annular dilation does not usually cause important functional mitral regurgitation: comparison between patients with lone atrial fibrillation and those with idiopathic or ischemic cardiomyopathy. J Am Coll Cardiol. 2002;39:1651–6.

25. Zhou X, Otsuji Y, Yoshifuku S. Impact of atrial fibrillation on tricuspid and mitral annular dilatation and valvular regurgitation. Circulation journal : official journal of the Japanese Circulation Society. 2002;66:913–6.

26. Machino-Ohtsuka T, Seo Y, Ishizu T, Sato K, Sugano A, Yamamoto M, Hamada-Harimura Y, Aonuma K. Novel mechanistic insights into atrial functional mitral regurgitation- 3-dimensional echocardiographic study. Circulation journal : official journal of the Japanese Circulation Society. 2016;80:2240–8.

27. Kagiyama N, Hayashida A, Toki M, Fukuda S, Ohara M, Hirohata A, Yamamoto K, Isobe M, Yoshida K. Insufficient leaflet remodeling in patients with atrial fibrillation: association with the severity of mitral regurgitation. Circ Cardiovasc Imaging. 2017 Mar;10(3)

28. Salgo IS, Gorman JH 3rd, Gorman RC, Jackson BM, Bowen FW, Plappert T, St John Sutton MG, Edmunds LH Jr. Effect of annular shape on leaflet curvature in reducing mitral leaflet stress. Circulation 2002;106:711–717.

29. Boltwood CM, Tei C, Wong M, Shah PM. Quantitative echocardiography of the mitral complex in dilated cardiomyopathy: the mechanism of functional mitral regurgitation. Circulation. 1983;68:498–508.

30. Yiu SF, Enriquez-Sarano M, Tribouilloy C, Seward JB, Tajik AJ. Determinants of the degree of functional mitral regurgitation in patients with systolic left ventricular dysfunction: a quantitative clinical study. Circulation. 2000;102:1400–6.

31. Dal-Bianco JP, Levine RA. Anatomy of the mitral valve apparatus: role of 2d and 3d echocardiography. Cardiol Clin. 2013;31:151–64.

32. Perloff JK, Roberts WC. The mitral apparatus. Functional anatomy of mitral regurgitation. Circulation. 1972;46:227–39.

33. Maréchaux S, Pinçon C, Poueymidanette M, Verhaeghe M, Bellouin A, Asseman P, Le Tourneau T, Lejemtel TH, Pibarot P, Ennezat PV. Elevated left atrial pressure estimated by doppler echocardiography is a key determinant of mitral valve tenting in functional mitral regurgitation. Heart. 2010;96:289–97.

34. Bruch C, Grude M, Müller J, Breithardt G, Wichter T. Usefulness of tissue doppler imaging for estimation of left ventricular filling pressures in patients with systolic and diastolic heart failure. Am J Cardiol. 2005;95:892–5.

35. Chugh SS, Havmoeller R, Narayanan K, Singh D, Rienstra M, Benjamin EJ, Gillum RF, Kim YH, McAnulty JH Jr, Zheng ZJ, Forouzanfar MH, Naghavi M, Mensah GA, Ezzati M, Murray CJ. Worldwide epidemiology of atrial fibrillation: a global burden of disease 2010 study. Circulation. 2014;129:837–47.

36. Takahashi Y, Abe Y, Sasaki Y, Bito Y, Morisaki A, Nishimura S, Shibata T. Mitral valve repair for atrial functional mitral regurgitation in patients with chronic atrial fibrillation. Interact Cardiovasc Thorac Surg. 2015;21:163–8.

37. Feldman T, Young A. Percutaneous approaches to valve repair for mitral regurgitation. J Am Coll Cardiol. 2014;63:2057–68.

38. Lee AP, Acker M, Kubo SH, Bolling SF, Park SW, Bruce CJ, Oh JK. Mechanisms of recurrent functional mitral regurgitation after mitral valve repair in nonischemic dilated cardiomyopathy: importance of distal anterior leaflet tethering. Circulation. 2009;119:2606–14.

28

Long-term follow-up in adults after tetralogy of Fallot repair

Natalia Dłużniewska[1], Piotr Podolec[1], Maciej Skubera[1], Monika Smaś-Suska[1], Jacek Pająk[2], Małgorzata Urbańczyk-Zawadzka[3], Wojciech Płazak[1], Maria Olszowska[1] and Lidia Tomkiewicz-Pająk[1*]

Abstract

Background: Tetralogy of Fallot (ToF) is the most common cyanotic congenital heart disease and the population of ToF repair survivors is growing rapidly. Adults with repaired ToF develop late complications. The aim of this study was to describe and analyze long-term follow-up of patients with repaired ToF.

Methods: This is a retrospective cohort study. Consecutive 83 patients with repaired ToF who did not undergo pulmonary valve replacement were included. Mean age of all patients was 30.5 ± 10.7. There were 49 (59%) male. Patients were divided into two groups according to the time since the repair (< 25 years and ≥ 25 years). The electrocardiographic (ECG), cardiopulmonary exercise testing (CPET), echocardiographic and cardiac magnetic resonance (CMR) data were reviewed retrospectively.

Results: In CPET values were not significantly different in the two groups. In CMR volumes of left and right ventricles were not significantly different in the two groups. There were no differences between the groups in ventricular ejection fraction, mass of ventricles, or pulmonary regurgitation fraction. Among all the patients, ejection fraction and left and right ventricle mass, indexed pulmonary regurgitation volume measured by CMR did not correlate with the time since repair. In ECG among all the patients, ejection fraction of the RV, measured in CMR, negatively correlated with QRS duration ($r = -0.43$; $p < 0.001$). There was a positive correlation between QRS duration and end diastolic volume of the RV ($r = 0.30$; $p < 0.02$), indexed end diastolic volume of the RV ($r = 0.29$; $p = 0.04$), RV mass ($r = 0.36$; $p < 0.001$) and left ventricle mass ($r = 0.26$; $p = 0.04$).

Conclusion: Long-term survival and clinical condition after surgical correction of ToF in infancy is generally good and the late functional status in ToF – operated patients could be excellent up to 25 years after the repair. QRS duration could be an utility and easy factor to assessment of right ventricular function.

Keywords: Tetralogy of Fallot, Long term follow up, Cardiac magnetic resonance, Echocardiography cardiopulmonary exercise test

Background

Tetralogy of Fallot (ToF) is the most common cyanotic congenital heart disease [1, 2]. Surgical correction of ToF has become the treatment of choice over four decades ago [3] and is well established [4]. As a result, survival has improved significantly and the population of ToF repair survivors is growing rapidly [1], with a 20–30-year survival rate at near 90% [1, 2, 5]. Nevertheless, survival at 30 years is lower than in the normal population [2], and the risk of death in the third postoperative decade is more than triple [5]. Adults with repaired ToF develop late complications, such as progressive exercise intolerance, arrhythmias, and heart failure [4, 6]. These complications are mainly due to pulmonary regurgitation, which leads to right ventricle dysfunction [7]. Previous studies have focused on outcomes of pulmonary valve replacement [8, 9] and risk factors assessment for adverse events [2, 10], but few have

* Correspondence: ltom@wp.pl
[1]Department of Cardiac and Vascular Disease, Collegium Medicum, Jagiellonian University, John Paul II Hospital, Krakow, Poland
Full list of author information is available at the end of the article

reported a long-term symptomatic status of patients after ToF repair.

The primary aim of this study was to describe and analyze long-term follow-up of patients with repaired ToF. The secondary aim was to assess the patients' exercise capacity and type and frequency of complications.

Methods

Patient population

This is a retrospective cohort study. Consecutive patients with repaired ToF were included from the outpatients registry if they were > 18 years of age. Patients were referred for clinical assessment as part of routine clinical follow-up at the Department of Cardiac and Vascular Diseases, Institute of Cardiology Jagiellonian University College of Medicine, in the John Paul II Hospital, in Krakow. A main diagnosis was determined for every patient from hospital records, and patients were included in the study if they had only ToF as the primary diagnosis (ToF variants were excluded). To the further analysis 83 patients who did not undergo PVR were included. Patients were divided into two groups according to the time since the repair (< 25 years and ≥ 25 years). In patients population who did undergo PVR the data were obtained after PVR.

Study protocol

All clinical and demographic variables were extracted from the patients' medical records. Body mass index (BMI) was computed as weight/ height^2 expressed in kg/m$^{2.}$ [11]. Information on cardiac malformations, type of previous cardiac operations, age at surgical repair, reoperations, and current medications were recorded. The electrocardiographic (ECG), cardiopulmonary exercise testing (CPET), echocardiographic and cardiac magnetic resonance (CMR) data for the patients who did not undergo pulmonary valve replacement were reviewed retrospectively.

The study protocol was approved by the local Ethics Committee (license number 122.6120.88.2016). Each participant provided informed consent to participate in the study. All procedures were conducted in accordance with the ethical standards of the institutional and/or national research committee and with the 1964 Declaration of Helsinki and its later amendments, or comparable ethical standards. The study was funded by Jagiellonian Universtiy Collegium Medicum (CMUJ K/ZDS/007189; CMUJ K/ZDS/007820).

ECG and Holter monitoring

Standard (25 mm/s speed and 1 mV/cm) 12-lead surface ECGs were analysed for rhythm, PQ interval and QRS duration (defined as the maximal QRS length in any lead from the first inflection to the final sharp vector crossing the isoelectric line). ECGs in patients with a pacemaker were excluded from this comparison. Twenty-four-hour Holter monitoring, performed with a Pathfinder SL version 1.7.1.4557, was analysed for rhythm and conduction abnormalities.

Cardiopulmonary exercise testing

CPET was performed on a treadmill with a modified Bruce protocol (Reynolds Medical System, ZAN-600) as previously described [12]. To avoid pharmacologic influence, beta blockers were discontinued before CPET. Oxygen saturation and 12-lead ECG were continually monitored during the test, and blood pressure was measured manually every two minutes. Oxygen consumption (VO$_2$) and carbon dioxide production (VCO$_2$) were measured with computerized breath-by-breath analyzer. Peak oxygen uptake (VO$_2$ peak) was defined as the highest value at peak workload, expressed in ml/kg/min and as % of predicted value.

Echocardiography

During echocardiographic examination, ejection fraction of the left and right ventricle, according to the European Society of Cardiology guidelines, was measured [13]. Valves regurgitations and stenoses were evaluated with continuous wave Doppler and pulsed- wave Doppler. To estimate the severity of pulmonary stenosis, pulmonary gradient with continuous wave Doppler was measured. The severity of pulmonary and tricuspid regurgitation was estimated with the color Doppler. A quantitative assessment of the severity of pulmonary regurgitation was based on the deceleration velocity of the regurgitant flow, known as pressure half time (PHT). The PHT was measured with continuous wave Doppler. Function of the right heart was assessed by tricuspid annular-plane systolic excursion (TAPSE). Values of TAPSE lower than 18 mm were indicative of right ventricular longitudinal dysfunction [14]. Tissue Doppler imaging technique was applied at the tricuspid annulus to measure its systolic velocity (S'). The presence or absence of atrial and ventricle septal defect was checked. Images were obtained with Vivid 7 GE Medical System, USA.

Cardiac magnetic resonance: imaging protocol

Breath-hold, ECG-gated imaging was performed by use of cardiac phased-array coil on 1.5 T whole-body scanner (Magnetom Sonata Maestro Class, Siemens, Erlangen, Germany) in left and right ventricle short-axis and axial views. After scout imaging was performed, cine biventricular imaging, using breath-hold steady-state free precision gradient echo technique, and flow-sensitive imaging at the pulmonary valve level, using free-breathing phase-contrast technique, were acquired. The imaging plane for a flow sequence was oriented perpendicularly to the main pulmonary artery at the pulmonary valve level. The velocity encoding was set at 100–550 cm/sec to avoid an aliasing artefact.

Cardiac magnetic resonance: image analysis

Cine and flow images were assessed off-line with dedicated software package (MASS Medis, Leiden, the Netherlands). Left ventricular and right ventricular end-diastolic volume, end-systolic volume, ejection fraction, and myocardial mass were computed. End-diastolic volume, end-systolic volume and pulmonary regurgitation fraction were indexed to body surface area.

Flow images

The forward flow and backward flow were calculated. Backward flow was considered to represent the volume of pulmonary regurgitation. Based on the forward and backward flow volumes, the fraction of pulmonary regurgitation (PRF) was calculated.

Statistical analysis

Data were analyzed by use of statistical software package StatSoft STATISTICA 12.5. A p value of < 0.05 was considered statistically significant. Continuous variables are presented as mean $\pm$ SD or median with range. Student's unpaired t-test and Mann-Whitney U test were used for comparison of continuous variables. All categorical variables were compared by use of the χ^2 test. The age difference between the groups according to the time after the surgery was compensated for in statistical analysis. To assess the effects of the time-dependent covariates, repeated multivariate analyses of variance were performed. In case of significant results of these analyses, post-hoc testing was applied. Correlations between nominal variables were tested with Spearman's rank correlation coefficient test or Pearson's rank correlation coefficient test, depending on the distribution of interval variables.

Results

Population characteristics

The total cohort of ToF patients was 109. The median age of all patients was 28 years (interquartile range 19–64). There were 64 (59%) male. 57 (52.3%) of patients were in I NYHA class, 38 (34.9%) in II NYHA class and 14 (12.8%) in III NYHA class. The corrective surgery was performed between 1964 and 2012; the median patients age of intracardiac repair was 3.0 years (interquartile range 0.0–31.0 years). The mean time from repair to study was 26.1 ± 8.3 years. Twenty (18%) patients had received a palliative shunt (Blalock-Taussig repair) prior to complete repair. The most common surgical procedure was transannular patch, performed in 54 (49%) patients. Twenty-six patients were qualified for reoperation

according to European Society of Cardiology guidelines [15] and underwent pulmonary valve replacement. The median age at PVR was 30.5 (interquartile range 19–53). To the further analysis 83 patients (76%), of median age of 26 years (interquartile range 19–64), who did not undergo PVR were included. None of the patients of this population had the criteria for reintervention at the time of the study. Patients were divided into two groups according to the time since the repair (< 25 years and ≥ 25 years). Table 1 illustrates the demographics and surgical characteristics of patients who did not undergo PVR after ToF repair.

Cardiopulmonary exercise testing

The results of cardiopulmonary exercise test are presented in Table 2. Patients who were ≥ 25 years since the repair had significantly lower peak heart rate. Other values were not significantly differe in the two groups.

Echocardiography

Echocardiography was completed in all patients. The results of echocardiography are presented in Table 3. Moderate or severe pulmonary regurgitation was present in 69 subjects (83%), and severe tricuspid regurgitation was present in 4 (5%). Hemodynamically insignificant residual ventricular septal defect, was present in 16 patients (19%).

The patients with less than 25 years since the repair had significantly smaller right and left atria than did the patients operated before that time.

Cardiac magnetic resonance

The results of cardiac magnetic resonance are presented in Table 4. Volumes of left and right ventricles were not significantly different in the two groups. Also, there were no differences between the groups in ventricular ejection fraction, mass of ventricles, or pulmonary regurgitation fraction.

Among all the patients, ejection fraction and left and right ventricle mass, indexed pulmonary regurgitation volume measured by CMR did not correlate with the time since repair.

ECG and Holter monitoring

Patients' ECG and Holter monitor findings are illustrated in the figure below (Fig. 1). Among all the patients, 77 (93%) had sinus rhythm, 6 (7%) had persistent atrial fibrillation, which was the most common arrhythmia. Most of the patients (69, 83%) had right bundle branch block; 13 (17%) had episodes of ventricular tachycardia, 9 (11%) atrioventricular block; and 40 (48%) were treated with beta blocker.

Ventricular tachycardia and the need to use beta blocker medications were significantly less frequent in

Table 1 Baseline demographics and surgical characteristics of patients who did not undergo PVR

	All patients (n = 83)	Group 1 < 25 years since repair (n = 51)	Group 2 ≥ 25 years since repair (n = 32)	P values
Median age with interquartile range (yr)	26 (19–64)	25 (19–49)	37 (21–64)	< 0.001
Male/female	49/34	32/19	17/15	0.39
Height	168.3 ± 10.8	169.9 ± 12.2	165.8 ± 7.7	0.11
Weight	64.7 ± 14.8	63.5 ± 15.4	66.6 ± 14.0	0.40
BMI	22.8 ± 4.4	21.9 ± 4.5	24.1 ± 4.0	0.04
BSA	1.7 ± 0.2	1.7 ± 0.2	1.7 ± 0.2	0.94
Median age with interquartile range at ToF repair (yr)	3 (0–30)	3 (0–30)	3 (0–30)	0.66
Time since ToF repair (yr)	23 (6–53)	21 (6–24)	31 (25–53)	< 0.001
Number with prior Blalock – Taussig shunt	17	6	11	0.02
Number with transannular patch	39	29	10	0.02
NYHA functional class	NYHA I – 56	NYHA I – 38	NYHA I – 18	0.23
	NYHA II – 23	NYHA II – 13	NYHA II – 10	NYHA I – 0.08
	NYHA III – 4	NYHA III – 0	NYHA III – 4	NYHA II – 0.38
	NYHA IV – 0	NYHA IV –0	NYHA IV –0	NYHA III – 0.98

BMI Body mass index, *BSA* Body surface area, *NYHA* New York Heart Association

patients who were < 25 years since the repair as compared to operated later (13 vs 70; *p* = 0.002 and 40 vs 43; *p* = 0.003, respectively). There were no statistically significant differences between these groups in PQ interval duration (176 ms vs 191 ms; *p* = 0.3) or QRS interval duration (138 ms vs 132 ms; *p* = 0.5).

Among all the patients, ejection fraction of the right ventricle, measured in CMR, negatively correlated with QRS duration (*r* = – 0.43; *p* < 0.001). There was a positive correlation between QRS duration and end diastolic volume of the right ventricle (*r* = 0.30; *p* < 0.02), indexed end diastolic volume of the right ventricle (*r* = 0.29; *p* = 0.04), right ventricle mass (*r* = 0.36; *p* < 0.001) and left ventricle mass (*r* = 0.26; *p* = 0.04).

Discussion

The main finding of the study is to show that the late functional status in ToF – operated patients could be excellent up to 25 years after the repair. However, after more than 25 years since the repair, significant changes can occur, manifesting itself as progressive RV dilation and dysfunction or clinical arrhythmia.

Good functional status up to 25 years after the operation corresponds with other reports of excellent long-term outcomes [17–19]. Most prior studies focused on risk factors for pulmonary valve regurgitation and preoperative or postoperative testing. In contrast with some studies [16], we did not evaluate patients who had undergone reoperation; thus, our data are unique in this regard.

Table 2 Results of patients' cardiopulmonary exercise testing of patients who did not undergo PVR

CPET variable	Mean value ± SD (n = 83)	Group 1 < 25 years since repair (n = 43)	Group 2 ≥ 25 years since repair (n = 40)	p value
T [min]	16.3 ± 3.3.4	16.9 ± 3.6	15.5 ± 2.8	0.08
HR peak [beat/min]	157 ± 29	164 ± 29	146 ± 26	< 0.001
HR peak [%N]	70 ± 33	71 ± 29	69 ± 35	0.27
SBP peak [mmHg]	141 ± 23	141 ± 18	141 ± 30	0.96
DBP peak [mmHg]	73 ± 12	71 ± 12	75 ± 12	0.23
VO2 peak	1.8 ± 0.7	1.9 ± 0.7	1.7 ± 0.6	0.42
VO2 peak [%N]	69.1 ± 23.0	67.1 ± 23.5	72.0 ± 22.3	0.39
VO2/kg peak [ml/min*kg]	27.6 ± 8.2	28.6 ± 8.6	25.9 ± 7.5	0.18
VO2max/kg [%N]	76.3 ± 22.1	73.4 ± 22.3	80.5 ± 21.5	0.19
VCO2 peak	2.0 ± 0.8	2.0 ± 0.9	1.9 ± 0.7	0.34
VCO2 peak [%N]	57.5 ± 18.3	56.8 ± 19.5	58.4 ± 16.8	0.72
RER peak	1.1 ± 0.2	1.1 ± 0.2	1.1 ± 0.1	0.84

T Time, *HR* Heart rate, *SBP* Systolic blood pressure, *DBP* Diastolic blood pressure, *VO2peak* Peak oxygen uptake, *VO2peak/kg* Peak oxygen uptake per kilogram, *VCO2peak* Peak carbon dioxide uptake, *RER* Respiratory exchange ratio

Table 3 Results of patients' echocardiography of patients who did not undergo PVR

Echocardiography parameter	Mean value ± SD ($n = 83$)	Group 1 < 25 years since repair ($n = 51$)	Group 2 ≥ 25 years since repair ($n = 32$)	p value
RVOT prox [mm]	30.5 ± 6.7	29.6 ± 5.8	31.9 ± 7.9	0.14
RDVs [mm]	36.1 ± 8.9	37.7 ± 9.3	33.9 ± 7.7	0.10
RDVd [mm]	71.6 ± 9.9	72.4 ± 10.6	70.3 ± 8.8	0.41
LVD [mm]	44.3 ± 5.9	43.9 ± 6.1	44.9 ± 5.6	0.45
LVS [mm]	28.2 ± 6.0	28.5 ± 4.7	27.7 ± 7.6	0.54
RA area [cm^2]	19.3 ± 7.2	17.9 ± 4.9	21.5 ± 9.4	0.04
LA area[cm^2]	14.9 ± 5.3	12.8 ± 2.3	17.8 ± 6.6	< 0.001
EF [%]	58.7 ± 20.3	57.9 ± 20.1	60.0 ± 20.8	0.64
PV gr.max [mmHg]	24.3 ± 21.2	22.5 ± 16.3	27.2 ± 27.1	0.33
PV gr.mean [mmHg]	14.0 ± 12.9	12.7 ± 8.6	16.0 ± 17.6	0.26
PV PHT	104.3 ± 58.9	91.1 ± 42.0	126.2 ± 75.2	0.01
Tricuspid annulus [mm]	36.5 ± 7.3	36.0 ± 7.6	37.4 ± 6.8	0.57
TAPSE [mm]	21.2 ± 4.3	21.3 ± 4.1	21.2 ± 4.5	0.94
S' [cm/s]	11.7 ± 2.0	11.8 ± 1.9	11.4 ± 2.1	0.43
RVSP (mmHg)	38.8 ± 16.5	36.0 ± 12.3	42.2 ± 20.4	0.20

RVOT Right ventricle outflow track, *RDVs* Right ventricle dimension at end systole, *RDVd* Right ventricle dimension at end diastole, *LVD* Left ventricle diastolic dimension, *LVS* Left ventricle systolic dimension, *LA* Left atrium, *RA* Right atrium, *EF* Ejection fraction, *PV gr max* Maximal pulmonary valve gradient, *PV gr min* Minimal pulmonary valve gradient, *PV PHT* Pulmonary valve pressure half time, *TAPSE* Tricuspid annular plane systolic excursion, *S'* Systolic velocity of tricuspid annulus, *RVSP* Right ventricular systolic pressure

Table 4 Results of patients' cardiac magnetic resonance of patients who did not undergo PVR

CMR parameter	Mean value ± SD ($n = 83$)	Group 1 < 25 years since repair ($n = 51$)	Group 2 ≥ 25 years since repair ($n = 32$)	p value
LA area [cm^2]	20.2 ± 5.1	19.6 ± 5.4	21.1 ± 4.5	0.18
RA area [cm^2]	26.3 ± 8.2	24.9 ± 7.2	28.4 ± 9.2	0.06
RV area [cm^2]	41.9 ± 10.3	43.2 ± 11.0	40.3 ± 9.4	0.42
LVD [cm]	4.8 ± 0.5	4.7 ± 0.5	4.8 ± 0.5	0.47
LVS [cm]	3.2 ± 0.5	3.2 ± 0.5	3.2 ± 0.5	0.72
RV EF [%]	50.7 ± 9.9	50.2 ± 8.9	51.5 ± 11.3	0.57
RV EDV [ml]	197.4 ± 61.9	202.6 ± 58.0	189.0 ± 67.8	0.33
RV EDV indexed [ml/m^2]	112.9 ± 33.8	118.4 ± 28.4	103.8 ± 40.0	0.07
RV ESV [ml]	104.0 ± 47.8	95.4 ± 35.8	122. ± 65.5	0.17
RV ESV indexed [ml/m^2]	59.8 ± 27.9	55.9 ± 16.8	66.7 ± 41.5	0.39
RV mass [g]	46.3 ± 19.5	47.3 ± 19.6	44.9 ± 19.5	0.59
RV mass indexed [g/m^2]	27.5 ± 10.6	28.8 ± 10.6	25.7 ± 10.4	0.23
LV EF [%]	57.7 ± 7.6	56.6 ± 7.5	59.3 ± 7.4	0.11
LV EDV [ml]	129.8 ± 35.1	129.9 ± 36.9	129.6 ± 32.5	0.97
LV EDV indexed [ml/m^2]	76.3 ± 17.0	76.3 ± 16.1	76.3 ± 18.7	0.99
LV ESV [ml]	56.1 ± 17.9	59.5 ± 18.9	49.7 ± 14.7	0.19
LV ESV indexed [ml/m^2]	31.6 ± 8.2	33.6 ± 8.7	28.7 ± 6.6	0.19
LV mass [g]	100.9 ± 31.2	99.6 ± 33.4	102.8 ± 27.9	0.66
LV mass indexed [g/m^2]	58.3 ± 14.8	58.3 ± 16.7	58.3 ± 11.8	0.98
PRV [ml]	54.4 ± 30.5	53.7 ± 26.8	55.6 ± 37.0	0.84
PRV indexed [ml/m^2]	30.0 ± 17.2	28.0 ± 13.1	34.3 ± 23.7	0.30
PRF [%]	42.0 ± 10.3	42.6 ± 10.7	40.9 ± 10.1	0.67

CMR Cardiac magnetic resonance, *LA* Left atrium, *RA* Right atrium, *RV* Right ventricle, *LVD* Left ventricle diastolic dimension, *LVS* Left ventricle systolic dimension, *RVEDV* Right ventricle end-diastolic volume, *RVESV* Right ventricle end-systolic volume, *RVEF* Right ventricle ejection fraction, *RV mass* Right ventricle mass, *LVEF* Left ventricle ejection fraction, *LVEDV* Left ventricle end-diastolic volume, *LVESV* Left ventricle end-systolic volume, *LV mass* Left ventricle mass, *PRV* Pulmonary regurgitation volume, *PRF* Pulmonary regurgitation fraction

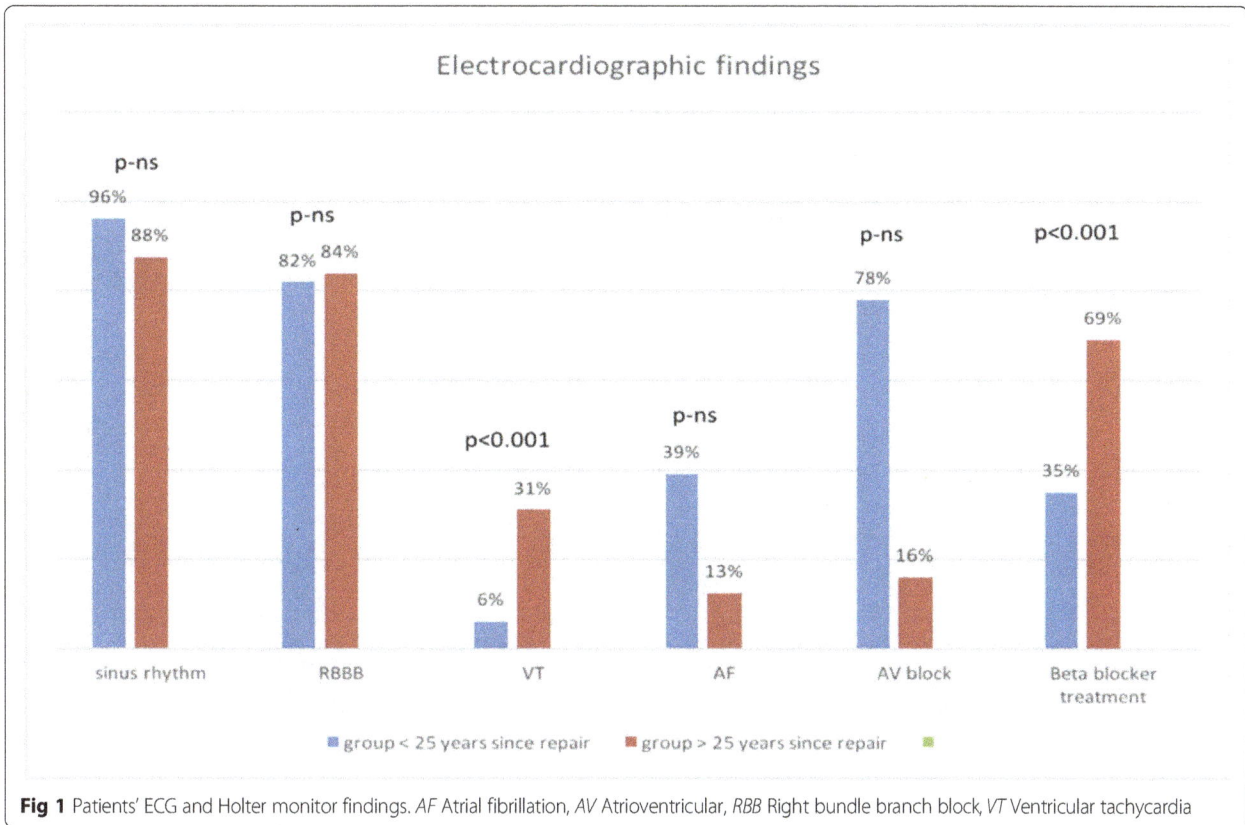

Fig 1 Patients' ECG and Holter monitor findings. *AF* Atrial fibrillation, *AV* Atrioventricular, *RBB* Right bundle branch block, *VT* Ventricular tachycardia

In our cohort, exercise performance in both groups did not have significant differences in regard to time since repair. O'Meagher et al. [21] found that the age at ToF repair did not explain the disparity in exercise capacity. Others [20] have reported that patients after ToF repair have markedly depressed exercise capacity but in comparison with healthy controls.

Chronic right ventricular overload due to pulmonary valve insufficiency can lead to right ventricle dilatation, dysfunction of both ventricles and arrhythmias [19, 21–23]. Although previous studies documented that pulmonary regurgitation can be well tolerated for many years [24, 25], our data extend these observations and showed, as did Bacha et al. [23], that right ventricular volume can be preserved without deterioration for more than 25 years.

QRS duration is strongly associated with right ventricular function [10], as was first recognized by Gatzoulis et al. [26], and QRS prolongation has been correlated with the presence of ventricular arrhythmias [19]. In contrast to previous findings [10], we found that QRS interval was not correlated with the length of follow-up and was not prolonged after 25 years from date of operation, even though the presence of ventricular tachycardia increased with time. This should be obviously noted that beta blockers may affect the QRS.

The relationship between QRS duration and right ventricular enlargement and mass was found primarily in studies of Book et al. [27] and Neffke et al. [28]. In our study, we confirmed a significant correlation between QRS duration and right ventricular mass and end diastolic volume in patients with ToF; also, we made the new finding of a strong negative relationship between QRS duration and right ventricular ejection fraction.

Supraventricular and ventricular tachycardia are well-documented complications of ToF repair [6, 24]. We found an increasing incidence of these arrhythmias with time from the repair. Abnormal right atrial size has been shown as a strong predictor of tachyarrhythmia [6], and we found significant increases in right atrial area with time since the repair.

Pulmonary regurgitation is a frequent late consequence of repair in ToF patients [25] is associated with right ventricle dilatation. In natural history, pulmonary regurgitation leads to ventricular dysfunction and heart failure developing over time [29]. Our study did not confirm time related impairment both ventricles ejection fractions and relationship to pulmonary regurgitation volume. This finding supports those of studies which showed that the right ventricle fails after 40 years of successful adaptation [19]. Moreover, in our study, in both groups right ventricle parameters were not adequate according to current guidelines to meet criteria of pulmonary valve replacement or right ventricular failure.

In conclusion, long-term survival and clinical condition after surgical correction of ToF in infancy is generally good. Our observations indicate an optimistic clinical function and exercise capacity in the patients operated more than 25 years ago. QRS duration could be an utility and easy factor to assessment of right ventricular function. Additionally longer prospective follow up is still needed and may provide a clearer understanding of this group.

Study limitations

The limitations of the study should be mentioned. First, the small sample of patients population and retrospective cohort study. Second, this is a cross sectional study and the parameters and the history of adverse event was collected at the time of patient enrollment.

Abbreviations

CMR: Cardiac magnetic resonance; CPET: Cardiopulmonary exercise testing; ECG: Electrocardiographic; PHT: Pressure half time; PVR: Pulmonary valve replacement; TAPSE: Tricuspid annular-plane systolic excursion; ToF: Tetralogy of Fallot; VO_2 peak: Peak oxygen uptake

Acknowledgements

None of the authors contributed towards the study by making substantial contributions to conception, design, acquisition of data, or analysis and interpretation of data. All authors are working for Jagiellonian University College of Medicine, John Paul II Hospital, Krakow, Poland.

Funding

Project number CMUJ K/ZDS/007189; CMUJ K/ZDS/007820.

Authors' contributions

ND acquisition of data, analysis of data and major contributor in writing the manuscript; PP involved in revising manuscript critically for important intellectual content; MS involved in revising manuscript; MSS- involved in revising manuscript; JP involved in revising manuscript; MUZ involved in revising manuscript; WP involved in revising manuscript critically for important intellectual content; MO involved in revising manuscript critically for important intellectual content; LTP made substantial contributions to conception and design, interpretation of data and involved in giving final approval of the version to be published. All authors read and approved the final manuscript.

Authors' information

Not applicable.

Consent for publication

Not applicable.

Competing interests

All authors declare that they have no competing interests.

Author details

Department of Cardiac and Vascular Disease, Collegium Medicum, Jagiellonian University, John Paul II Hospital, Krakow, Poland. [2]Paediatric Heart Surgery Department and General Paediatric Surgery Department, Medical University of Warsaw, Warsaw, Poland. [3]Department of Radiology and Diagnostic Imaging, John Paul II Hospital, Krakow, Poland.

References

1. Geva T. Indications and timing of pulmonary valve replacement after ToF repair. Semin Thorac Cardiovasc Surg Pediatr Card Surg Annu. 2006;9(1):11–22.
2. Cuypers JAAE, Menting ME, Konings EEM, Opiü P, Utens EMWJ, Helbing WA, et al. The unnatural history of ToF: prospective follow-up of 40 years after surgical correction. Circulation. 2014;130:1944–53.
3. Gatzoulis MA, Balaji S, Webber SA, Siu SC, Hokanson JS, Poile C, et al. Risk factors for arrhythmia and sudden cardiac death late after repair of ToF: a multicentre study. Lancet. 2000;356(9234):975–81.
4. Oechslin EN, Harrison DA, Harris L, Downar E, Webb GD, Siu SS, et al. Reoperation in adults with repair of ToF: indications and outcomes. J Thorac Cardiovasc Surg. 1999;118:245–51.
5. Geva T, Sandweiss BM, Gauvreau K, Lock JE, Powell AJ. Factors associated with impaired clinical status in long-term survivors of ToF repair evaluated by magnetic resonance imaging. J Am Coll Cardiol. 2004;43(6):1068–74.
6. Dennis M, Moore B, Kotchetkova I, Lynne Pressley RC, DSC. Adults with repaired tetralogy: low mortality but high morbidity up to middle age. Open Heart. 2017;4:e000564.
7. Babu-Narayan SV, Diller G-P, Gheta RR, Bastin AJ, Karonis T, Li W, et al. Clinical outcomes of surgical pulmonary valve replacement after repair of ToF and potential prognostic value of preoperative cardiopulmonary exercise testing. Circulation. 2014 Jan;129(1):18–27.
8. Therrien J, Siu SC, McLaughlin PR, Liu PP, Williams WG, Webb GD, et al. Pulmonary valve replacement in adults late after repair of ToF: are we operating too late? J Am Coll Cardiol. 2000;36:1670–5.
9. Lee C, Kim YM, Lee C-H, Kwak JG, Park CS, Song JY, et al. Outcomes of pulmonary valve replacement in 170 patients with chronic pulmonary regurgitation after relief of right ventricular outflow tract obstruction. J Am Coll Cardiol. 2012;60(11):1005–14.
10. Scherptong RWC, Hazekamp MG, Mulder BJM, Wijers O, Swenne CA, Van Der Wall EE, et al. Follow-up after pulmonary valve replacement in adults with ToF: Association between QRS duration and outcome. J Am Coll Cardiol. Elsevier Inc.;. 2010;56(18):1486–92.
11. Must A, Dallal GE, Dietz WH. Reference data for obesity: 85th and 95th percentiles of body mass index (wt/ht2) and triceps skinfold thickness. Am J Clin Nutr. 1991 Apr;53(4):839–46.
12. Tomkiewicz-Pajak L, Podolec P, Kostkiewicz M, Tracz W. Lung function and exercise tolerance in patients with heart failure. Acta Cardiol. 2002; 57(1):80–1.
13. Lang RM, Badano LP, Mor-Avi V, Afilalo J, Armstrong A, Ernande L, et al. Recommendations for Cardiac Chamber Quantification by Echocardiography in Adults: An Update from the American Society of Echocardiography and the European Association of Cardiovascular Imaging. EHJ - Cardiovasc Imaging. 2015;16(3):233–71.
14. O'Meagher S, Seneviratne M, Skilton MR, Munoz PA, Robinson PJ, Malitz N, et al. Right ventricular mass is associated with exercise capacity in adults with repaired ToF. Pediatr Cardiol Springer US. 2015;36(6):1225-31.
15. Michael A, Gatzoulis U, Gohlke C, Baerwolf GH, Kilner P, et al. ESC Guidelines for the management of grown-up congenital heart disease (new version 2010). The Task Force on the Management of Grown-up Congenital Heart Disease of the European Society of Cardiology (ESC). Eur Heart J. 2010; 31(23):2915–57.
16. Cavalcanti PEF, Barros MP, Sá O, Cecília Y, Santos A, et al. Pulmonary valve replacement after operative repair of ToF meta-analysis and meta-regression of 3,118 patients from 48 studies. J Am Coll Cardiol. 2013;62:2227–43.
17. Katz NM, Blackstone EH, Kirklin JW, Pacifico AD, Bargeron LM. Late survival and symptoms after repair of ToF. Circulation. 1982;65(2):403–10.
18. Murphy JG, Gersh BJ, Mair DD, Fuster V, McGoon MD, Ilstrup DM, et al. Long-term outcome in patients undergoing surgical repair of ToF. N Engl J Med. 1993;329(9):593–9.
19. Nollert G, Fischlein T, Bouterwek S, Böhmer C, Klinner W, Reichart B. Long-term survival in patients with repair of ToF: 36-year follow-up of 490 survivors of the first year after surgical repair. J Am Coll Cardiol. 1997;30(5): 1374–83.
20. Dłużniewska N, Podolec P, Miszalski-Jamka T, Krupiński M, Banyś P, Urbańczyk M, et al. Effect of ventricular function and volumes on exercise capacity in adults with repaired ToF. Indian Heart J. 2018;70(1):87–92.
21. O'Meagher S, Munoz PA, Alison JA, Young IH, Tanous DJ, Celermajer DS, et al. Exercise capacity and stroke volume are preserved late after tetralogy repair, despite severe right ventricular dilatation. Heart. 2012;98(21):1595–9.

22. Sabate Rotes A, Johnson JN, Burkhart HM, Eidem BW, Allison TG, Driscoll DJ. Cardiorespiratory response to exercise before and after pulmonary valve replacement in patients with repaired tetralogy of Fallot: A retrospective study and systematic review of the literature. Congenit Heart Dis. 2015;10(3):263–70.

23. Bacha EA, Scheule AM, Zurakowski D, Erickson LC, Hung J, Lang P, et al. Long-term results after early primary repair of ToF. J Thorac Cardiovasc Surg. 2001;122(1):154–61.

24. Discigil B, Dearani JA, Puga FJ, Schaff HV, Hagler DJ, Warnes CA, et al. Late pulmonary valve replacement after repair of ToF. J Thorac Cardiovasc Surg. 2001;121(2):344–51.

25. Hickey EJ, Veldtman G, Bradley TJ, Gengsakul A, Manlhiot C, Williams WG, et al. Late risk of outcomes for adults with repaired ToF from an inception cohort spanning four decades. Eur J Cardio-Thoracic Surg Oxford University Press. 2009;35(1):156–64.

26. Gatzoulis MA, Till JA, Somerville J, Redington AN, Cordina R, Celermajer DS. Mechanoelectrical interaction in ToF. QRS prolongation relates to right ventricular size and predicts malignant ventricular arrhythmias and sudden death. Circulation. Archives of Disease in childhood. 1995;92(2):231–7.

27. Book WM, Parks WJ, Hopkins KL, Hurst JW. Electrocardiographic predictors of right ventricular volume measured by magnetic resonance imaging late after total repair of ToF. Clin Cardiol. 1999;22(11):740–6.

28. Neffke JGJ, Tulevski II, Van Der Wall EE, Wilde AAM, Van Veldhuisen DJ, Dodge-Khatami A, et al. ECG determinants in adult patients with chronic right ventricular pressure overload caused by congenital heart disease: relation with plasma neurohormones and MRI parameters. Heart. 2002;88:266–70.

29. Bove T, Vandekerckhove K, Devos D, Panzer J, Groote K, De Wilde H, et al. Functional analysis of the anatomical right ventricular components: should assessment of right ventricular function after repair of ToF be refined? Eur J Cardio-thoracic Surg. 2014;45(2):6–12.

Permissions

The contributors of this book come from diverse backgrounds, making this book a truly international effort. This book will bring forth new frontiers with its revolutionizing research information and detailed analysis of the nascent developments around the world.

We would like to thank all the contributing authors for lending their expertise to make the book truly unique. They have played a crucial role in the development of this book. Without their invaluable contributions this book wouldn't have been possible. They have made vital efforts to compile up to date information on the varied aspects of this subject to make this book a valuable addition to the collection of many professionals and students.

This book was conceptualized with the vision of imparting up-to-date information and advanced data in this field. To ensure the same, a matchless editorial board was set up. Every individual on the board went through rigorous rounds of assessment to prove their worth. After which they invested a large part of their time researching and compiling the most relevant data for our readers.

The editorial board has been involved in producing this book since its inception. They have spent rigorous hours researching and exploring the diverse topics which have resulted in the successful publishing of this book. They have passed on their knowledge of decades through this book. To expedite this challenging task, the publisher supported the team at every step. A small team of assistant editors was also appointed to further simplify the editing procedure and attain best results for the readers.

Apart from the editorial board, the designing team has also invested a significant amount of their time in understanding the subject and creating the most relevant covers. They scrutinized every image to scout for the most suitable representation of the subject and create an appropriate cover for the book.

The publishing team has been an ardent support to the editorial, designing and production team. Their endless efforts to recruit the best for this project, has resulted in the accomplishment of this book. They are a veteran in the field of academics and their pool of knowledge is as vast as their experience in printing. Their expertise and guidance has proved useful at every step. Their uncompromising quality standards have made this book an exceptional effort. Their encouragement from time to time has been an inspiration for everyone.

The publisher and the editorial board hope that this book will prove to be a valuable piece of knowledge for researchers, students, practitioners and scholars across the globe.

Contributors

Martina Chantal de Knegt, Tor Biering-Sørensen, Jacob Sivertsen and Jan Skov Jensen
Herlev and Gentofte Hospital, Department of Cardiology, Faculty of Health Sciences, University of Copenhagen, Copenhagen, Denmark

Peter Søgaard
Department of Cardiology, Centre for Cardiovascular Research, Aalborg University Hospital, Aalborg, Denmark

Rasmus Møgelvang
Rigshospitalet, Department of Cardiology, Faculty of Health Sciences, University of Copenhagen, Copenhagen, Denmark

Zahraa Alsafi, Andreas Malmgren and Magnus Dencker
Department of Medical Imaging and Physiology, Skåne University Hospital, Lund University, Malmö, Sweden

Petri Gudmundsson
Department of Biomedical Science, Malmö University, Malmö, Sweden

Martin Stagmo
Department of Cardiology, Skåne University Hospital, Lund University, Lund, Sweden

Bálint Lakatos, Márton Tokodi, Alexandra Doronina, Annamária Kosztin, Attila Kovács and Béla Merkely
MTA-SE Cardiovascular Imaging Research Group, Heart and Vascular Center, Semmelweis University, Városmajor St. 68, H-1122 Budapest, Hungary

Zoltán Tősér
Department of Software Technology and Methodology, Eötvös Loránd University, Budapest, Hungary

Denisa Muraru and Luigi P. Badano
Department of Cardiac, Thoracic and Vascular Sciences, University of Padova, Padova, Italy

Yu Wang, Wei Sun, Xue Sun, Wenjia Lei and Ying Zhang
Department of Sonography, Shengjing Hospital of China Medical University, Heping District, Shenyang, China

Miao Fan
Department of Radiology, The first Affiliated Hospital of Sun Yat-sen University, Guangzhou, China

Faiza Amber Siddiqui
Department of Entomology, The Pennsylvania State University, University Park, PA 16802, USA

Meilian Wang
Department of Entomology, The Pennsylvania State University, University Park, PA 16802, USA
Department of Microbiology and Parasitology, College of Basic Medical Sciences, China Medical University, Heping District, Shenyang, China

Hyukjin Park, Young Joon Hong, Hyung Wook Park, Ju Han Kim, Youngkeun Ahn and Myung Ho Jeong
Department of Cardiovascular Medicine, Chonnam National University Hospital, 42 Jaebong-ro, Donggu, Gwangju 501-757, South Korea

Hyun Ju Yoon, Kye Hun Kim, Jae Yeong Cho, Jeong Gwan Cho and Jong Chun Park
Department of Cardiovascular Medicine, Chonnam National University Hospital, 42 Jaebong-ro, Donggu, Gwangju 501-757, South Korea
Translational Research Center on Aging, Chonnam National University Hospital, 42 Jaebong-ro, Donggu, Gwangju 501-757, South Korea

Johannes Scherr and Lars Pollmer
Department of Prevention and Sports Medicine, Klinikum rechts der Isar, Technische Universitaet Muenchen, Georg-Brauchle-Ring 56, D-80992 Munich, Germany

Martin Halle
Department of Prevention and Sports Medicine, Klinikum rechts der Isar, Technische Universitaet Muenchen, Georg-Brauchle-Ring 56, D-80992 Munich, Germany
Munich Heart Alliance, Munich, Germany

Philip Jung
Medizinische Klinik und Poliklinik I, Klinikum der Universität München, Munich, Germany

Tibor Schuster
Department for Medical Statistics and Epidemiology, Klinikum rechts der Isar, Technische Universitaet Muenchen, Munich, Germany

Gert Eisele and Franz Goss
Heart Center "Alter Hof", Munich, Germany

Jens Schneider
Universitäts Herz-Zentrum Freiburg - Bad Krozingen, Klinik für Kardiologie und Angiologie II, Bad Krozingen, Germany

Jacek Pająk and Michał Buczyński
Pediatric Heart Surgery and General Pediatric Surgery Department, Medical University of Warsaw, ul. Żwirki i Wigury 63A, 02-091 Warszawa, Poland

Piotr Stanek, Grzegorz Zalewski and Marek Wites
Pediatric Heart Surgery Department, The Independent Public Clinical Hospital no. 6 of the Medical University of Silesia, Katowice, Poland

Lesław Szydłowski and Bogusław Mazurek
Department of Pediatric Cardiology, Medical University of Silesia, Katowice, Poland

Lidia Tomkiewicz-Pająk
Institute of Cardiology, Jagiellonian University, Medical College and John Paul II Hospital, Krakow, Poland

Christina Tan, David Rubenson, Ajay Srivastava, Rajeev Mohan, Michael R. Smith, Kristen Billick, Samuel Bardarian and J. Thomas Heywood
Fellow, Scripps Clinic Cardiology, 10666 N. Torrey Pines Road, La Jolla, CA 92037, USA

Wouter M. van Everdingen, Mathias Meine, Arco J. Teske and Maarten J. Cramer
Department of Cardiology, University Medical Centre Utrecht, P.O. Box 855500, 3508, GA, Utrecht, The Netherlands

Alexander H. Maass, Bastiaan Geelhoed, Michiel Rienstra and Isabelle C. Van Gelder
Department of Cardiology, Thoraxcenter, University of Groningen, University Medical Centre Groningen, Groningen, The Netherlands

Kevin Vernooy
Department of Cardiology, Maastricht University Medical Centre, Maastricht, The Netherlands

Cornelis P. Allaart
Department of Cardiology, VU University Medical Centre, Amsterdam, The Netherlands

Frederik J. De Lange
Department of Cardiology, Academic Medical Centre, Amsterdam, The Netherlands

Marc A. Vos
Department of Medical Physiology, University of Utrecht, Utrecht, The Netherlands

Ibadete Bytyçi
Clinic of Cardiology, University Clinical Centre of Kosova, "Rrethi i Spitalit", p.n., Prishtina, Kosovo

Artan Ahmeti, Edmond Haliti and Arlind Batalli
Clinic of Cardiology, University Clinical Centre of Kosova, "Rrethi i Spitalit", p.n., Prishtina, Kosovo
Medical Faculty, University of Prishtina, Prishtina, Kosovo

Gani Bajraktari
Clinic of Cardiology, University Clinical Centre of Kosova, "Rrethi i Spitalit", p.n., Prishtina, Kosovo
Medical Faculty, University of Prishtina, Prishtina, Kosovo
Department of Public Health and Clinical Medicine, Umeå University and Heart Centre, Umeå, Sweden

Pranvera Ibrahimi
Clinic of Cardiology, University Clinical Centre of Kosova, "Rrethi i Spitalit", p.n., Prishtina, Kosovo
Department of Public Health and Clinical Medicine, Umeå University and Heart Centre, Umeå, Sweden

Shpend Elezi
Medical Faculty, University of Prishtina, Prishtina, Kosovo

Michael Y. Henein
Department of Public Health and Clinical Medicine, Umeå University and Heart Centre, Umeå, Sweden
Molecular and Clinical Sciences Research Institute, St George University London, London, United Kingdom

Michał Podgórski, Piotr Grzelak and Ludomir Stefańczyk
Department of Radiology and Diagnostic Imaging, Medical University of Lodz, 22, Kopcińskiego St., Barlicki Hospital, Lodz, Poland

Monika Winnicka and Michał Polguj
Department of Angiology, Chair of Anatomy, Medical University of Lodz, 60, Narutowicza St, Lodz, Poland

Maciej Łukaszewski
Department of Diagnostic Imaging, Polish Mother's Memorial Hospital Research Institute, 281/289, Rzgowska St, Lodz, Poland

Ayse Selcan Koc
Department of Radiology, University of Health Sciences - Adana Health Practices and Research Center, Adana, Turkey

Hilmi Erdem Sumbul
Department of Internal Medicine, University of Health Sciences - Adana Health Practices and Research Center, Adana, Turkey

Agostino Buonauro
Hypertension Research Center, Federico II University Hospital of Naples, Via Pansini 5, bld #1, 80131 Naples, Italy

Costantino Mancusi
Hypertension Research Center, Federico II University Hospital of Naples, Via Pansini 5, bld #1, 80131 Naples, Italy
Department of Advanced Biomedical Science, Federico II University Hospital, Naples, Italy

Maria Viviana Carlino and Giovanni de Simone
Hypertension Research Center, Federico II University Hospital of Naples, Via Pansini 5, bld #1, 80131 Naples, Italy
Department of Traslational Medical Science. Federico II University Hospital, Naples, Italy

Alfonso Sforza
Hypertension Research Center, Federico II University Hospital of Naples, Via Pansini 5, bld #1, 80131 Naples, Italy Emergency Department, Bufalini Hospital, Cesena, Italy

Marco Barozzi, Giuseppe Romano and Sossio Serra
Emergency Department, Bufalini Hospital, Cesena, Italy

Talal Dahhan
Department of Medicine, Division of Pulmonary, Allergy and Critical Care Medicine, Duke University, Durham, NC, USA
Center for Pulmonary Vascular Disease, Box 102351, DUMC, Durham, NC 27710, USA

Irfan Siddiqui
Department of Medicine, East Carolina University, Greenville, NC, USA

Victor F. Tapson
Department of Medicine, Division of Pulmonary and Critical Care Medicine, Cedars Sinai Medical Center, Los Angeles, CA, USA

Eric J. Velazquez and Zainab Samad
Department of Medicine, Division of Cardiology, Duke University, Durham, NC, USA

Sudarshan Rajagopal
Department of Medicine, Division of Cardiology, Duke University, Durham, NC, USA
Center for Pulmonary Vascular Disease, Box 102351, DUMC, Durham, NC 27710, USA

Stephanie Sun and Clemontina A. Davenport
Department of Biostatistics and Bioinformatics, Duke University Medical Center, Durham, NC, USA

Hyo-Suk Ahn, Gee-Hee Kim, Jung Sun Cho, Sang-Hyun Ihm, Hee-Yeol Kim, Chan Seok Park and Ho-Joong Youn
Divisions of Cardiology, College of Medicine, Catholic University of Korea, 222 Banpo-daero, Seocho-gu, Seoul 06591, Republic of Korea

Yong-Kyun Kim, Ho Chul Song and Euy Jin Choi
Nephrology, College of Medicine, Catholic University of Korea, Seoul, South Korea

Juan Cong, Zhibin Wang, Wugang Wang, Kun Gong, Yuanyuan Meng and Yong Lee
Department of Echocardiography, The Affiliated Hospital of Qingdao University, Qingdao, Shandong Province, China

Hong Jin
Department of Cardiology, The Affiliated Hospital of Shandong Medical College, Linyi, Shandong Province, China

William A. Teeter
University of North Carolina, Raleigh, North Carolina, USA

Bianca M. Conti
Department of Anesthesiology, Division of Trauma Anesthesiology, University of Maryland School of Medicine, Baltimore, MD, USA

Dawn Parsell and Phil J. Wasicek
Department of Surgery, University of Maryland School of Medicine, Baltimore, MD, USA

Jonathan J. Morrison
Department of Surgery, Program in Trauma, University of Maryland School of Medicine, Baltimore, MD, USA

Bryan Gamble
Department of Surgery, Walter Reed National Medical Center, United States Army, Bethesda, MD, USA

Melanie R. Hoehn
Department of Surgery, Emory University, Atlanta, GA, USA

Thomas M. Scalea
University of Maryland, Program in Trauma, Baltimore, MD, USA

Samuel M. Galvagno Jr
Department of Anesthesiology, Divisions of Critical Care Medicine and Trauma Anesthesiology, University of Maryland School of Medicine, Baltimore, MD, USA

Raúl Franco-Gutiérrez, Alberto José Pérez-Pérez, Ana María Testa-Fernández, Rafael Carlos Vidal-Pérez, Víctor Manuel Puebla-Rojo, Melisa Santás-Álvarez and Carlos González-Juanatey
Department of Cardiology, Hospital Universitario Lucus Augusti (HULA), Avenida doctor Ulises Romero n° 1, 27003 Lugo, Spain

Virginia Franco-Gutiérrez
Department of Otolaryngology, Hospital Universitario Marqués de Valdecilla, Avenida Valdecilla n° 25, Santander 39008, Spain

Manuel Lorenzo López-Reboiro
Department of Internal Medicine, Hospital Universitario Lucus Augusti (HULA), Avenida doctor Ulises Romero n° 1, Lugo 27003, Spain

María Generosa Crespo-Leiro
Department of Cardiology, Complejo Hospitalario Universitario A Coruña (CHUAC), As Xubias de Arriba n° 84, A Coruña 15006, Spain
Intituto de Investigación Biomédica A Coruña (INIBIC), Xubias de Arriba n° 84, A Coruña 15006, Spain
Universidad de La Coruña (UDC), Calle de la Maestranza n° 9, A Coruña 15001, Spain

Vicente Mora, Ildefonso Roldán, Elena Romero, Javier Bertolín, Carmen Pérez-Olivares and Jana Pérez-Gozalbo
Cardiology Department, Hospital Dr Peset, Valencia, Spain

Diana Romero, Natalia Ugalde, Melisa Rodriguez-Israel and Jorge A. Lowenstein
Cardiodiagnosis Department Medical Research of Buenos Aires, Buenos Aires, Argentina

Eugenio Picano, Michele De Nes, Marco Paterni and Clara Carpeggiani
CNR, Institute of Clinical Physiology, Biomedicine Department, Pisa, Italy

Quirino Ciampi
CNR, Institute of Clinical Physiology, Biomedicine Department, Pisa, Italy Cardiology Division, Fatebenefratelli Hospital, Benevento, Italy

Bruno Villari
Cardiology Division, Fatebenefratelli Hospital, Benevento, Italy

Rodolfo Citro
Cardiology Department and Echocardiography Lab, University Hospital "San Giovanni di Dio e Ruggi d'Aragona", Salerno, Italy

Paolo Colonna
Cardiology Hospital, Policlinico of Bari, Bari, Italy

Marco Fabio Costantino
Cardiology Department, San Carlo Hospital, Potenza, Italy

Lauro Cortigiani
Cardiology Department, San Luca Hospital, Lucca, Italy

Antonello D'. Andrea and Sergio Severino
Cardiology Department, Echocardiography Lab, Monaldi Hospital, Second University of Naples, Naples, Italy

Claudio Dodi
Casa di Cura Figlie di San Camillo, Cremona, Italy

Nicola Gaibazzi
Cardiology Department, Parma University Hospital, Parma, Italy

Maurizio Galderisi
Department of Advanced Biomedical Sciences, Federico II University Hospital, Naples, Italy

Andrea Barbieri
Cardiology Department, Modena University Hospital, Modena, Italy

Ines Monte
Cardio-Thorax-Vascular Department, Echocardiography lab, Policlinico Vittorio Emanuele, University of Catania, Catania, Italy

Fabio Mori
Cardiology Department, Careggi Hospital, Florence, Italy

Barbara Reisenhofer
Cardiology Division, Pontedera-Volterra Hospital, ASL Toscana 3 Nord-Ovest, Florence, Italy

Federica Re
Cardiology Department, San Camillo-Forlanini Hospital, Rome, Italy

Fausto Rigo
Cardiology Department, Ospedale dell'Angelo Mestre-Venice, Venice, Italy

Maria Chiara Scali
Cardiology Department, Nottola Hospital, Siena, Italy Cardiothoracic Department, University of Pisa, Pisa, Italy

Eduardo Bossone and Francesco Ferrara
Cardiology Department, Ospedale santa Maria Incoronata dell'Olmo, cava de' Tirreni, Salerno, Italy

Paolo Trambaiolo
Department of Cardiology, Sandro Pertini Hospital, Rome, Italy

Miguel Amor
Cardiology Department, Ramos Mejia Hospital, Buenos Aires, Argentina.

Pablo Martin Merlo and Jorge Lowenstein
Cardiodiagnosticos, Investigaciones Medicas, Buenos Aires, Argentina

Clarissa Borguezan Daros
Cardiology Division, Hospital San José, Criciuma, Brasília, Brazil

José Luis de Castro e Silva Pretto
Hospital Sao Vicente de Paulo e Hospital de Cidade, Passo Fundo, Brazil

Marcelo Haertel Miglioranza
Cardiology Institute of Rio Grande do Sul, Porto Alegre, Brazil

Marco A. R. Torres and Clarissa Carmona de Azevedo Bellagamba
Hospital de Clinicas de Porto Alegre - Universidade Federal do Rio Grande do Sul, Porto Alegre, Brazil

Daniel Quesada Chaves
Hospital San Vicente de Paul, Heredia, Costa Rica

Iana Simova
Acibadem City Clinic Cardiovascular Center, University Hospital, Sofia, Bulgaria

Albert Varga
Institute of Family Medicine, University of Szeged, Szeged, Hungary

Jelena Čelutkienė
Centre of Cardiology and Angiology, Vilnius University Hospital Santaros Klinikos, Faculty of Medicine, Vilnius University, State Research Institute for Innovative Medicine, Vilnius, Lithuania

Jaroslaw D. Kasprzak, Karina Wierzbowska-Drabik, Piotr Lipiec, Paulina Weiner-Mik, Eva Szymczyk and Katarzyna Wdowiak-Okrojek
Chair of Cardiology, Bieganski Hospital, Medical University, Lodz, Poland

Branko Beleslin and Ana Djordjevic-Dikic
Cardiology Clinic, Clinical Center of Serbia, Medical School, University of Belgrade, Belgrade, Serbia

Milica Dekleva
Clinical Hospital Zvezdara Belgrade, Belgrade, Serbia

Ivan Stankovic and Aleksandar N. Neskovic
Department of Cardiology, Clinical Hospital Center Zemun, Faculty of Medicine, University of Belgrade, Belgrade, Serbia

Angela Zagatina
Cardiology Department, University Hospital, Saint Petersburg, Russian Federation

Giovanni Di Salvo
Pediatric Cardiology Department, Brompton Hospital, London, UK

Julio E. Perez
Washington University School of Medicine, Barnes-Jewish Hospital, St. Louis, MO, USA

Ana Cristina Camarozano
Hospital de Clinicas UFPR, Medicine Department, Federal University of Paranà, Curitiba, Brazil

Anca Irina Corciu38
Department of Cardiology, IRCCS Policlinico San Donato Clinic, Milan, Italy

Alla Boshchenko
Cardiology Research Institute, Tomsk National Research Medical Center of Russian Academy of Sciences, Tomsk, Russia

Luis Ignacio Martin Leal and Fabio Lattanzi
Cardiothoracic Department, University of Pisa, Pisa, Italy

Carlos Cotrim
Heart Center, Hospital da Cruz Vermelha, Lisbon and Medical School of University of Algarve, Faro, Portugal

Paula Fazendas
Cardiology Department, Hospital Garcia de Orta, Almada, Portugal

Maciej Haberka
Department of Cardiology, School of Health Sciences, Medical University of Silesia, Katowice, Poland

Bozena Sobkowic
Department of Cardiology, Medical University of Białystok, Białystok, Poland

Wojciech Kosmala and Tomasz Witkowski
Department of Cardiology, Wroclaw Medical University, Wroclaw, Poland

Piotr Gosciniak
Department of Cardiology, Provincial Hospital, Szczecin, Poland

Alessandro Salustri
Hamad Medical Corporation, Heart Hospital, Doha, Qatar

Hugo Rodriguez-Zanella
Instituto Nacional de Cardiologia Ignacio Chavez, Mexico City, Mexico

Alexandra Nikolic
Institute for Cardiovascular Diseases, Dedinje, Belgrade, Italy

Miodrag Ostojic
Institute for Cardiovascular Diseases, Dedinje, Belgrade, Italy
University Clinical Center, Banja Luka, Republic of Srpska, Bosnia and Herzegovina

Suzana Gligorova
Cardiology Division Ospedale Casilino, Rome, Italy

Madalina-Loredana Urluescu
Cardiology Department, County Hospital Sibiu, Invasive and Non-Invasive Center for Cardiac and Vascular Pathology in Adults - CVASIC Sibiu, Faculty of Medicine, Sibiu, Romania

Maria Fiorino
Cardiology Division Ospedale Civico Di Cristina Benfratelli, Palermo, Italy

Giuseppina Novo
Cardiology Division, University Hospital, Palermo, Italy

Tamara Preradovic-Kovacevic
University Clinical Center, Banja Luka, Republic of Srpska, Bosnia and Herzegovina

Xin Huang, Lu Liu, Yanqi Di, Shasha Sun, Li Fan and Jian Cao
Department of cardiology, Nanlou Division, Chinese PLA General Hospital, National Clinical Research Center for Geriatric Diseases, Beijing 100853, China

Yan Yue
Department of medical administration, Chinese PLA General Hospital, Beijing 100853, China

Yinmeng Wang
Department of Respiration, Clifford Hospital, Guangzhou 511495, China

Yujiao Deng
Department of Ultrasound, Chinese PLA General Hospital, Beijing 100853, China

Deyou Chen
Department of Outpatient, Chinese PLA General Hospital, Beijing 100853, China

Jakub Kaczynski, William and David E. Newby
British Heart Foundation Centre for Cardiovascular Science, University of Edinburgh, Chancellor's Building, 49 Little France Crescent, Edinburgh EH16 4SA, UK

Rachel Home
College of Medicine and Veterinary Medicine, University of Edinburgh, 47 Little France Crescent, Edinburgh EH16 4TJ, UK

Karen Shields
Stroke Unit, Queen Elizabeth University Hospital, 1345 Govan Road, Glasgow G51 4TF, UK

Matthew Walters
College of Medical, Veterinary and Life Sciences, Wolfson Medical School Building, University of Glasgow, University Avenue, Glasgow G12 8QQ, UK

Whiteley and Joanna Wardlaw
Royal Infirmary of Edinburgh, 51 Little France Crescent, Old Dalkeith Road, Edinburgh EH16 4SA, UK

Mustafa Adem Yılmaztepe and Fatih Mehmet Uçar
Department of Cardiology, School of Medicine, Trakya University, 22030 Edirne, Turkey

Eugenio Picano and Clara Carpeggiani
Institute of Clinical Physiology, National Council Research, Via Giuseppe Moruzzi 1, 56124 Pisa, Italy

Quirino Ciampi
Fatebenefratelli Hospital of Benevento, Viale Principe di Napoli, 12, 82100 Benevento, Italy

Karina Wierzbowska-Drabik
Department of Cardiology, Medical University of Lodz, Bieganski Hospital, Ul Kniaziewicza 1/5, 91-347 Lodz, Poland

Mădălina-Loredana Urluescu
CVASIC Research Center Sibiu, "Lucian Blaga" University of Sibiu, Sibiu, Romania

Doralisa Morrone
Cardiothoracic department, Cisanello Hospital, University of Pisa, Pisa, Italy

Patrizia Aruta, Denisa Muraru, Niccolò Ruozi, Chiara Palermo, Sabino Iliceto and Luigi P. Badano
Department of Cardiac, Thoracic and Vascular Science, University of Padua, Via Giustiniani 2, 35128 Padua, Italy

Andrada Camelia Guta
Department of Cardiac, Thoracic and Vascular Science, University of Padua, Via Giustiniani 2, 35128 Padua, Italy
University of Medicine and Pharmacy "Carol Davila", Bucharest, Romania

Sorina Mihaila
University of Medicine and Pharmacy "Carol Davila", Bucharest, Romania

Basma Elnagar
Tanta University Hospital, Tanta, Egypt

Andreea Motoc, Bram Roosens1, Esther Scheirlynck, Benedicte Heyndrickx, Steven Droogmans and Bernard Cosyns
Centrum Voor Hart-en Vaatziekten (CHVZ), Department of Cardiology, UZ Brussel, Laarbeeklaan 101, 1090 Brussels, Belgium

Juan-Pablo Abugattas, Carlo de Asmundis and Gian-Battista Chierchia
Heart Rhythm Management Centre, UZ Brussel, Laarbeeklaan 101, 1090 Brussels, Belgium

Tao Cong, Zhijuan Shang, Yinghui Sun, Qiaobing Sun, Hong Wei, Na Chen, Siyao Sun and Tingting Fu
Department of Cardiology, The First Affiliated Hospital of Dalian Medical University, Dalian 116000, Liaoning, China

Jinping Gu
Department of Intensive Care Unit, The Second Affiliated Hospital of Dalian Medical University, Liaoning, China

Alex Pui-Wai Lee
Division of Cardiology, Department of Medicine and Therapeutics, The Prince of Wales Hospital of Chinese University of Hong Kong, Hong Kong, China

Natalia Dłużniewska, Piotr Podolec, Maciej Skubera, Monika Smaś-Suska, Wojciech Płazak, Maria Olszowska and Lidia Tomkiewicz-Pająk
Department of Cardiac and Vascular Disease, Collegium Medicum, Jagiellonian University, John Paul II Hospital, Krakow, Poland

Jacek Pająk
Paediatric Heart Surgery Department and General Paediatric Surgery Department, Medical University of Warsaw, Warsaw, Poland

Małgorzata Urbańczyk-Zawadzka
Department of Radiology and Diagnostic Imaging, John Paul II Hospital, Krakow, Poland

Index

www.ingramcontent.com/pod-product-compliance
Lightning Source LLC
Chambersburg PA
CBHW080457200326
41458CB00012B/3995